THE SHOULDER

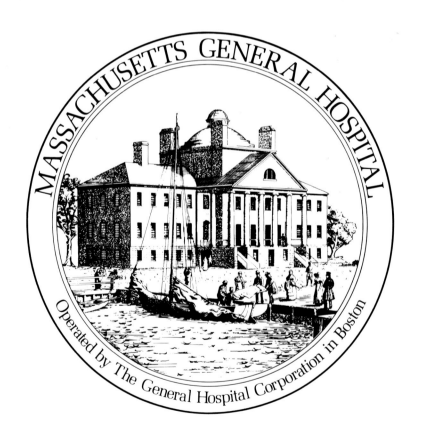

MASSACHUSETTS GENERAL HOSPITAL

Operated by The General Hospital Corporation in Boston

THE SHOULDER

Edited by

Carter R. Rowe, M.D.

Associate Clinical Professor (Emeritus)
Department of Orthopaedic Surgery
Harvard Medical School
Senior Surgeon
Department of Orthopaedics
Massachusetts General Hospital
Boston, Massachusetts

With illustrations by Laurel Cook

Churchill Livingstone
New York, Edinburgh, London, Melbourne   1988

Library of Congress Cataloging in Publication Data

The Shoulder.
   Includes bibliographies and index.
   1. Shoulder—Surgery.   I. Rowe, Carter R.
[DNLM: 1. Shoulder.   WE 810 S5586]
RD557.5.S48   1988   617′.572   87–20828
ISBN 0–443–08457–2

Accurate indications, adverse reactions, and dosage schedules for drugs are provided in this book, but it is possible that they may change. The reader is urged to review the package information data of the manufacturers of the medications mentioned.

Acquisitions Editor: *Robert A. Hurley*
Copy Editor: *Ozzievelt Owens*
Production Designer: *Melanie Haber*
Production Supervisor: *Jane Grochowski*

Printed in the United States of America

First published in 1988

This book is dedicated to Ernest Amory Codman, a man of intellect, courage, conviction, controversy, and irrepressible honesty. He was a surgeon far ahead of his time, whose legacy to the medical world has been the establishment of the "End-Result Idea" for doctors and hospitals, the initiation of the Registry of Bone Sarcomas, and the publication of his classic book, *The Shoulder,* in 1934, from which came the inspiration for this book.

Contributors

William P. Barrett, M.D.
Former Fellow, Department of Orthopaedic Surgery, Brigham and Women's Hospital, Boston, Massachusetts; Staff Surgeon, Valley Medical Center, Renton, Washington

Thomas Bilko, M.D.
Former Research and Clinical Fellow in Sports Medicine, Department of Orthopaedics, Massachusetts General Hospital, Boston, Massachusetts; Medical Director, Nanticoke Sports Medicine Center, Nanticoke Hospital, Nanticoke, Pennsylvania; Orthopaedic Staff, Mercy Hospital, Wilkes-Barre, Pennsylvania

John J. Boyle, M.D.
Clinical Instructor, Department of Orthopaedic Surgery, Harvard Medical School; Clinical Associate, Department of Orthopaedics, Massachusetts General Hospital, Boston, Massachusetts; Director of Sports Medicine, Performance Center, Beverly, Massachusetts

Mark Colville, M.D.
Former Research and Clinical Fellow in Sports Medicine, Department of Orthopaedics, Massachusetts General Hospital, Boston, Massachusetts; Assistant Professor, Department of Surgery, Division of Orthopaedics and Rehabilitation, Oregon Health Sciences University School of Medicine, Portland, Oregon

Michael G. Ehrlich, M.D.
Associate Professor, Department of Orthopaedic Surgery, Harvard Medical School; Chief, Pediatric Orthopaedic Service, Massachusetts General Hospital, Boston, Massachusetts

Mark C. Gebhardt, M.D.
Clinical Instructor, Department of Orthopaedic Surgery, Harvard Medical School; Assistant in Orthopaedic Surgery, Departments of Orthopaedics, Massachusetts General Hospital and The Children's Hospital, Boston, Massachusetts

Bette Ann Harris, M.S., P.T.
Assistant Professor, Program in Physical Therapy, Massachusetts General Hospital Institute of Health Professions; Clinical Research Associate, Department of Rehabilitation, Massachusetts General Hospital, Boston, Massachusetts

Newton E. Hyslop, Jr., M.D.
Professor, Department of Medicine, Tulane University School of Medicine; Chief, Infectious Disease Section, Tulane University Medical Center, New Orleans, Louisiana

Robert D. Leffert, M.D.
Associate Professor, Department of Orthopaedic Surgery, Harvard Medical School; Chief, Surgical Upper Extremity Rehabilitation Unit and the Department of Rehabilitation Medicine, Massachusetts General Hospital, Boston, Massachusetts

Henry J. Mankin, M.D.
Edith M. Ashley Professor, Department of Orthopaedic Surgery, Harvard Medical School; Orthopaedist-In-Chief, Department of Orthopaedics, Massachusetts General Hospital, Boston, Massachusetts

Richard A. Marder, M.D.
Assistant Professor, Department of Orthopaedic Surgery, University of California, Davis, School of Medicine, Davis, California

John A. Mills, M.D.
Associate Professor, Department of Medicine, Harvard Medical School; Physician, Massachusetts General Hospital, Boston, Massachusetts

Jacquelin Perry, M.D.
Professor, Department of Orthopaedics, University of Southern California School of Medicine, Los Angeles, California; Chief, Pathokinesiology, Rancho Los Amigos Medical Center, Downey, California; Consultant, Biomechanical Laboratory, Centinela Hospital, Inglewood, California

Chadwick C. Prodromos, M.D.
Clinical Instructor, Department of Orthopaedic Surgery, Northwestern University Medical School, Chicago, Illinois; Orthopaedic Surgeon, St. Francis Hospital, Evanston, Illinois; Orthopaedic Surgeon, Highland Park Hospital, Highland Park, Illinois

Daniel I. Rosenthal, M.D.
Associate Professor, Department of Radiology, Harvard Medical School; Director, Bone and Joint Radiology, Massachusetts General Hospital, Boston, Massachusetts

Carter R. Rowe, M.D.
Associate Clinical Professor (Emeritus), Department of Orthopaedic Surgery, Harvard Medical School; Senior Surgeon, Department of Orthopaedics, Massachusetts General Hospital, Boston, Massachusetts

Alan L. Schiller, M.D.
Associate Professor, Department of Pathology, Harvard Medical School; Consultant Pathologist, Massachusetts General Hospital, Boston, Massachusetts; Professor, Department of Pathology, New York University School of Medicine, New York, New York; Chief of Pathology, Booth Memorial Medical Center, Flushing, New York

Thomas S. Thornhill, M.D.
Assistant Professor, Department of Orthopaedic Surgery, Harvard Medical School; Orthopaedic Surgeon, Brigham and Women's Hospital; Orthopaedic Surgeon, New England Baptist Hospital, Boston, Massachusetts

Bertram Zarins, M.D.
Asssitant Clinical Professor, Department of Orthopaedic Surgery, Harvard Medical School;
Chief, Sports Medicine Unit, Department of Orthopaedics, Massachusetts General Hospital,
Boston, Massachusetts

Foreword

In 1893, a student at the Harvard Medical School spent his third year studying in Europe. It was during this time that Dr. E. A. Codman's attention was first attracted to the "subdeltoid bursa" and his lifelong interest in the shoulder began. His subsequent studies of the shoulder cumulated in the private printing and publication of his book *The Shoulder*. This, the first and only book on the human shoulder at that time (1934), was in large measure the result of work done at the Massachusetts General Hospital. It therefore seems especially fitting that some 50 years later another "shoulder" book should come from this institution, edited and in large measure written by an orthopaedic surgeon who at the Massachusetts General Hospital as a resident had known Dr. Codman as a teacher.

Dr. Rowe's interest in the shoulder began in his World War II experiences overseas (1942–45), where he encountered a great variety of injuries to the shoulder, particularly instabilities. Following World War II, Dr. Rowe returned to the Massachusetts General Hospital, where his contributions have continued. It was quite fitting that in 1980 he was invited to give the first Codman Lecture at the Inaugural International Conference on the shoulder at the Royal National Orthopaedic Hospital, London, England. Since the first book on the shoulder by Codman in 1934, many have been published, but this very comprehensive volume, with its ties to the beginnings of "shoulder surgery," is a welcome edition.

Thornton Brown, M.D.

Preface

This book is written in response to questions, general and specific, from medical students, residents, and practicing orthopaedic surgeons. Emphasis is given to new techniques and investigative aids, as well as to procedures that have withstood the test of time. Every effort has been made to support conclusions with follow-up study.

The text begins with chapters that present basic information about the shoulder: its biomechanics, the muscles that control and stabilize the shoulder joint, the recommended procedures for examining the shoulder, and present-day diagnostic techniques, including methods of imaging, tomography, arthroscopy, and electrodiagnosis. The usual disturbing problems of the subacromial area are grouped together, including impingement syndromes, rotator cuff injuries, "frozen" shoulder, and calcific tendinitis.

One of the most challenging chapters of the book concerns instabilities of the shoulder. The commonly used procedures are carefully analyzed and discussed, leaving the reader free to make his or her own choice. A section is allotted to specific suggestions in the number of ways the Bankart procedure can be made an easier, safer, and stronger repair.

Special attention is given to the embarrassing, and at times catastrophic, problems of failed surgical procedures, and of unusual complications, such as severe Hill-Sachs lesions or severe fractures of the glenoid rim. Successful reoperations will depend on detailed identification and correction of the lesions. Combination of procedures are at times indicated. The newly evolving types of multidirectional instabilities are reviewed in which a Bankart, or other traumatic lesions, are absent, and some type of capsulorrhaphy is indicated.

Today, the orthopaedic surgeon is faced with an increasing problem of shoulder salvage, resulting from unsuccessful surgery, disease, or trauma, for which joint replacement has been one of the major advances in modern medicine. It is especially important to know what to do when a replacement prosthesis cannot be used. The techniques and positions of the arm at the shoulder for arthrodesis have been redesigned for a much stronger, more comfortable, and more acceptable operation. These are designed particularly for a patient who is required to do heavy construction or farm work.

Septic complications involving the shoulder often are given too little attention in the literature or in symposia. Although infections occur infrequently, prompt and correct steps are necessary to avoid disaster. The appropriate procedures for the identification of the organisms and the selection of the most effective antibiotics are reviewed. The relative merits of arthroscopy and arthrotomy for joint drainage and debridement are also considered.

A special feature of this volume is the chapter on tumors about the shoulder. Emphasis is placed on comprehensive teamwork, involving the orthopaedic surgeon, the pathologist, the oncologist, and the radiologist. An orderly approach from biopsy to definitive care is put in concise sequence for the reader.

In addition, there are chapters on the rehabilitation of the shoulder and the changing role of physical therapy, the rating of results after treatment of the shoulder, and, finally, a chapter on unusual shoulder conditions.

Sports medicine brings attention to the demands of athletes from grade school to the professional ranks.

Chapters on fractures and growth disturbances deal with problems of the child and the needs of the adult. Complications of trauma, including nerve injuries, are presented in recent investigations.

Lastly, it should be noted that our intent in this book is to cover the shoulder problems that fall within the purview of most orthopaedic surgeons in active clinical practice and to provide useful information that is readable and convenient.

Carter R. Rowe, M.D.

Acknowledgment

We are most grateful to all who have made this book possible: busy surgeons, special secretaries, our publisher and editors, and always our families.

Contents

Introduction

An engineer with a blueprint of the structural setup for the shoulder and a list of the functional demands required of the shoulder would perhaps pronounce the human shoulder completely inadequate to withstand the numerous assignments of daily living. In many ways, the engineer would be correct. How could the glenohumeral joint remain stable, without a bony socket like the hip or strong supporting ligaments like the knee, when exposed to excessive strain and trauma in all positions? The limited contact between the large humeral head and a smaller shallow glenoid fossa, secured only by a fibrous capsule and overlying musculocutaneous rotator cuff, would perhaps doom the shoulder to failure when exposed to contact, stress, and the leverage demands of the upper extremity.

One may ask, how then has nature provided for a stable joint, with complete range of motion in the face of such obvious mechanical deficits? There are several unique adjustments that nature has built into the shoulder to provide stability.

A MOVABLE BASE FOR THE HUMERAL HEAD

The glenoid fossa, although small in comparison to the humeral head, makes up for its limited size by continuous adjustments to optimal mechanical positions. As the arm is raised to complete elevation, the glenoid fossa smoothly and effectively positions itself beneath the humeral head for increased mechanical stability (Fig. I-1). We may liken this to a seal balancing a ball on its nose (Fig. I-2). This is made possible by the synchronous teamwork of the entire shoulder girdle, the acromioclavicular, the sternoclavicular, and the scapulothoracic joints.

THE RECOIL MECHANISM OF THE SCAPULA (FIG. I-3)

An important factor adding stability to the shoulder is the subtle and effective recoil mechanism of the scapula. The glide of the scapula along the chest wall absorbs the impact to the shoulder from falls, and direct and indirect blows to the shoulder, as well as the strain of forceful pushing, pulling, and lifting. This is a major protective mechanism to the shoulder. Unlike the hip, in which the force of the femur is expended against a fixed acetabulum, the scapula provides an excellent *shock absorber*, little appreciated by anatomists.

COMPENSATING MOTION

The shoulder possesses subtle adjustments for loss of motion of one of its four joints. When, for instance, glenohumeral motion is lost from trauma or arthrodesis, the scapula

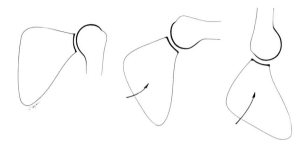

FIG. I-1 The scapula acts as a movable base to the shoulder, adjusting to positions of mechanical advantage. (Rowe CR, Sakellarides HT: Factors related to recurrences of anterior dislocations of the shoulder. Clin Orthop 20:41, 1961.)

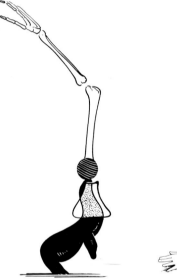

FIG. I-2 The glenoid fossa functions much like the nose of a seal in balancing a ball.

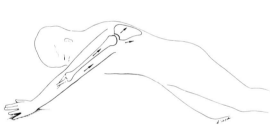

FIG. I-3 The recoil mechanism of the scapula absorbs impacts of blows to the shoulder, a mechanism that the hip joint lacks. (Rowe CR, Sakellarides HT: Factors related to recurrences of anterior dislocations of the shoulder. Clin Orthop 20:41, 1961.)

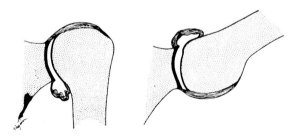

FIG. I-4 The capsule and labrum constitute the primary stabilizing elements of the shoulder. (Rowe CR, Sakellarides HT: Factors related to recurrences of anterior dislocations of the shoulder. Clin Orthop 20:41, 1961.)

supplies needed motion by its glide and rotation along the chest wall, to allow elevation of the arm to the head or above, as well as gliding motion in adduction and abduction.

THE CAPSULE

A stable shoulder must have a strong adjustable capsule, particularly in positions of elevation. In this position, the rotator cuff muscles glide upward, leaving protected the inferior capsule and capsular ligament (Fig. I-4). With avulsion of the capsule from the glenoid rim, or excess laxity of the capsule, stability of the shoulder is lost.

Thus, without a clear understanding of the complex anatomy of the shoulder girdle, the engineer would perhaps be left wondering how the structure of the shoulder would respond to the multiple demands made upon it. Were the shoulder a mechanical unit, it would most likely come apart.

We have invited Jacqueline Perry to help develop our concepts of the anatomic and biochemical aspects of the shoulder.

Biomechanics of the Shoulder

1

Jacquelin Perry

The shoulder is a highly mobile and dynamic junction between the arm and trunk. In sports it contributes essential propulsive and precise motions. Most industrial occupations and household chores depend on the shoulder's lifting capability. Basic self-care utilizes the shoulder's three-dimensional mobility to reach all parts of the body. Performance of these functions involves several clinically significant biomechanical characteristics that are unique to the shoulder because of its anatomical complexity. The areas of concern are its patterns and magnitude of motion (kinematics) and the forces involved (kinetics).

MECHANICAL STRUCTURE

Structurally, the arm is suspended from the scapula, which in turn lies at the end of the clavicle. Hence, shoulder motion involves three joints in series, with the point of origin on the trunk being the sternum (Fig. 1-1).

Mobility

The most mobile joint is the junction of the humerus and scapula. Vast three-dimensional mobility is provided by the skeletal characteristics of this artic-ulation. The humeral articular surface is a superio-medially oriented hemisphere (diameter 35 to 55 mm).[18,21] Opposing this is the small, shallow glenoid fossa of the scapula, which has half the contour and one-third the surface area.[14] Glenoid area and depth are enlarged by a fibrocartilaginous labrum. This increases the humeral contact areas to 75 percent vertically and 56 percent transversely.[23] The effect is enhanced joint stability without impeding mobility from hard bony edges (Fig. 1-2). As a result, the humerus has a wide range of motion in all three planes. Supplementing this is the gliding of the scapula on the thorax as it rotates with the clavicle about the sternal point of origin. The dominance of mobility over stability is even evident in the arm's resting posture.

Resting Alignment

The functional resting posture of the shoulder places the arm at the side of the body. With the subject standing, the arm is dependent and the humerus is grossly vertical. Detailed analysis of humeral alignment demonstrated minor differences in the study groups, with the men's mean values varying from vertical by $+2.5°$ (abduction) to $-1°$ (adduction).[8,10,21] Individual humeral position ranged from $+9°$ to $-3°$. The women averaged more abduction: $5.2°$ to $+3.5°$.

Within the scapula, the significant alignment of the

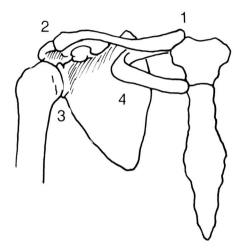

Fig. 1-1. Sites of motion within the shoulder complex. (1) Sternoclavicular joint, (2) acromioclavicular joint, (3) glenohumeral joint, (4) scapulothoracic interface.

glenohumeral joint is the plane of the glenoid fossa. Both Walker and Freedman, on roentogenographic studies, found the mean alignment to be 5° downward (Fig. 1-2). Considerable individual variability was evi-

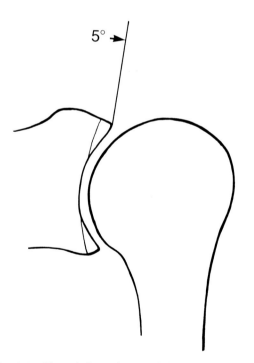

Fig. 1-2. Glenoid fossa deepened by fibrous labrum. In the dependent resting position of the arm, the glenoid fossa is tilted downward 5°.

denced by the range between −11° and +10°. Calculations with a double protractor designed to align with the body's vertical axis, scapular spine, and humerus showed a more neutral alignment (0.3° + 4.0°).

The neutral to slightly downward tilt of the scapula demonstrated by direct measurement implies an absence of skeletal support for the humeral head. These findings contradict Basmajian's[1] assumption that the glenoid face invariably tilts upward to provide a supporting surface for the humerus.

MOTION

Shoulder mobility is classified by three patterns of motion: elevation, internal/external rotation, and horizontal flexion and extension.

Elevation

Raising the arm from the side of the body to its peak overhead position is a theoretical 180° arc. Few men (4 percent) and less than one-third of women (28%) actually attain this range. The men's mean range was 167° and the women's 171°.[8,10] These values still display the shoulder as the most mobile joint in the body. Posterior elevation or extension is about 60°.[19]

Arm elevation is a complex action that is best analyzed as three functional modes: planes of motion, scapulohumeral rhythm, and centers of rotation.

Planes of Motion

Neutral elevation of the arm occurs in the plane of the scapula (Fig. 1-3). This is angled approximately 30° anterior to the body's coronal plane.[25] Exact alignment is determined by the contour of the thoracic wall on which the scapula rests.[24a]

This alignment of the glenoid fossa is matched by 30° retroversion of the head of the humerus on its shaft (measured in relationship to the intercondylar line at the elbow) (Fig. 1-4). Hence, the glenohumeral joint is designed to follow the plane of the scapula.

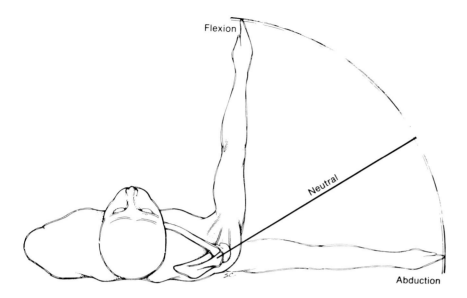

Fig. 1-3. Planes of arm elevation: neutral, flexion, abduction.

As the arm is raised in the scapular plane, the path of the humerus is perpendicular to the face of the glenoid: the joint is in neutral alignment. Johnston[17] noted that the inferior capsule remained without tor-

sion only when the humerus was raised in the scapular plane.

Flexion is sagittal plane elevation (Fig. 1-3). Placing the arm in this plane includes significant horizontal

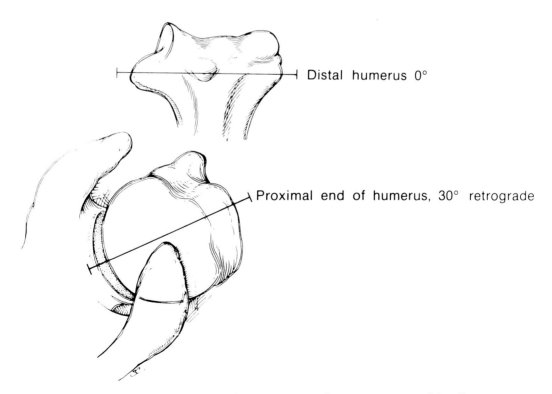

Fig. 1-4. Humeral head retroversion 30° compared to transverse axis of the elbow.

flexion. Hence, the path of the humerus is oblique to the face of the scapula. The inferior joint capsule twists to accommodate this path of arm elevation.[17]

Abduction raises the arm in the coronal plane (Fig. 1-3). This introduces two limitations. An element of horizontal extension is included in the elevation motion. More significant is the potential for impingement of the greater tuberosity against the acromion since normal clearance is so minimal that there is no space for tendon thickening (Fig. 1-5). This can be avoided by adding external rotation to the abduction motion.

The difference in joint alignment has been reflected in the available range of arm elevation. Among a group of men Boone found mean abduction to be 10 percent greater than average flexion.[3] This may reflect greater scapular freedom as Doody and Freeman[8] found that scapular plane elevation equaled Boone's flexion value (167°).

Differences in the two ranges of motion have necessitated dual testing since there have been no guidelines for selecting one over the other. Awareness of the scapular plane representing neutral joint alignment resolves this indecision. Clinical experience indicates that it is the simplest path of motion. Patients with limited strength spontaneously choose the scapular plane when asked to raise their arm overhead. Based on such anatomical and clinical findings it is recommended that the scapular plane be used for basic testing of arm elevation capability. Accepting this practice will facilitate outcome comparisons among studies.

Scapulohumeral Rhythm

Total arm elevation is the sum of motion at two areas: the glenohumeral joint and gliding of the scapula on the thorax[5] (Fig. 1-6). In gross terms the ratio is 2:1 but more precise analysis has shown considerable variability.[8,10,23]

At the onset of arm elevation, scapular participation has proved to be highly variable. It may be absent, minimal, or even reversed.[16] This lag in scapular motion persisted through the first 60° of flexion and 30° abduction. Once the scapula started to participate, both segments (humerus and scapula) moved continuously and synchronously. Relative humeral and scapular motion was identified by Inman et al.[16] as a 2:1 ratio. Other investigators have found both higher and lower ratios (2.5:1 to 1.25:1).[8,10,21,23] The average among all the studies is 1.5:1.[25] Hence, there is ap-

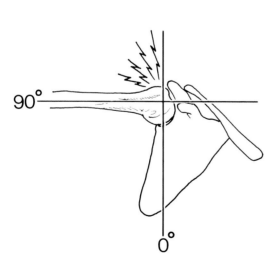

Fig. 1-5. Coronal plane abduction without external rotation allows greater impingement of the tuberosity against the acromion.

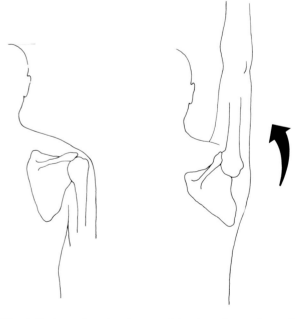

Fig. 1-6. Arm elevation is a combination of scapular and humeral rotation.

proximately 3° of glenohumeral motion for each 2° occurring at the scapula.

Dividing the total arc into segments helps to identify inconstant rates of motion for both bones (Fig. 1-7). Of particular significance was a relative slowing in scapular motion in the terminal arc (120° to maximum).[8] As this analysis related to the scapular plane elevation, the terminal differences may represent a passive limitation in scapular mobility. The clinical significance relates to the potential for humeral impingement against the acromion in high overhead motions, as are used in swimming.

Instant Centers of Motion

Each joint has its own pattern of motion. This is defined by its path of instant centers.

Excursion of the humeral head on the glenoid has been described as both gliding and rolling. The marked disparity in curvature between the humerus and glenoid led some investigators to assume that the found humeral head rolled across the glenoid face from one margin to the other (i.e., rolling motion).[9,23] Direct roentgenologic analysis of glenohumeral joint contradicted this assumption. It demonstrated intraarticular displacement to be minimal. At the onset of arm elevation (0° to 30°) Walker[25] found a 3 mm upward shift that could be interpreted as rolling along the joint's surface. This action appears to be correction of arm sag from its dependent position. During the rest of the elevation range the point of glenohumeral contact remained within 1 mm of the center of the fossa (Fig. 1-8). Hence, rolling is not a significant element of shoulder motion.[9,23] Instead, an intact labrum forms a sufficiently deep socket to keep the humeral head centered, making gliding of the humeral surface on that of the glenoid fossa the dominant type of motion within the joint.

The axis of glenohumeral joint rotation also is quite consistent. Calculation of the instant centers for each 30° arc of arm elevation placed these points within 5 mm of the center of the humeral head (Fig. 1-8). Hence, the glenohumeral joint acts as true ball and socket. Similar assessment of persons with a painful shoulder showed half of them to have abnormal mechanics.[21] Both humeral head excursion and in-

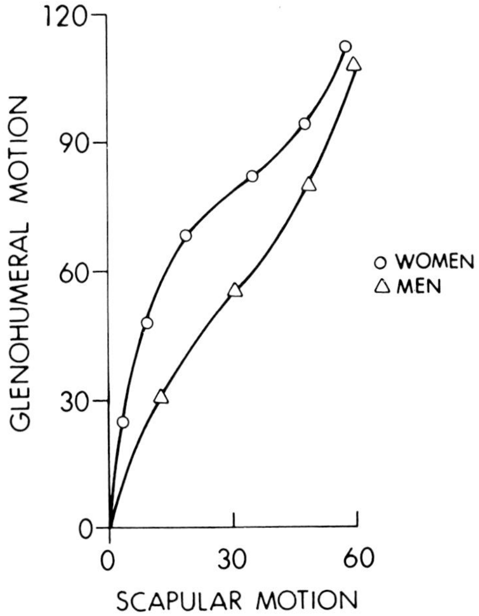

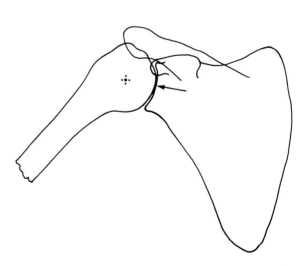

Fig. 1-7. Scapulohumeral rhythm variability and relative humeral and scapular rotation throughout the range of arm elevation.

Fig. 1-8. Pattern of humeral motion. Axis of rotation within 5 mm (small dots) of humeral head center (large dots). Consistent area of humeral contact at midpoint of glenoid fossa (arrows).

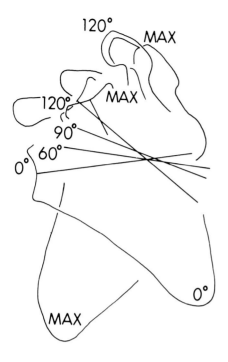

Fig. 1-9. Centers of scapular rotation during arm elevation tend to cluster about two points. Base of scapular spine (0° to 90°). Base of coracoid process (120° to max).

stant center displacement were increased, with the greater change occurring in excursion. Only 2 of these 15 patients had altered scapulohumeral ratios.

The scapula was found to follow a more complex path of motion. During its initial setting stage (the first 60°), either there was no motion or the scapula joggled around a center of rotation in the lower part of the blade. Subsequent scapular rotation was grossly centered near to the base of the scapular spine until the arm reached 120°. As illustrated by the intersection of the instant joint axes during the final arc, the center of rotation shifted to a point near the base of the glenoid (Fig. 1-9). This marked change in instant

center location can be related to scapula motion arising first in the sternoclavicular (SC) and then the acromioclavicular (AC) joints (Fig. 1-10). During the first 30° arc of arm elevation there might be a jog (5°) of AC rotation but the major arc of motion relating to the scapula is clavicular elevation at the SC joint until the arm reached the 120° position. Beyond this point scapular rotation depends on two actions: motion at the AC joint and 40° of clavicular rotation about its longitudinal axis. The latter action uses the concave curvature of the clavical lateral end to lengthen functionally the coracoclavicular ligaments so that scapular motion can continue.[15] Three-dimen-

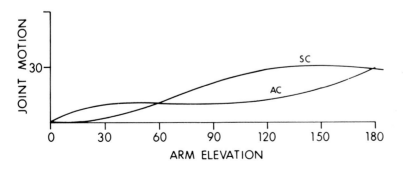

Fig. 1-10. Sternoclavicular (SC) and acromioclavicular (AC) motion during arm elevation.

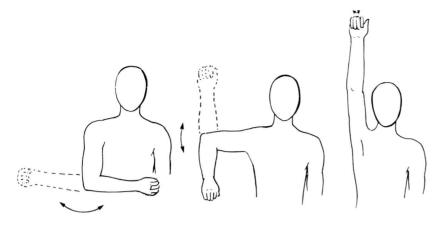

Fig. 1-11. Arm external/internal rotation ranges available with shoulder at 0°, 90°, and full elevation.

sional mobility of the clavicle is therefore a significant component of complete scapular rotation and, consequently, full arm elevation.[16] Clinically, surgeons have found good arm function can be restored despite some compromise in clavicular rotation.[19] Conversely, the clavicle is not an indispensible bone but its presence adds stability for heavy, overhead arm use.[15]

Scapular rotation also is reflected by the path of the coracoid, while the acromion remains relatively fixed.[25]

Axial Rotation

Internal and external rotation of the arm is a function of the glenohumeral joints. Due to change in relative capsule length, the range varies with arm

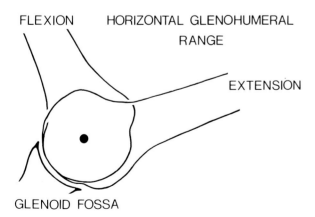

Fig. 1-12. Horizontal flexion and extension. Posterior humeral motion is limited by glenoid margin.

position (Fig. 1-11). Maximum rotation of approximately 180° is present with the arm at the side of the body (adducted).[2] The larger portion of that range (108° or 60 percent) is external rotation.[3] Abduction of the arm to 90° reduces the total arc to 120°. Within this range there is more internal than external rotation.[2] At peak elevation (by either flexion or abduction) no more than a jog of rotation is possible.

Horizontal Flexion/Extension

These motions also have been called horizontal adduction/abduction. Within the normal 180° arc, only 45° or 24 percent is horizontal extension behind the coronal plan.[3] Most of the motion is glenohumeral. As was true in the scapular plane the humeral head remains centrally located in the glenoid fossa (unpublished data). The limitation of this motion is the edge of the humeral articular surface. Further effort leads to impingement between the posterior rims of the glenoid fossa and humeral head as wedging replaces gliding (Fig. 1-12).

Scapular rotation also is reflected by the path of the coracoid, while the acromion remains relatively fixed.[25]

FORCES

Muscles create the force needed to lift the arm and move it from one position to another. Incidental to that action forces are created within the joint. Some contribute to stability while others threaten joint integrity. The balance of joint forces depends on arm position and the pattern of responding muscles.

Arm Torque

To understand the relationships between arm function and muscle action, some simple rules of mechanics must be appreciated.

The arm weighs approximately 5 percent of the total body weight.[7,8] For a 70 kg (154 lb) person, arm weight is 3.3 kg. Within the arm there is a point of balance where the weight of the tissues on either side is equal. The center of gravity point (C/G) is used to represent the location of arm weight in space. In the dependent position the arm's C/G lies on the same vertical line as the shoulder joint center. The weight of the arm creates a downward traction on the supporting ligaments but induces no motion. Raising the arm from the side of the body moves its C/G away from this neutral line. A moment arm (or lever) has been created. (The word moment is an engineering synonym for torque, i.e., the tendency to produce motion, to rotate). This is seen as a demand torque to which the muscles must respond. As arm elevation increases, the functional lever is lengthened leading to a correspondingly greater demand torque (Fig. 1-13).

The ability of a body segment to create motion passively is identified by its torque using the relationship that torque equals force times lever length: $T = F \times L$. Hence, force (or weight) is only one element of motion. The other is the distance between the segment's C/G and the fulcrum of motion.

For the arm the center of motion is the shoulder joint. Its anatomical lever length is the distance between this point and the arm's C/G. For the fully extended arm (elbow and wrist straight) the typical length is 32 cm.[21] In the 90° position (arm horizontal) this also is the arm's momentary functional lever length. Other shoulder positions move the C/G closer to the joint center and thus reduce the arm's functional lever. These changes follow the cosine law of trigonometry. In 30° elevation the arm lever is 50 percent of maximum (Fig. 1-13). At 45° it is 71 percent. Hence, arm torque is 108.5 kg·cm (31 cm × 3.5 kg) with the arm abducted 90°. It decreases to 77 kg·cm in the 30° posture. The significance of these

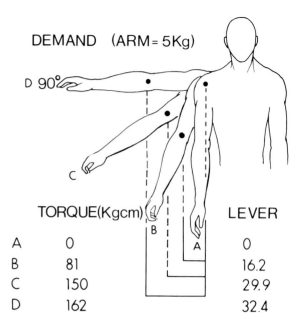

Fig. 1-13. Shoulder torque introduced by arm position. Weight is consistent but leverage increases with greater elevation. *A*=0°, *B*=30°, *C*=45QoW, *D*=90°.

numbers relates to the changing demands arm weight places on the shoulder's abducting musculature.

Arm torque can be reduced by flexing the elbow. Each segment of the arm (upper arm, forearm, hand) introduces a torque depending on its weight and C/G point. Due to its semiconical shape the average location of the segment's C/G is 43 percent distal from its proximal end rather than in the middle.[7] The distance from this point to the shoulder joint is the segment's lever length. With the elbow and wrist in neutral extension the C/G of each segment is proportionally farther from the shoulder (humerus, 14.7 cm; forearm, 44.7; hand, 66.3 cm) (Fig. 1-14). The sum of their torques for an average man's arm is 108 kg·cm (Table 1-1).

Flexing the elbow 90° moves the C/G of the forearm and hand to the level of the elbow (33.8 cm) while the humeral lever length remains the same (Fig. 1-14B). Now the arm is only 84 kg·cm., a 22 percent reduction. There would be a further decrease with full elbow flexion. These postural changes, however, moved forearm and hand weight anterior to the humeral axis, introducing an internal rotation torque. Hence, while the deltoid demand was lessened, a need for infraspinatus activity was added. Such pos-

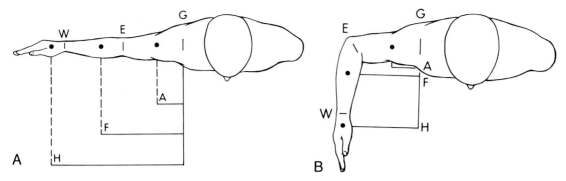

Fig. 1-14. Shoulder torque variations with arm alignment. (**A**) Elbow extended. Lever length of each more peripheral segment is progressively increased. *G*, glenohumeral joint axis; *E*, elbow; *W*, wrist; *dot*, mass center of that bony segment; *A*, upper arm mass center lever length; *F*, forearm mass center lever length; *H*, hand mass center lever length. (**B**) Elbow flexed 90°. Upper arm lever length is unchanged. The forearm and hand masses center levers now equal to the length of the humerus. Forearm and hand masses also are anterior to the shoulder joint axis.

tural variations can be used in the design of therapeutic exercises, performance of a sport or for basic daily use.

Muscle Forces

Muscles provide the body's active force to create or restrain motion. They function through bony levers. As a result, muscle strength also is a torque (F × K = T), as was arm demand. Both muscle force and lever lengths are modified by joint position.

The maximum force a muscle can produce is proportional to the number of motor cells it contains. These slender fibers (50 μm diameter) are counted indirectly by measuring the muscle's physiologic cross-section (the sum of all the perpendicular areas of the variously oblique muscle fiber bundles). Muscle force/cm^2 has been calculated at various levels, ranging between 3.9 and 9.2 (female, 7.2).[6] A commonly accepted value is 4 kg/cm.[2,13] Arrangement of the contracting fibers within a muscle determines its dominant function. Longitudinal fiber presents maximal muscle shortening for speed. The oblique fiber pattern allows more muscle cells to be included in the same volume, resulting in increased power. A muscle's fiber pattern also determines the ease of identifying its physiological cross-section. If all the fibers have a longitudinal arrangement, a simple transverse (anatomical) section is sufficient. Pennate muscles have oblique fibers (Fig. 1-15). This means one must count several bundles to attain the perpendicular areas of all its fibers, a task that can only be done by detailed anatomical dissection. Hence, muscle sizes quoted

Table 1-1. Arm Torque at Shoulder (Demand on Muscles)

	Weight (kg)	Lever (cm)	Torque (kg·cm)
Elbow Extended = 108 kg·cm			
Humerus	1.9	14.7	27.9
Forearm	1.2	44.7	53.6
Hand	0.4	66.3	26.5
Elbow Flexed = 84 kg·cm			
Humerus	1.9	14.7	27.9
Forearm	1.2	33.8	40.6
Hand	0.4	33.8	15.5

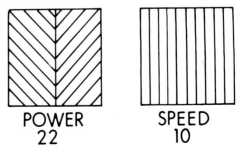

Fig. 1-15. Relationship of muscle fiber alignment to the potential power and speed (force of fiber pattern).

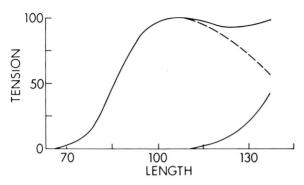

Fig. 1-16. Length tension relationships of muscle. Top curve, total tension; dotted line, active tension; lower curve, passive tension as muscle is pulled beyond resting length (100 percent).

in this chapter represent research data.[26] Clarity of modern computed tomography is encouraging definition of muscle size with the use of transverse sections.[12] Use of this technique must be approached with caution. It can indicate relative changes in a muscle under changing circumstances. Comparisons between muscles, however, will not be accurate unless the differences in muscle fiber direction and distribution are considered.

As the arm is used, each muscle creates just enough force to meet the demand. Arm position, type of contraction, and speed of motion are the derminants of the amount of muscle action that occurs.

For each muscle, an optimal fiber length yields maximum actin/myosin bonding within the chain of sarcomeres and, hence, force. Both lengthening and shortening of the fiber from this "resting length" by a change in joint position reduce the available force (Fig. 1-16). The effect of fiber length on muscle strength can only be determined indirectly. It repre-

sents the difference between measured strength and calculated muscle lever length.

The type of muscle action is a second strength variable. Isometric contractions provide the basic force. This value is modified by whether the motion is eccentric or concentric.[4] Eccentric action (contraction versus passive lengthening) has been found to produce the same amount of use.[24] In these two forms of muscle action (isometric and eccentric) the resulting force is a combination of both active and passive tension (Fig. 1-16). The latter arises from the collagenous sheaths enveloping each muscle fiber.[11] Concentric (shortening) contractions lack the advantage of passive tension and thus produce proportionally less force (13 to 20 percent).[24]

Speed further reduces concentric force. Motion at 214°/second decreases maximum strength by 50 percent.[20]

Lever length is the final determinant of muscle effectiveness. The greater leverage a muscle has, the more effective its force. Available lever length is the perpendicular distance between the muscle's line of pull and the fulcrum of motion (Fig. 1-17). The latter point really is the site of contact between the two joint surfaces (humeral head against the glenoid fossa). Because this point often is difficult to define, the custom of using a joint center of rotation has been substituted. The differences are sufficiently small to be an acceptable compromise under most circumstances.

Lever length for most muscles is modified by joint position. Hence, as the arm is raised muscle effectiveness varies. This is particularly true for the deltoid[22] (Fig. 1-17). Arm elevation progressively moves the muscle's humeral insertion from below to above the center of shoulder rotation. Lever length is increased proportionally. Due to their differences in points of

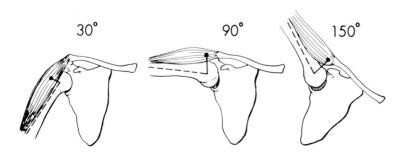

Fig. 1-17. Mechanical lever of the muscle equals the distance between the longitudinal muscle axis and center of glenohumeral rotation. It is modified by the degree of arm elevation.

MUSCLE LEVERS

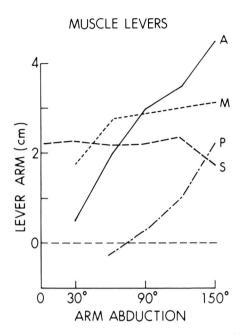

Fig. 1-18. Pattern of abductor muscle lever lengths throughout arm elevation. *A*, anterior deltoid; *M*, middle deltoid; *P*, posterior deltoid; *S*, supraspinatus. (Adapted from Poppen NK, Walker PS; Forces at the glenohumeral joint in abduction. Clin Orthop 136:165, 1978.)

origin, each head of the deltoid (anterior, middle, posterior) has its own lever length pattern.

At the onset of arm elevation in the scapular plane, only the middle deltoid has an effective lever among the three muscles (1.7 cm at 30°) (Fig. 1-18). Abduction to 60° increases the muscle's leverage to 2.6 cm. It then remains relatively stable (20 percent gain by 150°).[21] The anterior deltoid, with much of its origin on the clavicle, starts with an insignificant abduction lever (0.5 cm at the 30° position) but rapid and continual arm elevation moves a greater proportion of the muscle lateral to the joint center. At 60° of scapular plane abduction, the muscle's leverage is 2 cm. By 90° it has surpassed that of the middle deltoid (2.8 versus 2.6 cm) and reaches a final value of 4.5 cm at 150°. In the resting position the origin of the posterior deltoid on the scapular spine places most of the muscle mass medial to the shoulder joint center. This alignment does not significantly improve until the arm has abducted 120° These various improvements in mechanical leverage counter the effects or shorten muscle fiber (sarcomere) length. They also accommo-

date the increase in arm demand so that elevation strength is maintained. In contrast, lever length for the supraspinatus remains fairly constant, averaging 2.2 cm throughout the range of arm elevation (Fig. 1-18). This means there is no leverage advantage available to compensate for the reduction in muscle fiber length. Consequently, the supraspinatus becomes progressively less effective.

Joint Forces

As the muscles act to control the arm they create forces within the joint. These forces are classified by their alignment to the joint surface as either compression or shear (Fig. 1-19). Those directed towards the center of the joint (i.e., perpendicular to the plane of the glenoid fossa) are called compression. Shear forces are parallel to the joint surface.[22]

The line of pull of most shoulder muscles is oblique to the plane of the glenoid fossa. As a result, both compression and shear forces accompany muscle action. The compressive forces contribute to joint stability as they drive the humeral head into the glenoid socket. In contrast, shear forces threaten the stabilizing tissues by the sliding strains created. The absolute

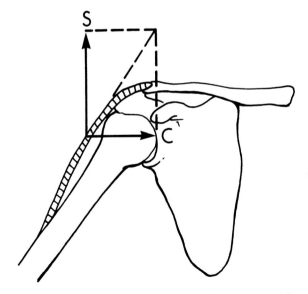

Fig. 1-19. Joint forces induced by muscle action (middle deltoid is the model). *C*, compression (perpendicular to plane of joint); *S*, shear (parallel to joint).

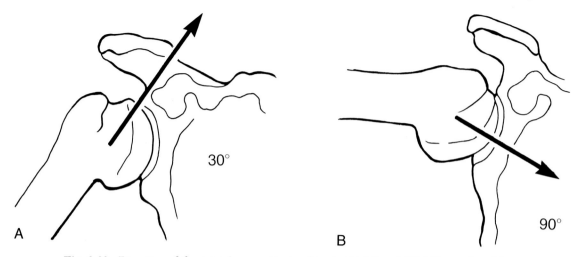

Fig. 1-20. Direction of the joint forces with shoulder in (**A**) 30° and (**B**) 90° scapular abduction.

magnitude of the forces is determined by the intensity of muscle action. Relative amounts of shear and compression vary as the muscle's alignment changes.

During arm function the forces within the shoulder joint are related to two major forces within the shoulder joint related to two major muscle groups: deltoid and rotator cuff. They differ markedly in their patterns of compression and shear.

DELTOID

The deltoid changes from a vertical to horizontal muscle as the arm is elevated. This alters the relative dominance of shear and compression force produced. During scapular plane abduction the force patterns of the anterior and posterior components are similar to that of the middle head. All three have a point of origin just above and external to the glenoid joint surface (acromion, lateral clavicle, or scapular spine) and insert into the midpoint of the humeral shaft (deltoid tuberosity).

With the arm at rest, the middle deltoid's line of pull is 27° to the glenoid face. As a result, at the initiation of abduction the dominant direction of deltoid pull is vertical, creating significant upward shear (89 percent of the muscle's total force, compared to a compression value of 45 percent) (Fig. 1-20A). Further elevation progressively makes the muscle's line of pull more horizontal, because the humeral insertion is raised. Shear is correspondingly reduced and

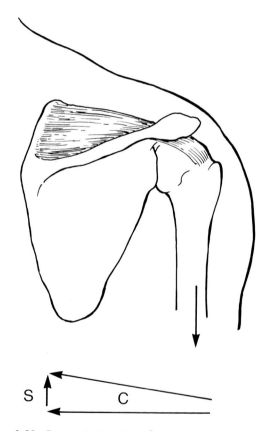

Fig. 1-21. Supraspinatus joint forces, compression dominant.

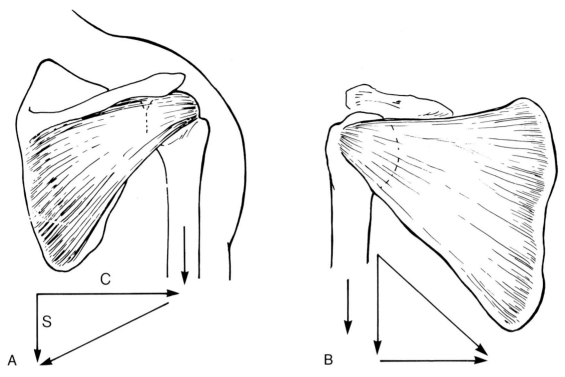

Fig. 1-22. Depressor muscles of the rotator cuff: shear force is strong and downward. **(A)** Infraspinatus. **(B)** Subscapularis.

compression increased. By 60° abduction the shear and compression values are equal. Above this position, compression dominates (Fig. 1-20B).

Independent deltoid action, thus leads to upward displacement of the humerus on the glenoid during the initial 45° of arm elevation. As this is the range commonly used, it represents a significant clinical threat. The effect can be impingement of the rotator cuff against the acromion.

ROTATOR CUFF

Rotator cuff muscle force patterns contrast sharply with the deltoid. Their dominant directions are horizontal and downward. The supraspinatus, extending from the supraspinous fossa to the greater tuberosity, is basically horizontal (Fig. 1-21). It has 70° angle with the glenoid face. As a result, compression (93 percent) is the dominant joint force generated. There is a much smaller vertical shear, equalling 4 percent of the muscle force.

All three of the other rotator cuff muscles have a mean downward alignment (Fig. 1-22). While their precise alignment has not been measured, it approximates 45° for the intraspinatus and subscapularis and 55° for the teres minor.[20] Their inferior shear force (71 percent to 82 percent) would counteract that of the deltoid.[15] Inman noted that during routine arm elevation the deltoid and rotator cuff contracted synchronously. He termed this action the shoulder force coupled with the upward and downward forces balance (Fig. 1-23). Inman also postulated that arm abduction could not occur without rotator cuff coordination.

The combined effect of such muscle action was calculated by Inman et al.[16] as creating a shoulder joint compression force equaling 10.2 times the arm's weight. Since they estimated the arm as 9 percent of the body (rather than Demster's[7] anatomically determined 5 percent) this force approximated the one times body weight value of Poppen and Walker.[22]

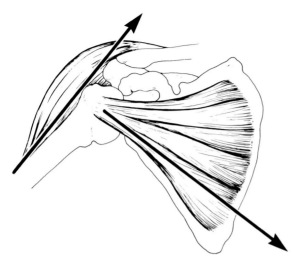

Fig. 1-23. Inman force couple between deltoid and depressor muscles in the rotator cuff.

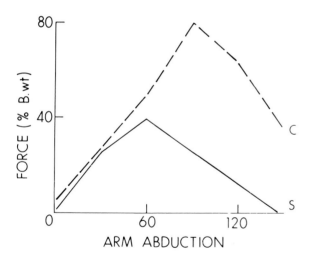

Fig. 1-24. Shoulder joint force pattern during scapular plane arm elevation. *C*, compression; *S*, shear. (Poppen NK, Walker PS: Forces at the glenohumeral joint in abduction. Clin Orthop 136:165, 1978.)

These authors also found that peak joint force occurred at 90° while maximum shear was at the 60° position (Fig. 1-24). Hence, activities with the shoulder elevated to 90° offers optimum joint stability.

SUMMARY

Shoulder versatility lies in its vast three-dimensional mobility. Arm elevation to approximately 180° is the basic motion. This is supplemented by axial rotation and horizontal flexion/extension. Neutral arm elevation occurs in the plane of the scapula (30 to 45° anterior to the coronal plane). Flexion and abduction introduce supplementary motion and twisting of the interior capsule.

Normal function combines humeral and scapular motion for arm elevation. Their relative contributions approximate a 2:1 ratio. This includes a scapular lag at both the initial and terminal 30° arcs. Athletes, such as swimmers, who drive the arm to maximum range have a special functional challenge.

As virtually all arm function is antigravity, direct muscular control is needed. The intensity of such action is proportional to the demands imposed by arm weight and position plus the added effects of any object held. Arm weight gains leverage as it is raised from the body plane, thereby increasing the demand torque (torque = force × lever length). The force of the muscular response it must exert depends on its available lever length. For the deltoid, leverage changes markedly with joint position, while that of the supraspinatus remains about the same.

Shear and compression joint forces are created as the muscles contract. Compression contributes to joint stability, while shear tends to induce humeral displacement. The deltoid, in particular, creates upward shear forces greater than its compression until the arm is horizontal. Counterbalancing downward forces are provided by the infraspinatus and subscapularis. The supraspinatus, with its horizontal alignment, reduces the work of the deltoid. It also provides a compressive force that tends to centralize the humeral head within the glenoid socket. Joint stability thus depends on balanced muscle forces.

REFERENCES

1. Basmajian JV, Bazant, FG: Factors preventing downward dislocation of the adducted shoulder—an electromyographic and morphological study. J Bone Joint Surg 41A:1182, 1959

2. Bechtol CO: Biomechanics of the shoulder. Clin Orthop 146:37, 1980

3. Boone DC, Azen SP: Normal range of motion of joint in male subjects. J Bone Joint Surg 61A:756, 1979

4. Carlson BR: Relationship between isometric and isotonic strength. Arch Phys Med Rehabil 51:176, 1970

5. Codman EA: The Shoulder. G Miller, New York, 1934

6. DeLuca CJ, Forrest WJ: Force analysis of individual muscles acting simultaneously on the shoulder joint during isometric abduction. J Biomech 6:385, 1973

7. Demster W: Space requirements of the seated operator. WADC Technical Report 55–159, Washington, D.C., Office of Technical Services, U.S. Dept. of Commerce, 1955

8. Doody SG, Freedman L, Waterland JC: Shoulder movements during abduction in the scapular plane. Arch Phys Med Rehabil 51:595, 1970

9. Dvir Z, Berme N: The shoulder complex in elevation of the arm: a mechanism approach. J Biomech 11:219, 1978

10. Freedman L, Munro R: Abduction of the arm in the scapular plane: scapular and glenohumeral movements. J Bone Joint Surg 48A:1503, 1966

11. Garfin SR, Tipton CM, Mubark SJ et al: Role of fascia in maintenance of muscle tension and pressure. J Appl Physiol 51(2):317, 1981

12. Haggmark T, Jansson E, Svane B: Cross-sectional area of the thigh muscle in man measured by computed tomography. Scan J Clin Lab Invest 38:355, 1978

13. Haxton HA: Absolute muscle force in the ankle plantar flexors of man. J Physiol (London) 103:267, 1944

14. Kent BE: Functional anatomy of the shoulder complex. Phys Ther 51:867, 1971

15. Inman VT, Saunders JBDeCM: Observations on the function of the clavicle. Calif Med 65:158, 1946

16. Inman VT, Saunders JBDeCM, Abbott LC: Observations on the function of the shoulder joint. J Bone Joint Surg 42:1, 1944

17. Johnston TB: The movements of the shoulder joint. Br J Surg 25:252, 1937

18. Maki S, Gruen T: Anthropometric study of the glenohumeral joints. Trans Orthop Res Soc 1:173, 1976

19. Matsen FA III: Biomechanics of the shoulder. In Frankel VH, Nordin M (eds): Basic Biomechanics of the Skeletal System. Lea & Febiger, Philadelphia, 1980

20. Perry J: Anatomy and biomechanics of the shoulder in throwing, swimming, gymnastics and tennis. Clin Sports Med 2:2:247, 1983

21. Poppen NK, Walker PS: Normal and abnormal motion of the shoulder. J Bone Joint Surg 58A:195, 1976

22. Poppen NK, Walker PS: Forces at the glenohumeral joint in abduction. Clin Orthop 136:165, 1978

23. Saha AK: Mechanics of elevation of glenohumeral joint. Acta Orthop Scand 44:668, 1973

24. Schmidt GL: Biomechanical analysis of knee flexion and extension. J Biomech 6:79, 1973

24a. Steindler A: Kinesiology of the Human Body. Charles C Thomas, Springfield, 1964

25. Walker PS. Human Joints and Their Artificial Replacements. Charles C Thomas, Springfield, IL, 1977

26. Weber EF: Ueber die langenderhaltnisse der fleischfasen der muskeln im allgemeinen. Berlin Verh K Sach Ges Wissensch Math-Phys 63, 1851

Muscle Control of the Shoulder 2

Jacquelin Perry

Muscles act to create motion, restrain passive motion, or maintain a stationary posture. In these capacities they serve as accelerators, decelerators, and stabilizers, respectively. The immediate muscular synergy is determined by the action desired, the force required, and the position of the body in space.

Shoulder function most commonly relates to lifting, moving, or propelling an object. Conversely, by stabilizing the arm, the shoulder muscles also may be used to move the body.

During the course of these activities the arm imposes three demands on its controlling muscles: postural stability, dynamic stability, and selective motion. Because the arm and shoulder girdle are suspended from the body at the sternum both the glenohumeral and scapulothoracic muscles must meet all demands. Arm function presents a vigorous challenge to the tissue. Optimal protection depends on appropriate muscle strength and coordination.

Clinical concerns relating to muscle control raise two questions. What muscle strength is needed to meet functional demand? How is injury avoided? At the shoulder the particular problems are pathologic impingement and subluxation. These questions will be answered by focusing on the most relevant motion patterns.

GLENOHUMERAL JOINT

Twelve muscle units control the glenohumeral joint.[39] This number includes the anterior, middle, and posterior deltoid as well as the clavicular and sternal components of the pectoralis major as functionally distinct muscles. Their unique origins provide different lines of pull across the joint even though the muscles coalesce into common tendons of insertion. Anatomically the twelve muscles fall into three functional groups: superficial, deep, and peripheral.[27]

The superficial muscle group is dominated by the three heads of the deltoid (Fig. 2-1). Their primary function is arm elevation. Anteriorly the deltoid is supplemented by three additional muscles: the clavicular pectoralis major, coracobrachialis, and long head of the biceps brachii.[23]

Four muscles constitute the deep group. Due to the blending of their tendons about the humeral head, they are called the *rotator cuff*.[21] Included are the supraspinatus, subscapularis, infraspinatus, and teres minor. (Fig. 2-2). They are characterized by short muscle fibers, close proximity to the joint, and coalescence of their tendons into a fibrous cuff. These muscle have two functions: rotation and joint stabilization.

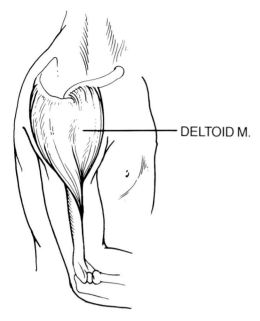

Fig. 2-1. Deltoid, the dominant superficial muscle, positioned to elevate the arm. It is composed of anterior, middle, and posterior heads.

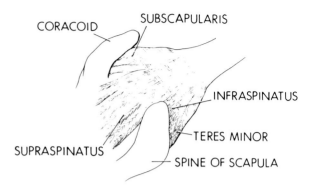

Fig. 2-2. Rotator cuff, the deep shoulder muscle group composed of the subscapularis, supraspinatus, infraspinatus, and teres minor. (Adapted from Jobe FW, Moynes DM, Tibone JE, Perry J: An EMG analysis of the shoulder in throwing and pitching. A preliminary report. Am U Sports Med 11:3, 1983.)

The peripheral muscles are unique because they originate on the thorax rather than the scapula yet insert on the humerus. Anteriorly there is the sternal pectoralis major and posteriorly the latissimus dorsi (Fig. 2-3). Both are large sheets of long muscle fibers arising from broad sites of origin. Their architecture allows for a large arc of forceful depression. In arm function, this provides rapid descent. The same muscles also are the means of raising the trunk with the arms. Blending with the tendon of the latissimus dorsi is the teres major, which arises from the scapula. As its humeral actions are the same as the larger muscle it has been included in this peripheral group even though there is no trunk attachment.

POSTURAL STABILITY

In the standing position the arm at rest is suspended by soft tissues because the bony shelf is too shallow to provide an adequate supporting surface.

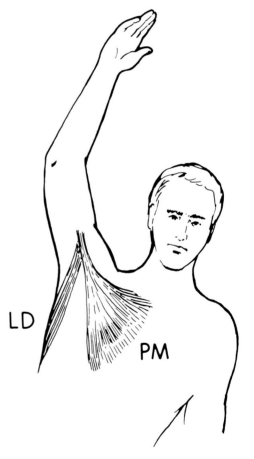

Fig. 2-3. The latissimus dorsi (*LD*) and pectoralis major (*PM*) constitute the peripheral muscle group.

Glenohumeral relations are similar to a cup against a vertical saucer. Persistent ligamentous tension causes relative ischemia, pain, and eventual stretch.[29] Muscular protection is needed, at least intermittently, to relieve the ligaments of their strain so that tissue integrity is preserved. The pattern of such protection varies between quiet standing and walking.

Quiet Standing

In the relaxed, erect posture, none of the muscles about the shoulder joint has been found to display any EMG activity. When the dynamic suspensory system is challenged, however, by a downward tug on the arm or a weight in the hand there is a strong response in the supraspinatus and a weak reaction by the posterior deltoid (Fig. 2-4). No activity has been identified in the middle deltoid, triceps, or biceps.[6] The difference between the responding and inactive muscle groups is their fiber alignment and hence the direction of their force. Compression is the dominant force produced by the horizontally oriented supraspinatus[28] (70° angle with the glenoid fossa). Much of the posterior deltoid also has an oblique orientation of its fibers and thus also would provide a compressive force. In contrast, shear is the primary force produced by the other muscles since their primary alignment is longitudinal. Their action would raise the humerus yet not place the head into the glenoid socket. This simple experiment strongly implies that compression is the stabilizing force for the glenohumeral joint. Only by pressing the ball into the shallow socket can the narrow rim inhibit shear.

Walking

Arm swing while subject walked on a treadmill shows a similar but more intense pattern of muscle action.[3] Throughout each stride there was almost continuous supraspinatus activity (Fig. 2-4). Both the posterior and middle deltoids were active during the period of backward arm swing and at the termination of the arm's forward motion (the time of ipsilateral heel strike). Middle deltoid began slightly earlier. Deceleration of forward swing was assisted by the latissimus dorsi and teres major. There intensity of action was 5 to 10 percent of maximum. The anterior deltoid biceps and triceps were quiet during deceleration.

DYNAMIC STABILITY

Rotator cuff strength is the key to dynamic glenohumeral stability. The function of this muscle group is to reduce the shearing strain experienced by the joint, which they accomplish both by fiber alignment and immediate proximity of their insertion sites to the joint margin. Contouring of the tendons around the humeral head is the basis of a restraining force

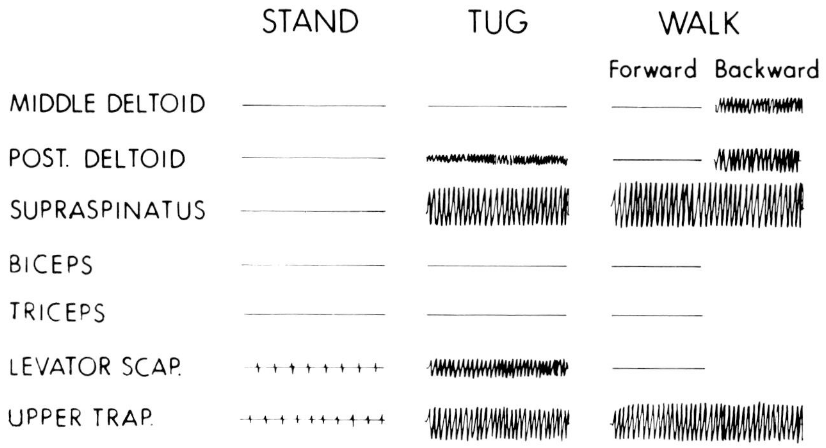

	STAND	TUG	WALK	
			Forward	Backward
MIDDLE DELTOID	———	———	———	∿∿∿∿∿
POST. DELTOID	———	∿∿∿∿∿	———	∿∿∿∿∿
SUPRASPINATUS	———	∿∿∿∿∿∿∿	∿∿∿∿∿∿∿	
BICEPS	———	———	———	
TRICEPS	———	———	———	
LEVATOR SCAP.	+ + + + + + + +	∿∿∿∿∿∿∿	———	
UPPER TRAP.	+ + + + + + + + +	∿∿∿∿∿∿∿	∿∿∿∿∿∿∿∿∿	

Fig. 2-4. Muscle support for the dependent arm.

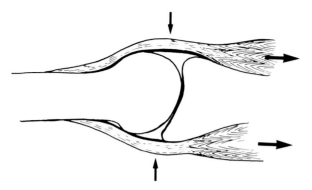

Fig. 2-5. Rotator cuff muscle action creates compressive and encircling shear forces to stabilize the humeral head on the glenoid fossa.

as muscle action transforms the tissue into straighter, tense bands (Fig. 2-5). Both compression and shear forces are created to stabilize the humeral head on the glenoid.

Alignment of the deltoid induces a significant shear force as the muscle elevates the arm.[28] This is true for all three heads. Synchronous action by the supraspinatus, infraspinatus, and subscapularis can provide protective counterforces.[16,21] The synergy between the rotator cuff and deltoid will be detailed in the following discussion of the different patterns of motion.

MOTION

Raising the arm from its resting position is the basic shoulder motion. Versatility in hand placement or the path of dynamic arm propulsion is accomplished by varying the plane of arm elevation and supplementing the action with horizontal and rotatory motion. This represents a vast number of possible movement combinations. A simple personal experiment demonstrated that normal selective control is so precise that the arm can be repositioned within 1° of the first position. Applying this level of control to the average ranges of shoulder motion indicates that the normal person has the potential to place the hand selectively in 16,000 positions.[26] The fine artist or champion athlete very probably has more precise con-

trol and hence a greater number of options available. To allow interpretation of the patterns of muscle control, however, the basic motion patterns will be considered separately.

Elevation

Two sources of control are used to raise the arm: the superficial muscle group and the underlying supraspinatus. Within the superficial musculature, the deltoid is dominant. The exact pattern of muscle action varies with the plane of motion selected.

DELTOID

While the deltoid is a continuous muscular sheet wrapped around the shoulder, it functions as three distinct muscles: anteriorly, middle, and posterior.

The middle deltoid is dominant: it participates in all arm elevation activities.[24,36] Supplementing its action are the anterior and posterior heads. They may act synergistically to add an abductor force or assume primary responsibility for arm elevation in their direction (flexion or extension). Hence, the pattern of deltoid action varies with the plane of motion used. Middle deltoid dominance in most arm elevation actions is enhanced by its larger size (12 cm^2 compared to 9 cm^2 for the anterior and posterior deltoids).

Scapular plane elevation is provided by combined

ARM ELEVATION

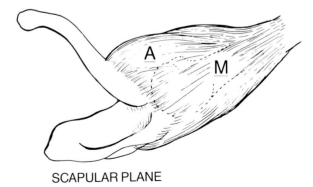

SCAPULAR PLANE

Fig. 2-6. Muscles providing neutral arm elevation (scapular plane). *A*, anterior deltoid; *M*, middle deltoid.

action of the middle and anterior deltoids[24,36] (Fig. 2-6). Their relative effectiveness, however, varies with arm position. In the lower arc of motion (30°) the middle deltoid has the better leverage (1.7 versus 0.5 cm).[28] As the arm reaches 60°, anterior deltoid lever length become equals to that of the middle muscle (3 cm). At 90° and above the anterior deltoid has the greater leverage, reaching 4.5 cm by 150° while the middle deltoid experiences little change (3.2 cm). EMG studies[19,24] confirm the simultaneous action of the anterior and middle deltoids throughout arm elevation.

Participation of the posterior deltoid in scapular plane elevation is less consistent. By roentgenologic analysis an abduction lever was not identified until the arm reached the 90° position.[28] This increased rapidly as the arm was raised but reached only moderate effectiveness (2.5 cm). Various EMG studies are in conflict. Jones[18] found that the posterior deltoid did not become active until the arm was above 60°. Nuber and Gowan,[24] however, recorded significant

activity throughout the range, though peak intensity was lower (49 percent compared to 71 percent and 60 percent, respectively, for the middle and anterior deltoids). Hence, all three deltoid muscles can make significant contribution to neutral arm elevation.

For flexion, the anterior deltoid is the primary muscle. It is assisted by the clavicular pectoralis major, coracobrachialis, and biceps brachii as well as the middle deltoid (Fig. 2-7). While only the EMG activity of the clavicular pectoralis major (CPM) has been studied in detail,[16,32,36] participation by the other muscles has been confirmed. Relative EMG activity of the CPM and deltoid indicated that these superficial muscles provided about 30 percent of the arm elevation effort.

Abduction in the coronal plane adds significant posterior deltoid action to that of the anterior and middle components[24,32] (Fig. 2-8). Conversely, participation of the anterior deltoid is less. This difference is particularly apparent in the arc of motion below 90°.

Hyperextension, or posterior elevation, is dominated by the posterior deltoid. There also is strong participation by the middle deltoid but the anterior muscle is silent.[36]

Effectiveness of the deltoid muscles depends on their functional fiber length. It is greatest with the arm in the dependent rest period and shortest with full glenohumeral elevation (Fig. 2-9).[22] Anatomically, this represents a 33 percent reduction in the length of the muscle.[22] Functionally, the muscle becomes weaker. With the scapula held rigid by body straps,

ARM ELEVATION

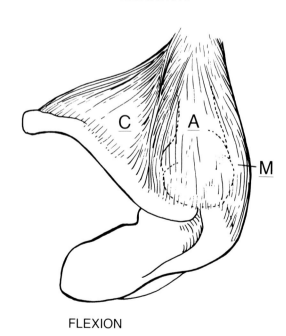

FLEXION

Fig. 2-7. Muscles providing arm flexion (sagittal plane elevation). *C*, clavicular head of the major; *A*, anterior deltoid; *M*, middle deltoid.

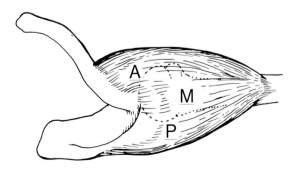

ABDUCTION

Fig. 2-8. Muscle providing arm abduction (coronal plane elevation). *A*, anterior deltoid; *M*, middle deltoid; *P*, posterior deltoid.

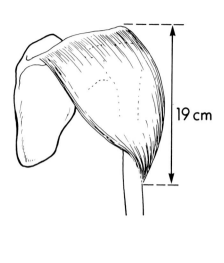

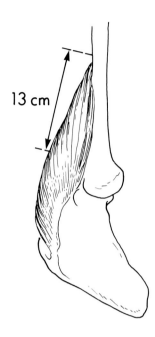

Fig. 2-9. Change in deltoid muscle length between the resting position and full arm elevation. (Adapted from Lucas DB: Biomechanics of the shoulder joint. Arch Surg 107:425, 1973.)

the arm can only be raised 90°, though an additional 30° of passive range (120° elevation) is available.[15] Also, strength in the 90° position is insufficient to accept any additional resistance.[22] Such loss of deltoid strength normally is avoided by scapular rotation. This synergy not only preserves deltoid force but also reduces the demand by placing the glenoid under the humeral head for support. Hence, deltoid function is very dependent on scapulohumeral rhythm.

The deltoid is anatomically capable of initiating, as well as completing, arm elevation independently due to its mass, even though the leverage at 30° is very low. A strenuous effect (about 54 percent of maximal) would be required, however, with a corresponding limit in endurance (Fig. 2-10).

SUPRASPINATUS

This muscle is active in all patterns of arm elevation.[16,24,36] Its short leverage (2.2 cm) and modest size (6 cm²)[28] limit the torque that can be produced, however. Maximum effort (calculated as 98 percent) could accomplish arm elevation to 30° but not higher (Fig. 2-10B). As this intensity of action would leave no endurance for a second effort, assistance, not initiation of abduction, is its role.

DELTOID–SUPRASPINATUS RELATIONSHIPS

Common to all three patterns of arm elevation is combined deltoid and supraspinatus action.[15,16,18,24,31,36] The relative responsibility of these two muscles, however, still is in doubt.

It has been commonly assumed that abduction of the arm is initiated by the supraspinatus and continued by the deltoid.[14]

Codman[9] believed that the deltoid could not abduct the arm without the supraspinatus. This interpretation is based on clinical experience with large rotator cuff ruptures.[9] Such a lesion deprives the person of the ability to lift the arm, yet once the arm has been passively raised to the horizontal the patient can maintain that arm position, though strength is reduced.[9]

Three findings contradict the probability that abduction is initiated by the supraspinatus: muscle size, EMG patterns, and cuff mechanics.

As described in Chapter 1, the muscle is anatomically too small to lift the arm independently. While it could accomplish the first 30°, a 200 percent effort would be required to reach the horizontal position. In contrast, the size and leverage of the deltoid would allow the arm to be raised with an effort of 55 percent of maximum.

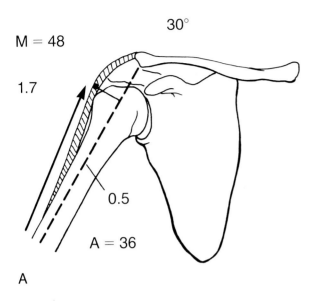

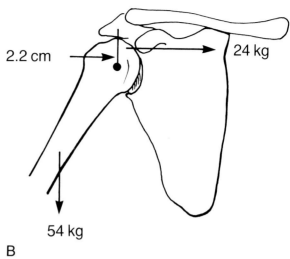

A

B

Fig. 2-10. Relative effectiveness of deltoid and supraspinatus in arm elevation. (**A**) Independent deltoid action at 30° equals 54 percent of maximum capability. (**B**) Independent supraspinatus capability equals 98 percent of available torque. 2.2 cm = lever length; 24 kg = muscle force; 54 kg = demand torque by arm weight. Shoulder position = 30° abduction. (**C**) Combined deltoid (*D*) and supraspinatus (*S*) action reduces effort to 35 percent for each muscle. Arrows indicate direction of dominant muscle force.

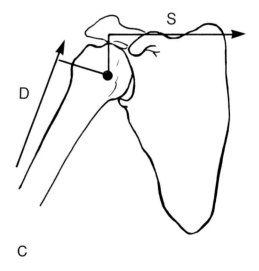

C

Dynamic EMG shows that the middle and anterior deltoids and supraspinatus function synchronously.[15,24,36] Through such a combined action, the calculated intensity of each muscle is 35 percent of maximum strength (Fig. 2-10C). This level of muscular effort would be compatible with long endurance demands.

Participation by the other rotator cuff muscle also has been identified. Presumably they contribute to the force couple that facilitates arm elevation.[16,24,36]

GLENOHUMERAL FORCE COUPLE

Dynamic EMG studies of the four rotator cuff muscles and the deltoid during arm elevation in flexion, abduction, or scapular plane elevation have shown that all were active throughout the full range,[16,24,31,36] though their intensities varied (Fig. 2-11). Inman et al.[16] interpreted this as an obligatory multidirectional force couple to counteract the effect of the deltoid's longitudinal alignment.

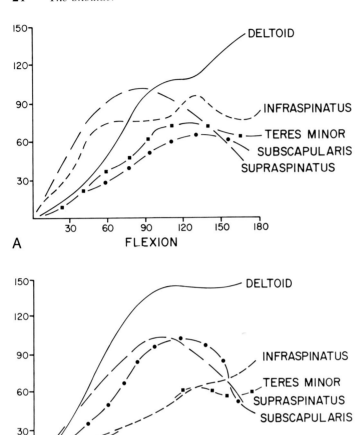

Fig. 2-11. Relative intensity of deltoid and rotator cuff muscle action during arm elevation (dynamic EMG values) for **(A)** flexion and **(B)** abduction. Vertical scale, microvolts of EMG; horizontal scale, degrees of arm elevation.

Acting independently, the vertical alignment of the deltoid would introduce upward displacement of the humerus (Fig. 2-12). This could lead to the cuff impinging against the acromion.[28] Also, the lack of articular cartilage presents a less efficient fulcrum, so joint motion would be impeded.[9]

Synergistic action of the supraspinatus leads to better joint function. The muscle's horizontal alignment combined with a tension band effect of its tendon tends to direct the humeral head towards the glenoid (Fig. 2-10C), thereby improving the fulcrum. Accompanying action of the subscapularis and infraspinatus offers a downward pull that would most specifically counter the deltoid-induced displacement.[16] (Fig. 2-13). Mechanically, the combination of upward, horizontal, and downward muscle pull results in optimal arm elevation as well as joint centralization.[16] This

theory is very compatible with the loss of abduction by a massive cuff tear.

Electromyography of rapid motions, such as pitching a baseball, fail to display this presumably obligatory synergy. While the deltoid and supraspinatus show similar timing and intensity, the subscapularis and infraspinatus act independently.[15,18,19]

Nerve block studies also have demonstrated that synergistic action between the deltoid and supraspinatus muscles is not essential for full arm elevation, though about 50 percent of normal strength was lost[10,11] (Fig. 2-14). Suprascapular anesthesia that inhibited both the supraspinatus and infraspinatus muscles left two other components of the rotator cuff intact because both the subscapularis and teres minor have other innervation. With the cuff structurally intact, these two remaining muscles might provide a mini-

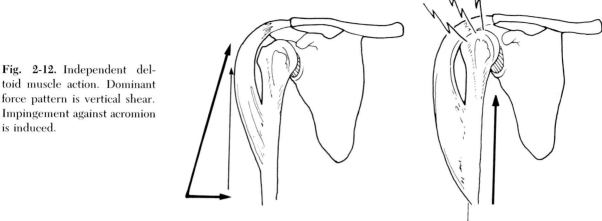

Fig. 2-12. Independent deltoid muscle action. Dominant force pattern is vertical shear. Impingement against acromion is induced.

mally adequate counterforce to preserve humeral head alignment. As this would be lost with a major cuff rupture, the experimental situation did not truly mimic the clinical problem.

The axillary nerve blocks to deactivate the deltoid also allowed complete arm abduction.[10,11] Again, the strength loss was approximately 50 percent of normal. This situation is similar to natural pathologic conditions. There are several reports in the literature of patients recovering full arm elevation despite complete paralysis of the deltoid.[35,37] A substitution we have observed is external rotation of the arm as elevation is attempted. This would favorably position the biceps on the lateral side of the joint for optimal lever-

age. Muscle force would be adequate because the cross-sectional size of the biceps is approximately two-thirds of the middle deltoid. Also, the coracobrachialis might assist because it has the same line of pull as the short head of the biceps.

Simultaneous axillary and suprascapular blocks removed the subject's ability to raise the arm.[10] The investigators considered that this finding confirmed that only the supraspinatus and deltoid were functionally significant in arm abduction. A more cautious interpretation of these experimental findings is indicated, however, since neither side of the force couple was completely eliminated. It would have been appropriate to have said that accessory muscles by them-

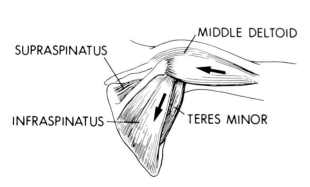

Fig. 2-13. Synergistic action of infraspinatus and supraspinatus provides a depression force to counteract the deltoid's upward shear.

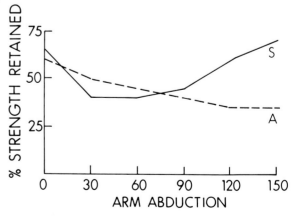

Fig. 2-14. Reduction in arm abduction force following suprascapular and axillary nerve blocks.

selves are insufficient but the lack may have been borderline due to the high torque requirement presented by the arm.

The results of these studies lead to five clinically significant conclusions:

1. A strong person can attain full arm elevation with only minimal assistance from one side of the force couple because there is sufficient extra strength to accommodate the inefficiency. This means athletes may have a disabling rotator cuff tear without losing the ability to complete arm elevation.
2. Conversely, patients lacking full arm elevation may have any of three contributing factors. They may be naturally weak (due to their life style), they might have developed disuse atrophy from a chronic pathologic condition, or they may have a very massive lesion. As a result, they lack the substitutive capacity to accommodate force couple imbalance.
3. All four muscles constituting the force couple need not work in synergy with the deltoid. The supraspinatus may be sufficient assistance if it is of adequate strength.
4. The patient's total motor control picture must be considered, not just the deltoid, when arm elevation is being assessed.
5. Relative strength also is highly significant, not just a "yes–no" capability.

INFRASPINATUS AND SUBSCAPULARIS

The normal,[16,24,31,36] athletic,[6,18] and nerve block[10,11] studies leave the role of the infraspinatus and subscapularis during arm elevation in question. Electromyographically, the infraspinatus is the next most active rotator muscle after the supraspinatus muscle while the subscapularis is more selective.[15,17,18] Because of their potential contribution to glenohumeral joint stability, enhancing their participation in arm elevation is very desirous. The basic function of these two muscles and the teres minor is humeral rotation on the glenoid.[36]

Infraspinatus activity is stimulated by elevating the arm with some degree of elbow flexion. This introduces an internal rotation torque that must be restrained if hand position is to be preserved. The teres minor would also participate in this action. EMG

studies[15,18] indicate that the infraspinatus is the more active muscle in this pair.

Subscapularis activity relates to its ability to provide internal rotation. Deceleration of external rotation is a common stimulus.[15] It often functions in company with the other internal rotators of the shoulder, such as the pectoralis major, teres major, and latissimus dorsi.

BICEPS BRACHII

Between its origin on the superior rim of the glenoid and passage through the bicipital groove on the humeral shaft, the long head of the biceps lies across the top of the humeral head. Contraction of the biceps muscle would thus appear to be a useful humeral head depressor. Limitations to its effectiveness result from its distal attachment to the radius, hence it is an elbow muscle. EMG analysis of pitching confirmed that the need for elbow control was the stimulus for biceps action, not humeral elevation. Also, peak activity of the biceps was only 36 percent of its maximum capacity. with a 9 cm^2 cross-section and only half of the muscle related to the long head, the humeral force is small. It seems doubtful that this is a significant stabilizing force at the glenohumeral joint.

Horizontal Extension and External Rotation

This motion synergy is commonly used to create a propulsive force in sports. It provides the cocking[2,14] phase of pitching,[15,18] throwing,[2] and tennis serve[1] as well as being a significant part of most strokes in swimming.[7,30,34] Both posterior impingement and anterior subluxation are likely complications.

As the middle and anterior deltoids support arm weight, the posterior deltoids increases its activity to draw the humerus backwards (horizontal extension) (Fig. 2-15). Two force patterns result: compression and anterior shear.

At the beginning of posterior deltoid action, the muscle's line of pull is primarily longitudinal, making compression the major force. Alignment of the muscle tends to concentrate the force at the posterior margins of the humeral head and glenoid fossa. During rapid motion this can be an abrupt and destructive impact of considerable intensity.

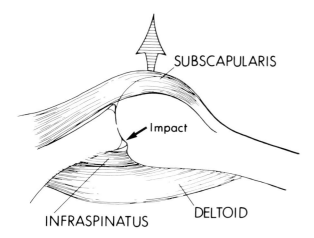

Fig. 2-15. Horizontal extension and external rotation. Posterior deltoid induced impact (small arrow) and anterior shear (large arrow) countered by infraspinatus and subscapularis muscle action.

The muscle's origination along the length of the scapular spine and insertion at the midhumeral shaft places the posterior deltoid's line of pull a considerable distance behind the glenohumeral joint center. This distance increases as horizontal extension becomes greater. This induces an anterior shear force that increases in intensity as hyperextension proceeds. External rotation accentuates the anterior subluxation tendency by directing the angulated humeral head against the anterior capsule.

Protective forces are available from three rotator cuff muscles: infraspinatus, teres minor, and subscapularis. The infraspinatus is a primary motor for both external rotation and hyperextension. Hence it can reduce the intensity of posterior deltoid action. Also, because it lies adjacent to the joint margin its actions prevent humeral subluxation. The teres minor, as an external rotator, also reduces the deltoid response.

Subscapularis activity at the end of the hyperextension/external rotation effort provides an anterior restraint against humeral displacement. This synergistic sequence is displayed in the EMG analysis of a baseball pitch (Fig. 2-16). The sternal pectoralis major also provides a protective force as its tendon crosses the anterior joint surface when the arm is both hyperextended and externally rotated. Hence, initiation of the motion combined with decelerating forces involves a complex synergy and sequence of muscle action (Fig. 2-16B).

Internal Rotation and Horizontal Flexion

Acceleration to complete the throwing or propulsive act and then follow-through are performed by the following sequence of cocking, acceleration, and follow-through. Muscle activity is stimulated by tension at the end of the cocking phase. EMG recordings

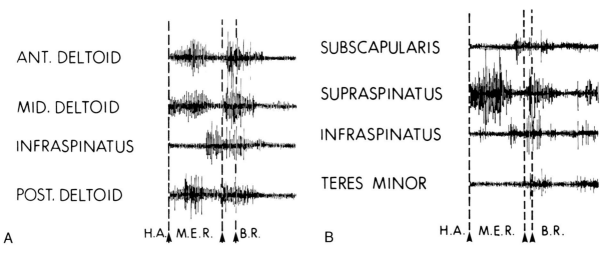

Fig. 2-16. Muscle action during a typical baseball pitch. (**A**) Deltoid. (**B**) Rotator cuff. Phases of pitching: *HA*, hands apart; *MER*, maximum external rotation; *BR*, ball release.

show that the major muscle contributing to acceleration is the subscapularis.[15,18] Participation of the sternal pectoralis major and latissimus dorsi was less consistent. The latter muscle was strongly used by professional pitchers while the amateurs called on the pectoralis major.[13] Athletic use of the teres major has not been assessed but EMG studies of basic arm function identified its action in internal rotation and adduction.[36] This implies that the teres major would be a logical participant in the acceleration to follow-through motion sequence.

During follow-through the weight of the arm creates a distractive force at the shoulder from the pendulous momentum present. Antagonistic action identified in the infraspinatus, teres minor supraspinatus, and latissimus dorsi[13] to decelerate the force would serve to maintain shoulder joint integrity.

SCAPULOTHORACIC ARTICULATION

Five muscles directly control the scapula. Functional division of the trapezius into upper, middle, and lower units expands the number to seven. Because the actions of the pectoralis minor can only be guessed at, its actions will not be discussed. Also, the major and minor rhomboids will be considered as one. Hence, functional concern revolves around six muscle units: levator scapulae; upper, middle, and lower trapezius; rhomboids; and serratus anterior. Synergistic action of the muscles varies with the scapular motion desired (Fig. 2-17).

Among the scapula's six potential functions two are of major clinical concern: upward rotation in conjunc-

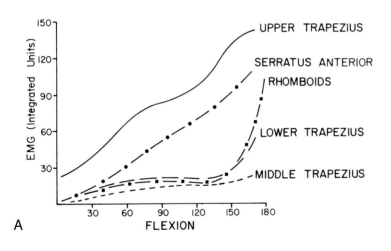

A   FLEXION

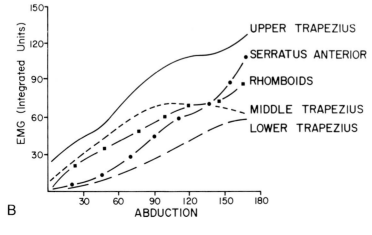

B   ABDUCTION

Fig. 2-17. Synergistic action of the major muscles controlling the scapula during arm elevation. (**A**) Flexion. (**B**) Abduction. (Adapted from Inman et al: Observation on the function of the shoulder joint. J Bone Joint Surg 26:3, 1944.)

tion with arm elevation and postural support of the scapula. The other actions complete the arm's versatility with their significance varying according to the person's occupation or sport.

Postural Support

With the trunk upright (sitting or standing), arm weight tends to draw the scapula downward. Passive suspension is available from the deep fascia of the neck, which extends from head to clavicle and spine of the scapula, enclosing the trapezius and sternocleidomastoid muscles within its span. The deep fascia of the back also contributes to scapular stability.

Active suspension is available from two vertically oriented muscles: the levator scapulae and upper trapezius (Fig. 2-18). Visibility of the latter muscle has led most people to assume that the upper trapezius was the major source of support but the underlying levator scapulae is the larger muscle mass.[38] As was identified at the glenohumeral joint, no consistent muscle action is required during quiet standing though low levels of EMG activity have been noted.[5,8] The possibility of this minimal action being a continuation of initial positioning is implied by its cessation following conscious relaxation.[8]

Adding a load to the hand or active elevation of the scapula initiates a brisk response by the levator scapulae[12] and upper trapezius.[8] Relative dominance

between the levator scapulae and upper trapezius has not been assessed by a common study.

The rhomboid and serratus anterior muscles also have been assumed to assist scapular suspension, as their fibers have an obliquely vertical orientation.[5,12] EMG studies of active scapula elevation, however, have failed to demonstrate any participation of either the rhomboid or serratus. Hence, the initial assumption is incorrect. A closer look at fiber alignment identifies that neither muscle has a dominantly vertical orientation and hence mechanically they would be very inefficient as scapular elevators.[12,36]

During walking, virtually continuous activity of the upper trapezius has been recorded.[3] Participation by the levator scapulae has not been assessed but the trend to accentuate the static posture during walking suggests it is active at a low level.

Tension on the two suspensory muscles (levator scapulae and upper trapezius) varies with the resting position of the scapula. This, in turn, is influenced by trunk alignment. In the normal erect posture the scapula's superior angle lies opposite the second vertebra. The vertebral border is 7 to 8 cm from

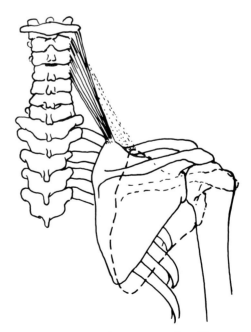

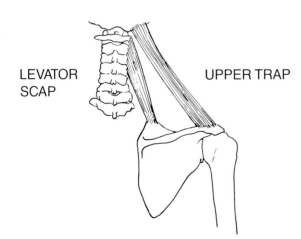

Fig. 2-18. Active suspension of the scapula with the arm dependent.

Fig. 2-19. Levator scapulae tension induced by passive forward droop of the scapula.

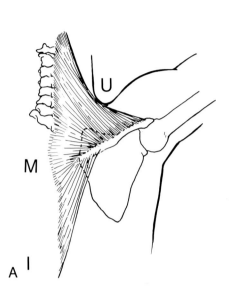
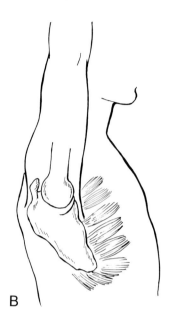

Fig. 2-20. Dominant rotators of the scapula during arm elevation. (**A**) Trapezius. *U*, upper; *M*, middle; *I*, inferior. (**B**) Serratus anterior.

the midline and rests on the relatively flat, posterior surface of the rib cage.[4] The root of the scapular spine is opposite the sternoclavicular joint. Forward trunk lean (thoracic slump) allows arm weight to pull the scapula down as well as laterally along the more oblique surface of the ribs. The suspensory muscles (levator scapulae in particular) are put on stretch (Fig. 2-19). Such tension can be relieved by scapular retraction. As the middle trapezius and rhomboids pull the scapulae towards the midline, they automatically also cause it to ascend the rib channel. Chronic forward posturing leads to contracture of the anterior pectoral fascia, which may require stretching before the desired alignment can be attained.

Motion

Although each scapular motion can be performed independently for testing, they normally are an integral component of arm function.

Upward Rotation

Rotation of the scapula is defined by the direction the glenoid moves. Upward rotation is an essential component of arm elevation. Two muscles are recog-

nized as the upward rotators of the scapula: trapezius and serratus anterior (Fig. 2-20). Inman et al.[16] also included the levator scapulae. Normally, the trapezius and serratus act together but either also can accomplish scapular rotation independently, though the strength of arm elevation will be less.

Inman et al.[16] identified a force couple in each muscle comprised of upper and lower segments that produced upward rotation of the scapula (Fig. 2-21). For the serratus anterior the levator scapulae was considered to be the upward force unit, rather than the proximal segments of the serratus. Phylogenetically these two muscles are a common sheet (Fig. 2-22). This is confirmed by De Freitas,[12] who recently showed strong EMG activity of the levator scapulae during abduction and moderate action during flexion. Consistent activity of the fifth and sixth digitations of the serratus anterior during both patterns of arm elevation designates this as the primary lower force.[16] The most distal digitations (seven and eight) displayed less participation in the latter range of abduction, allowing the inferior scapular angle to remain in the coronal plane. Our unpublished study of the serratus showed that the upper (transverse) fibers of the serratus also participated in upward rotation of the scapula.[20]

Within the trapezius, Inman et al.[16] found that only

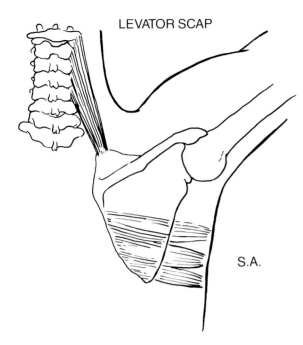

LEVATOR SCAP

S.A.

Fig. 2-21. Serratus force couple: upper force = levator scapulae; lower force = digits 5, 6 of serratus anterior (*SA*).

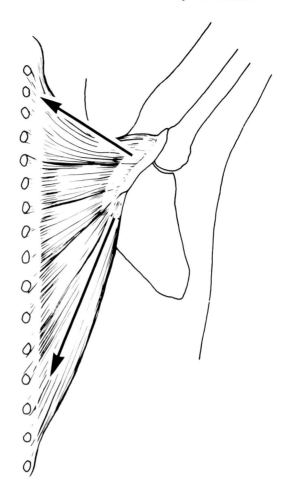

Fig. 2-22. Trapezius force couple: upper force = upper trapezius; lower force = lower trapezius.

the upper segment displayed consistent action in both abduction and flexion (Fig. 2-22). Reduced participation by the lower trapezius in all but the last segment of flexion leaves the scapula free to move anteriorly. Consistent with its transverse alignment and posterior location, the middle trapezius showed significant activity only in abduction. These two limitations in the trapezius's contribution to flexion places an added burden on the serratus anterior. This is particularly true in swimming where maximum upward reach is used to increase one's stroke.

Rhomboid muscle action was found to be similar to that of the middle trapezius but less intense. Its participation in any arm elevation suggests that the downward obliquity of the fibers is functionally less significant than their horizontal component, which contributes to medial stabilization during abduction. As the scapula rotates upward, rhomboid fiber alignment would become more favorable.

Upward rotation of the scapula serves three functions. It provides stabilizing base for the humerus by moving the glenoid underneath the arm as it is raised. Deltoid fiber length is preserved as acromial–humeral distance is maintained. Upward rotation of

the acromial arch also lessens the potential for humeral impingement at the end of the arm range.

To attain maximum scapular rotation, both the trapezius and serratus anterior must be effective. EMG analysis of swimming demonstrates that the serratus worked at 75 percent of its maximum muscle test capability.[25] This is too strenuous for a lengthy effort. A similar high level of activity was identified during voluntary arm elevation in all three basic planes whether the elbow was flexed or extended.[24] Raising the arm to 90° averaged 41 percent of maximum while reaching full elevation increased the effort to 66 percent of maximum. The relative intensity of the serratus consistently was greater than that of the trapezius, which progressed from 34 to 42 percent maximum.

According to Weber's data[38] the two muscles are of equivalent size (12.8 and 12.6 cm²) and thus should have similar force potentials. The greater effort by the serratus suggests that it is less well developed to meet the functional demands imposed on it. Adequate training, thus, is particularly significant if one is to lessen the threats of impingement. Maximum overhead reach puts all the muscles in a relatively inefficient situation due to fiber shortening. Activities in flexion reduce the ability of the lower trapezius to contribute, resulting in a higher demand on the serratus. A 75 percent effort by the serratus cannot be maintained during lengthy swimming sessions, hence better training is indicated.

Retraction (Adduction)

Drawing the scapula back towards the vertebral midline accentuates horizontal extension of the arm. A synonym for this action is scapular adduction. The cocking phase of pitching and pulling relies on such assistance. Several swimming strokes also use this action.

Direct muscle control is provided by the middle trapezius and rhomboids. The latissimus dorsi also retracts the scapula incidental to complete arm extension.

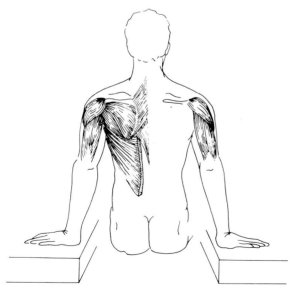

Fig. 2-23. Scapular depression used to lift body weight.

Protraction (Abduction)

Advancement of the scapula anteriorly on the thorax has been termed both protraction and scapular abduction (moving away from the vertebral column). The latter term, however, leads to confusion when scapular and humeral motions are considered together. Hence, the older term *protraction* is being adopted again. Protraction is the function of the serratus anterior. There also may be some assistance by the sternal pectoralis major as it horizontally flexes the arm. Follow-through in throwing,[2] pitching,[6] tennis serve, and crawl strokes[9,34] include scapular protraction.

Depression

Descent of the scapula is used to elevate the trunk while the arms are stabilized. The site of arm fixation varies. During gymnastics an overhead bar, ring, or underlying platform is used. Patients commonly rely on scapular depression to rise from a chair.[33]

Immediate muscular control is provided by the inferior digitations of the serratus anterior and the lower trapezius. Additional force of considerable magnitude is gained from the two large thoracohumeral muscles: sternal pectoralis major and latissimus dorsi (Fig. 2-23).

SUMMARY

Normal muscular control of the glenohumeral joint provides three functions: postural and dynamic stability and willful motion. The 12 available muscles are classified into three groups: arm elevators (deltoid and supraspinatus), joint stabilizers (rotator cuff), and peripheral movers (pectoralis major, latissimus dorsi, and teres major).

Arm elevation capability of the deltoid and supraspinatus differs markedly. The deltoid can meet the demand independently, while the supraspinatus cannot. Synergistic action reduces the intensity either muscle must exert. Additional action by the infraspinatus and subscapularis also balances the shear forces, leading to further muscular efficiency as well as protection of the joint. Participation of the depressor rotator cuff muscles is not obligatory, hence they must be selectively strengthened. Horizontal extension and external rotation introduce considerable potential for shear by the dominant posterior deltoid action. Action of the infraspinatus and subscapularis reduces the threat to the joint.

Upward rotation of the scapula as part of arm elevation is provided by synergistic action of the trapezius and serratus anterior. The muscles serve two roles: increasing the range of motion and moving the acromial arch away from the rising humerus. Independent action by either muscle is possible but less efficient. Serratus development appeared less optimal, with the overhead swimming action displaying an effort 75 percent of maximum. This is inconsistent with good endurance. Thus, adequate strength must be developed in all the glenohumeral and scapular muscles and will not necessarily occur without a special training program.

REFERENCES

1. Anderson MB: Comparison of muscle patterning in the overarm throw and tennis serve. Res Q 50:541, 1979
2. Atwater AE: Biomechanics of overarm throwing movements and of throwing injuries. P. 43. In Hutton RS, Miller DI (eds): Exercise and Sport Sciences Reviews. Franklin Inst Press, Philadelphia, 1979
3. Ballesteros MLF, Buchthal F, Rosenfalck P: The pattern of muscular activity during the arm swing of natural walking. Acta Physiol Scand 63:296, 1965
4. Basmajian JV: Primary Anatomy. Williams & Wilkins, Baltimore, 1964
5. Basmajian JV: Muscles Alive, 4th ed. Williams & Wilkins, Baltimore, 1979
6. Basmajian JV, Bazant FJ: Factors preventing downward dislocation of the adducted shoulder joint. J Bone Joint Surg 41A:1182–1186, 1959
7. Batterman C: Mechanics of the crawl arm stroke. Swimming World 7:4, 1966
8. Bearn JG: An electromyographic study of the trapezius, deltoid, pectoralis major, biceps and triceps muscles during static loading of the upper arm. Anat Rec 140, 1961
9. Codman EA: The Shoulder. G. Miller, Brooklyn, NY, 1934
10. Colachis SC, Jr., Strom BR: Effects of suprascapular and axillary nerve blocks on muscle force in the upper extremity. Arch Phys Med Rehabil 52:22, 1971
11. Colachis SC, Jr., Strom BR, Brecher VL: Effects of axillary nerve blocks on muscle force in the upper extremity. Arch Phys Med Rehabil 50:647, 1969
12. De Freitas V, Vitti M, Furlani J: Electromyographic study of levator scapulae and rhombodius major muscles in movements of the shoulder and arm. Electromyog Clin Neurophysiol 20:205, 1980
13. Gowan ID, Jobe FW, Tibone JE et al: A comparative EMG analysis of the shoulder during pitching: professional vs amateur pitchers. Am J Sports Med (in press)
14. Hollingshead WH: Anatomy for Surgeons. The Back and Limbs, vol. 3. Hoeber-Harper, New York, 1958
15. Inman VT, Saunders JBDeCM: Observations on the function of the clavicle. Calif Med 65:158, 1946
16. Inman VT, Saunders JBDeCM, Abbott LeR C: Observations on the function of the shoulder joint. J Bone Surg 26:3–32, 1944
17. Jobe FW, Moynes DM, Tibone JE, Perry J: An EMG analysis of the shoulder in pitching. A second report. Am J Sports Med 12:218, 1984
18. Jobe FW, Tibone JE, Perry J, Moynes D: An EMG analysis of the shoulder in throwing and pitching. A preliminary report. Am J Sports Med 11:3, 1983
19. Jones DW, Jr.: The role of shoulder muscles in the control of humeral position (an electromyographic study). Masters Thesis, Case Western Reserve University, 1970
20. Katz DR: EMG comparison of two serratus anterior manual muscle tests, a pilot study. University of Southern California, Physical Therapy Department, 1983
21. Kent B: Functional anatomy of the shoulder complex. Phys Ther 51:867, 1971
22. Lucas DB: Biomechanics of the shoulder joint. Arch Surg 107:425, 1973
23. Matsen FA: Biomechanics of the shoulder. In Bateman JE (ed): The Shoulder and Neck, 2nd ed. W.B. Saunders, Philadelphia, 1978
24. Nuber GW, Bowan ID, Perry JP et al: EMG analysis of classical shoulder motion. Trans Orthop Res Soc 11: 1986
25. Nuber GW, Jobe FW, Perry J et al: Fine wire EMG analysis of the shoulder during swimming. Am J Sport Med 14:7, 1986
26. Perry J: Normal upper extremity kinesiology. Phys Ther 58:265, 1978
27. Perry J: Anatomy and biomechanics of the shoulder in throwing, swimming, gymnastics and tennis. Clin Sports Med 2:247, 1983

28. Poppen NK, Walker PS: Forces at the glenohumeral joint in abduction. Clin Orthop Rel Res 135:165, 1978

29. Rathburn JB, Macnab I: The microvascular pattern of the rotator cuff. J Bone Joint Surg 52B:540, 1970

30. Richardson AB, Jobe FW, Collins HR: The shoulder in competitive swimming. Am J Sports Med 8:159, 1980

31. Saha AK: Theory of Shoulder Mechanism: Descriptive and Applied. Charles C Thomas, Springfield, 1961

32. Shevlin MG, Lehmann JF, Lucci JA: Electromyographic study of the function of some muscles crossing the glenohumeral joint. Arch Phys Med Rehabil 50:264, 1969

33. Shoo MJ, Perry J: The shoulder girdle muscles in transfer, an electromyographic study. Resident Seminars, Rancho Los Amigos Hospital, 1978

34. Slater-Hammel AT: An action current study of contraction-movement relationships in the tennis stroke. Res Q 20:424, 1949

35. Staples OS, Watkins AL: Full active abduction in traumatic paralysis of the deltoid. J Bone Joint Surg 25:85, 1943

36. Sugahara R: Electromyographic study of shoulder movements. Jpn J Rehab Med 11:41, 1974

37. Van Linge B, Mulder JD: Function of the supraspinatus muscle and its relation to the supraspinatus syndrome. J Bone Joint Surg 45B:750, 1963

38. Weber EF: Ueber die langenderhaltnisse der fleischfasen der muskeln im allgemeinen. Berlin Verh K Sach Ges Wissensch Math-Phys 63, 1851

39. Williams PL, Warwick R: Gray's Anatomy, 36th ed. WB Saunders, Philadelphia, 1980

Surgical Approaches to the Shoulder

3

Carter R. Rowe

The anatomy of the shoulder allows for excellent surgical exposure, if it is properly understood. Each muscle layer can be turned back, leading to the next, in a symmetrical fashion down to the glenohumeral joint. There are strict rules, however, which, if not observed, will result in ugly scars, muscle damage, and, at times, nerve injury. There seems little reason to abuse the anatomical orderliness of the shoulder structures, yet a number of surgical approaches and operative techniques are guilty of this.

The first consideration in surgical approaches to the shoulder is to follow the skin "wrinkle" lines of Kraisal,[4] or Langer's lines[5] (Fig. 3-1) when possible, as this will give the least spread of the incision. In Figure 3-2A, the skin lines were crossed by a vertical incision resulting in a wide ugly scar. A minimal scar results when Langer's lines are followed (Fig. 3-2B). In Figure 3-3, a comparison of a correct and incorrect shoulder incision is shown.

In all exposures of the shoulder (except the sternoclavicular joint), one has to deal with the deltoid muscle, either by turning it down from its attachment or by splitting its fibers, safely down to the axillary nerve (a distance of four fingerbreadths). Some surgeons do not recommend turning the deltoid attachment down for fear that it will not reattach securely. They have good reason for this concern, since this

will occur if the procedure is not performed properly. It has been our experience that the deltoid attachment can be safely turned down, with its osteoperiosteal attachment, from the clavicle and the spine of the scapula without taking bone with the muscle. It is important that an osteoperiosteal flap of the muscle attachment be preserved for resuturing. There is only one place where this may not be adequate: over the curve of the lateral acromion, where the central tendon of the deltoid attaches. Here we have found it safer to osteotomize 0.5 cm of acromion, leaving the deltoid muscle attached to the osteotomized bone. Without the bony attachment, the deltoid may pull off and glide down the arm in an alarming manner. The osteotomized rim of acromion serves as a "handle" to the deltoid, and can be securely reattached through three or four drill holes in the acromion. We have never experienced a pull-off of the deltoid muscle using this technique.

The following approaches to the shoulder are described:

1. The horizontal "strap" incision (for calcific deposits and localized cuff injury)
2. The anterior deltoid muscle splitting approach (for localized rotator cuff tears or tuberosity fractures)
3. The "saber" anterior deltoid splitting approach (for

35

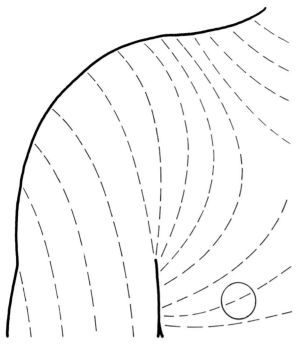

Fig. 3-1. Langer's lines originate in the axilla, and curve up and over the shoulder to the opposite axilla.

acromioclavicular arthroplasty and more extensive rotator cuff exposure)

4. The superior shoulder approach (for maximum rotator cuff exposure)
5. The anterior deltopectoral approach (for the anterior glenohumeral joint)
6. The total deltoid turndown approach (for anterior, lateral, and posterior approaches to the glenohumeral joint)
7. The posterior shoulder approaches (for posterior glenohumeral exposure)

HORIZONTAL "STRAP" INCISION

The horizontal "strap" incision (Fig. 3-4) is used primarily for removal of calcific deposits in the rotator cuff.

Skin Incision. The skin incision (Fig. 3-4A) is horizontal, just off the outer edge of the acromion, in line with the skin creases.

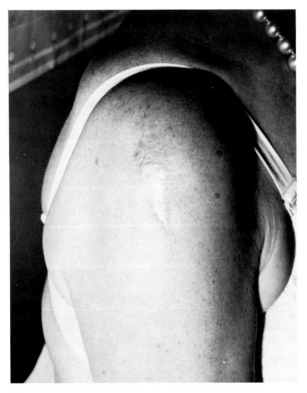

A

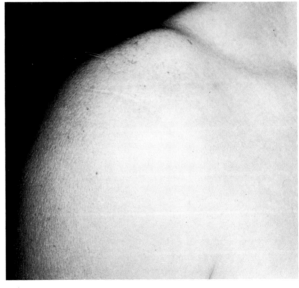

B

Fig. 3-2. (A) A verticle incision crossing Langer's lines results in an unsightly scar. **(B)** A minimal scar results when Langer's lines are followed.

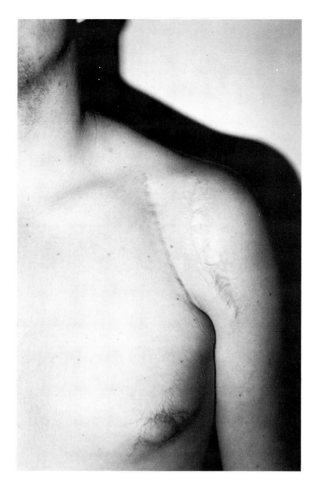

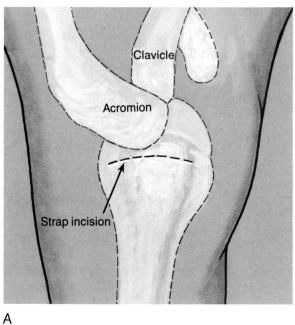

A

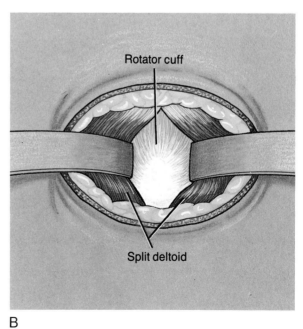

B

Fig. 3-3. Comparison of an incision following the skin lines from the axilla to an incorrect one crossing the skin lines down the arm.

Fig. 3-4. (A) Horizontal "strap" skin incision. (B) The deltoid muscle is split in the line of its fibers. The bursa is opened; by rotating the arm, much of the rotator cuff can be brought into view.

Muscle Approach.   The deltoid muscle is split in the line of its fibers, and retracted (Fig. 3-4B). This will expose the underlying subdeltoid bursa and rotator cuff. By rotating the arm, excellent exposure of the rotator cuff is obtained through the muscle "window."

LIMITED ANTERIOR DELTOID MUSCLE-SPLITTING APPROACH

The limited anterior deltoid muscle-splitting approach (Fig. 3-5) exposes the largest amount of rotator cuff with minimal soft tissue dissection, and is used primarily for localized rotator cuff tears, for avulsed tuberosity fractures, and for Rush rod stabilization of the humeral head. The deltoid is not released from the acromion or clavicle.

Skin Incision.   The skin incision extends from the acromioclavicular joint 6 to 8 cm over the greater curvature of the head and anterior deltoid.

Muscle Approach.   The deltoid muscle is split, with care being taken to avoid the axillary nerve. The exposure limits one to the anterior and superior humeral head. It is particularly effective in athletes, when minimal muscle release is desired.

"SABER" INCISION

The "saber" incision (Fig. 3-6) approach is used to expose the greater part of the rotator cuff, the subacromial space, and the acromioclavicular joint.

Skin Incision.   The skin incision extends over the outer end of the clavicle, acromioclavicular joint, and down the anterior deltoid for approximately four fingerbreadths. Two options are available: one over the anterior shoulder; the other over the greater curvature of the humeral head.

Muscle Approach.   The anterior deltoid muscle is split, with care being taken to avoid the axillary nerve.

The deltoid osteoperiosteal attachment can be removed from the distal clavicle and anterior acromion as needed. The coracoacromial ligament is resected. If greater exposure is needed for the infraspinatus and teres minor, the distal end of the clavicle is removed.

SUPERIOR SHOULDER APPROACH

The superior shoulder approach (Fig. 3-7) has given us greater exposure of the humeral head and rotator cuff from the subscapularis to the teres minor. It also gives an excellent exposure for transplantation of the infraspinatus muscle into a severe Hill-Sachs lesion. The only drawback of this incision is that it crosses the natural skin lines of the shoulder, and may cause some spread of the incision.

Skin Incision.   The skin incision begins over the distal clavicle and acromioclavicular joint, and extends out along the anterior border of the acromion and out over the greater curvature of the humeral head. The deltoid, with its osteoperiosteal attachment, is removed from the distal clavicle and anterior acromion by sharp dissection down to bone; its strong periosteal and muscle attachments are preserved. This must be done very carefully to retain strength in closure. The deltoid muscle is then split over the greater curvature of the humeral head for a distance of three to four fingerbreadths. For greater exposure, the leading edge of the anterior acromion can be removed along with the distal centimeter of the clavicle. This allows an excellent exposure of the dome of the humeral head, especially the infraspinatus and teres minor. Closure is carried out by suturing the periosteal flaps of the deltoid back to the acromion and distal clavicle. An option is to osteotomize the leading edge of the acromion, in very muscular patients, and reattach it through several holes in the acromion. The anterior deltoid is closed with interrupted absorbable sutures. We have not found it necessary to make holes in the anterior acromion or spine of scapula when removing the deltoid, if a thick osteoperiosteal layer is preserved. We warn the surgeon, however, when turning down the deltoid from the

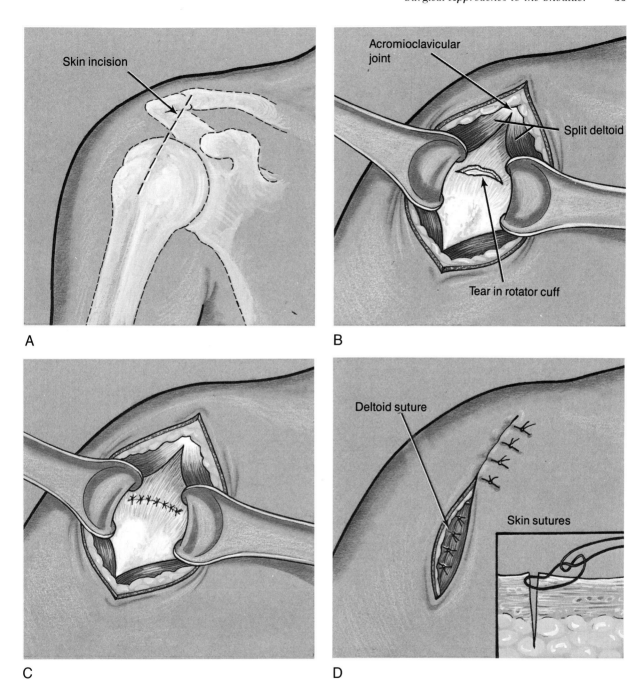

Fig. 3-5. The limited anterior deltoid muscle-splitting incision. (**A**) Skin incision from the acromioclavicular joint 6 cm down the anterior deltoid. (**B**) The deltoid is split. (**C**) Repair of cuff rupture. The approach is limited and posterior infraspinatus and teres minor are poorly exposed. (**D**) Closure.

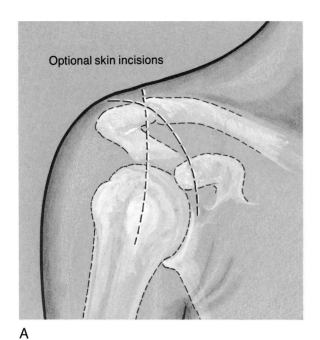

Optional skin incisions

A

Fig. 3-6. The "saber" incision. (**A**) Skin incision extends from over the acromioclavicular joint, 6 to 8 cm down the anterior deltoid. Optional incision is over the deltopectoral junction. (**B**) The coracoacromial ligament is resected. (**C**) A portion of the deltoid attachments can be removed from the distal clavicle and anterior acromion, and the distal centimeter of the clavicle removed for additional exposure if necessary.

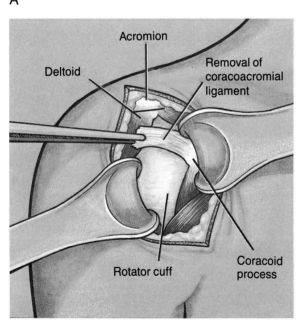

Acromion

Deltoid

Removal of coracoacromial ligament

Rotator cuff

Coracoid process

B

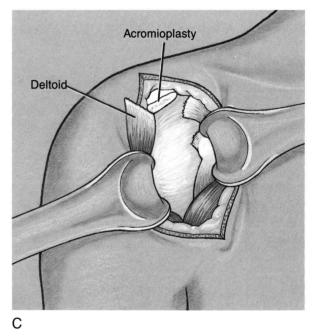

Acromioplasty

Deltoid

C

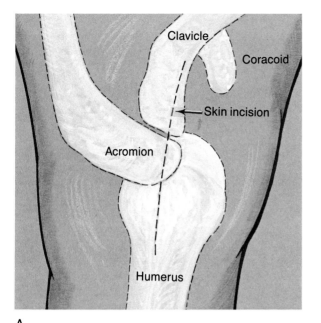

A

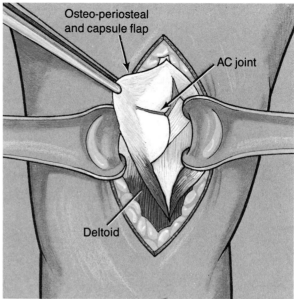

B

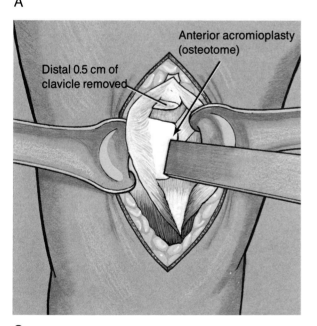

C

Fig. 3-7. The superior shoulder approach (excellent exposure of the anterior, superior, and posterior rotator cuff). **(A)** Skin incision extends over the distal clavicle, the acromioclavicular joint, and down the lateral deltoid 6 cm. **(B)** The deltoid is turned down with a strong osteoperiosteal flap from the distal clavicle and anterior acromion. **(C)** Resection of the anterior edge of acromion increases the exposure. Excision of distal clavicle is optional (*Figure continues.*)

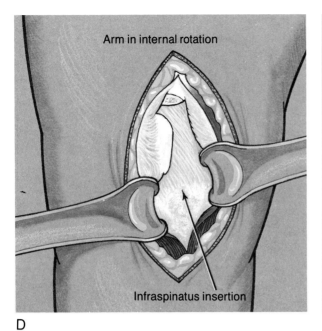

Arm in internal rotation

Infraspinatus insertion

D

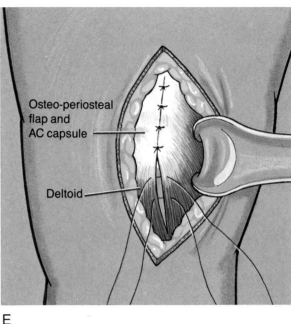

Osteo-periosteal flap and AC capsule

Deltoid

E

Fig. 3-7 (*Continued*). (**D**) Deltoid muscle is split 4 to 6 cm with excellent exposure of the rotator cuff. (**E**) The osteoperiosteal flaps are closed over the clavicle and acromion.

lateral acromion, that it is necessary to osteotomize 0.5 cm of acromion leaving the deltoid attached for resuturing. Otherwise, the deltoid will pull off and glide down the arm.

Kessel's[3] superior approach (Fig. 3-8A; a modification of Debeyre's approach,[2] Fig. 3-8B) to the rotator cuff, in which the acromion is transected and retracted open, gives an excellent exposure to the superior shoulder. In closure, the acromion is stabilized by suturing the osteoperiosteal flaps of the trapezius and deltoid together. Kessel has not found that internal fixation is necessary.

ANTERIOR DELTOPECTORAL APPROACH

The anterior deltopectoral approach (Fig. 3-9) exposes the anterior glenohumeral joint and is used chiefly for anterior recurrent dislocations of the shoulder, fractures of the shoulder, or joint replacements.

Skin Incision. For the average man, a slightly curved incision is made from the coracoid process to the axilla following the anatomical skin lines. In women, the incision can be shorter.

Muscle Approach. The interval between the deltoid and the pectoralis major muscles is developed. The interval is identified by a fat pad, under which lies the cephalic vein. It is not necessary to ligate the cephalic vein or to detach the deltoid attachment from the clavicle. Osteotomizing the coracoid process is optimal. It allows the short head of biceps and coracobrachialis to be retracted medially, and will eliminate the need for traction on the common tendon and possible injury to the musculocutaneous nerve. It also allows better exposure of the seam between the supraspinatus and subscapularis attachments. By external rotation of the arm, the subscapularis muscle is exposed and can be removed from the anterior capsule, thus completely exposing the capsule. In the anterior approach to the shoulder, the surgeon should be mindful of two very important nerves: the musculocutaneous nerve, which enters the common tendon of the coracoid in varying distances from the coracoid;

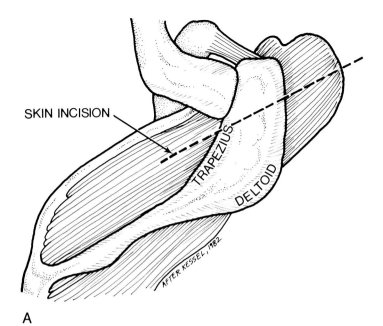

SKIN INCISION

TRAPEZIUS

DELTOID

AFTER KESSEL, 1982

A

Fig. 3-8. (**A**) Kessel's superior approach to the shoulder (a modification of Debeyre's approach). The osteotomized acromion is spread open, giving an excellent exposure of the rotator cuff. Closure of the osteoperiosteal flaps are sufficient to stabilize the acromion, without pins or screws. (**B**) Debeyre's superior approach to the rotator cuff.

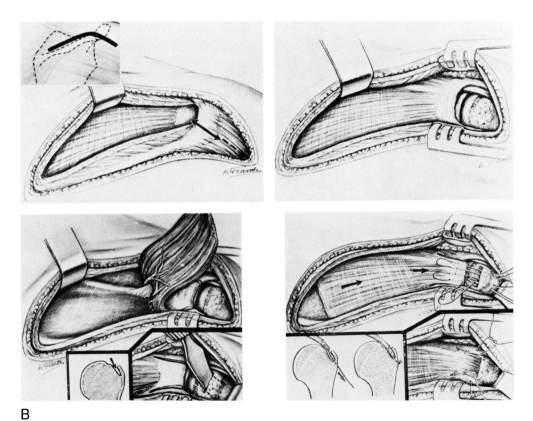

B

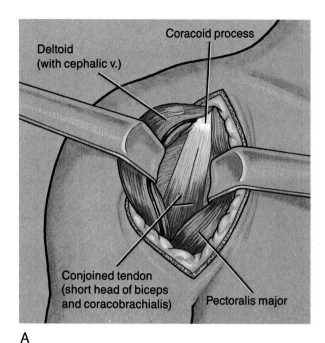

A

Fig. 3-9. **(A)** The anterior deltopectoral approach. **(B)** The surgeon should be constantly aware of two important nerves: the musculocutaneous and the axillary.

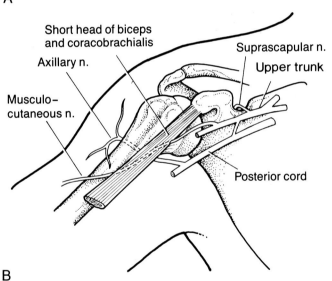

B

and the axillary nerve, which courses over the lower subscapularis muscle attachment to enter the quadrilateral space (Fig. 3-9B). When one dissects under the subscapularis muscle in separating it from the capsule, the axillary nerve is turned back and protected. The musculocutaneous nerve should be protected by careful traction on the common tendon, or by osteotomizing the coracoid and allowing the tendon to relax medially. This incision can be enlarged down the arm for joint replacement procedures or proximal humeral fractures.

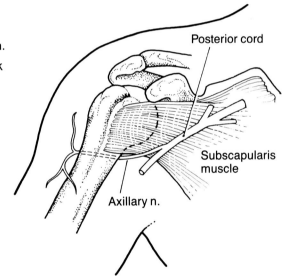

TOTAL DELTOID TURN-DOWN APPROACH

We have used the total deltoid turn-down approach (Fig. 3-10) for total anterior, lateral, and posterior exposure of the shoulder joint. It has been most helpful for chronic unreduced posterior shoulder dislocations of long duration, in which the humeral head should be carefully removed from the glenoid rim and reduced. We find that there is less damage to

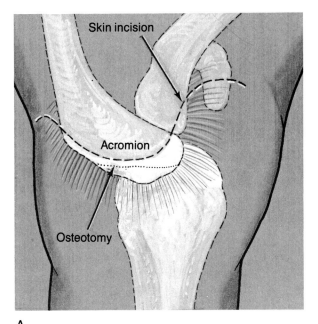

A

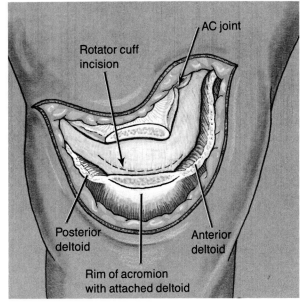

B

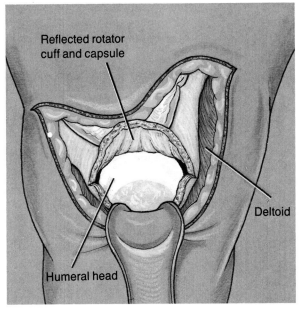

C

Fig. 3-10. The total deltoid turn-down approach. (**A**) Skin incision, with dotted line indicating osteotomy of acromion. (**B**) The deltoid muscle turned down with rim of acromion, exposing rotator cuff. (**C**) Incision of rotator cuff attachment to humeral head, exposing the head and glenoid. (*Figure continues.*)

the vulnerable humeral head, and less chance of vascular or nerve injury from displaced anatomy and scar tissue, when an adequate anterior as well as posterior exposure is used. In long-standing chronic dislocations, the humeral head may be osteoporotic, and can be easily damaged if exposure is limited, and the head difficult to reduce. Cubbins et al.[1] appreciated the complete exposure of the humeral head in 1934 and, although our techniques differ, the principle is the same.

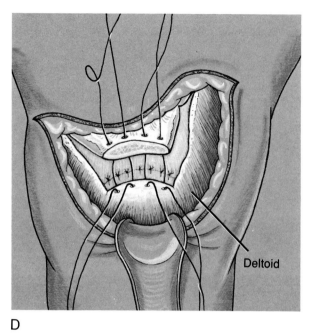

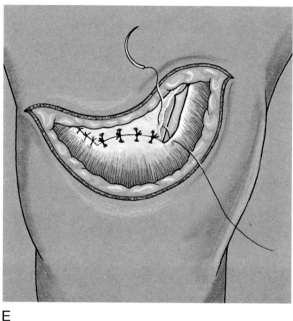

D   E

Fig. 3-10 (*Continued*). (**D**) Reattachment of osteotomized acromion to the acromion. (**E**) The osteoperiosteal flaps of deltoid sutured back to clavicle and spine of scapula.

Skin Incision.   The skin incision extends along the spine of the scapula out around the curvature of the acromion, along the distal clavicle, and then down over the anterior deltoid.

Muscle Approach.   The deltoid is turned down by sharp dissection of the muscle from the distal clavicle and spine of the scapula, leaving an osteoperiosteal flap to the muscle. The lateral rim of the acromion (0.5 cm thick) is osteotomized, leaving the deltoid muscle attached. The deltoid is split posteriorly and anteriorly enough to allow the muscle to be turned down. The humeral head is approached by sharp dissection through the rotator cuff attachments of the supraspinatus and infraspinatus tendons. If more exposure is needed, portions of the subscapularis and teres minor may be incised. This will give complete anterior, lateral, and posterior exposure of the humeral head, which are so important in the safe, atraumatic reduction of chronic dislocations of 4 to 6 months' duration. Closure is carried out by direct suture of the rotator cuff to its attachments. The lateral deltoid is reattached by making three to four holes in the acromion to which the osteotomized border is resutured. The osteoperiosteal flaps of deltoid are resutured to the spine of the scapula and the distal clavicle.

POSTERIOR APPROACHES TO THE SHOULDER

Usual Posterior Approach

The usual posterior approach to the shoulder consists of turning down the posterior deltoid muscle from the spine of the scapula[8] (Fig. 3-11).

The skin incision extends along the spine of the scapula and 3 cm down the lateral deltoid muscle. Care must be taken to avoid incising the infraspinatus muscle, which lies just below the spine. Extending the incision to the lateral deltoid muscle allows the muscle to be turned down. The capsule of the joint can be reached either by separating the infraspinatus

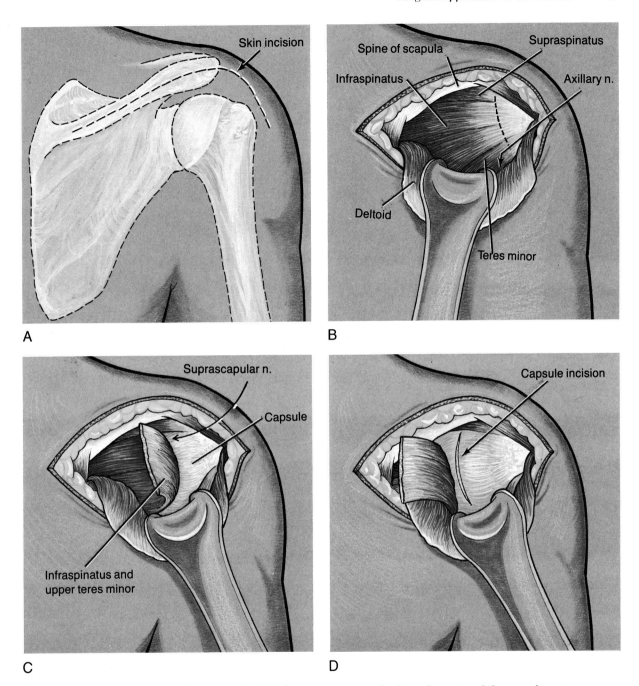

Fig. 3-11. Posterior shoulder approach. (**A**) Skin incision: extends along the spine of the scapula out over the lateral deltoid. (**B**) Deltoid muscle is turned down from the spine of scapula and split laterally over the curvature of the humeral head. (**C**) The infraspinatus and teres minor may be separated from the capsule by sharp dissection. (**D**) Incision into the joint. (*Figure continues.*)

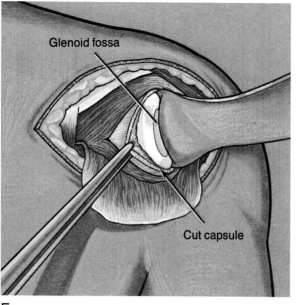

E

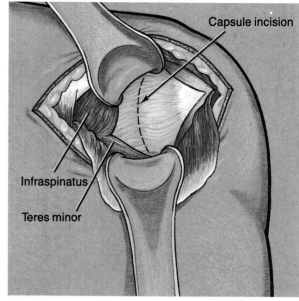

F

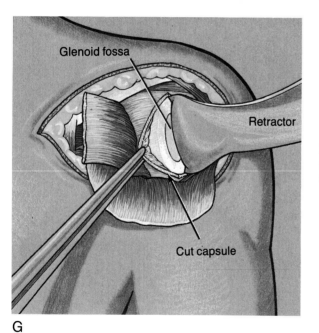

G

Fig. 3-11 (*Continued*). (**E**) The joint is opened with a vertical incision. (**F**) The infraspinatus and teres minor may be separated, exposing the capsule. (**G**) The joint is opened.

and a portion of the teres minor muscles from the capsule, much as it is done anteriorly with the subscapularis (Fig. 3-11B–D), or by separating the interval between the infraspinatus and the teres minor (Fig. 3-11F,G). In either instance, the surgeon should be mindful of the supraspinous nerve and the axillary nerve. In closing, the infraspinatus is reattached to the greater tuberosity and the deltoid to the spine of the scapula. This approach is safe and gives adequate posterior exposure to the shoulder.

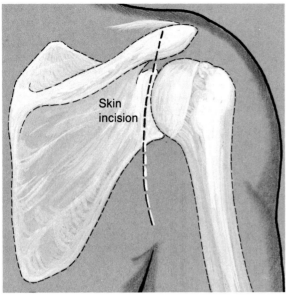

A

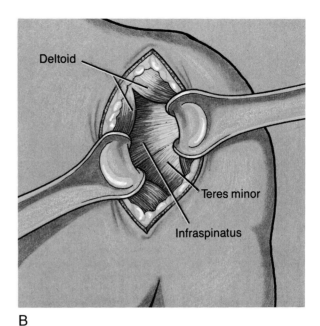

B

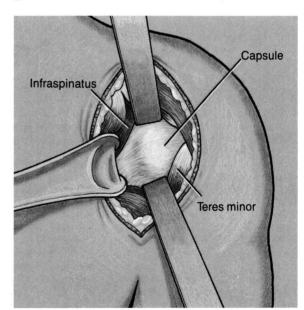

C

Fig. 3-12. The Rockwood posterior approach to the shoulder. (**A**) The skin incision is vertical from spine of scapula to the posterior axilla. (**B**) The deltoid muscle is split, with care being taken to avoid the axillary nerve. (**C**) The capsule is exposed by separating the infraspinatus and the teres minor, as in Figure 3-11. (Moseley HF: Shoulder Lesions. E&S Livingstone, Edinburgh and London, 1969.)

Rockwood Posterior Approach to the Shoulder

Rockwood[7] uses a very ingenious approach to the posterior shoulder through a vertical deltoid splitting incision.

Skin Incision. The skin incision (Fig. 3-12A) extends from the spine of the scapula down to the axillary crease.

Muscle Exposure. The posterior deltoid is split vertically in the line of its fibers (Fig. 3-12B), from the spine of the scapula down 10 cm toward the posterior axillary crease, exposing the infraspinatus and teres minor. Take care to protect the quadrilateral space and axillary nerve. The capsule is then exposed by either resecting off the infraspinatus and teres minor or resecting horizontally through the infraspinatus–teres minor interval (Fig. 3-12C).

OTHER SURGICAL EXPOSURES OF THE SHOULDER GIRDLE

Exposure of the Clavicle

Skin Incision.   A linear incision (Fig. 3-13) is made in line with the clavicle, just inferior or superior to the bone. The incision should not be placed directly over the clavicle.

Muscle Exposure.   The periosteum of the clavicle is incised along the interval of the deltoid and the trapezius muscles. The bone is exposed subperiosteally. Care should be taken to remain within the periosteal sleeve. In this way, the underlying vessels and nerves will be protected. If it is necessary to remove the entire clavicle, the incisions can be extended and the clavicle filleted out of the periosteal sleeve. The sleeve is then resutured, to preserve the attachment of the trapezius and deltoid.

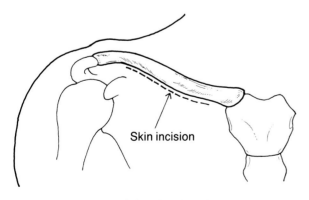

Fig. 3-13. Exposure of the clavicle. The incision should be in line with the clavicle, either just above or below the bone.

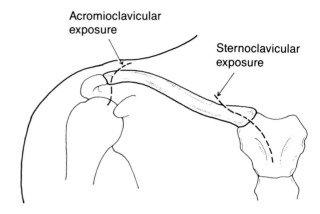

Fig. 3-14. Exposure of the acromioclavicular and sternoclavicular joints. The alternatives to the curved incisions are straight incisions over the joint; however, the exposure is less with the latter.

Sternoclavicular Joint

Skin Incision.   The skin incision (Fig. 3-14) has a tendency, in this area, to spread and may be a concern to the patient. The usual approach is a curved incision over the inner clavicle down the border of the manubrium. A straight incision in line with the clavicle and over the sternoclavicular joint spreads less, although its exposure is less.

Muscle Exposure.   The medial few centimeters of clavicle are exposed by subperiosteal release of the sternocleidomastoid, pectoral, and subclavius insertions. This gives an adequate exposure of the joint. Remain in the periosteal sleeve of the clavicle to avoid damage to the underlying nerves and vessels.

Disarticulation of the Shoulder

This is discussed in more detail in Chapter 7.

REFERENCES

1. Cubbins WR, Callahan JJ, Scuderi CS: Reduction of old or irreducible dislocation of the shoulder. Surg Gynecol Obstet 58:129, 1934

2. Debeyre J, Patte D, Elmelik E: Repair of rupture of rotator cuff of the shoulder. J Bone Joint Surg 47B:36, 1965
3. Kessel L: Clinical Disorders of the Shoulder. Churchill Livingstone, London, 1982
4. Kraisal CJ: The selection of appropriate lines for elective surgical incisions. Plast Reconstr Surg 8:1, 1951
5. Langer, K: Ueber die Spaltbarkeit der Cutis. Sitzungsber Akad Wissenseh Wein Abt 44:19, 1861
6. Moseley HF: Shoulder Lesions. E & S Livingstone, Edinburgh and London, 1969
7. Rockwood CA, Jr., Green DP: Fractures in Adults, 2nd ed. J.B. Lippincott, Philadelphia, 1975
8. Rowe CR, Yee BK: A posterior approach to the shoulder joint. J Bone Joint Surg 26:580, 1944

Examination of the Shoulder

4

Carter R. Rowe

HISTORY

In obtaining the history of a shoulder complaint, it is important to adhere to a definite and logical sequence of questioning: when? where? and how? Several general notations should be made in taking the history, such as the patient's age, occupation (whether an office worker, laborer, or athlete), physical type, arm dominance, duration of complaint, and the mechanism of injury.

It is a good plan to start at the very beginning of the patient's complaint, by asking "When was it that your shoulder felt perfectly normal? What were the initiating factors relative to the onset of pain, discomfort, or weakness? Was it due to an activity, to overuse of the shoulder, to the position in which the shoulder was used, or was the onset spontaneous?" These are the "specifics" needed in obtaining the history. Often a simple routine activity may be the causative factor, such as excessive serving in tennis, pitching, swimming, or polishing the car on a Sunday afternoon. However, this information may sometimes be difficult to obtain from the patient. I recall a very high powered business executive who was seen because of chronic unexplained and unrelieved pain of his right shoulder. His problem seemed mechanical, but we were unable to find a clue as to the cause. Review

of his systems and radiograms were normal. Finally, I began with his waking hours. "What is the first thing you do when you awake in the morning?" His response was prompt, "I roll out of bed and do 50 push-ups!" At last, there was the answer to his chronic shoulder pain. He did not relate the push-ups to his painful shoulder, as he had done these "for 20 years." It was explained to him that his rotator cuff was finally beginning to show wear and tear with secondary subacromial bursal reactions and impingement from the push-ups. Thus, his shoulder was sending warning signals to him to omit the push-ups. He was surprised and delighted when his shoulder pain subsided, without the usual routines of medications, injections, and physical therapy, but merely by identifying and eliminating the cause.

Character of Pain

The character of the patient's pain should be evaluated. It should be noted whether the pain is dull and constant, sharp and intermittent, present during the day or night, or produced by some type of activity. The factors that aggravate or alleviate the patient's pain should be identified. The distribution of the pain should be known: whether local or radiating down

53

the arm. The pathway of its radiation should be made clear: whether over C5-C6 or C7-T1.

Response to Treatment

The history should include also a record of the patient's previous treatment, and particularly the response to previous treatment. Much can be learned from the patient's account of previous evaluation and treatment. Did the treatment help or aggravate the shoulder problem? Was surgery performed, and if so, what did the operative report reveal? What was the patient's response to the surgical procedure? Were there soft tissue, vascular or neurologic complications? A careful review of the patient's response to treatment may also reveal very valuable information about the patient's personality, motivation, pain level, cooperation, or level of resentment. At this point, it is most important to be careful in one's response or reaction to the previous doctor's treatment or judgment. An expression of surprise, amazement, disagreement, or suggestion that the previous doctor's treatment was incorrect, or not indicated, may lead to malpractice action by the patient. Information should be obtained without comment or response. Often the patient may be angered, emotionally upset, exhausted, frustrated, and depressed from chronic unrelieved pain. The patient may be helped by an understanding, unhurried, and thorough examination, with time being taken to listen to the patient. The busy orthopaedist is apt to brush through his interview because of an overloaded schedule, and send the patient off to physical therapy, without an explanation of the pain problem, or the purpose of therapy.

Surgery of other parts of the body should be noted, for instance, the prostate, the pelvis, breast, kidney, or intestine. The pathologic report from previous surgery is important, as a malignant tumor may have been removed without the patient's knowledge.

Consistencies and Inconsistencies

In putting all the information from the history together, one should note consistencies and inconsistencies. Did the cause and effect form a reasonable sequence, or did the patient complain of pain, yet exhibit complete range of painless motion on examination? In these instances, one should be mindful of referred pain, whether neurologic, vascular, or visceral.

Unexplained pain may be due also to brachial neuritis or viral neuritis of the upper extremity such as winged scapula (long nerve of Bell), selected nerves of the brachial plexus, or herpes zoster. Also, one should be mindful of metastatic disease.

PHYSICAL EXAMINATION

It is important that both shoulders and upper body be exposed so that one shoulder can be compared to the other. Men should be stripped to the waist, and women should have a towel or gown around the chest with both shoulders exposed (Fig. 4-1). The physical type of the patient should be noted, and the degree of generalized ligament laxity graded; this may have a direct bearing on diagnosis and treatment (Fig. 4-2).

Some surgeons prefer to examine the patient sitting, others prefer the patient standing. We prefer to begin our examination with the patient standing so that we may walk around the patient, noting his or her postural stance, general ligament laxity, and coordination of the shoulder joints (Fig. 4-3A–E). In the standing position the patient will exhibit the presence or absence of rhythmic shoulder motion much more clearly than in the sitting position. The sitting position should be used, however, for above shoulder level observation of the contour of the shoulders, or checking range of motion. The supine position may be used for additional tests of relaxation of the shoulders, and for specific ranges of motion.

Surface Anatomy

The symmetry of the trapezius muscle is noted. The supra- and infraspinatus fossae are checked for possible atrophy. The contour of the humeral head should be anterior to the acromion. The prominence and stability of the acromioclavicular and sternoclavicular joints are tested. The skin is observed for blemishes or for possible vesicles that may reveal early herpes zoster. Palpation of the tender areas

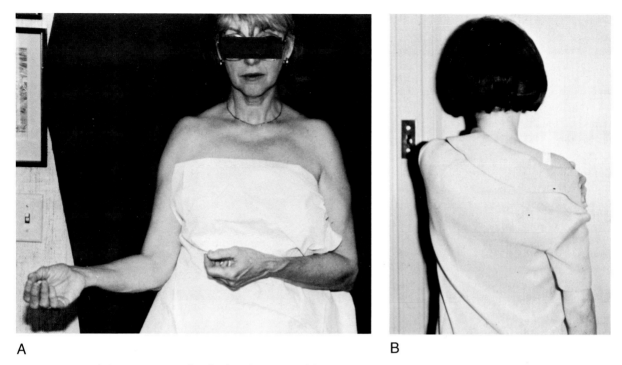

Fig. 4-1. (A) Correct attire for the female patient. **(B)** Incorrect exposure of shoulder for the female patient.

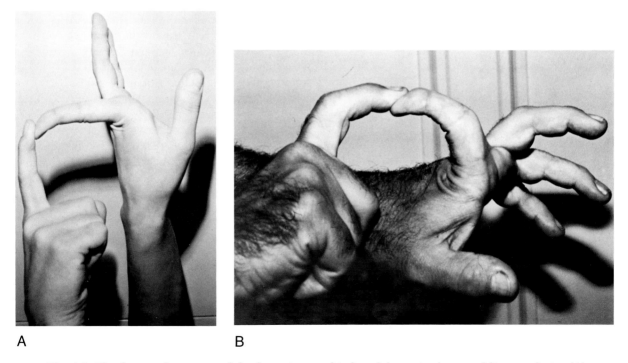

Fig. 4-2. The degree of extension of the finger is a good index of the patient's general ligament laxity. **(A)** Normal extension. **(B)** Severe laxity.

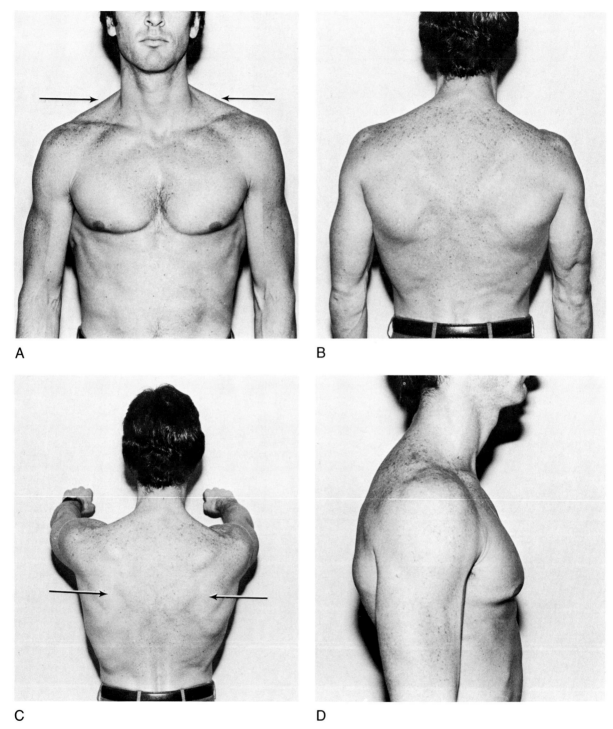

Fig. 4-3. (A) Anterior: note the anatomical landmarks, the symmetry of the trapezius muscles (arrows), the acromioclavicular and sternoclavicular joints. **(B)** Posterior: note areas of atrophy of the scapula fossae, and level of the scapulae. **(C)** Forward flexion: note the stability of the scapulae (arrows), with its rhythmic motion. **(D)** Side view: the prominence of the humeral head should be anterior. Note the deltoid contour. (*Figure continues.*)

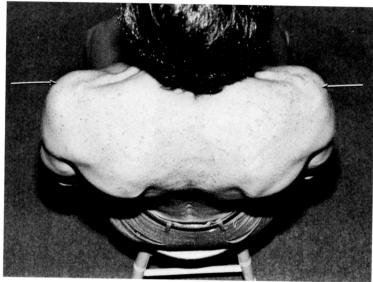

Fig. 4-3 (*Continued*). (**E**) Above: again note the anterior prominence of the humeral head and deltoid contour (arrows).

E

should be carried out carefully. If the patient's shoulder is painful, it is important to have the patient point to the area of pain first, rather than pressing too abruptly, and hurting the patient. By gentle maneuvers, one can find out much more than with a hurried abrupt motion. When indicated, the chest expansion should be noted, since early rheumatoid spondylitis may be identified. Abnormal pulsations of the carotids and radial arteries should be noted, and, when indicated, auscultation of the lungs. Areas of hypesthesia, anesthesia, or hyperesthesia are noted. A limited neurologic examination should be carried out when indicated.

Motions

Motions of the shoulder are recorded as recommended by the American Academy of Orthopaedic Surgeons' booklet, *The Measuring and Recording of Joint Motion* (Fig. 4-4).

In 1959, the Executive Committee of the American Academy of Orthopaedic Surgeons appointed a committee to study the measuring and recording of joint motions, to obtain a standard "agreed upon" method. This was accepted by the American Academy of Orthopaedic Surgeons[3] in 1962. In 1964, the method proposed was accepted by the six English Speaking Orthopaedic Associations, and internationally by Society International of Orthopaedic Surgery and Traumatology (SICOT) in Mexico City in 1969. This method is based on accepted neutral zero positions. The concept of shoulder motion should be global. Vertical motion of the shoulder is abduction and forward flexion. The positions in which vertical motion occurs can be noted in the horizontal plane. Rotation in external (outward) or internal (inward) direction is recorded with the arm at the side of the body, and in 90° of abduction. Internal rotation can also be recorded where the thumb reaches the greater trochanter, the sacrum, and along the lumbar spine to the scapula.

The use of a goniometer is recommended for consistency in measuring joint motion. "Normal" ranges of motion will depend on the physical build of the patient, and should be compared to the patient's opposite shoulder (if normal). As a check to recording motion in the standing position, the supine position of the patient may be used, as recommended by the American Shoulder and Elbow Surgeons.

Active Motions

By standing behind the patient, one can observe true glenohumeral and combined scapulothoracic motions of both shoulders. Limitations of motions and muscle guarding are recorded.

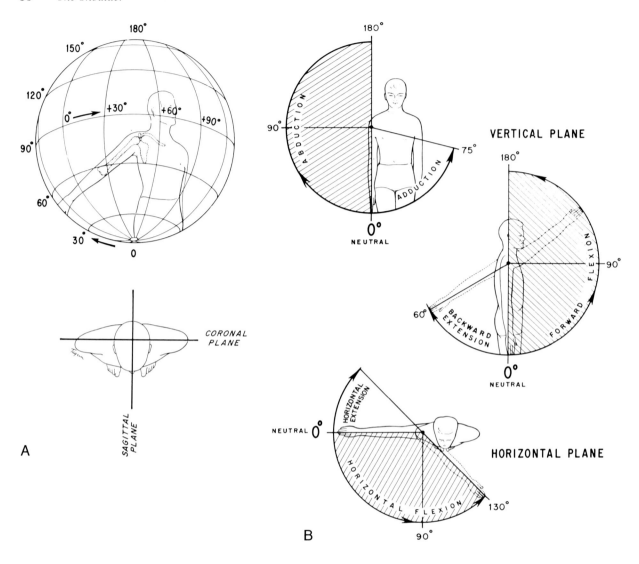

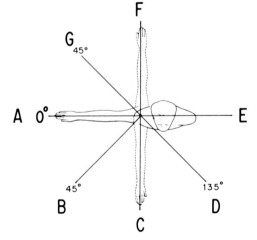

Fig. 4-4. The method of measuring and recording of joint motion as accepted by the American Academy of Orthopaedic Surgeons. (**A**) Global shoulder motion. (**B**) Vertical and horizontal motion. (**C**) Method of identifying positions of elevation of the arm. *A*, neutral abduction; *B*, abduction in 45° of horizontal flexion; *C*, forward flexion; *D*, adduction in 135° of horizontal flexion; *E*, neutral adduction; *F*, backward extension; *G*, abduction in 45° of horizontal extension. (*Figure continues.*)

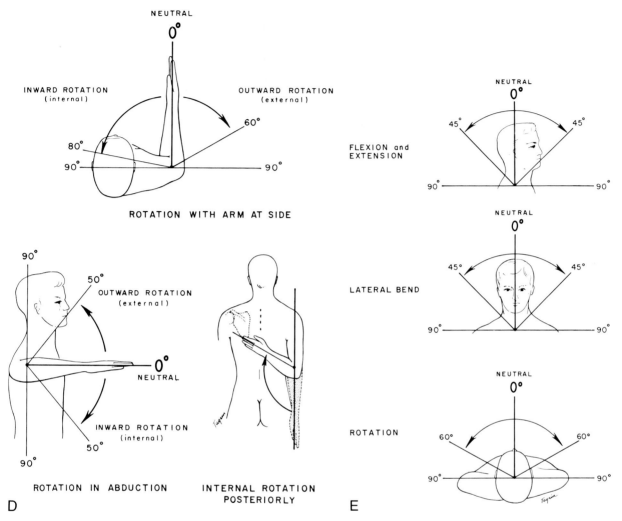

Fig. 4-4 (*Continued*). (**D**) Recording of inward (internal) and outward (external rotation). (**E**) Motions of the cervical spine. (*Figure continues.*)

Passive Motions

To record true glenohumeral motion, the lower angle of the scapula is grasped between the index finger and thumb, and the arm slowly elevated (Fig. 4-4G). This motion should be free (without motion of the scapula) up to 60 to 70° of elevation. This is true glenohumeral motion. Beyond this, the angle of the scapula will move a 1:2 ratio of the humerus. This is referred to as "combined glenohumeral and scapulothoracic motion." Rotation is also recorded with the arm at the side of the body, and the elbow flexed 90°. Starting from the neutral zero postion, both arms are rotated in internal rotation (inward rotation) and in external rotation (outward position). The motions of the affected arm should be compared to the opposite extremity. Signs of subacromial impingement, instability of the glenohumeral joint, acromioclavicular, and sternoclavicular joints are noted (see appropriate chapter for specific details). Examination of the shoulder motions should never be complete until motions of the cervical spine have been checked. Also, a measurement of the patient's chest expansion is indicated to rule out early rheumatoid spondylitis.

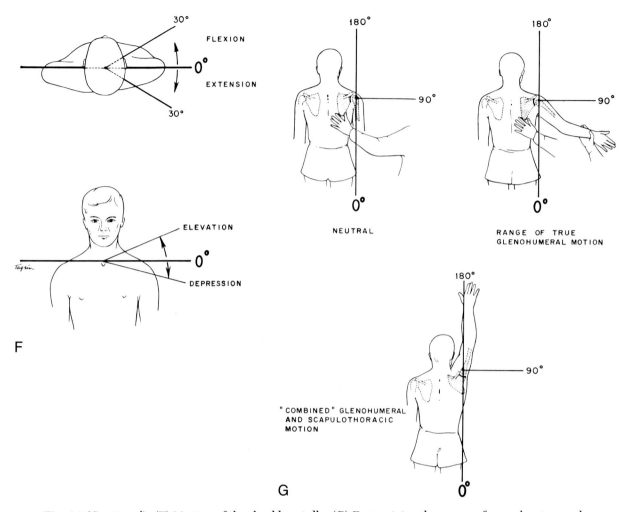

F

G

Fig. 4-4 *(Continued)*. **(F)** Motions of the shoulder girdle. **(G)** Determining the ranges of true glenohumeral motion and combined scapulothoracic motion.

DIAGNOSIS

One should differentiate between a diagnosis and an impression. A *diagnosis* is the definite identification of a disease or injury from its signs and symptoms, such as a fractured tibia. An *impression* is the possible existence of a disease or injury, such as an impingement syndrome.

As a rule, the history and physical findings of mechanical problems of the shoulder should be consistent. Pain of an impingement of the rotator cuff, hypertrophied bursa, or rupture of the rotator cuff, for instance, is reproduced by elevating the arm in abduction, and rotating it under the acromial arch, which should be consistent with the patient's history and physical findings, when he or she uses the arm in an elevated position. The arm may be pronated and elevated in forward flexion, thus jamming the greater tuberosity under the acromial arch (the "impingement position"), whereas there is little or no discomfort if the arm is supinated and elevated in forward flexion, thus allowing the greater tuberosity to rotate away from the acromial arch. In instances of instability, the patient will describe sudden pain, "at the top of

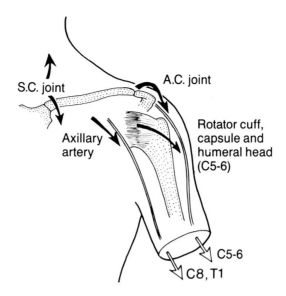

Fig. 4-5. Referred pain from the shoulder is usually over the pathway of C5-6.

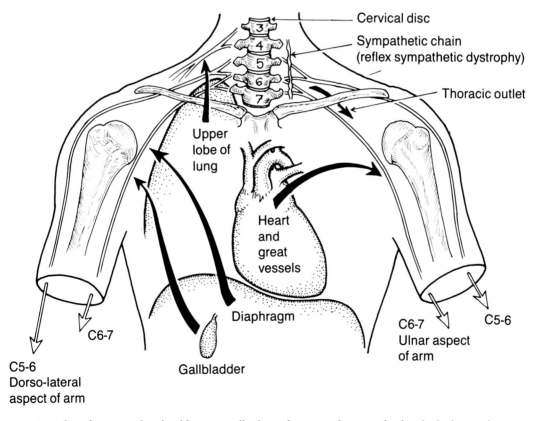

Fig. 4-6. Referred pain to the shoulder is usually from the cervical spine, the brachial plexus, the upper lobe of the lung, or from the vascular rupture.

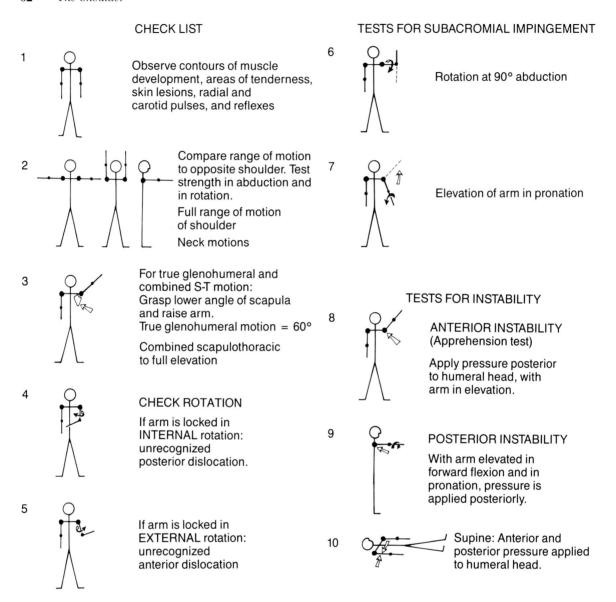

CHECK LIST

1. Observe contours of muscle development, areas of tenderness, skin lesions, radial and carotid pulses, and reflexes

2. Compare range of motion to opposite shoulder. Test strength in abduction and in rotation.
   Full range of motion of shoulder
   Neck motions

3. For true glenohumeral and combined S-T motion:
   Grasp lower angle of scapula and raise arm.
   True glenohumeral motion = 60°
   Combined scapulothoracic to full elevation

4. CHECK ROTATION
   If arm is locked in INTERNAL rotation: unrecognized posterior dislocation.

5. If arm is locked in EXTERNAL rotation: unrecognized anterior dislocation

TESTS FOR SUBACROMIAL IMPINGEMENT

6. Rotation at 90° abduction

7. Elevation of arm in pronation

TESTS FOR INSTABILITY

8. ANTERIOR INSTABILITY (Apprehension test)
   Apply pressure posterior to humeral head, with arm in elevation.

9. POSTERIOR INSTABILITY
   With arm elevated in forward flexion and in pronation, pressure is applied posteriorly.

10. Supine: Anterior and posterior pressure applied to humeral head.

Fig. 4-7. A checklist of shoulder motions.

my serve" in tennis, or, in throwing a ball, when the arm is in full elevation and outward rotation. A consistent physical finding would be a positive "apprehension" test, which is reproduced with the arm in elevation and external rotation and pressure applied posteriorly to the humeral head. In this position, the muscles of the shoulder are aligned upward, leaving only the inferior capsule to stabilize the humeral head. Figure 4-5 is an outline of pain radiation from the shoulder. Figure 4-6 shows areas that may radiate pain to the shoulder.

Diagnosis becomes more difficult when the history and physical findings are inconsistent; for instance, when the patient's pain or weakness cannot be reproduced by the patient or by the examiner. In these instances, a further search must be made for the source of the patient's pain. Very careful neurologic, vascular, and visceral searches are indicated. The cause of the pain may be due to referred pain to the shoulder and arm from the cervical spine (usually C5-6), or from the heart or diaphragm (usually to the clavicular area or down the medial aspect of the arm, C6-7). The pain of a Pancoast's tumor of the upper lobe of the lung is usually referred to the anterior or posterior aspect of the shoulder girdle and scapula area. Occasionally, the pain may radiate down the medial aspect of the arm. Horner's syndrome may be present. Metastatic or primary lesions of the scapula, or upper humeral shaft, will give local pain usually with little loss of motion. Other sources of severe referred pain to the shoulder region are viral neuritis syndromes.[1] Winging of the scapula (paralysis of the long nerve of Bell) has a very painful prodromal period of a week to 10 days, after which the pain diminishes with the onset of weakness of the arm and winging of the scapula. Involvement of the axillary and suprascapular nerves reveals motor weaknesses of their respective muscles. Herpes zoster (shingles) should be considered when there is severe burning pain in the shoulder region or down the arm, particularly when there is no limitation of motion or aggravation of the pain by movements of the arm. Characteristic skin vesicles will appear over the involved dermatome to establish the diagnosis. Occasionally, herpes zoster is associated with muscular weakness of the upper or lower extremity.[2] Further evaluation of shoulder pain is discussed in Chapter 6.

Figure 4-7 shows a checklist of motions. It will be helpful to keep these in mind.

REFERENCES

1. Dillin L, Hoaglund FT, Scheck M: Brachial neuritis. J Bone Joint Surg 67A:878, 1985
2. Grant B, Rowe CR: Motor paralysis of the extremities in herpes zoster. J Bone Joint Surg 43A:885, 1961
3. American Academy of Orthopaedic Surgeons: Joint Motion—Method of Measuring and Recording. Chicago, 1965

5

INVESTIGATIVE TECHNIQUES

Radiologic Techniques

Daniel I. Rosenthal

RADIOGRAPHIC SCREENING EXAMINATION

Perhaps because it is the most mobile joint in the body, the shoulder can be examined with the greatest variety of radiographic views and projections. There is no consensus on what constitutes an adequate radiographic examination of the shoulder. In many departments routine shoulder radiography consists only of internal and external rotation views (Fig. 5-1A,B). This practice violates a basic precept of radiology: the need for orthogonal projections. Although the humerus is seen in two different projections using internal and external rotations, only one projection of the scapula and glenoid is seen using these views. Several studies have recently been undertaken to determine which combination of views is optimal.

An AP view with the humerus in external rotation seems to be the single most informative view. This is probably true in patients both with and without acute shoulder trauma.[11,12,14,18] A minority opinion holds that it is preferable to rotate the patient into a 40° posterior oblique view (Fig. 5-2). This orientation provides a true tangential view of the glenohumeral joint, and may allow more accurate diagnosis of joint pathology.[34] Because of the oblique position of the torso, this projection gives an external rotation view of the humerus and therefore presumably allows the same sensitivity to detection of rotator cuff calcifications as the AP-external rotation view.

The choice of a second view is more contentious. The axillary view, originally described by Lawrence,[25] offers the greatest amount of additional anatomical information, and is preferred whenever it can be obtained[12,18] (Fig. 5-3). However, positioning for the axillary view may be difficult and painful, especially in patients who have sustained acute shoulder injuries. In such patients, the anterior oblique projection ("Y" view) has been shown to be a suitable alternative[11,14] (Fig. 5-4).

VIEWS FOR SPECIAL PURPOSES

To evaluate shoulder *instability*, *subluxation*, and *dislocation*, it is necessary to assess the degree of anterior or posterior displacement of the humerus with respect to the glenoid. This can be done most directly using lateral or axial views. It can also be done using AP or PA images with cranial or caudal beam angulation.

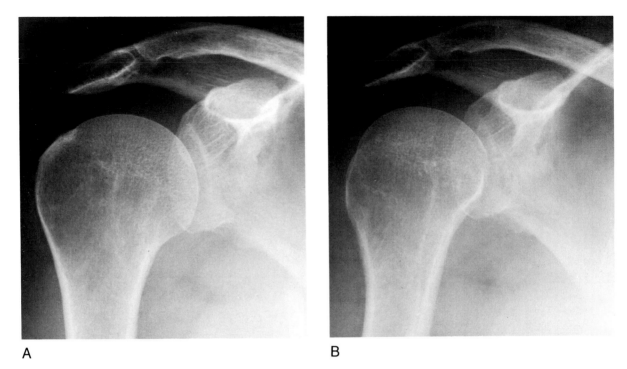

Fig. 5-1. (**A**) An AP view of the shoulder with the humerus in external rotation. The position of the humerus can be recognized by the lateral position of the greater tuberosity and the demonstration of the humeral neck-shaft angle. The lucency projected through the surgical neck in two different planes represents the open growth plate, an appearance that can sometimes be mistaken for a fracture. (**B**) AP view of the shoulder with the humerus in internal rotation. The position of the humerus is recognizable by the medial projection of the lesser tuberosity and the super imposition of the humeral shaft over the humeral head, obscuring the neck-shaft angle.

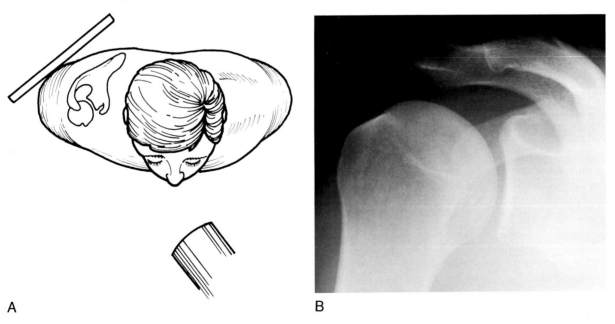

Fig. 5-2. (**A**) Technique of the posterior, oblique view. The patient is rotated 40° from the AP projection with the affected shoulder turned toward the film. (**B**) A posterior, oblique view of the shoulder demonstrating a true-lateral projection of the glenohumeral joint.

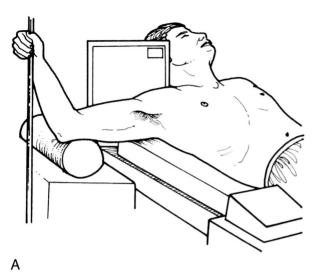

A

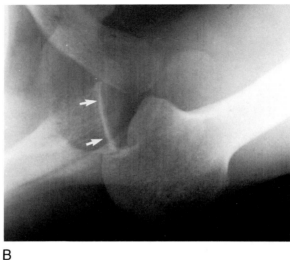

B

Fig. 5-3. (A) Technique of performing the axillary view. The arm is abducted 90°. The central beam is directed into the axilla, with a cassette placed above the shoulder. This projection can also be achieved with a vertical beam and a cassette placed under the axilla. (B) Axillary view of the shoulder reveals posterior dislocation of the humeral head with respect to the glenoid fossa (arrows). There is fracture deformity of the humerus (reverse Hill-Sachs lesion).

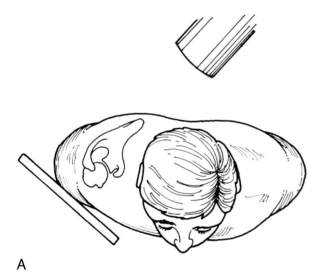

A

Fig. 5-4. (A) Technique of the anterior, oblique view. The patient is rotated approximately 50° from the PA projection with the affected shoulder turned towards the film. This gives a true "en-face" projection of the glenohumeral joint. (B) Anterior, oblique view of the shoulder demonstrates anterior dislocation of the humeral head. The glenoid fossa is found in the "crotch" formed by the coracoid, acromion, and body of the scapula ("Y" view).

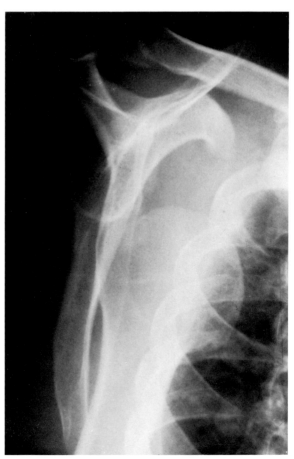

B

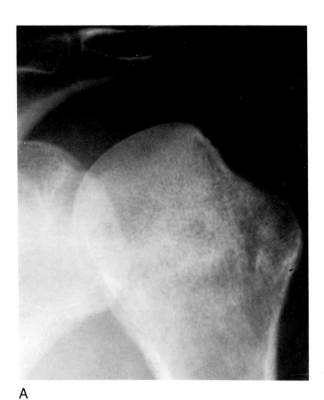

A

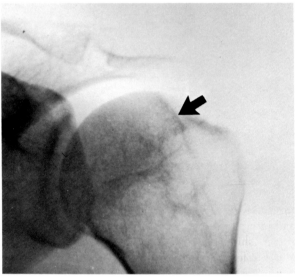

B

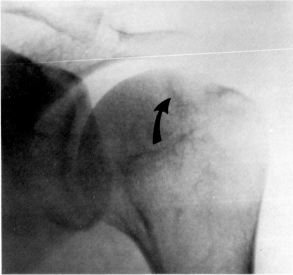

C

Fig. 5-5. **(A)** A marked Hill-Sachs lesion is demonstrated in this internal rotation view (60°). **(B)** A subtle Hill-Sachs lesion can be seen when the humerus is internally rotated as a flattened lateral profile of the humeral head (arrow). **(C)** In external rotation, the Hill-Sachs lesion (arrow) is projected over the humeral head and is more difficult to identify. (*Figure continues.*)

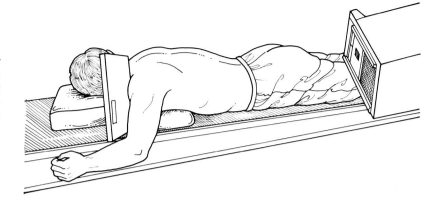

Fig. 5-5 (*Continued*). (**D**) A prone axillary, or "West Point" view. The arm is abducted 90° and rotated so that the anterior surface is facing the cassette. The beam is angled 25° medially and 25° cephalad.

Transthoracic Lateral View

An anterior or posterior dislocation of the shoulder can be recognized using a transthoracic lateral view. However, because of overlap with the thoracic structures the glenoid may be difficult to demonstrate, and interpretation may depend upon recognizing the relationship of the humeral head to the scapular body. We find few applications for this view.

Axillary Projection

The axillary projection offers a better definition of anatomy, but, as we have indicated, it may be difficult to position the acutely injured patient for such a view. For this reason, several modifications of the axillary view have been devised. The lateral recumbent axillary view requires the patient to lie on the unaffected side. The cassette is placed above the shoulder and the x-ray tube is angled into the axilla.[6] This requires less abduction of the arm than the conventional axillary view. The Velpeau axillary view can be performed with the patient's arm in a sling. The patient stands or sits in an upright position and leans backward over a cassette which is placed flat on the x-ray table. A vertical x-ray beam is used with the tube placed above the patient's shoulder.[3] This method requires a limber torso, but almost no glenohumeral motion. It results in considerable image magnification.

Anterior Oblique View

The scapula "Y" view (Fig. 5-4) has been shown to be an effective method of diagnosing dislocation.

Correctly performed, the humeral head projects over the crotch of the "Y" formed by the body of the scapula, the coracoid process, and the scapular spine. Anterior or posterior displacement is thus readily recognized (Fig. 5-4A).

Other Views

Modifications of the AP view using angled beams can also be employed to demonstrate shoulder dislocations. The *angle-up* view of Bloom uses 35° of cranial beam angulation.[3] An anteriorly displaced humeral head will be projected further cranially than the glenoid. Posterior displacement results in apparent caudal displacement. The *apical oblique* view makes use of a caudally angled x-ray beam in the posterior oblique projection.[16] With this technique, anterior dislocation results in apparent caudal displacement of the humeral head.

Demonstration of the Hill-Sachs Lesion, the Coracoid Process, and the Acromioclavicular and Sternodavicular Joints

The Hill-Sachs lesion may be very difficult to demonstrate on routine radiographs (Fig. 5-5A to C). The reported frequency of this finding in patients who have sustained shoulder dislocations varies from 27 to 100 percent.[21] Perhaps some of this variability results from the degree of diligence that is employed in efforts to demonstrate the lesion. We have had excellent results with the AP view in 60° of internal rotation. An experimental study performed by Danzig et al indicated that the most useful views for visualization of the Hill-Sachs lesion are the AP view in internal rotation, the Stryker notch view, and the modified Didier view, listed in order of efficacy.[8] Both Goldman[19] and Pavlov et al[30] recommend addition of the modified "West Point" axillary view originally described by Rokous[32] (Fig. 5-5D). Other authors also employ the tangential *Hermoddson* view, the *Miller* view (done with the patient supine and 30° of caudal beam angulation),[15] and the apical oblique view.[16] Computed tomography (CT) is also highly effective in demonstrating the Hill-Sachs lesion.[9]

Fracture of the anterior glenoid, which may accompany a Bankart lesion, is most consistently observed on the modified West Point axial and Didier views.[30] The conventional axillary view and the AP view in external rotation are also useful for this lesion, as is CT.[9] Since many Bankart lesions are primarily or exclusively cartilaginous in nature, arthrography is necessary for demonstration in many cases.[19]

The acromioclavicular (AC) joint can be best evaluated using AP views obtained with cephalad beam angulation. Two views have been suggested by Zanka,[31] one angled 12° to 15°, and the other angled 30° to 35° toward the head. These project the AC joint away from the scapular body (Fig. 5-6). Upright views obtained with the patient holding weights may be helpful for diagnosis of type 2 AC joint separations. The distal clavicle and AC joint are usually well demonstrated on axillary views.

The coracoid process can be difficult to see on AP views. Most authors recommend the use of axillary projections for demonstration of coracoid fractures. Views with 30° to 35° of cephalad angulation[31] or 20° of cephalad angulation and 20° of posterior obliquity[17] have been shown to be effective in diagnosing fractures of the base of the coracoid.

The sternoclavicular joints can be extremely difficult to demonstrate. Fifty degree oblique and lateral views can be helpful. However tomography and CT are frequently required.

ARTHROGRAPHY

Shoulder arthrography is a well-established technique for use in the diagnosis of rotator cuff tear. It can also be used to demonstrate the size and shape of the joint capsule. An abnormally small and tight joint capsule is characteristic of adhesive capsulitis. Previous shoulder dislocation results in the anterior portion of the capsule becoming abnormally lax and redundant. Inflammatory synovitis produces a markedly nodular and irregular capsular outline. The articular cartilage of the humerus and glenoid and the fibrocartilaginous glenoid labrum can also be demonstrated using arthrography.

Arthrography can be performed with either single or double contrast technique. For single contrast arthrography, approximately 10 to 15 ml of positive contrast is injected into the shoulder joint. We recommend that approximately 2 to 3 ml of local anesthetic

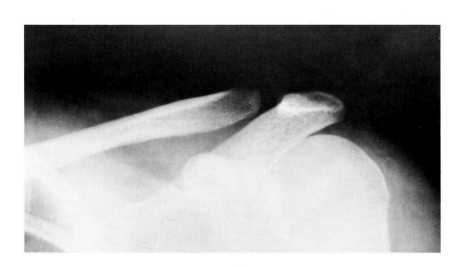

Fig. 5-6. An AP view of the acromioclavicular joint obtained with 30° of cephalad beam angulation.

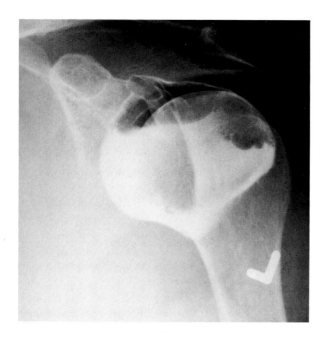

Fig. 5-7. An AP view of a normal double contrast arthrogram. There is contrast and air filling the normal synovial recesses along the biceps tendon sheath, the subcoracoid joint extension and the axillary fold. The upper surface of the joint marks the lower boundary of the rotator cuff which appears to be smooth and intact. There is no contrast or air in the subdeltoid bursa.

be included in the contrast mixture, as distension of the capsule can be painful. Double contrast arthrography is done with 1 to 3 ml of positive contrast (including 1 ml of anesthetic) and approximately 10 ml of air (Fig. 5-7).

In general, double contrast arthrography studies are more satisfactory than single contrast studies. The morbidity from a double contrast study is substantially less than that of a single contrast study, owing to a lower incidence of joint irritation provoked by smaller volumes of positive contrast.[22] Joint irritation from shoulder arthrography is relatively frequent with single contrast studies, and can be clinically significant. The pain begins 6 to 12 hours after the procedure, is poorly localized, and may last for several days. It can be distinguished from infection by its early onset and the fact that maximum severity is reached within 12 to 20 hours after the procedure. In our experience pain control with ice packs, aspirin, or other mild analgesics may be insufficient and narcotics are sometimes needed.

Adhesive capsulitis is probably the one remaining indication for single contrast arthrography. Adhesive capsulitis can be suspected if the joint capacity is less than 10 ml (Fig. 5-8). Accurate measurements of volume are more easily performed with liquid con-

Fig. 5-8. Adhesive capsulitis of the shoulder is demonstrated by a small, somewhat irregular, and "tight"-appearing joint capsule. There is no filling of the biceps tendon sheath or of the subcoracoid recess and the axillary fold appears smaller than normal. Total joint capacity in this case was only 3 ml.

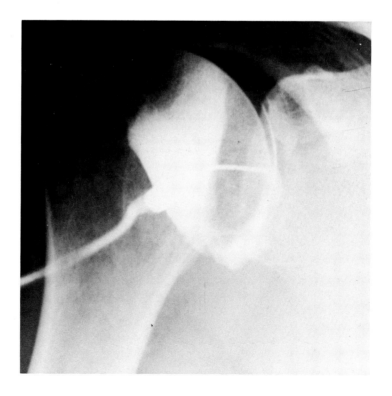

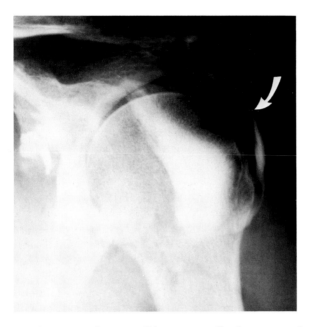

Fig. 5-9. A complete tear of the rotator cuff is demonstrated by extravasation of contrast and air from the shoulder joint into the subacromial bursa (arrow).

trast than with air. Furthermore, use of air contrast frequently leads to early and rapid extravasation in patients with adhesive capsulitis, resulting in a less satisfactory examination. Distension of the shoulder capsule by single contrast arthrography can actually improve the symptoms of adhesive capsulitis.[2,29]

The respective abilities of single and double contrast arthrography to detect tears of the rotator cuff appear comparable. Some authors believe that the double contrast technique allows more precise measurement of the size of the rotator cuff defect,[20] but there is some dispute as to whether such measurements are accurate.[1] In either case, upright films should be obtained both before and after exercising the shoulder, as tears of the rotator cuff that appear incomplete prior to exercise may be shown to be complete following exercise.

Complete tear of the rotator cuff is seen as communication of contrast material between the glenohumeral joint and the subacromial–subdeltoid bursa (Fig. 5-9). Partial tears of the inferior surface of the rotator cuff appear as small ulcerations filled with air or contrast on the lower surface of the rotator cuff. Partial

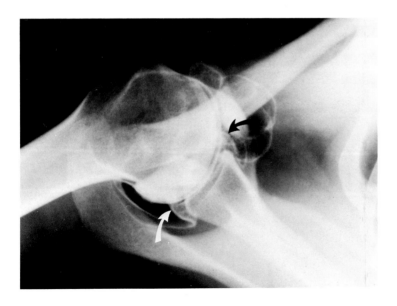

Fig. 5-10. Axillary view following double contrast arthrography with very small quantities of contrast and a large amount of air demonstrate the cartilaginous glenoid labrum (arrows). The anterior labrum is somewhat longer and more pointed than the posterior labrum, which appears blunt and round in this normal patient.

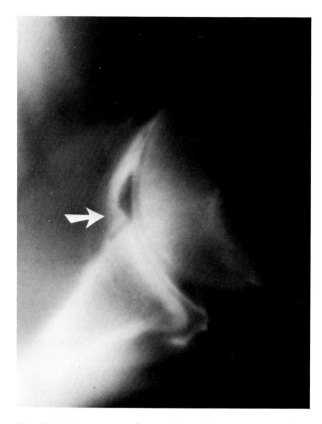

Fig. 5-11. Tomogram taken in the axillary projection demonstrates tear of the anterior glenoid labrum. The cartilaginous fragment is seen as a triangular shadow anterior to the glenoid.

tears of the upper surface of the rotator cuff are invisible by arthrography.

Lesions of the articular cartilage and glenoid labrum are best demonstrated by double contrast arthrography. In fact, very small volumes of positive contrast are desirable.[5] Prone and supine axillary views should be added to the routine films for evaluation of the anterior and posterior glenoid. These views will demonstrate the anterior and posterior labrum outlined with both air and contrast (Fig. 5-10).[28]

Tomograms may be helpful to supplement the arthrographic findings. Upright tomograms can be done to better define the size of the rotator cuff defect. Oblique tomograms have been advocated to demonstrate the glenoid labrum.[5] However, for this purpose we prefer tomograms done in the axillary position (Fig. 5-11).[13] Recently, CT has been shown to be a highly sensitive and relatively convenient method of demonstrating the glenoid labra (Fig. 5-12).[24]

OTHER SPECIAL TECHNIQUES

Subacromial bursography has recently been described as a technique that is useful for the diagnosis of impingement syndrome.[26,35] Bursography is rela-

Fig. 5-12. Computed tomography scan taken following shoulder arthrography demonstrates tear of the anterior glenoid labrum (arrow). The transaxial projection necessary for demonstration of the glenoid labrum is easily accomplished with CT but can be performed only with difficulty using conventional tomography.

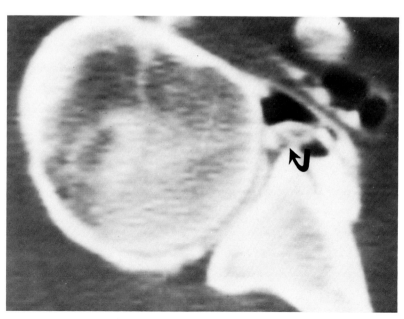

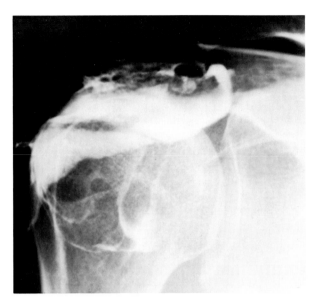

Fig. 5-13. A normal subacromial bursagram. Notice that the bursa is a large structure and that its lateral portions extend over the greater tuberosity in the subdeltoid region.

tively simple to perform. The subacromial bursa is a large potential space, accepting between 5 and 10 ml of air or contrast (Fig. 5-13). Either anterior or lateral approaches can be used. In our experience, the lateral approach is somewhat easier and less painful. Filling of a normal bursa helps to exclude the possibility of impingement syndrome.[35] In some cases, it will be impossible to opacify the bursa, presumptive evidence of adhesions, or obliteration due to impingement. In other cases of impingement, deformity of the lateral aspect of the bursa occurs during abduction of arm.[26] Although tears of the upper surface of the rotator cuff are theoretically demonstrable by this technique, this has not yet been demonstrated to be a clinically useful tool.

Arthrography of the acromioclavicular joint is technically feasible.[36] Although it has been reported to be useful in the diagnosis of AC ligamentous tears,[37] it has not found a widespread clinical application. We have occasionally used AC joint arthrography to confirm that the AC joint is the source of patient

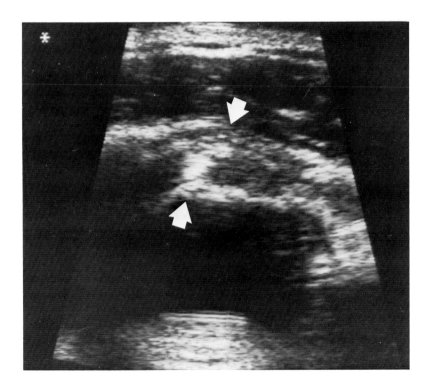

Fig. 5-14. Ultrasound scan of the rotator cuff demonstrates a tear as an echogenic focus extending through the cuff to the humeral head.

complaint. By mixing local anesthetic with our contrast, intraarticular injection alleviates patients symptoms.

Special low voltage *soft tissue radiographs* of the shoulder can demonstrate edema of the rotator cuff in patients with acute tendonitis.[10] This ability may be important because although soft tissue calcification is common in patients with shoulder pain,[38] it is also seen in patients without symptoms.[4]

The newest imaging modality, *magnetic resonance imaging* (MRI), is especially promising in that it can produce images in any plane, has the potential of demonstrating articular cartilage without the use of contrast material, and is extremely sensitive to bone marrow disorders such as avascular necrosis. MRI is extremely sensitive to soft tissue contrast and can define the presence of soft tissue tumors better than any other radiographic modality. It is also highly sensitive to inflammation; we have seen examples of calcific tendonitis in which inflammatory changes in muscle have been demonstrated adjacent to a focus of calcification. Unfortunately, at the present time there is no certain method for distinguishing between inflammation and tumor.

Ultrasonography has recently been shown to have several applications in studying the shoulder. It is capable of demonstrating the presence of intra-articular effusions,[33] and can be used to directly demonstrate the presence of rotator cuff tears.[7,27]

A 10-MHz small parts scanner is needed for best results. Rotator cuff tears are seen as echogenic foci within the rotator cuff (Fig. 5-14) or as central echogenic bands. Very large tears may result in complete nonvisualization of the cuff, as in arthrography.[27] Ultrasonography is quite sensitive (93 percent). Although some false positives may be encountered, it appears to be an objective screening technique.

REFERENCES

1. Ahovuo J, Paavolainen P, Slatis P: The diagnostic value of arthrography and plain radiography in rotator cuff tears. Acta Orthop Scand 55:220, 1984
2. Andren L, Lundberg BJ: Treatment of rigid shoulders by joint distension during arthrography. Acta Orthop Scand 36:45, 1965
3. Bloom MH, Obata WG: Diagnosis of posterior dislocation of the shoulder with use of velpeau axillary and angle-up roentgenographic views. J Bone Joint Surg 49A:943, 1967
4. Bosworth BM: Deposits in shoulder and subacromial bursitis. JAMA 116:2477, 1941
5. Braunstein EM, O'connor G: Double contrast arthrotomography of the shoulder. J Bone Joint Surg 64A:192, 1982
6. Clements RW: Adaptation of the technique for radiography of the glenohumeral joint in the lateral projection. Radiol Technol 51:305, 1979
7. Crass JR, Craig EV, Thompson RC, Feinberg SB: Ultrasonography of the rotator cuff: surgical correlation. J Clin Ultrasound 12:487, 1984
8. Danzig LA, Greenway G, Resnick D: The Hill-Sachs lesion: an experimental study. Am J Sports Med 8:328, 1980
9. Danzig L, Resnick D, Greenway G: Evaluation of unstable shoulders by computed tomography. A preliminary study. Am J Sports Med 10:138, 1982
10. Deiehgraber E, Olsson B: Soft tissue radiography in painful shoulders. Acta Radiol (Diagn) 16:393, 1975
11. DeSmet AA: Anterior oblique projection in radiography of the traumatized shoulder. AJR 134:515, 1980
12. DeSmet AA: Axillary projection in radiography of the nontraumatized shoulder. AJR 134:511, 1980
13. El-Khoury GY, Albright JP, Monzer M et al: Arthrotomography of the glenoid labrum. Radiology 131:333, 1979
14. Flinn RM, MacMillan CL Jr, Campbell PR, Fraser DR: Optimal radiography of the acutely injured shoulder. J Can Assoc Radiol 34:128, 1983
15. Fodor J III, Malott JC: The radiographic evaluation of the dislocated shoulder. Radiol Technol 55:154, 1984
16. Garth WP, Slappey CE, Ochs CW: Roentgenographic demonstration of instability of the shoulder: The apical oblique projection. J Bone Joint Surg 66A:1450, 1984
17. Goldberg RP, Vicks B: Oblique angled view for coracoid fractures. Skeletal Radiol 9:195, 1983
18. Golding FC: The shoulder—The forgotten joint. Br J Radiol 35:149, 1962
19. Goldman AB: Shoulder Arthrography. p. 209. In Goldman AB (ed): Procedures in Skeletal Radiology. Grune & Stratton, Orlando, 1984
20. Goldman AB, Ghelmen B: The double-contrast shoulder arthrogram. Radiology 127:655, 1978
21. Greenway GD, Danzig LA, Resnick D, Haghighi P: The painful shoulder. Med Radiogr Photogr 58 (2):21, 1982
22. Hall F, Rosenthal DI, Goldberg RP, Wyshak G: Morbidity from shoulder arthrography: etiology, incidence, and prevention. AJR 136:59, 1981

23. Kilcoyne RF, Matsen FA III: Rotator cuff measurement by arthropneumotomography. AJR 140:315, 1983

24. Kinnard P, Tricoire JL, Levesque R, Bergeron D: Assessment of the unstable shoulder by computed arthrography. A preliminary report. Am J Sports Med 11:157, 1983

25. Lawrence WS: A method of obtaining an accurate lateral roentgenogram of the shoulder joint. Am J Roentgenol 5:193, 1918

26. Lie S, Mast WA: Subacromial bursography. Radiology 144:626, 1982

27. Middleton WD, Edelstein G, Reinus WR et al: Sonographic detection of rotator cuff tears. AJR 144:349, 1985

28. Mink JH, Richardson A, Grant TT: Evaluation of the glenoid labrum by double contrast arthrography. AJR 133:883, 1979

29. Older MW, McIntyre JL, Lloyd GJ: Distension arthrography of the shoulder joint. Can J Surg 19:203, 1976

30. Pavlov H, Warren RF, Weiss CB, Dines DM: The roentgenographic evaluation of anterior shoulder instability. Clin Orthop 194:153, 1985

31. Protass JJ, Stampfli FV, Osmer JC: Coracoid process fracture diagnosis in acromioclavicular separation. Radiology 116:61, 1975

32. Rokous JR, Feagin JA, Abbott HG: Modified axillary roentgenogram. Clin Orthop 82:84, 1972

33. Seltzer SE, Finberg HJ, Weissman BN et al: Arthrosonography: Gray scale ultrasound evaluation of the shoulder. Radiology 132:467, 1979

34. Slivka J, Resnick D: An improved radiographic view of the glenohumeral joint. J Can Assoc Radiol 30:83, 1979

35. Strizak AM, Danzig LA, Jackson DW et al: Subacromial bursography. J Bone Joint Surg 64A:196, 1982

36. Weston WJ: Arthrography of the acromio-clavicular joint. Australas Radiol 18:213, 1974

37. Zachrisson BE, Ejeskar A: Arthrography in dislocation of the acromioclavicular joint. Acta Radiol (Diagn) 20:81, 1979

38. Zanca P: Shoulder pain. Involvement of the acromioclavicular joint. Am J Roentgenol 112:493, 1971

Shoulder Arthroscopy and Arthroscopic Surgery

Bertram Zarins
John J. Boyle

Arthroscopic visualization of the glenohumeral and acromioclavicular (AC) joints and the subacromial bursa yields a much higher degree of diagnostic accuracy of shoulder conditions than has been possible in the past. Arthroscopic surgery of the shoulder is in a developmental stage, but has already radically altered techniques used to treat certain shoulder conditions. In this chapter, we discuss the ways arthroscopy can be used to improve diagnostic accuracy in patients who have shoulder problems and explain current applications of arthroscopic surgery to treat some of these conditions.

HISTORY OF SHOULDER ARTHROSCOPY

In 1931, Burman experimented with anterior and posterior approaches for shoulder arthroscopy in cadavers.[5] Tagaki reportedly performed shoulder arthroscopy on a patient in 1935.[27] World War II interrupted progress in the development of arthroscopy. Watanabe et al, in 1973,[27] and Ikeuchi, in 1978,[14] published their clinical experiences with shoulder arthroscopy. Recent reports on shoulder arthroscopy have been published by Lloyd,[17] Johnson,[11,15,16] Wiley,[28] Caspari,[7] Cofield,[8] Rojvanit,[25] Andrews,[3] Lombardo,[18] Eriksson,[12] and Zarins.[29]

At present, diagnostic shoulder arthroscopy is a well-established technique that has a definite place in the diagnosis of shoulder conditions. Arthroscopic visualizations of the AC joint and subacromial bursa have recently been developed into standard techniques although these are less frequently used than is glenohumeral arthroscopy. Operative arthroscopy has demonstrated its usefulness in procedures such as loose body removal, synovial biopsy, and joint culture and irrigation. Its usefulness in correcting problems such as certain types of glenoid labrum tears, subacromial impingement, and calcific supraspinatus tendinitis is encouraging. The safety and efficacy of arthroscopic surgical techniques to correct glenohumeral instability and rotator cuff tears has not been clearly demonstrated yet and is still at an experimental stage.

79

INDICATIONS FOR USE

Shoulder pain can be caused by a variety of pathologic conditions that affect the shoulder joint or adjacent structures. The physician must take into consideration the possibility that shoulder pain is caused by disorders of structures other than the glenohumeral joint, its surrounding capsule, and the rotator cuff. Referred pain to the shoulder joint commonly comes from the AC joint, cervical spine, brachial plexus, thorax, or abdomen. Information acquired from history, physical examination, and radiographs usually is enough to make an accurate diagnosis. In instances in which the diagnosis is not clear using standard clinical methods, arthroscopy can be a valuable adjunct for arriving at the correct diagnosis.

Indications for performing shoulder arthroscopy are

1. To diagnose the cause of pain, clicking, or other symptoms in the glenohumeral joint.
2. To determine the direction of glenohumeral instability in patients who have a history of probable dislocation or subluxation. This is useful if multidirectional instability is suspected.
3. To inspect the rotator cuff from above (by viewing the subacromial bursa) and from below (by viewing the glenohumeral joint) in patients who have painful subacromial impingement.
4. To confirm or rule out the glenohumeral joint as the site of pathology in patients who have atypical shoulder pain.
5. To obtain tissue or fluid under direct visualization for culture or histologic examination. This is useful to diagnose pathologic conditions such as rheumatoid arthritis, infection, pigmented villonodular synovitis, and synovial osteochondromatosis.
6. To treat certain shoulder conditions, such as removal of loose bodies, using arthroscopic methods.

DIAGNOSTIC SHOULDER ARTHROSCOPY—TECHNIQUE

Shoulder arthroscopy is performed in the operating room usually using general anesthesia. Arthroscopy can be performed under local anesthesia but this method requires considerable expertise on the part of the operating surgeon and cooperation and muscle relaxation on the part of the patient.

Patient Position

The patient is positioned in the lateral decubitus position (Fig. 5-15). Adhesive tape 4 inches wide is placed across the iliac crest and is secured to the operating table to stabilize the pelvis. The arm of the shoulder to be examined using the arthroscope is positioned upward. Foam rubber-backed straps or moleskin straps are wrapped onto the forearm using elastic bandages. These are used to apply traction to the extremity. Bony prominences at the wrist are wrapped with padding to prevent injury from excess pressure. Skin traction is applied to the upper extremity using a rope that attaches, via a pulley, to a 10-lb weight. The shoulder is positioned at approximately 45° abduction and 20° forward flexion.

The shoulder is prepared and draped in the usual sterile manner. A sterile towel is used to cover the forearm which is wrapped with a sterile gauze bandage. A Steridrape is then used to cover the forearm.

Introducing Arthroscope Through a Posterior Portal

A posterior portal is the best approach for visualizing the glenohumeral joint (Fig. 5-16). The portal is located 1½ cm distal to the acromial angle in a "soft spot." The examiner's thumb and index finger are placed on the anterior and posterior aspects of the acromion process, respectively. The acromion process is the best landmark for locating the glenohumeral joint. An 18-gauge spinal needle is passed parallel to the line connecting the finger tips at a distance 1½ cm distal to the acromion. The direction of the tip of the needle is the coracoid process anteriorly.

The spinal needle is first introduced into the glenohumeral joint. Rotating the humerus is helpful when locating deep bony landmarks and the joint. The joint is distended with 50 ml saline or Ringer's lactate. Backflow of fluid through the spinal needle is confirmation that the glenohumeral joint has been distended. Prior to withdrawing the spinal needle, attach a syringe containing bupivicaine 0.5 percent with epi-

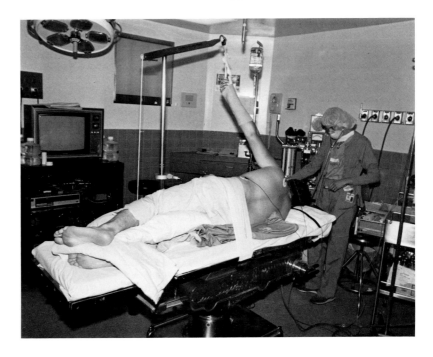

Fig. 5-15. Patient positioning for arthroscopy of the left shoulder. Four-inch wide tape stabilizes the pelvis in a lateral position. A pillow is placed between the knees. The left arm is suspended in skin traction and connected to a ten pound weight via pulleys.

nephrine 1–200,000. This solution is infiltrated into the soft tissues for the entire distance from the shoulder joint to the skin as the spinal needle is withdrawn. The epinephrine helps reduce the amount of bleeding along the tract created by the arthroscope. The local

anesthetic also keeps the shoulder painless during the first several hours after the arthroscopy. The direction of the spinal needle (in reference to the acromion process) is noted; this will be the future direction of the arthroscope).

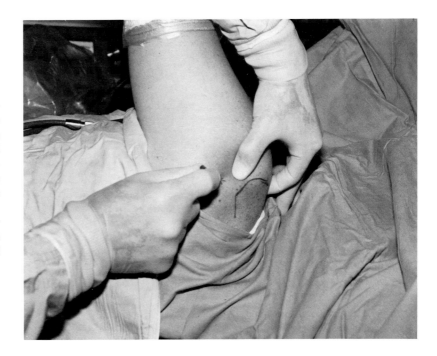

Fig. 5-16. Introducing a spinal needle into the posterior aspect of the left shoulder. The thumb and index finger are placed on the posterior and anterior aspects of the acromion process respectively. The spinal needle passes below a line connecting the tips of the thumb and index finger, approximately 2 cm below the inferior surface of the acromion process. The tip of the needle is directed toward the coracoid process anteriorly.

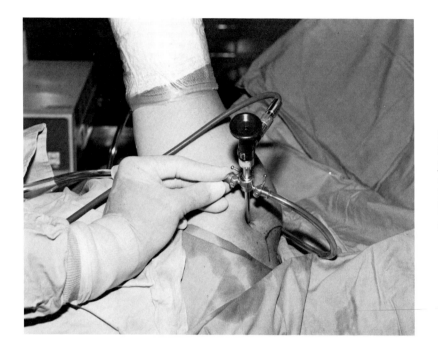

Fig. 5-17. The arthroscope has been introduced into the glenohumeral joint through a posterior portal. Ringer's lactate inflow and suction have been connected to the sheath. A fiber-optic light cable has been connected to the telescope.

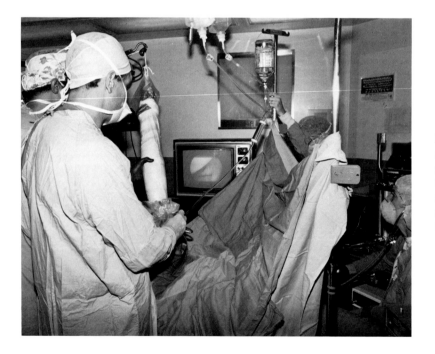

Fig. 5-18. Arthroscopic visualization of the left shoulder through a posterior portal. A video camera displays the image on a monitor placed on the opposite side of the table from the surgeon. The assistant applies traction and rotation to the arm.

A 5-mm long skin incision is made in the posterior soft spot at the site of needle entry. A 5-mm diameter arthroscope sheath is introduced with the aid of a sharp obturator. It is usually safe to pop directly through the posterior joint capsule using the sharp obturator if the joint has been distended. Occasionally it is safer to switch to a rounded obturator so that articular surfaces will not be damaged, but the capsule is thick and is difficult to penetrate. Introducing the arthroscope into the glenohumeral joint is usually the most difficult part of shoulder arthroscopy. If the tip of the blunt obturator cannot be moved about freely, it is still in soft tissues around the shoulder joint rather than inside the joint. The instrument should be redirected, usually in a proximal direction and aimed towards the inferior surface of the acromion process. This is only a short distance above the superior aspect of the glenohumeral joint. The top of the glenohumeral joint is bounded by the supraspinatus tendon. Only the thin subacromial bursa separates the supraspinatus tendon from the acromion process. If the arthroscope cannot be introduced into the glenohumeral joint via this posterior portal, it is usually possible to get into the joint using the superior portal (described below).

The telescope is then inserted into the sheath and inflow and suction are connected to the two stopcocks (Fig. 5-17). The joint is distended with Ringer's lactate.[23] An assistant pulls on the forearm to distract the joint—the patient is given a muscle relaxant to allow better distraction of the glenohumeral joint. The arm can also be rotated and moved into different positions to bring various intra-articular structures into view. A video camera can be connected to the arthroscope so that the procedure can be viewed on a television monitor (Fig. 5-18).

Diagnostic Arthroscopy

The inside of the glenohumeral joint should be inspected in a systematic manner.[16,19] The intra-articular portion of the biceps brachii tendon is the most useful landmark to use to get oriented within the joint (Fig. 15-19). The supraspinatus tendon is located superior to the biceps tendon. The superior, posterior, and inferior glenoid recesses are located below the level of the glenoid cavity articular cartilage. Loose bodies can collect in these recesses.

The glenoid labrum is visualized for the entire circumference at the margin of the glenoid cavity. There is variability in the size of the labrum and how much of a meniscus-type appearance it has. Slight irregularities are a common normal finding especially on the posterior part. The glenoid cavity articular cartilage is inspected. Note the synovium.

With the patient relaxed apply traction to the arm to distract the humeral joint. This exposes the anterior aspect of the joint. Note the superior border of the subscapularis tendon and the adjacent opening into the subscapularis bursa (recess). The middle glenohumeral ligament obliquely crosses the medial edge of the subscapularis tendon. The inferior glenohumeral ligament is in a plane slightly posterior to the middle

Fig. 5-19. Diagram of shoulder anatomy from posterior aspect with patient in lateral position as for shoulder arthroscopy. The subacromial bursa separates the supraspinatus tendon from the inferior surface of the acromion process. The superior aspect of the glenohumeral joint lies just below the supraspinatus tendon. The biceps brachii tendon is the most useful landmark for gaining orientation within the glenohumeral joint. (Zarins B: Arthroscopy of the shoulder: technique. p. 76. In Zarins B, Andrews JR, Carson WG (eds): Injuries to the Throwing Arm. WB Saunders, Philadelphia, 1985. Reprinted with permission from WB Saunders Co.)

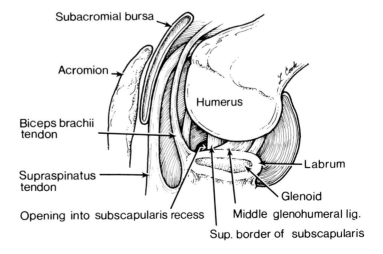

glenohumeral ligament and is continuous with the anterior–inferior portion of the glenoid labrum.

The posterior two thirds of the humeral head can be seen if the humeral head is rotated. There is an area at the posterior humeral head at the junction of the articular cartilage with the synovium that can normally be devoid of articular cartilage. One or more blood vessels penetrate the bone in this area.

INTRODUCING A PROBE THROUGH AN ANTERIOR PORTAL

Once the arthroscope has been introduced into the glenohumeral joint through the posterior portal, the light from the arthroscope can be used to transilluminate the skin as an aid in selecting sites for additional portals. Intraarticular landmarks can also be visualized through the arthroscope and used as a guide to portal placement.[20] The intraarticular site of entry of the anterior portal is within a triangle bounded by the biceps tendon (proximally), the superior border of subscapularis tendon (distally), and the rim of the anterior glenoid (medially) (Plate 5-1). The portal should enter the skin at a point lateral to the coracoid process, which can be palpated anteriorly.

The light of the arthroscope is shined through the center of the triangle described above and the skin is transilluminated in the anterior deltoid area. Palpate the coracoid process. Staying lateral to the coracoid process, the tip of an 18-gauge spinal needle should be aimed toward the light. The interior of the joint is viewed as the tip of the needle enters the joint within the triangle. The needle must pass easily in a straight line into the center of the triangle. The direction of needle passage is noted (Fig. 5-20).

Bupivicaine 0.5 percent with epinephrine is then infiltrated into the needle tract as the needle is withdrawn and then a small stab incision using a #11 knife blade is made. A probe, instrument or inflow cannula is introduced through the anterior portal. The arthroscope can also be introduced through the anterior portal for visualization.

An alternate method for establishing an anterior portal has been described by Detrisac and Johnson, who credit Wissinger for the idea.[11] This is a retrograde method. The anterior triangle[20] is located by arthroscopic visualization and the tip of the arthroscope is placed against the synovium. The telescope is withdrawn from the sheath. A long, thin metal rod is passed through the sheath and pushed anteriorly into the subcutaneous tissues. A small skin incision is made over the tip of the rod and a cannula is

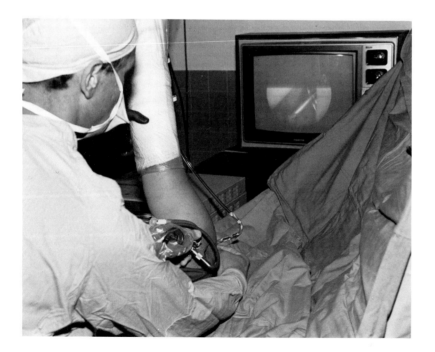

Fig. 5-20. The arthroscope has been introduced from a posterior portal. A needle is being directed from the anterior aspect of the left shoulder and enters the joint within the triangular space bounded by the biceps tendon, superior margin of the subscapularis tendon, and glenoid rim.

passed over the rod in a retrograde manner. Be careful not to place the rod too medial using this method.

SUPERIOR PORTAL

Using the shoulders of a cadaver, Rojvanit simulated a superior portal located at the anterior angle of the acromion process.[24] He concluded that this approach could injure the supraspinatus tendon and recommended against its use.

A superior portal located medial to the acromion process that pierces the supraspinatus muscle instead of the tendon was described by Nevaiser.[11] The portal is located posterior to the distal clavicle and anterior to the scapular spine (Fig. 5-21). The supraspinatus nerve and artery are medial to the path of the incision for this portal.

ADDITIONAL PORTALS

A second anterior portal can be made slightly distal to the first. This must be located distal and lateral to the coracoid process. The retrograde method using a rod passed from a posterior portal should not be used to establish an additional anterior portal because of risk of injuring the musculocutaneous nerve.[11] A second posterior portal placed distal to the first can be used, but is risky because of the location of the axillary nerve.

ANATOMY AND PATHOLOGY OF THE GLENOHUMERAL JOINT

This section describes the arthroscopic appearance of normal intraarticular structures and common pathologic entities.

Biceps Tendon

The intraarticular portion of the long head of the biceps brachii tendon originates from the supraglenoid tubercle at the 12-o'clock position of the glenoid cavity (Plate 5-2). It is continuous posteriorly with the posterior glenoid labrum. Externally rotating the arm allows an additional segment of the tendon to be seen as it exits the shoulder near the insertion of the supraspinatus tendon and enters the intertubercular groove. The biceps tendon has been reported to be bifid on occasion,[9] as well as extrasynovial.[24]

Pathologic changes that can involve the biceps tendon are fraying, partial rupture, and other degenerative processes. The tendon of the long head of biceps can rupture leaving a 2-cm long stump of tendon still attached to the supraglenoid tubercle within the joint. This stump can cause symptoms of painful clicking with shoulder motion and can be resected using arthroscopic surgical methods. Rotator cuff tears can occur in conjunction with biceps tendon disruptions.

Supraspinatus Tendon/Rotator Cuff

The superior boundary of the glenohumeral joint is the supraspinatus tendon. Anteriorly, the tendon is separated from the superior border of the subscapularis tendon by a small synovial-lined interval and the opening into the subscapularis bursa (recess). The posterior border of the supraspinatus tendon blends with the superior border of the infraspinatus. This area can be seen from an anterior portal.

The supraspinatus tendon can tear partially or completely due to acute trauma without being affected by a prior disease process. This usually occurs in young people. However, more commonly tearing of the rotator cuff occurs because the tendons are weakened by a degenerative process. This process can be caused by overuse or aging.

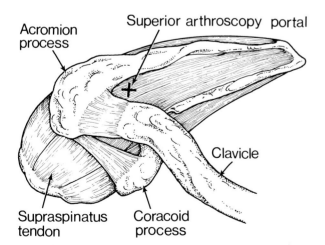

Fig. 5-21. Superior view right shoulder showing location (X) of superior portal for shoulder arthroscopy.

If the rotator cuff tear is incomplete, it can be seen only from within the joint (Fig. 5-22) or the subacromial bursa depending upon the location of the tear. If the tear is complete, the arthroscope can be passed from the glenohumeral joint into the subacromial bursa (Plate 5-3A). If the tear is massive and the edges of the cuff have retracted, the humeral head appears to be "bald" (Plate 5-3B).

Calcification within the supraspinatus tendon can often be seen by viewing laterally in the subacromial bursa. Shoulder "bursitis" is actually supraspinatus tendinitis in most instances.

Synovium

The synovial membrane lines the inside of the capsule as well as the capsular thickenings (glenohumeral ligaments). It also lines the subacromial bursa (recess) and the intraarticular portion of the biceps tendon. Along the peripheral edge of the articular surface of the humeral head is a several millimeters wide rim of humeral head bone that is covered by synovium

and can appear to be "bare." This is a normal finding and should not be confused with Hill-Sachs lesion.

The synovial membrane can be afflicted by a variety of pathologic conditions. It can respond by an acute or chronic inflammatory reaction. The result is usually an acute or chronic nonspecific synovitis. Other pathologic synovial conditions that can be seen within the shoulder joint include synovial osteochondromatosis, pigmented villonodular synovitis, crystalline synovitis (gout or pseudogout), and rheumatoid arthritis.

Arthroscopic findings in patients with adhesive capsulitis or "frozen shoulder" have been reported.[13] The capacity of the glenohumeral joint was smaller than normal in more than half of the patients. No intraarticular adhesions were noted. The authors concluded that the clinical syndrome of "frozen shoulder" is not due to visible intraarticular pathology. Detrisac and Johnson also found the joint capacity to be one half normal in patients with adhesive capsulitis. Synovitis was usually present at the exit of the biceps tendon. They noted marked synovitis at the opening into the subscapularis bursa and in the region of the superior glenohumeral ligament. No intraarticular adhesions were seen.

Articular Cartilage

The round humeral head and oval glenoid cavity are lined by hyaline cartilage. Acute chondral or osteochondral fragments can fracture from the surfaces when the humeral head dislocates or subluxates (Fig. 5-23). With anterior glenohumeral instability, the humeral head lesion will be on the posterior aspect of the humeral head, the Hill-Sachs lesion (Plate 5-4).

The articular surface and underlying bone can also be afflicted by a variety of inflammatory and degenerative conditions such as osteoarthritis, rheumatoid arthritis, calcium pyrophosphate deposition, pyogenic arthritis, and osteonecrosis.

Capsule and Glenohumeral Ligaments

The capsule is attached to the entire circumference of the glenoid cavity. Anteriorly, three separate thickenings of the capsule can be identified and are named.

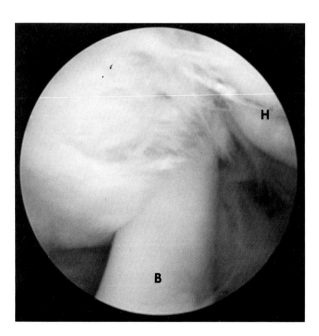

Fig. 5-22. Arthroscopic view right shoulder showing frayed inferior surface of supraspinatus tendon insertion. This is a partial thickness tear of the inferior surface of the rotator cuff. B, biceps tendon; H, humeral head.

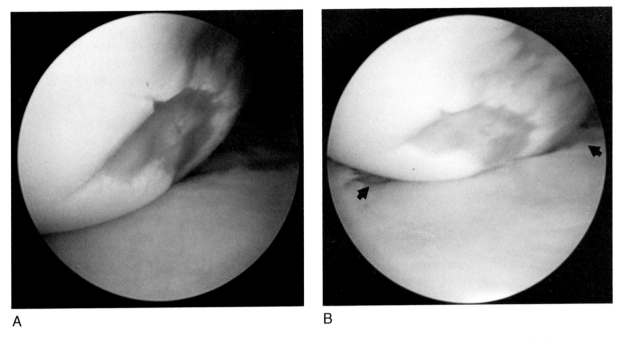

A   B

Fig. 5-23. (**A**) Posterior inferior humeral head, chondral fracture (posterior arthroscopic view). (**B**) The arm has been moved into a position of abduction and external rotation. The humeral head is sliding forward. The humeral head defect is sliding over the anterior glenoid rim and labrum. The patient has a large Bankart lesion (arrows).

The *superior glenohumeral ligament* is attached to the superior tubercle of the glenoid fossa anterior to the long head of the biceps origin. It blends with the coracohumeral ligament and inserts into the fovea capitis of the humerus. The superior middle glenohumeral ligament is difficult to visualize arthroscopically. The *middle glenohumeral ligament* is attached to the supraglenoid tubercle just below the superior glenohumeral ligament attachment, as well as to the upper half of the glenoid and neck of the scapula. When viewed arthroscopically, the middle glenohumeral ligament appears to cross the superior border of the subscapularis at an angle of approximately 60° (Plate 5-5). Laterally, the middle glenohumeral ligament is attached to the anterior humeral neck just medial to the lesser tuberosity. The *inferior glenohumeral ligament* is in a plane more posterior to the plane of the middle glenohumeral ligament. It attaches to the middle of the anterior glenoid rim. It courses distally to attach to the medial aspect of the surgical neck of the humerus. The inferior glenohumeral ligament appears to be continuous with the inferior portion of the anterior glenoid labrum.

In a patient who has recurrent anterior shoulder dislocation or subluxation, the anterior glenoid labrum and/or capsule can be torn from the rim of the glenoid (Bankart lesion). The pathologic changes in the patient with recurrent anterior shoulder instability can vary from anterior capsule stretching to a fracture of the anterior glenoid rim.[26] The glenoid labrum can be torn in a circumferential manner but without disruption of the capsule from the bony glenoid rim (Plate 5-6). The glenoid labrum and capsule can tear away from the bone (the "classic" Bankart lesion) (Plate 5-7).[4] The anterior rim of the glenoid fossa can fracture to a greater or lesser extent.

When viewed arthroscopically, the Bankart lesion does not appear to be a disruption of the middle or inferior glenohumeral ligament. Rather, the lesion seen in shoulders that are unstable in an anterior direction appears to be a tearing of the labrum and capsule from the glenoid rim.

Detrisac and Johnson have reported that the "anterior capsule" described in surgical procedures for recurrent shoulder dislocation is really the middle glenohumeral ligament.[11] The inferior glenohumeral ligament is difficult to visualize when approaching the shoulder from an open anterior approach since it blends with the glenoid labrum and is obscured by the middle glenohumeral ligament.

Since there is considerable variation in the size and appearance of the middle glenohumeral ligament, it is often difficult to distinguish anatomical variations from pathologic absence of ligaments. The middle glenohumeral ligament can be a very thin structure with large openings above and below the ligament into the subscapularis bursa (Plates 5-3 and 5-4). This anatomical variation should not be confused with disruption of the middle glenohumeral ligament or a Bankart lesion.[21]

Glenoid Labrum

The glenoid labrum is a narrow band of fibrocartilaginous tissue located at the junction of the shoulder capsule and the rim of the glenoid fossa. There is considerable variation in the size and shape of the glenoid labrum in various sections of its circumference. Increasing age is associated with progressive degenerative changes in the glenoid labrum.[10]

Detrisac and Johnson[11] have described five variations in labral anatomy and have classified these as types A through E. The *type A* labrum has a meniscus type labrum located only at the superior segment of the glenoid rim. The *type B* labrum is a large meniscus type labrum located only in the posterior segment of the glenoid rim. The *type C* labrum appears to have a meniscus shape in the anterior segment only. The *type D* labrum is a combination of types A and C and consists of a large labrum that extends from the posterosuperior to the anteroinferior segment of the glenoid rim. The *type E* labrum is shaped like a circumferential meniscus extending around the entire circumference of the glenoid cavity.

Glenoid labrum tears can be classified into two general categories, although complex types of tears can be seen. *Circumferential* (vertical longitudinal) tears are caused by subluxation or dislocation of the humeral head over the margin of the glenoid fossa. This is analogous to the meniscus tearing when the tibia

subluxates in relation to the femur (such as with a torn anterior cruciate ligament). The location of the glenoid labrum tear is a clue to the direction of humeral head instability. For example, a circumferential tear of the inferior glenoid labrum suggests inferior humeral head instability (Plate 5-8).

A second type of glenoid labrum tear is a *radial* tear. This is usually found in the anterior superior quadrant of the glenoid fossa just anterior to the origin of the biceps brachii tendon from the supraglenoid tubercle (Plate 5-9). This type of glenoid labrum tear is reportedly not associated with glenohumeral instability.[1,22] Andrews believes that when the arm is in the overhead position excess traction of the biceps tendon can tear the anterior superior labrum.[2]

A *flap* tear of the labrum is a complete tear consisting of radial and circumferential components and is usually located in the anterior superior quadrant (Fig. 5-24).

Subacromial Bursa

The arthroscope can be used to visualize the subacromial bursa. The superior surface of the rotator

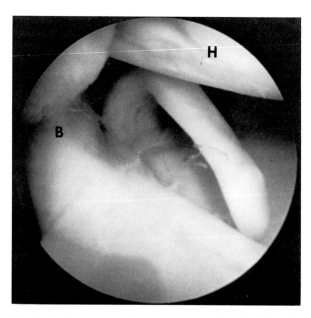

Fig. 5-24. Posterior arthroscopic view right shoulder. The patient has a large superiorly based flap tear of the anterior glenoid labrum. H, humeral head; B, biceps tendon.

cuff (supraspinatus tendon) as well as the inferior surface of the acromion process and coracoacromial ligament can be seen (Fig. 5-25).

TECHNIQUE

Following arthroscopic visualization of the glenohumeral joint, the tip of the arthroscope is placed above the biceps tendon at the inferior surface of the supraspinatus tendon. The telescope is withdrawn from the sheath and a sharp obturator is introduced. The sheath and obturator are withdrawn from the glenohumeral joint a distance of 1 cm. The tip of the sheath is redirected in a superior direction to hit the inferior surface of the acromion process. Do this as far laterally as possible. The telescope is introduced and the bursa is visualized. A needle passed through the acromioclavicular joint into the bursa is a useful landmark while visualizing the bursa.

PATHOLOGY

Superior surface tears of the supraspinatus tendon can be seen from within the subacromial bursa. Calcific deposits in the supraspinatus tendon can often

be seen. The inferior surface of the acromion process can be visualized.

ARTHROSCOPIC SURGERY

Arthroscopic excision of the coracoacromial ligament and anterior-inferior acromion process are being performed arthroscopically. It is still uncertain whether the arthroscopic technique is superior over open resection of the coracoacromial ligament and anterior-inferior acromion process. Excessive bleeding following division of the coracoacromial ligament is a common problem.

Calcific deposits within the supraspinatus tendon can be removed using arthroscopic surgical techniques. This method leaves a hole in the supraspinatus tendon. Possibly this can heal with scar tissue. We do not have enough experience with this method to know whether open resection of the calcific mass and repair of the tendon is better than arthroscopic removal. If arthroscopic resection is performed, the patient should be treated postoperatively with oral nonsteroidal anti-inflammatory agents to decrease the inflammatory response of the tissues to released calcium.

Acromioclavicular Joint

The acromioclavicular joint can be visualized through an arthroscope. This can be done under local or general anesthesia. The joint can be entered from the superior or posterior aspect. Additional instruments for arthroscopic debridement can be introduced from a superior approach.

Arthroscopic debridement of posttraumatic conditions in the acromioclavicular joint should be viewed as temporary measures. It is likely that symptoms will recur following arthroscopic debridement and that surgical excision of the distal clavicle may be required.

Complications and Pitfalls

Shoulder arthroscopy is a procedure that has the potential to result in serious injury of neurovascular tissues. Excess traction on the arm of a patient whose muscles are relaxed under general anesthesia can injure the brachial plexus. Do not apply traction with

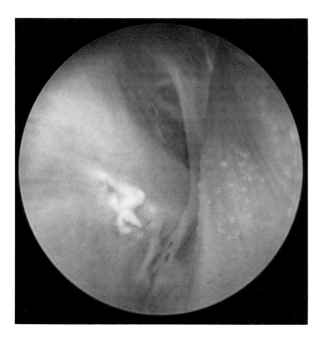

Fig. 5-25. Arthroscopic view, right subacromial bursa, showing coracoacromial ligament attachment to acromion process.

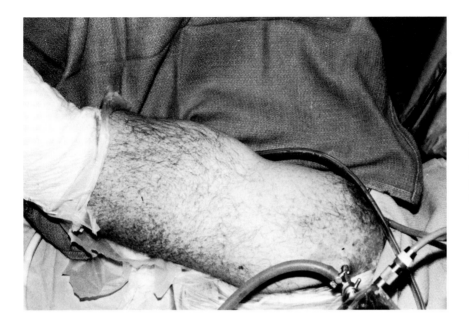

Fig. 5-26. Left shoulder arthroscopy showing marked distension of the arm at the completion of the procedure. The fluid resorbed uneventfully.

the arm in excessive elevation because of risk of injuring the brachial plexus.

Anterior portals should be placed lateral to the coracoid process to avoid injury to neurovascular structures.[20] The portals should not be placed distal to the coracoid process because of the location of the axillary nerve.[11]

Introducing the arthroscope into the shoulder joint can be difficult. The synovial membrane stretches. The arthroscope or operative instruments can be just outside the synovial membrane even though they feel free as if they have been introduced into the joint (Plate 5-10). It is often difficult to palpate bony landmarks.

Irrigating solution used for arthroscopy can extravasate into the soft tissues about the shoulder joint (Fig. 5-26). Therefore, arthroscopic procedures have a time limit because of soft tissue swelling.

REFERENCES

1. Andrews JR, Carson WG: The arthroscopic treatment of glenoid labrum tears in the throwing athlete. Orthop Trans 8:44, 1984
2. Andrews JR, Carson WG: Operative arthroscopy of the shoulder in the throwing athlete. p. 89. In Zarins B, Andrews JR, Carson WG (eds): Injuries to the Throwing Arm. WB Saunders, Philadelphia, 1985
3. Andrews JR, Carson WG: Shoulder joint arthroscopy. Orthopedics 6:1157, 1983
4. Bankart ASB: The pathology and treatment of recurrent dislocation of the shoulder joint. Br J Surg 26:23, 1938
5. Burman MS: Arthroscopy, or the direct visualization of joints: an experimental cadaver study. J. Bone Joint Surg 13:669, 1931
6. Carson G: Arthroscopy of the shoulder: normal anatomy. p. 83. In Zarins B, Andrews JR, Carson WG (eds): Injuries to the Throwing Arm. WB Saunders, Philadelphia, 1985
7. Caspari RB: Shoulder Arthroscopy: a review of the present state of the art. Contemp Ortho 4:523, 1982
8. Cofield RH: Arthroscopy of the shoulder. Orthop Trans 7:141, 1983
9. DePalma AF: Surgery of the Shoulder. Lippincott, Philadelphia, 1983
10. DePalma AF, Callery G, Bennett GA: Variational anatomy and degenerative lesions of the shoulder joint. p. 255. Vol. 6. In Instructional Course Lectures of the American Academy of Orthopaedic Surgeons, CV Mosby, St. Louis, 1949
11. Detrisac DA, Johnson LL: Arthroscopic Shoulder Anatomy. Pathologic and Surgical Implications. Slack, Thorofare, NJ, 1986
12. Eriksson E, Denti M: Diagnostic and operative arthroscopy of the shoulder and elbow joint. Ital J Sports Traumatol 7:165, 1985

13. Ha'Eri GB, Maitland A: Arthroscopic findings in the frozen shoulder. J Rheumatol 8:149, 1981
14. Ikeuchi H: Arthroscopy of the shoulder joint. Arthroscopy (Japn) 3:1, 1978
15. Johnson LL: Arthroscopy of the shoulder. Orthop Clin North Am 11:197, 1980
16. Johnson LL: Diagnostic and Surgical Arthroscopy, CV Mosby, St. Louis, 1981
17. Lloyd GJJ, Older MW, McIntyre JC: Distention arthroscopy of the shoulder joint. Can J Surg 19:203, 1976
18. Lombardo SJ: Arthroscopy of the shoulder. Clin Sports Med 2:309, 1983
19. Matthews LS, Vetter WL, Helfet DL: Arthroscopic surgery of the shoulder. In Advances in Orthopaedic Surgery. Williams & Wilkins, Baltimore, 1984
20. Matthews, LS, Zarins B, Michael RH, Helfet DL: Anterior portal selection for shoulder arthroscopy. Arthroscopy 1:33, 1985
21. Moseley HF, Overgaard B: The anterior capsular mechanism in recurrent anterior dislocation of the shoulder. J Bone Joint Surg 44B:913, 1962
22. Pappas AM, Goss TP, Kleinman PK: Symptomatic shoulder instability due to lesions of the glenoid labrum. Am J Sports Med, 11:279, 1983
23. Reagan BF, McInerney VK, Treadwell BV et al: Irrigating solutions for arthroscopy. J Bone Joint Surg, 65A:629, 1983
24. Rojvanit V: Arthroscopy of the shoulder joint: a cadaver and clinical study. Part 1: cadaver study. J Jpn Orthop 58:1035, 1984
25. Rojvanit V: Arthroscopy of the shoulder joint: a cadaver and clinical study. Part 2: clinical study. J Jpn Orthop 58:1047, 1984
26. Rowe CR, Zarins B: Recurrent transient subluxation of the shoulder. J Bone Joint Surg 63A:863, 1981
27. Watanabe M, Takeda S, Ikeuchi H: Atlas of Arthroscopy. 3rd Ed. Tokyo, Igaku-Shoin, 1978
28. Wiley AM, Older MWJ: Shoulder arthroscopy. Investigations with a fibrooptic instrument. Am J Sports Med 8:31. 1980
29. Zarins B: Arthroscopy of the shoulder: technique. p. 78. In Zarins B, Andrews JR, Carson WG (eds): Injuries to the Throwing Arm. WB Saunders, Philadelphia, 1985
30. Zarins B, Rowe CR: Current concepts in the diagnosis and treatment of shoulder instability in athletes. Med Sci Sports Exerc 16:444, 1984

COLOR PLATES

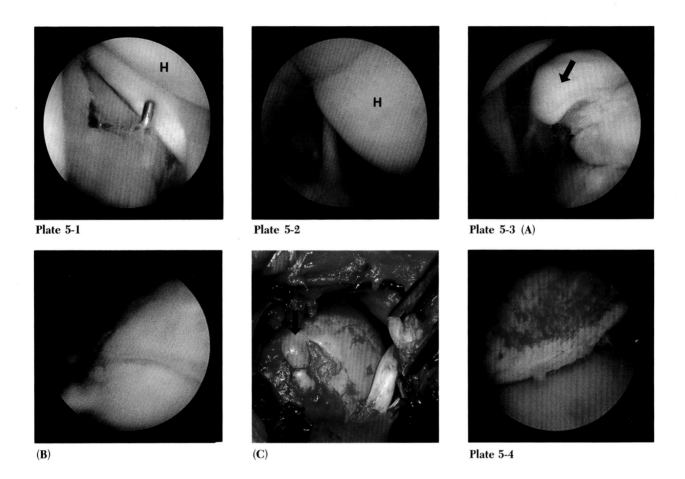

Plate 5-1

Plate 5-2

Plate 5-3 (A)

(B)

(C)

Plate 5-4

Plate 5-1. Intraarticular triangle that can be used as a landmark for locating an anterior portal. The probe enters between the biceps tendon (left), superior margin of subscapularis tendon (right), and anterior glenoid rim (below—not seen). Posterior view, left shoulder. H, humeral head.

Plate 5-2. Arthroscopic view, superior aspect, right shoulder viewed from a posterior portal. The supraspinatus tendon is on the left and humeral head (H) on the right. The biceps tendon takes origin from the supraglenoid tubercle (below) and is a useful landmark within the joint.

Plate 5-3. (A) Arthroscopic view, right shoulder, posterior approach. The patient has a complete tear of the rotator cuff. The stump of supraspinatus tendon attached to the humerus is in the upper right (arrow). (B) The superior aspect of the humeral head is "bald" and the arthroscope can be passed from the superior aspect of the glenohumeral joint (seen below) into the subacromial bursa (seen above). (C) Surgical exploration of this patient's right shoulder confirmed a complete tear of the rotator cuff. The stump of the supraspinatus tendon on the humeral head (seen in Plate 5-3A) is the center of the field (arrow). Two clamps on the right grasp the retracted edge of the torn rotator cuff. The biceps tendon can be seen.

Plate 5-4. Large Hill-Sachs lesion, left shoulder (posterior arthroscopic view).

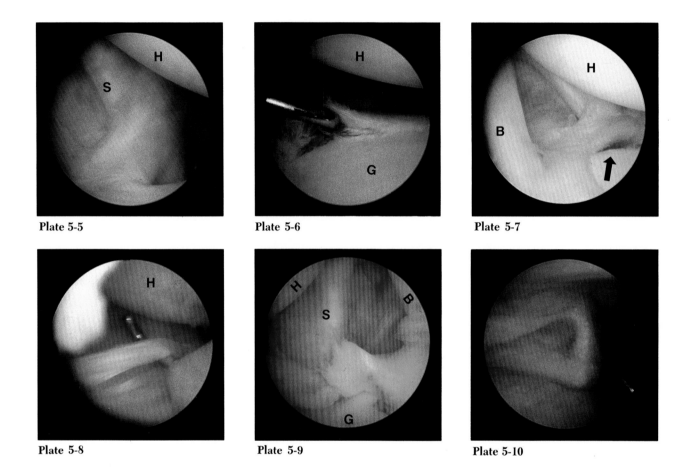

Plate 5-5

Plate 5-6

Plate 5-7

Plate 5-8

Plate 5-9

Plate 5-10

Plate 5-5. Right shoulder, posterior arthroscopic view. The middle glenohumeral ligament courses obliquely behind the subscapularis tendon (S) at an angle of 60°. Note two openings into the subscapularis bursa: one above and the second below the middle glenohumeral ligament. H, humeral head.

Plate 5-6. Grade one Bankart lesion, right shoulder. The anterior glenoid labrum is torn but the capsule has not been avulsed from the bony rim. The probe is in the tear. H, humeral head; G, glenoid fossa.

Plate 5-7. Posterior arthroscopic view, right shoulder. The superior border of subscapularis can be seen just at the edge of the humeral head (H). The anterior labrum and capsule have been avulsed from the anterior glenoid rim. B, biceps tendon; arrow, Bankart lesion.

Plate 5-8. Posterior arthroscopic view, right shoulder. The probe is passed through a circumferential tear of the inferior glenoid labrum. H, humeral head.

Plate 5-9. Posterior arthroscopic view, left shoulder, showing a radial tear of the anterosuperior glenoid labrum. H, humeral head; S, superior border subscapularis tendon; G, glenoid fossa; B, biceps tendon.

Plate 5-10. Left shoulder, posterior arthroscopic view. A probe has been introduced from an anterior portal but has not entered the joint. Note the thin synovial membrane preventing the tip of the probe from entering the joint.

Electrodiagnostic Studies

Robert D. Leffert

Electrodiagnosis has its basis in the fact that the electrical phenomena of depolarization and repolarization of the cell membranes of nerve and muscle parallel the muscle's mechanical contraction and relaxation. Despite the complexity of these neurophysiologic events, the minute electrical potentials that are generated by them can be amplified and displayed in a manner that is of great value to the clinician in diagnosing musculoskeletal problems in general[2] and, specifically, those about the shoulder.

These tests are essentially objective and therefore not under the patient's control with reference to their outcome. Although their results should be reproducible, technical errors and misinterpretations can sometimes lead to illogical and spurious conclusions. It is therefore necessary that they be placed in proper prospective by the surgeon caring for the patient with a shoulder problem. They must not be conceived of as a substitute for a thorough history and physical examination leading to formulation of a working diagnosis. These time-honored examinations must be completed prior to ordering and performing electrodiagnostic studies. If the tests are to be done by someone other than the surgeon, there must be clear communication of the clinical formulation, the reason for doing the test, and what questions are to be answered by it. The referring physician or surgeon must have sufficient knowledge of electrodiagnosis so that he is

able to sensibly interpret the results once they are available.

Basically, electrodiagnostic studies can indicate whether a muscle is normal or affected by a neurogenic or myopathic process. Information regarding the degree of acuity or chronicity of the process can be obtained and lesions can be localized along the neuromuscular axis from the spinal cord distally. What electrodiagnostic studies cannot do is provide an indication of etiology in the case of nerve or muscle injury.

The kinesiologic applications of electrodiagnosis allow us to know how a muscle actually functions in the living patient, rather than having to infer what it might have done under the artificial circumstances of the anatomy laboratory.

TYPES OF ELECTRODIAGNOSTIC STUDIES

The following studies are commonly in use today:

1. Electromyography
2. Nerve conduction velocity determination
3. F responses

93

4. Somatosensory evoked potentials
5. Nerve action potential determinations (intraoperative)

Chronaxie determinations, while of historic interest, are no longer routinely employed in clinical electrodiagnostic testing. They are not further described.

Electromyography

The basic electromyograph consists of a series of differential amplifiers that are capable of processing the minute electrical discharges from muscle, while rejecting the stray and spurious potentials to be found in most testing locations (Fig. 5-27). The examiner must choose between a surface electrode, usually

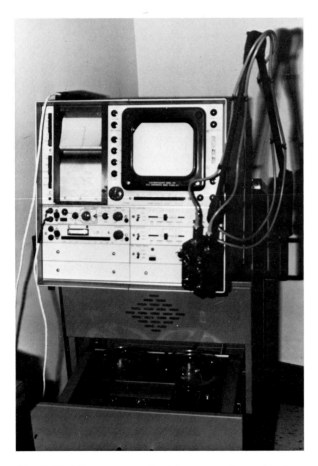

Fig. 5-27. Electromyograph with nerve and muscle stimulator, fiberoptic recording system, and tape recorder.

used for evaluation of larger muscle groups, and needle electrodes, which, although causing some discomfort with percutaneous insertion, are capable of defining the electrical activity not only of specific muscles but also small areas of muscle. The cathode ray tube of the electromyogram (EMG) machine can be calibrated so that the parameters of the wave forms that are observed can be accurately measured and subsequently documented.

A normally innervated muscle at rest ordinarily produces no change in the isoelectric baseline and is referred to as being "electrically silent." When voluntary contraction begins, the electrical discharge of single motor units can be observed as complex wave forms that generally range from 100 to 2000 μV in amplitude and between 2 and 10 msec in duration. With recruitment, the single motor units fall upon each other until the baseline is obliterated and the entire screen is filled with a recruitment or interference pattern. When the muscle contraction ceases, the isoelectric baseline returns. With axonal degeneration from any cause, Wallerian degeneration will result in muscle changes after 3 weeks; the degeneration can be observed electromyographically but not with the naked eye. The introduction of a needle electrode into a partially or completely denervated muscle will result in the appearance of low voltage *fibrillation potentials* and larger units called *sharp positive waves*. These are found in denervation and are not under the patient's voluntary control. They are often under 100 μV in amplitude and have a characteristic sound when heard through the EMG speaker system. If the muscle is totally denervated, there will be no voluntary potentials seen on attempted contraction, although partial denervation will demonstrate units under active control. With subacute or chronic denervation, the character of the voluntary units will become more polyphasic than normal and can be easily identified. So-called giant units may represent attempts at re-innervation of denervated muscle by adjacent motor units.

Muscle that has atrophied due to disuse, without the element of denervation, will not demonstrate fibrillation potentials and sharp positive waves at rest, nor will there be a high percentage of polyphasic units, as is seen in a muscle that is partially denervated. In this way, the atrophy of disuse may be defined from that due to interference with the nerve supply.

Nerve Conduction Velocity Determination

Localization of a nerve lesion along the course of the limb can be markedly facilitated by measurement of the velocity of conduction of peripheral nerves.[6,18,19] This is accomplished with the same basic equipment, including an electromyograph and a source of electrical stimulation that can trigger off impulses along the nerve. These can be subsequently measured so that the velocity of conduction may be determined for a specific length of nerve (Fig. 5-28).

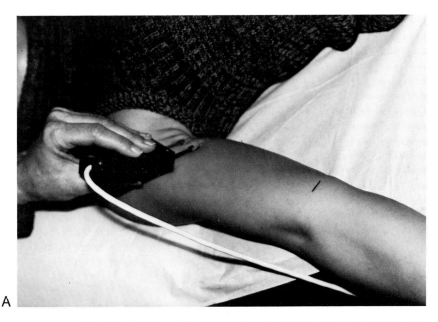

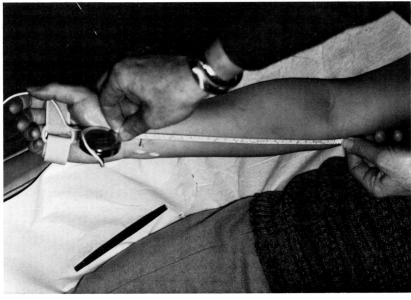

Fig. 5-28. Nerve conduction velocity determination. (**A**) Percutaneous stimulation of ulnar nerve at axilla. (**B**) Stimulation above elbow. Pickup electrode is needle in hypothenar muscles. (*Figure continues.*)

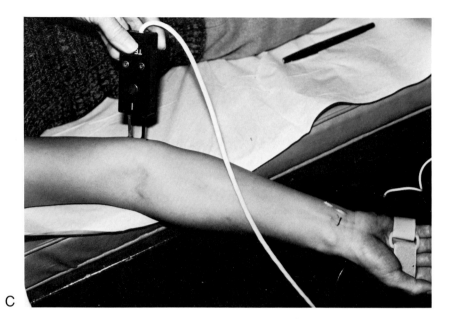

Fig. 5-28 (*Continued*). (C) Measurement of intervals for calculation of conduction velocity.

C

There exists a significant body of normative data for each nerve, both motor and sensory.[7–9,17] However, since individual laboratories may vary somewhat in their normals,[16] these must be used in interpretation of the data they generate. Because nerve conduction velocity determination requires percutaneous stimulation of the nerve at at least two points along its course, it is far more suited to use in the part of the limb that is below the axilla than that about the shoulder. Nevertheless, the determination of latency, the interval between stimulus of the nerve and the response from the muscle, may be of value if the patient's contralateral side is normal and can be used as an internal control.

the subject of some debate, but the impulse is then transmitted orthodromically down the motor nerve to the muscle. It is therefore a late potential, the latency of which depends on the length of nerve between the point of stimulation and the spinal cord. Since it may vary by a few milliseconds from one stimulus to the next, it requires multiple trials recorded on a storage oscilloscope. In combination with conventional nerve conduction velocity determination, it may be used to define the more proximal and largely inaccessible areas of the neuraxis, such as the brachial plexus and region of the spinal nerve roots.

The F Response

Because conventional nerve conduction studies have very limited application to proximal nerve lesions, motor conduction along this segment can be measured by use of the F wave. This is a late muscle potential that can be elicited from antidromically activated anterior horn cells. A supramaximal stimulus is applied transcutaneously to the motor nerve in the hand and travels centrally to the level of the anterior horn cell. Whether the response is a reflex or not is

H Reflex

The H reflex is an electrically elicited spinal monosynaptic reflex that may be elicited from the ulnar nerve of newborn infants and during the first year of life.[20] In adults it has a limited distribution and is elicited by a submaximal stimulus; although it is a measure of conduction velocity in the proximal segments of nerves, it has limited use about the shoulder. It increases in patients with polyneuropathies and with root compression.

Somatosensory Evoked Potentials

The use of spinal and scalp-recorded somatosensory evoked potentials (SEPs) allows us to assess the entire length of a peripheral nerve, including its proximal connections to and within the central nervous system.[16] Clinically, one may evaluate the proximal nerve segments from the axilla to the spinal cord; whereas the F wave is confined to motor fibers, the SEP is useful in brachial plexopathy or radiculopathy where there is involvement of sensory nerve fibers. It is necessary to employ considerably more electronic equipment than is used in conventional conduction velocity determination, and multiple channels, as well as a minicomputer and averager, are necessary.

Nerve Action Potential Measurement

The measurement of action potentials directly from the surface of the nerve is an intraoperative technique that is useful during the course of exploration of not only peripheral nerves, but of the brachial plexus as well.[10] It is particularly valuable in the evaluation of neuromas-in-continuity.

APPLICATION OF ELECTRODIAGNOSIS TO NEUROGENIC CONDITIONS INVOLVING THE SHOULDER

As has been described, electromyographic techniques can be of tremendous value in the clinical evaluation of weakness or muscle atrophy and may differentiate between the atrophy of disuse and that of denervation. They may also be used to identify those patients whose atrophy is due to intrinsic muscle disease such as muscular dystrophy. Particularly for patients with symmetrical muscle wasting about the shoulder girdles, such as is found in limb-girdle dystrophy, the absence of fibrillation potentials at rest and the reduction in the amplitude and duration of the voluntary motor units may, along with appropriate histologic studies, confirm a diagnosis that may be difficult to make, particularly if the atrophy is mild and asymmetrical (Fig. 5-29).

For patients for whom apparent lack of voluntary movement or power is unaccompanied by muscle atrophy, and who may not be exerting full effort during the course of examination, the EMG provides an extremely valuable test. Patients who are allegedly unable to normally activate muscles and who do not

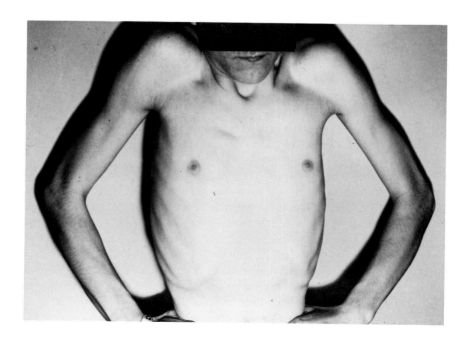

Fig. 5-29. Muscular dystrophy patient with deltoid atrophy and complete loss of pectorals.

have central nervous system lesions can be appropriately identified by their lack of electromyographic abnormalities.

In cases where pain and vague sensory disturbances are the focus of the patient's complaint, the presence or absence of definable peripheral neurologic dysfunction can be established by means of EMGs and nerve conduction studies.

SPECIFIC SHOULDER DYSFUNCTION AND ELECTRODIAGNOSIS

Brachial Plexus Injuries

In cases of traction injury to the brachial plexus where there is a suspicion of root avulsion, electromyography of the posterior cervical musculature can establish that the posterior primary rami have been denervated.[3] This is very strong presumptive evidence of root avulsion. The finding of fibrillation potentials in root collaterals such as the serratus anterior and rhomboids of such patients are additionally confirmatory. Motor and sensory nerve conduction velocity determinations, as well as somatosensory evoked potentials and F responses, can be employed to define a level of pathology in brachial plexus injury. These tests are ordinarily not indicated before the 3-week period necessary for Wallerian degeneration to occur.

Brachial Plexus Neuritis

Brachial plexus neuritis or neuralgic amyotrophy is a disease that causes pain and paralysis about the shoulder without obvious antecedent cause.[22] However, it may follow vaccinations or systemic infections. It is usually unilateral but occasionally may be bilateral and rarely is recurrent. Although the general outlook for recovery is good, there may be difficulty in diagnosing the condition and differentiating it from other causes of weakness about the shoulder. Very often the upper trunk of the brachial plexus is in-

volved but the long thoracic nerve and suprascapular nerve may also be selectively affected. Specific electromyographic changes of denervation can help to map the distribution, as can F responses. Usually the paraspinal muscles are uninvolved.

Thoracic Outlet Syndrome

Although it was claimed that the diagnosis of thoracic outlet compression of nerves could be specifically determined by means of nerve conduction velocity determination,[11,22] most investigators and clinicians now feel that the diagnosis is a clinical one. The technical problems involved in accurate measurement of nerves that are several centimeters beneath the surface make the potential for error very great. In some cases, F responses and somatosensory evoked

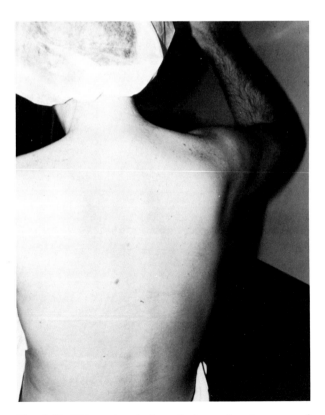

Fig. 5-30. This patient had marked atrophy of supra- and infraspinatus muscles with weakness of right shoulder due to suprascapular nerve lesion.

potentials may delineate the presence of compression of the plexus in the axilla or thoracic outlet, but not always. Care must be taken to position the arm in such a way as to cause compression during the course of the test.

Cervical Radiculopathy

In differential diagnosis, the common entity of cervical radiculopathy due to disc disease in the midcervical region must be considered in cases of otherwise unexplained weakness of the shoulder girdle musculature. Electromyography can be extremely helpful in validating the clinical diagnosis.

Suprascapular Nerve Versus Rotator Cuff Tear

In both a suprascapular nerve lesion and rotator cuff tear there may be aching pain in the shoulder and weakness of abduction accompanied by atrophy of the supra- and infraspinatus muscle (Fig. 5-30). Although in most cases the clinical diagnosis is evident and does not require further electrodiagnostic testing, this is not always the case. The finding of denervation potentials in the muscles supplied only by the suprascapular nerve and no other C5-6 innervated muscles essentially makes the diagnosis. Obviously, a positive arthrogram would identify a rotator cuff tear, and these tears are not ordinarily accompanied by denervation of the muscles, even in the presence of signifi-

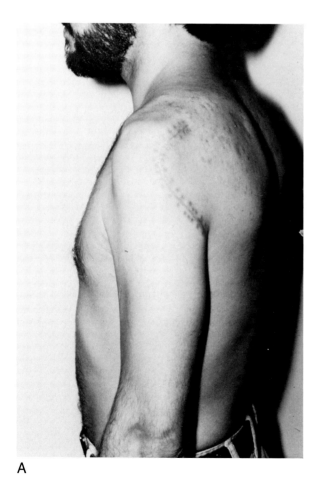
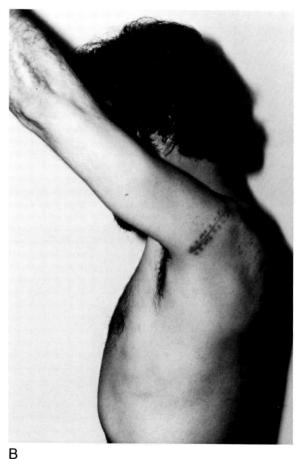

A   B

Fig. 5-31. (**A**) Patient with operatively verified complete laceration of left axillary nerve which could not be repaired. (**B**) He was able to raise his arm and maintain it against moderate resistance.

cant atrophy. Additionally, latency determinations for the susprascapular nerve may be made comparing the two sides of an otherwise intact individual.

Long Thoracic Nerve

Winging of the scapula caused by weakness or paralysis of the serratus anterior muscle may follow closed trauma or may develop as a manifestation of brachial plexus neuropathy. It may follow immunizations or generalized illnesses. In those cases where only evidence of denervation and no voluntary potentials are observed more than a year after the onset of the problem, the prognosis for functional recovery is, in my experience, poor.

Axillary Nerve

This nerve may be injured by closed dislocation or fracture dislocation of the glenohumeral joint either alone or in combination with other nerve injury of the infraclavicular brachial plexus. Although I formerly believed that the isolated injury had a poor prognosis,[14] experience has shown that that is not necessarily so. It may be difficult to establish whether or not the deltoid muscle is indeed functioning, since patients may exhibit remarkably good range of motion in the total absence of deltoid function, although they are not as strong as normal (Fig. 5-31). This situation may be sorted out by means of electromyography, but in cases where there is established denervation it is essential to have examined the posterior deltoid, as reinnervation occurs in that portion of the muscle before the other parts.

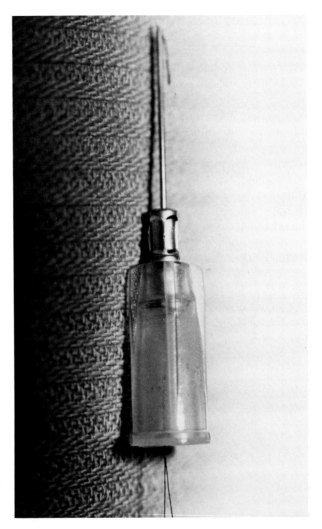

Fig. 5-32. The nichrome wire is introduced into the muscle with the number 25 needle, which is then withdrawn, leaving the flexible wires, which are then connected to the preamplifier of the electromyograph.

Spinal Accessory Nerve

The trapezius muscle is an essential elevator and stabilizer of the scapula, without which marked weakness and pain in the shoulder girdle are experienced. Closed injuries may occur, particularly with falls on the shoulder or weights dropped on it; although open injuries transecting the spinal accessory nerve are rare, those that occur during the course of surgical operations are not. In posttraumatic situations with apparent paralysis of the trapezius, electromyographic examination at 3 weeks can define those lesions that are degenerative and identify those in which some continuity of nerve exists. A treatment program can then be instituted on the basis of knowledge of the underlying nerve lesion.

Kinesiologic Problems About the Shoulder

Voluntary or habitual dislocation of the shoulder can be extremely difficult to deal with from the point of view of diagnosis and treatment. By the use of flexible wire EMG electrodes (Fig. 5-32) that do not inhibit motion, multiple simultaneous tracings of muscular activity may be recorded during the act of voluntary dislocation and reduction (Fig. 5-33). By this method, an individual therapeutic exercise program can be designed to strengthen the weakened muscles without activating those responsible for producing the muscle imbalance and instability. We have found the program to be extremely successful.[12]

Other kinesiologic puzzles, such as how a patient with complete deltoid paralysis can abduct the arm, can be clarified by EMG. EMG can also be quite helpful in preoperative evaluation of patients with muscles weakness prior to tendon transfer about the shoulder.[17]

It therefore behooves the shoulder surgeon to have more than a superficial knowledge of electrodiagnosis. Used properly, it can be extremely helpful.

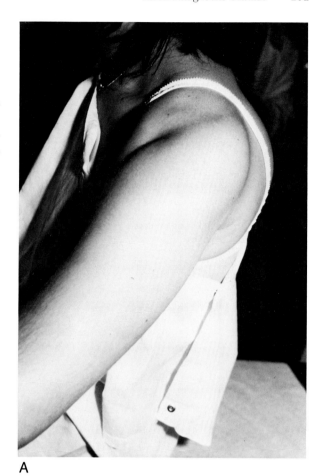

A

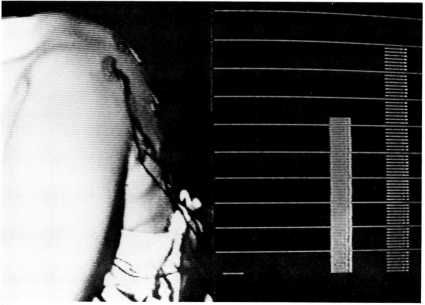

Fig. 5-33. (A) Voluntary inferior and posterior subluxation of the left shoulder. **(B)** Video-EMG done during dislocation. The bar histograms represent integrated EMG of supraspinatus and infraspinatus sampled with flexible wire electrode.

B

REFERENCES

1. Bonney G, Gilliatt RW: Sensory nerve conduction after traction lesions of the brachial plexus. Proc R Soc Med 51:365, 1958
2. Bouivens P: Electrodiagnostic definition of the site and nature of peripheral nerve lesions. Am Phys Med 5:149, 1960
3. Bufalini C, Pescatori G: Posterior cervical electromyography in the diagnosis and prognosis of brachial plexus injuries. J Bone Joint Surg 51B:627, 1969
4. Caldwell JW, Crane CR, Krusen UL: Nerve conduction studies in diagnosis of thoracic outlet syndrome. South Med J 64:210, 1971
5. Desmedt JE, Noel P: Cerebral evoked potentials. p. 480. In Dyck PJ, Thomas PK, Lambert EH (eds): Peripheral Neuropathy. WB Saunders, Philadelphia, 1975
6. Gilliatt RW: History of nerve conduction studies. p. 412. In Licht S (ed): Electrodiagnosis and Electromyography 3rd Ed. E Licht, New Haven, 1971
7. Jebsen RH: Motor conduction velocity in the median and ulnar nerves. Arch Phys Med Rehabil 48:185, 1967
8. Jebsen RH: Motor conduction velocity in proximal and distal segments of the radial nerve. Arch Phys Med Rehabil 47:597, 1966
9. Jebsen RH: Motor conduction velocity of distal radial nerve. Arch Phys Med Rehabil 47:12, 1966
10. Kline DG: Evaluation of the neuroma in continuity. p. 450. In Omer GE, Spinner M (eds): Management of Peripheral Nerve Problems. WB Saunders, Philadelphia, 1980
11. Lederman R: Thoracic outlet syndrome, letter to the editor. N Engl J Med 310(16):1052, 1984
12. Leffert RD, Rowe CR, Kozlowski B, Meister M: Treatment of voluntary dislocation of the shoulder by therapeutic exercise based on video-electromyographic analysis. J Bone Joint Surg 7:141, 1983
13. Leffert RD, Meister M: The phasic behavior of tendon transfers in the upper limb. J Hand Surg 1:181, 1976
14. Leffert RD, Seddon HJ: Infraclavicular brachial plexus injuries. J Bone Joint Surg 47B:9, 1966
15. Liberson WT, Gratze M, Zolis A, Grabinski B: Comparison of conduction velocities of motor and sensory fibres determined by different methods. Arch Phys Med Rehabil 47:17, 1966
16. Liberson WT, Kim KC: Mapping evoked potentials elicited by stimulation of the median and peroneal nerves. Electroencephalogr Clin Neurophysiol 15:721, 1963
17. Nelson RM, Currier DP: Motor nerve conduction velocity of musculocutaneous nerve. J Am Phys Ther Assoc 49:586, 1969
18. Smorto MP, Basmajian: Clinical Electroneurography: An Introduction to Nerve Conduction Tests. 2nd Ed. Williams & Wilkins, Baltimore, 1979
19. Staas WE Jr: Errors in interpretation of nerve conduction velocity. p. 331. In Hunter JM, Schneider LH, Mackin EJ, Bell J (eds): Rehabilitation of the hand. CV Mosby, St. Louis, 1978
20. Thomas JE, Lambert EH: Ulnar nerve conduction velocity and H reflex in infants and children. J Appl Physiol 15:1, 1960
21. Tsairis P: Brachial plexus neuropathies. p. 659. In Dyck PJ, Lambert Eh (eds): Peripheral neuropathy. WB Saunders, Philadelphia, 1975
22. Urschel HC Jr, Rassuk MA, Wood RE et al: Objective diagnosis (ulnar nerve conduction velocity) and current therapy of thoracic outlet syndrome. Am Thorac Surg 12:698, 1971

6

SUBACROMIAL SYNDROMES

Tendinitis, Bursitis, Impingement, "Snapping" Scapula, and Calcific Tendinitis

Carter R. Rowe

The term *Bursitis* is commonly used to describe the majority of painful conditions of the shoulder. Bursitis as a primary cause is perhaps an inaccurate term, as the bursa is merely an innocent bystander, positioned between the rotator cuff and the undersurface of the acromial arch, to protect the gliding surface of the cuff. Reaction of the bursa, except in rare instances of primary involvement, is secondary to overuse, misuse, or injury to the smooth surface of the tendinous rotator cuff. Thus, to be more exact, the term bursitis should be replaced by *tendinitis, with secondary bursal reaction.* This point of view has also been expressed by Uhthoff et al.[6,17]

ing" and a "snapping" sensation (Fig. 6-1). On occasion the bursa may be primarily involved due to rheumatoid arthritis, tuberculosis, or synovial chondromatosis (see Fig. 21-10B).

The reader will be surprised and interested in the discussion of the subdeltoid bursa by E.A. Codman[5] in 1906, in which he describes the different causes of tendinitis and bursitis, including the overuse of the rotator cuff giving pitchers a "glass arm" (our "dead arm" syndrome of today) and identifying the different stages of inflammation of the bursa.

PATHOLOGY

Normally, the subacromial bursa of the shoulder is a thin smooth membrane, lubricating the gliding surface of the rotator cuff. As stated, the bursa may become irritated, acutely inflamed from overuse of the arm in abduction, adduction, or forward flexion, and eventually chronically thickened, producing painful "catching" on motion of the shoulder, or "grind-

CAUSATIVE FACTORS RELATED TO IMPINGEMENT

Mechanical Use of the Shoulder: Soft Tissue Impingement; "Overuse" Syndrome

Whenever the arm is elevated, some degree of impingement of the rotator cuff and bursa may occur under the acromion and coracoacromial ligament (Fig. 6-1). The most vulnerable position of the shoul-

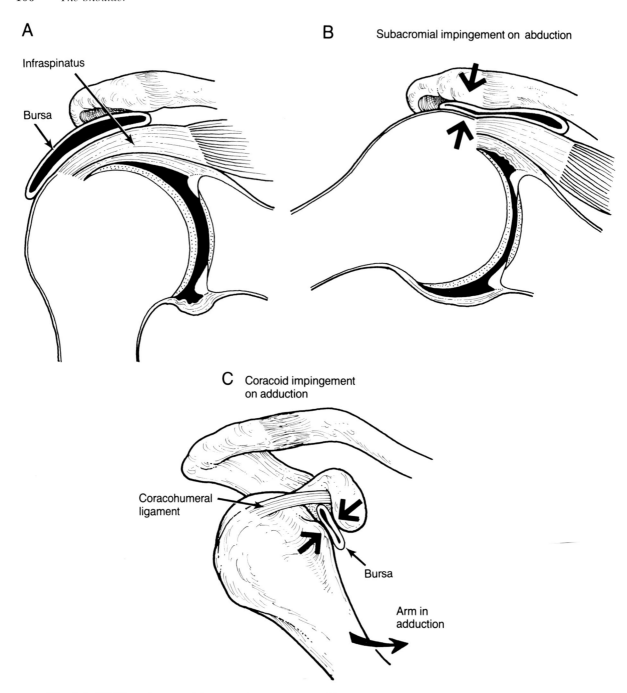

Fig. 6-1. **(A)** The subacromial bursa with arm in neutral position. **(B)** When the arm is abducted or flexed 90°, the rotator cuff and bursa are impinged under the acromial arch. **(C)** Repetition in adduction may produce impingement against the coracoid process. If the arm is elevated in forward flexion, the humeral head rolls away from the acromion.

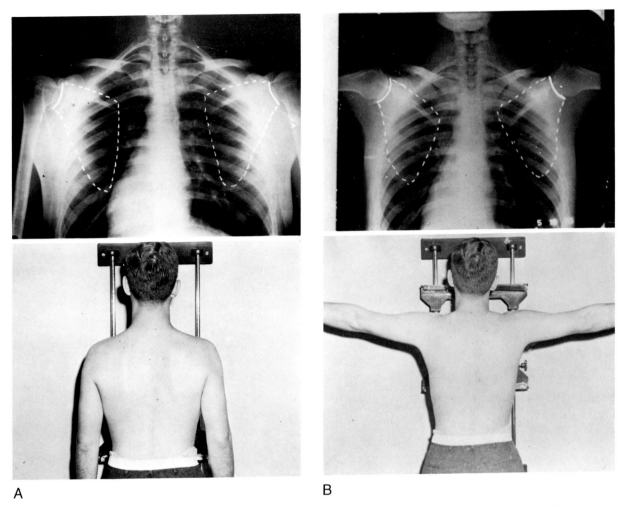

Fig. 6-2. Motions of the scapula. (**A**) In neutral position. (**B**) At 90° abduction the scapula has moved very little and remains in an impingement position. (*Figure continues.*)

der is at 90° of abduction (Fig. 6-1B), where the scapula has not rotated sufficiently to free the rotator cuff of the overhanging acromium and coracoacromial ligament. Another vulnerable position producing impingement is in adduction causing impingement against the coracoid process (Fig. 6-1C). Forward flexion of the arm, in pronation, will also jam the greater tuberosity up under the acromion, the coracoacromial ligament, and, at times, the coracoid process. However, if the arm is raised in supination, the greater tuberosity is turned away from the acromial arch, and the arm can be elevated without impingement.

I advise my colleagues to "supinate, don't operate." Were it not for the movable base of the rotating scapula, the rotator cuff would deteriorate very quickly (Fig. 6-2). We note that at 90° the scapula has moved very little (6-2B). This is the "impingement" position with the humeral head tight up under the acromial arch. With further elevation, the scapula and acromion roll away, freeing the humeral head and rotator cuff. The glenoid moves under the humeral head in a position of stability. In fact, the glenoid follows the humeral head, like a seal's nose under a ball (6-2D).

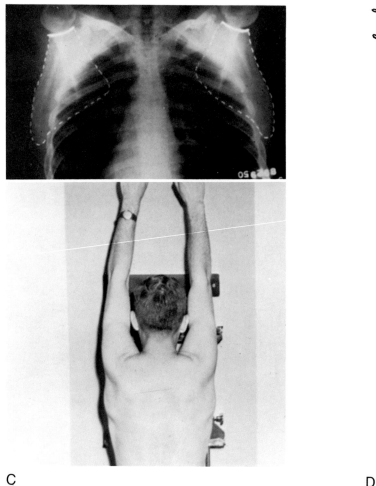

C

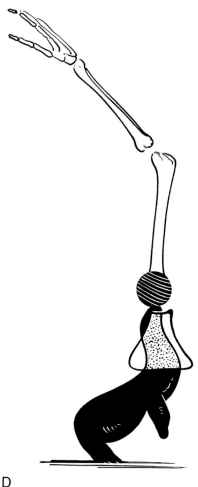

D

Fig. 6-2 *(Continued)*. **(C)** In full elevation the scapula rotates along the chest wall, thus eliminating the impingement of the acromion. The glenoid positions itself rhythmically under the humeral head for stability. **(D)** The glenoid fossa, like a seal with a ball on its nose, adjusts to the optimal position for the humeral head. The body should move with every shoulder motion, thus eliminating strain on the shoulder. (Figs. A–D from Rowe CR: Ruptures of the rotator cuff—selection of cases for conservative treatment. Surgery of the shoulder region. Surg Clin North Am 43:1531, 1963. Reprinted with permission from WB Saunders.)

Avoiding Impingement of the Shoulder

1. Keep the hands in front of the body.
2. When reaching upward, keep the elbow below the hands: avoid the "flying elbow" as frequently seen when polishing a car, washing a window, or working on an assembly line. If one drops the elbow and faces the object, strain and impingement are removed from the shoulder. Raising the arm in forward flexion and supination uses the short head of biceps and coracobrachialis muscles rather than the rotator cuff for elevation, (Fig. 6-3A, B).
3. Incorporate a body turn in every shoulder motion or when reaching. This relieves substantial strain from the shoulder.
4. Avoid "strengthening" exercises when strapped in the sitting position with forceful horizontal exercises at 90° of abduction, so frequently seen in health clubs. In this position, the scapula and the body are fixed, and the humeral head and rotator

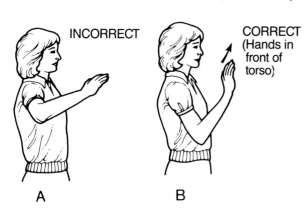

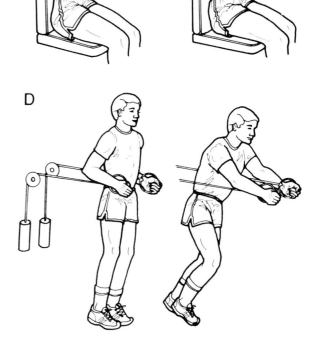

Fig. 6-3. (**A**) Avoid the "flying elbow" in use of the shoulder. In this position, the arm is at 90° and the head is impinged under the acromial arch. (**B**) Correct use of arm: keep elbows below the hands; avoid 90° impingement position; keep hands in front of body; use body turn with each shoulder motion. This lessens strain on the shoulder. (**C**) Forceful exercises with arms at 90° of abduction, in sitting position, uses the shoulder in the impinging position. The scapula has not rotated. The head grinds under the acromial arch. (**D**) Strengthening exercises may be done best standing with rhythmic body and leg motions. The elbows are down and the scapula is mobile. Impingement of shoulder is lessened.

cuff grind under the acromial arch producing hypertrophy of the subacromial bursa and attritional damage to the cuff tendons (Fig. 6-3C).

5. All strengthening exercises for the shoulder should be done standing with free scapula and body motion. Wall weights with free body and shoulder motion are more physiologic. Every tennis or golf pro will tell you that shoulder motion starts in the legs, with a body turn. This is lost in the sitting position; the same applies to "push-ups." The scapula is "locked" and free motion of the shoulder is eliminated (Fig. 6-3D).

Bony Impingement

1. Subacromial spurs may impinge on the rotator cuff (Fig. 6-4A, B).
2. Acromioclavicular joint enlargement may also produce impingement (Fig. 6-4C).

3. An enlarged coracoid process may impinge against the lesser tuberosity of the humeral head.

Primary Pathology

Primary pathologic abnormalities of the subacromial bursa may include rheumatoid arthritis, gout, pseudogout, tuberculosis, or synovial chondromatosis (see Chap. 14). Idiopathic adhesive capsulitis (frozen shoulder) is considered a primary capsular problem, but can secondarily involve the subacromial bursa with chronic adhesions.

Anatomical Abnormalities

In approximately 1 percent of shoulders the tendon of the pectoralis minor, instead of inserting on the coracoid process, passes over the process and inserts

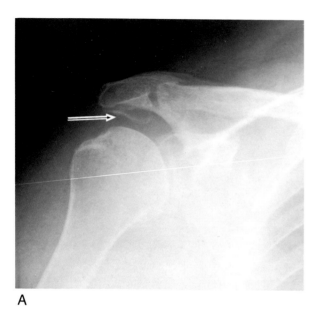

A

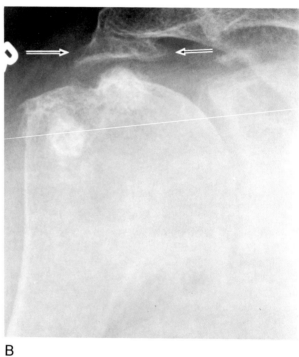

B

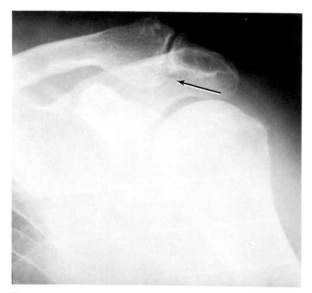

C

Fig. 6-4. (**A,B**) Subacromial spurs may also produce impingement and traumatize the rotator cuff (arrows). (**C**) An enlarged acromioclavicular joint may impinge on the rotator cuff (arrows).

onto the coracohumeral ligament and lesser tuberosity (as it does in the monkey) (see Chap. 22 and Fig. 6-1). A painful bursa may develop between the tendon and the coracoid process.

DIAGNOSIS

History

The majority of subacromial syndromes are due to disuse or poor mechnical use of the arm and shoulder. Specific information should be sought about the mechanical use of the patient's arm in his or her occupation, sports, or hobbies. Obtaining this information may prove difficult at times, as patients may not relate routine exercises or the occupational use of their arm to their pain. The hairdresser may not associate the elevation of the arms during a day's work, the musician to the abducted arm in long practice periods, the athlete to strengthening upper body exercises.

Although attention should be primarily on the shoulder area, do not become too concentrated on the shoulder per se. Consideration should be given to other areas of the body that may refer pain to the shoulder area, such as the cervical spine, the thoracic outlet, the lung, or the cardiovascular system.

Physical Examination

It is most important to have patients demonstrate the localization of the pain and the position of the shoulder that initiates or aggravates the pain, or which they tend to avoid. Both shoulders should be exposed for comparison. Rotation of the arm and shoulder at 90° of abduction, or forward flexion of the arm in pronation indicates subacromial impingement. Rotating the arm in adduction suggests impingements of the coracoid process. Degenerative cysts of the acromioclavicular joint may mimic subacromial impingement (see Fig. 22-7C, D). Tests for instability of the shoulder should be carried out also, because transient subluxation may mimic an impingement syndrome. A limited neurologic and vascular check of the extremity should be carried out.

Radiograph

In all patients with chronic shoulder pain, one anteroposterior view should be taken on a large film with the shoulder in neutral position including the entire humeral shaft, the lung field, the diaphragm, the shoulder girdle, and the lower cervical spine (Fig. 6-5). On a number of occasions, we have noted pathologic conditions in the lungs or humerus that would have been missed on a routine small or medium-sized film of the shoulder (Fig. 6-6). Additional films may be taken on a medium-sized film, with the shoulder in internal rotation (60°) and external rotation (60°). These views may reveal pathologic conditions that are not evident in the neutral position.

With patients who have *unrelieved* subacromial pain, one should always take a true axillary view. At

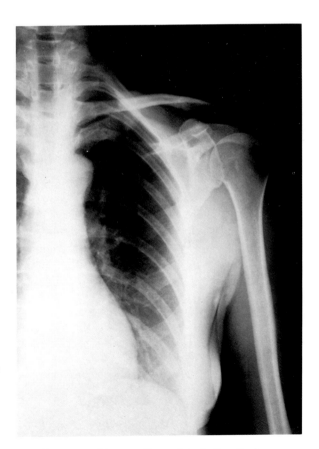

Fig.6-5. An initial large radiograph including the lower cervical spine, lung field, diaphragm, shoulder girdle, and humeral shaft is indicated in chronic pain syndromes.

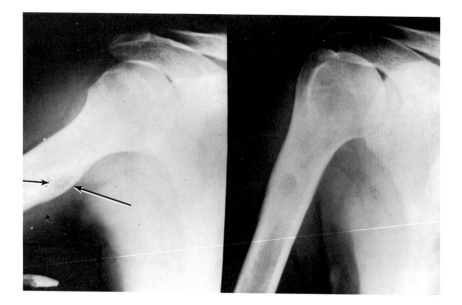

Fig. 6-6. This ostoid osteoma was missed initially on a small film of the shoulder joint. The patient had had unrelieved pain for over a year.

one time or another, the "frozen shoulder," the "chronic impingement," or "bicipital tendinitis" being treated, may turn out to be an unrecognized chronic posterior dislocation of the shoulder (Chapter 7—Posterior Dislocations).

Differential Diagnosis

It is important to remember with every patient who presents with shoulder pain that the source of the pain may be subacromial, subcoracoid, glenohumeral, bony, neurologic, circulatory, or referred to the shoulder from other sources, such as the cervical spine, lung, heart, or diaphragm. Once the cause is localized, steps to reproduce the pain, or relieve the pain are helpful.

If the subacromial or subcoracoid space is implicated, an injection of Novocain into the space, or into the acromioclavicular joint, will aid in localizing the source of pain. Injecting the attachment of the levator tendon to the scapula may prove helpful. If Novocain gives relief, this may be followed by one corticosteroid injection.

In instances in which the pain can not be relieved, we frequently give the patient a "road test," requesting that they reproduce or aggravate their pain syndrome. This information is helpful.

Further investigative study, EMG, and specific laboratory testing, is needed in unsolved instances such as bone scan, computed tomography.

TREATMENT

Conservative Treatment

A common fault in treating tendinitis, bursal hypertrophy, or impingement of the rotator cuff is to begin with treating the patient's symptoms, rather than first indentifying the initiating cause. Before one begins the rituals of anti-inflammatory drugs, injections, physical therapy, and pain medications, first identify and eliminate the specific cause of the irritated or abused rotator cuff. Relieving the symptoms, without eliminating the cause, invites recurrence of symptoms, and a disappointed patient.

The following three patients are typical of occupational causes.

Patient A (Fig. 6-7) had experienced chronic pain in her shoulders in spite of a long course of unrelieving conservative treatment. She was short of stature, necessitating elevation of her arms when operating an adding machine. Without further investigation, we had her chair raised, moved her closer to the

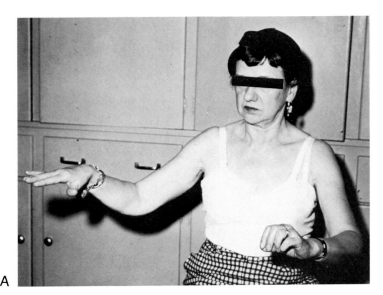

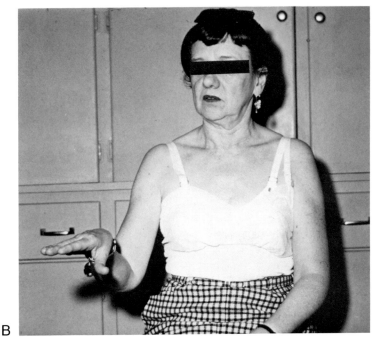

Fig. 6-7. (**A**) This patient had unrelieved pain and fatigue in running her computer with her arms suspended. (**B**) By raising her chair, moving closer to the keyboard, and dropping her elbow, her subacromial discomfort was relieved. No further treatment was necessary. (Rowe CR: Ruptures of the rotator cuff—Selection of cases for conservative treatment. Surgery of the shoulder region. Surg Clin North Am 43:1531, 1963. Reprinted with permission from WB Saunders.)

operating panel, and told her to "drop her elbows," thus relieving her shoulder of her suspended arms. This gave her complete and lasting relief of her pain. This was 20 years ago. She continues working pain-free. Her "treatment" consisted of eliminating the mechanical cause of her shoulder pain, rather than treating her symptoms and ignoring the specific cause.

Patient B (Fig. 6-8), a short-statured hairdresser, began to experience chronic pain and a fatigue of his shoulders at work to a point of disability. He had not responded to the usual routines of suppressive treatment and physical therapy. Our instruction was simply to keep his hands at the same level, but *lower* his elbows. This eliminated the impingement of the rotator cuff under the acromial arch at 90° of abduc-

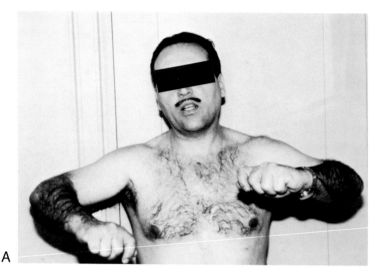

A

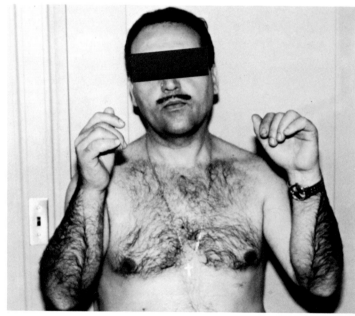

B

Fig. 6-8. (A) This short-statured hair dresser demonstrates the "flying" position of his elbows at work. Because of chronic pain in his shoulders, he was unable to work. **(B)** He was instructed to "drop" his elbows. After a week he was amazed that he no longer felt pain. "Why didn't I think of this?" He was no longer impinging his rotator cuff and bursa by the position of this arms.

tion, and the fatigue of suspending his arms while dressing his customers' hair. After a week, he exclaimed "Why didn't I think of this, I no longer have pain!" He continues busy, pain-free, and happy, without physical therapy, injections, or medications.

A 26-year-old cellist was seen because of fatigue and shoulder discomfort after long hours of practicing. We asked her to demonstrate the position of her arms when playing. Obviously, she was elevating her elbows too high while playing, a common source of

fatigue. We instructed her to lower her elbows, but keep her hands at the same level. Lowering the end-peg of the cello may also be helpful. Relaxing pendulum exercises were also advised during her rest periods. The fatigue in her arms and shoulder disappeared. She now practices and plays without the "nagging" discomfort of her shoulders and fatigue of her arms. I notice that Isaac Stern, the violinist, avoids elevating his elbows when playing. Rather, he keeps his elbows down and moves his body, to avoid the fatigue of sustained elevation of his arm. He has learned the secret, and continues playing professionally. With his economy of motion, he may play forever!

In sports, the side-arm jerky pitcher in baseball, as a rule, does not last as long at top performance as the rhythmic overhand pitcher such as Warren Spahn, Walter Johnson, or Jim Palmer. The side-arm pitcher delivers with his scapula fixed at 90°, thus grinding the rotator cuff under the acromion, whereas the overhand pitcher's scapula moves freely and adjusts to the position of the humeral head. We stress again that all forceful shoulder motions in throwing, serving in tennis, and pitching should be a part of a rhythmic free body motion. "Begin your stroke in your legs" is good advice. In so doing, the strain is eliminated in the shoulder and elbow, and the delivery is smoother and more accurate. When a pitcher begins "guiding" the ball, he tightens the shoulder muscles in his delivery. His shoulder problem begins and he loads the bases; the golfer slices; and the tennis player nets the ball.

Thus, in sports as well as in one's occupation, repeated attritional abuse of the rotator cuff can be eliminated first by analyzing and correcting the mechanical cause, rather than by treating the symptoms alone. Too often a patient whose shoulder problem was caused by repetitive overuse of the shoulder is sent to physical therapy, where routine "strengthening" exercises merely perpetuate the assault on the rotator cuff. Rather than benefitting, the patient complains "I hurt more after therapy, than I did before." The patient is correct. Exercises must be specific.

However, when pain and disability persist despite a careful search for and correction of mechanical factors, further investigation and treatment are indicated. Sources of referred pain must be ruled out (see Chap. 4). Bone scans are indicated to identify possible metastatic disease.

Complications of Shoulder Injections

The indications for corticosteroid injections of the subacromial space should be very specific (see below for injection technique).

A single injection may be diagnostic. If relief is

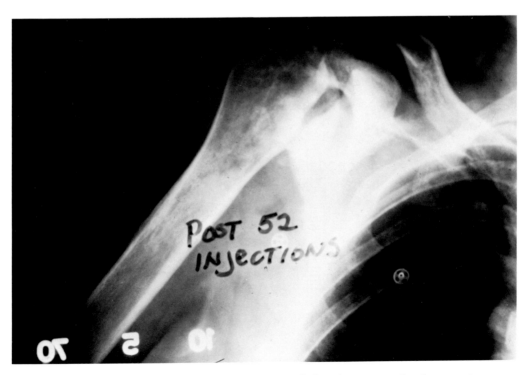

Fig. 6-9. Severe osteonecrosis of the humeral head after 52 injections for chronic pain.

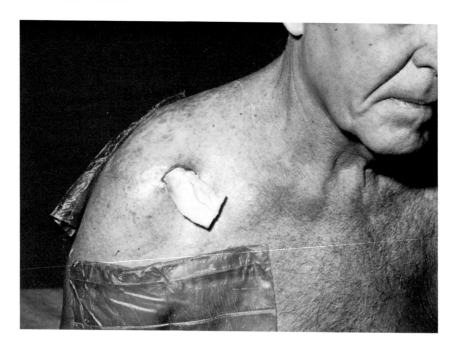

Fig. 6-10. Sepsis of the shoulder following 22 injections for "chronic bursitis."

obtained, the source of the pain is most likely a reactive bursa or subacromial problem. If relief is not obtained, the problem would be expected to be elsewhere. Injections should not be repeated often in an effort to subdue the problem. This may prove harmful to the shoulder and a disaster to the patient (Fig. 6-9). Repeated injections may also invite infection (Fig. 6-10). The effect of corticosteroid solutions on tendon and cartilage should be appreciated by every orthopaedist. A not uncommon complication

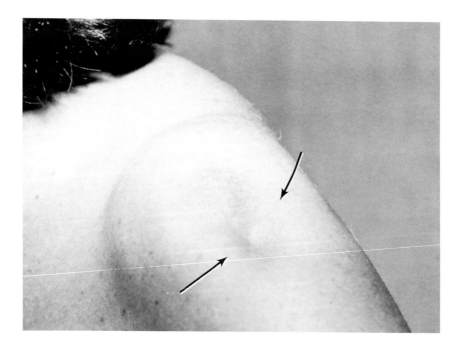

Fig. 6-11. Absorption of the subcutaneous fat and skin pigment may occur when the corticosteroid solution is injected subcutaneously.

is the absorption of subcutaneous fat and skin pigment when the corticosteroid solution is mixed with the Novocain (Fig. 6-11).

Surgical Procedures

Chronic unrelieved impingement of the subacromial space has been a subject of much concern among practitioners interested in shoulder problems over the past 15 years.

In 1972, Neer[13–15] brought this to the attention of orthopaedic surgeons by standardizing the surgical approach and emphasizing the principle of "decompression" of the subacromial space and giving the rotator cuff additional room in which to function. This is accomplished by one of the following procedures.

RESECTION OF THE CORACOACROMIAL LIGAMENT

This procedure is usually incomplete, although it has its limited indications.

ACROMIOCLAVICULAR ARTHROPLASTY

In an acromioclavicular arthroplasty (Fig. 6-12) the coracoacromial ligament is resected (it seems better to remove the entire ligament than merely to divide it), a partial anterior acromioplasty is performed, and any subacromial bony spurs are removed. The hypertrophied subacromial bursal tissue is also resected, and the rotator cuff repaired if damaged. The distal 1 cm of the clavicle is removed when additional exposure is needed or when there are degenerative changes of the acromioclavicular joint. The deltoid muscle is split for 4 cm for these procedures.

CAUTION IN REMOVING DISTAL CLAVICLE

When the acromioclavicular joint is damaged, the outer 1 cm of the clavicle is removed. Too often, too much clavicle is removed (Fig. 6-13). Seldom is it necessary to remove more than 1 cm of bone. Care should be taken to preserve the osteoperiosteal sleeve of the clavicle for closure, and to remove all capsule and bony irregularities, particularly inferiorly. Spurs may develop if these are not removed. It is important also to rongeur off the superior edge of the clavicle to ensure a smooth upper surface. The arm should be carried through a complete range of motion at

surgery to ensure that there is no contact between the end of the clavicle and the acromion. If more space is needed, a small portion of the medial surface of the acromion is removed, rather than more clavicle.

OSTEOTOMY

Gerber,[7] and more recently Warren,[18] recommend, in addition to routine acromioclavicular arthroplasty, resection of the tip or osteotomy of the coracoid.

Surgeons differ in their approach to the subacromial space (see Chap. 3) but the majority use an anterior approach with a muscle release of the deltoid from the outer clavicle and anterior acromion, and a limited splitting of anterior deltoid muscle. Leffert (personal communication) recommends approaching the subacromial space through the deltopectoral interval and Kessel by osteotoming the acromion from a superior approach[9] (Chap. 3).

ACROMIONECTOMY

There is general agreement among orthopaedic surgeons that total acromionectomy should not be performed except for tumor or osteomyelitis, due to the risk of the deltoid muscle pulling off and gliding down the arm (Fig. 6-14). This is a disturbing cosmetic and functional complication that will occur if the deltoid is removed without adequate attachment. Although the indications for acromionectomy are few, it is important to point out that it can be accomplished with much less cosmetic and functional defects by the following technique.

Allow the deltoid muscle to remain attached to the lateral rim of the acromion by osteotomy of a ¼ inch of acromion. This remains as a handle to the deltoid (see Chap. 3). Following the partial or total acromionectomy, the rim of acromion with the attached deltoid is reattached to the scapula and clavicle by holes drilled through the bone. This lessens the tendency of the deltoid to glide down the arm. Although the power of the deltoid may be weakened to some extent by the altered length–tension relationship of the muscle, it does not become avulsed and glide down the arm. Adequate time must be given, however, for union of the osteotomy.

Although Bosley[2] does not follow the above technique, his careful dissection of the osteoperiosteal layers from the acromion, which are double-breasted with the deltoid in a four-flap technique, has, in his

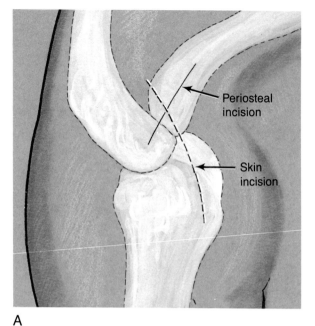

A

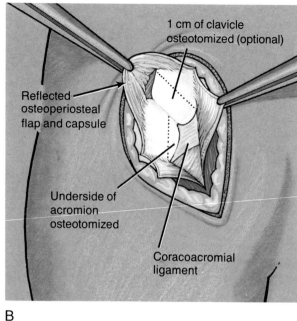

B

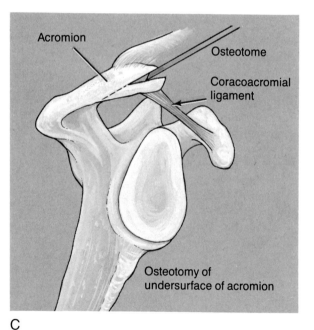

C

Fig. 6-12. Technique of acromioclavicular arthroplasty. (**A**) Through an anterior deltoid splitting incision, the leading edge of the acromion and the distal centimeter of the clavicle are exposed by turning down osteoperiosteal flaps. (**B**) The leading edge of the acromion is removed. Removal of the distal centimeter of the clavicle is optimal (for more exposure). (**C**) Osteotomy of the leading edge and undersurface of the acromion. (*Figure continues.*)

hands, been successful. He has carried out this technique on 30 patients with total acromionectomies with surprisingly good results. Hammond[8] has published a follow-up study of 65 total acromionectomies in 1971, in which 51 percent had no deformity after acromionectomy, 48 percent mild deformity, and 1

percent a moderate deformity. The objective results were excellent in 50, good in 18, fair in 4, and poor in 1. In a review of 30 acromionectomies ("performed elsewhere"), Neer[13] reports that 27 patients complained of persistent pain, "most of the patients complained of the appearance of their shoulder," and

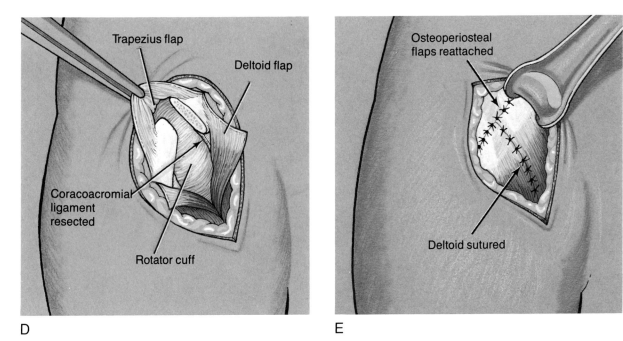

D   E

Fig. 6-12 *(Continued)*. **(D)** The coracoacromial ligament and hypertrophied bursal tissue are removed, giving good exposure of the rotator cuff. Any rotator cuff tears are repaired. **(E)** The deltoid and osteoperiosteal flaps are reattached.

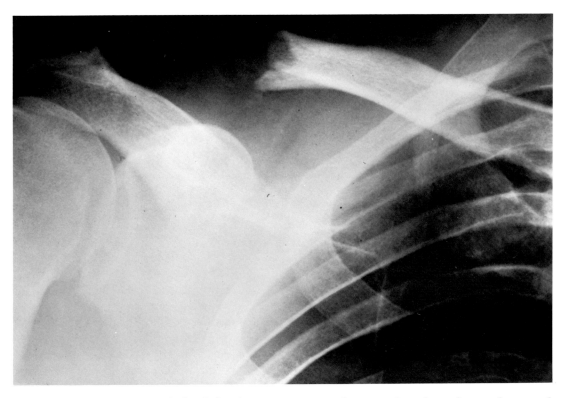

Fig. 6-13. Removal of too much distal clavicle is unnecessary and may result in discomfort, weakness, and a disturbing cosmetic result.

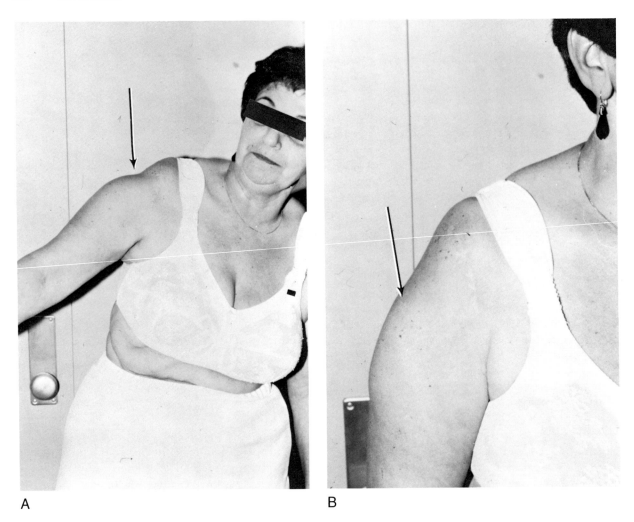

A   B

Fig. 6-14. Complication of total acromionectomy. (**A**) Note the pull-off of the deltoid muscle down the arm. (**B**) With weak abduction, this complication could be avoided if a section of acromion had been left attached to the deltoid muscle for reattachment.

manual muscle-testing showed "marked weakness in all shoulders." Serious postoperative wound complications "occurred in 8 of the 30 patients." Thus this is a surgical procedure not to be taken lightly or without study. The majority of orthopaedic surgeons avoid total acromionectomies. A minority have acceptable results following their specific techniques. While some approaches are adequate without removing the acromion, it would seem wise to avoid total acromionectomy unless there are strong indications for its use.

Summary

The success of acromioclavicular arthroplasties will depend on the accuracy of diagnosis and the proficiency of the technique. One must be certain that an impingement does, in fact, exist. Unfortunately, acromioclavicular arthroplasty has been mistakenly performed as treatment for other problems, such as transient subluxation of the shoulder, adhesive capsulitis, or thoracic outlet syndrome. As with many of the problems of the shoulder, one condition may mimic the other. Great care must be taken with accurate evaluation, and conservative treatment prior to deciding upon surgery. It is a mistake to resort to surgery, when correction of the shoulder's misuse may eliminate the patient's problem. Performing an acromioclavicular arthroplasty will not relieve the patient whose pain is due to chronic unresolved periarticular adhesions. In fact, this may make the patient worse by prolonging immobilization of the shoulder. This condition should be ruled out before surgery. Another cause of an unsuccessful procedure is technical, such as removing too much acromion or too much clavicle. Both of these are unnecessary, and may cause weakness of the shoulder as well as continued pain.

For better shoulders that may last longer and function with less strain and with greater efficiency, we emphasize again:

Keep the hands in front of the body.
Keep the elbows below the hands when reaching upward (avoid the "flying elbow").
Turn the body, with all shoulder motions, thus lessening strain on the shoulder.
Avoid strenuous repetitive exercises at 90° of abduction.

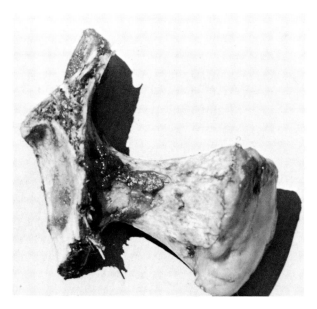

Fig. 6-15. A large osteochondroma removed from the undersurface of the scapula. On examination, there was a palpable thud on elevation of the arm, and a persistent mild degree of winging of the scapula.

"SNAPPING" OR "GRINDING" SCAPULA

A very bothersome and exhausting syndrome is the chronic "snapping" shoulder. This has also been identified by Codman.[4] These may be classified into two groups: those due to mechanical causes and those due to muscular tension.

Mechanical Causes

These may result from a large or small osteochondroma of the undersurface of the scapula, which is usually identified by oblique or profile views of the scapula. The large osteochondroma in Figure 6-15 caused a visible and palpable "thud" of the scapula when the arm was raised. It also produced a mild prominence of the scapula. Figure 6-16 shows a mass

of firm fibrous tissue removed from the lower angle of the scapula in a contact-sport athlete. This had produced a painful snapping of the rhythmic motion of his arm, and was evidently due to repeated trauma of the angle of the scapula. Irregularities of the rib cage secondary to malunited rib fractures, gunshot wounds, or chest surgery may also be a cause of irregularities of scapular motion.

Muscular Tension

A more common cause of snapping scapula is excessive tightening of the scapulothoracic muscles by the patient when initiating elevation of the arm. This may originate as protection against discomfort of the shoulder following an injury, or to an intentional muscular blocking of the rhythmic motion of the shoulder. One will note that as the patient begins to raise the arm, he first tightens the scapular muscles; thus, he "scrapes" or grinds the scapula along the rib cage. If repeated, this will produce irritation of the gliding surface of the scapula and bursal thickening. It is helpful to tell the patient when raising the arm "to leave the shoulder muscles out of it," and think only

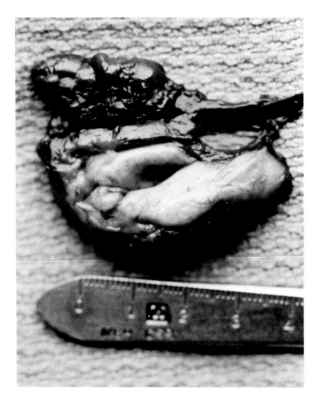

Fig. 6-16. A localized mass of thick fibrous bursal tissue removed from the gliding surface of the lower angle of the scapula, which had produced a painful snapping of the scapula.

of the hand moving: the shoulder muscles will perform better if not tightened. I compare this to "taking off the brakes, before stepping on the gas—otherwise you scrape your tires." Unfortunately, many of these patients have been sent to physical therapy for "strengthening exercises" which merely add to their problem rather than bringing relief. It is important to analyze the patient's problem carefully before prescribing treatment. The scapula could be lifted and the undersurface examined with an arthroscope to identify the presence or absence of bursal tissue or cartilaginous irregularities, if these are suspected.

A few of these patients are similar to voluntary dislocators and continue to "drag" their scapula along their rib cage, due to unidentified emotional or personality problems. The surgeon should be extremely careful to avoid surgery on these patients; one may find that not only have you not helped the patient, you have made the patient worse. Patients who can

voluntarily wing their scapula may also complain of a "snapping" shoulder (Chap. 22).

CALCIFIC TENDINITIS

Calcific deposits (amorphous calcium phosphate, oxalate, carbonate, or calcium hydroxyapatite) may occur in any tendon of the body, usually at its attachment. As well as at the shoulder, they have occurred in the tendons of the hand, wrist, elbow, knee, ankle, and, at times, the origin of the biceps femoris tendon at the ischial tuberosity of the pelvis. The shoulder, however, is the most common site. This is perhaps due to the stretching of the tendon over the humeral head, with repeated stress–trauma of the tendon under the acromial arch. It is interesting that calcific deposits are seldom seen before age 25 or after age 60. Eventually, all deposits absorb or disappear. The most common location in the shoulder is in the supraspinatus tendon as single deposits (Fig. 6-17A) or as multiple foci (Fig. 6-17B). The next most common locations are the infraspinatus, the teres minor, and, occasionally, in the subscapularis tendon (Fig. 6-17C). Rarely, they can be seen in the triceps tendon. Bosworth[3] reported that of 6,061 unselected employees of the Metropolitan Insurance Company in 1941, 2.7 percent were found to have calcific deposits in the shoulder. These were more frequently found in men than women. The supraspinatus tendon was the location in 51.5 percent.

Pathologic Characteristics

Codman[4] gives a detailed and extensive study of calcific deposits in the tendons of the shoulder. He stresses an important point: the deposits are in the tendon of the musculotendinous cuff and not in the bursa, although, at times, the calcific material may burst into the bursa during an acute attack. His study revealed that calcific material may consist of calcium phosphate, calcium oxalate, and, to a lesser degree, calcium carbonate localized in an area of hyalin tendon degeneration. Bateman[1] observed that the calcific deposits were usually in the tendon attachment, in a

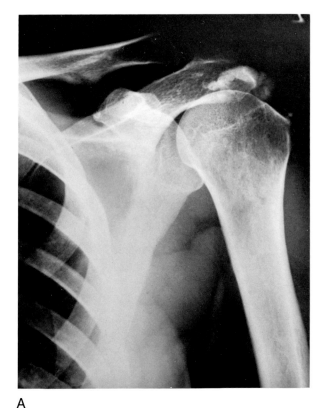

A

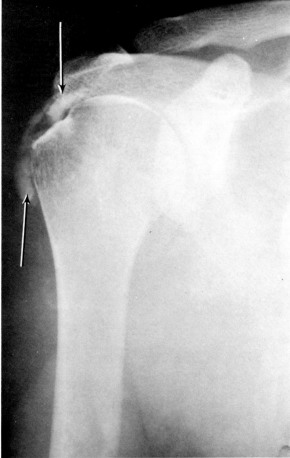

B

C

Fig. 6-17. (A) The most common site of calcific deposits in the shoulder is the supraspinatus tendon. The deposit may be a single foci, or **(B)** multiple foci deposits. **(C)** Occasionally, a deposit may occur in the subscapularis tendon.

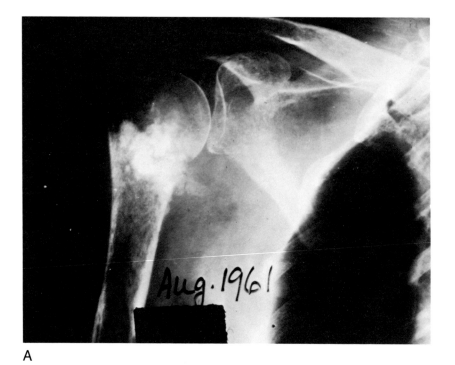

A

Fig. 6-18. (**A**) Calcific deposits in malignant tumors may mimic calcific tendinitis. (**B**) Appearance 1 month later.

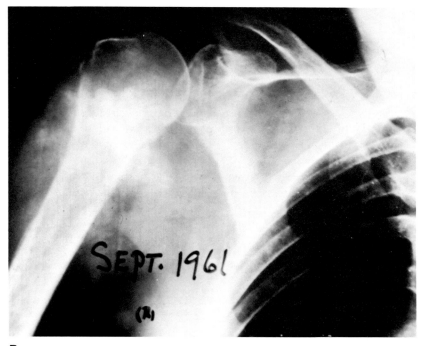

B

relatively avascular area, a "zone of stress," or the "critical zone." It was his opinion that "abnormal aging of the collagen fibers initiated the calcification mechanism." Moseley,[11,12] on the other hand, stated that "at operation, I have always noted that the tendon was well vascularized around the area of deposit and therefore, disagree with the idea that the calcium salts were precipitated in an area of previous disease with resultant ischemia." It may be fair to say that both investigators were right. Bateman was describing chronic calcific deposits, and Moseley the acute reactive calcific phase. More recent investigation of the pathology of calcific deposits in the tendons of the body is reported by Resnick and Resnick[16] with the use of polarizing microscopy. They point out that McCarty and Gatter[10] first implicated calcium hydroxyapatite. Their studies suggest still another theory of periarticular calcific formation: a metabolic rather than a local degenerative process may be the cause; the majority of patients with calcific lesions may indeed have calcium hydroxyapatite deposition disease.

Physical Characteristics

Clinically, calcific deposits may appear in one of three forms.

1. *Dry, Powdery Deposit*
   This is the chronic quiescent form.
2. *Soft, Putty-, or Toothpaste-like Deposit*
   This may produce a chronic discomfort that is painful when impinged under the acromion as the arm is abducted.
3. *Milky or Creamy Collection*
   This is usually under pressure and constitutes the acute, very painful phase. The deposit is surrounded by inflammation and an acute synovitis, with the appearance of an acute boil. As the material is released at surgery, the resident frequently asks whether the material should be "cultured" since its appearance is that of pus (see Fig. 6-20B).

Clinical Course

SILENT PHASE

Calcific deposits may remain as a painless accumulation for years and eventually become absorbed. Seldom is calcium seen in the shoulder in patients after 60 years of age or before 30 years of age. On the other hand, the deposit may slowly enlarge as a single deposit or in multiple foci in the tendon.

IMPINGEMENT PHASE

When the calcium deposit enlarges to the degree that it impinges under the acromial arch, it becomes painful on abduction or with forceful use of the arm in elevation and rotation. Discomfort can usually be controlled by avoiding impingement of the tendon or excessive use of the arm in abduction.

ACUTE OR RECURRENT PHASE

For some unknown reason, the chronic phase may suddenly burst into an acute, excruciatingly painful phase. This may occur at the most inopportune time, such as when one has just landed in Paris for a 2-week vacation, or 2 days before the marriage of one's favorite daughter. Patients who have experienced other painful conditions, such as an acute gallbladder attack, acute pancreatitis, or childbirth, say that the pain of an acute calcific tendinitis of the shoulder is the worst. Its clinical appearance resembles an acute infection. The shoulder is inflamed, hot, and extremely tender to lightest touch or motion. The patient enters the office holding the arm and wanting immediate help, preferably relief.

Differential Diagnosis

Although calcific deposits in the rotator cuff are seldom misdiagnosed, this may occur in rather embarrassing situations. In one of our patients, the "calcific mass," when exposed at surgery, turned out to be a piece of avulsed greater tuberosity. The symptoms and radiographic appearance were that of a chronic calcific deposit. Fortunately, the patient was relieved and happy. In other instances, early malignant tumors may have calcific foci that may be misinterpreted for calcific tendinitis (tumoral calcinosis) (Fig. 6-18). One should also be mindful of other conditions that may produce periarticular calcification, such as gout, hypervitaminosis D, hyperparathyroidism, renal osteodystrophy, collagen vascular disease, and pyrophosphate dehydrate crystals ("pseudogout").

Treatment

For the acute phase, the application of an ice cap every 2 hours plus codeine, with the arm supported in a sling, may bring some degree of relief. The pain may subside in 48 to 72 hours. Heat should not be applied at this stage; it will increase the pain. The calcific mass may rupture into the subacromial bursa with relief, or remain in the tendon and be gradually

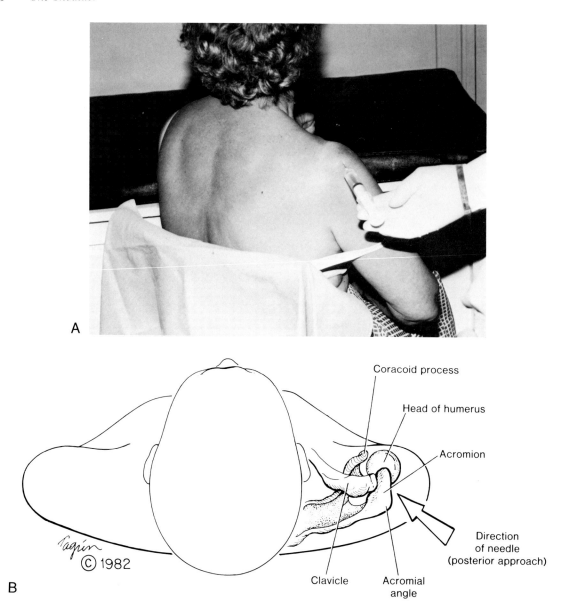

Fig. 6-19. Technique of injection into subacromial space. The injection should be made into the bursal space and *not* into the tendon. (**A**) The bursal space opens with the patient sitting with the arms relaxed in lap. The needle is inserted under the lateral posterior aspect of the acromion into the subacromial space. There is ample bursal space from this approach. (**B**) The needle will escape the tendon from this position. (*Figure continues.*)

absorbed. On the other hand, it may subside, only to strike again later with increased vigor.

A subacromial injection may be given initially for very severe pain. We do not recommend repeating the injections more than once or twice. Because the shoulder is quite painful, injecting over the painful area or in the anterior aspect of the shoulder, where there is so little space between the tendon and the coracoacromial ligament, may be extremely uncomfortable. We recommend the following technique.

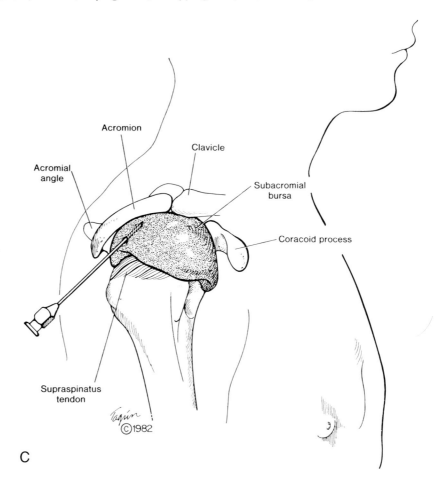

Acromion

Acromial
angle

Clavicle

Subacromial
bursa

Coracoid process

Supraspinatus
tendon

©1982

C

Fig. 6-19 (*Continued*). (**C**) This is much less painful than injecting anteriorly, where the bursal space is tight over the humeral head. (Wilkins EW, Jr: MGH Textbook of Emergency Medicine. 2nd Ed. p. 953. © 1983 The Williams & Wilkins Co., Baltimore.)

An effective and relatively painless method of injection is to have the patient sit in a chair, with the arm relaxed and hand in the lap (Fig. 6-19A). The shoulder is prepared with sterile technique; use sterile gloves and sterile technique in every respect. Care should be taken not to inject the solution into the tendons. The bursa can be entered very easily from the posterolateral aspect of the acromion, and without pain, where there is more space between the rotator cuff and acromial arch (Fig. 6-19B,C). Anteriorly the bursal space is limited and injections may go into the tendon instead of the bursa. We have found that it is not necessary to puncture the calcific deposits to obtain relief. Attempts to do this under local anesthesia, especially in one's office, may cause severe pain and produce a very unhappy patient. Entering the subacromial space without puncturing the calcific deposit has given satisfactory relief in our hands. Also, we do not recommend mixing the corti-

costeroid solution with the Novocain. Instead, the #22 needle with Novocain alone is first inserted under the acromion and the proper position of the needle determined. The syringe is then removed leaving the needle in situ, and 1 or 2 ml corticostertoid solution is drawn into the syringe. This is then inserted slowly through the in situ needle, to prevent injection into the tissues. This can be followed with another small amount of Novocain. Mixing the Novocain and steroid solution may cause an embarrassing complication of local atrophy of the subcutaneous fat, and loss of skin pigment (Fig. 6-11). Read the small print on the instructions that come with the corticosteroid solution; this complication is explained there in detail.

CHRONIC OR INTERMITTENT STAGE

As stated, the majority of acute attacks subside within 3 or 4 days; however, if the pain becomes chronic or intermittent, an additional injection may

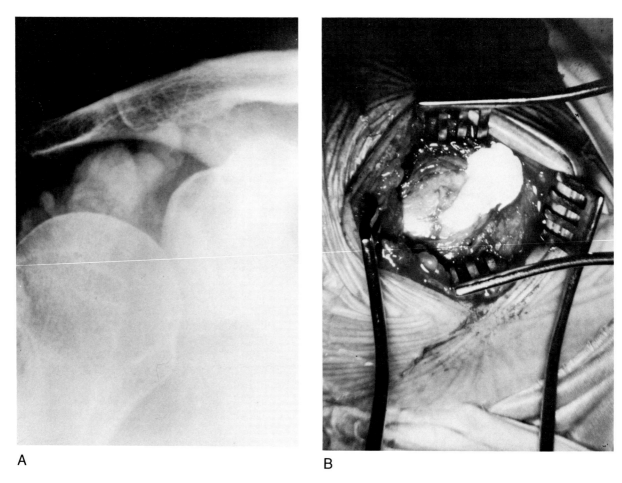

A   B

Fig. 6-20. (A) For a large multilocular calcium deposit, it is best to remove the calcium completely through a strap incision. (B) The calcific deposit is released, and the subacromial space irrigated. Large defects in the rotator cuff that which remain after the calcium is removed should be repaired.

be tried but further repeated injections are not recommended. If the pain continues or recurs, resection of the calcific deposits may be considered.

SURGICAL TECHNIQUE

A 5 cm horizontal strap incision is used over the greater curvature of the humeral head just beyond the edge of the acromion. A vertical skin incision is unsightly, and should be avoided (see Chap. 3). The deltoid muscle is split vertically in the line of its fibers, to expose the bursa and rotator cuff. Two thyroid pole retractors give good exposure. By rotating the arm, all sections of the rotator cuff will come in view through the muscular window. The exposure is ade-

quate to remove the calcium (Fig. 6-20). We recommend repairing the defect in the rotator cuff after removal of the calcium.

When multiple large calcium deposits in the tendon or the bursa have become chronically thickened causing a subacromial impingement, consideration should be given to decompressing the rotator cuff by resecting the coracoacromial ligament. Occasionally, patients who have experienced chronic recurrent attacks of calcific tendinitis over an extended period of time may develop the unfortunate complication of chronic adhesions. It is well to recognize this condition prior to surgical removal of the calcific deposits, and caution the patient that return of shoulder motion and relief of pain may be slow, even after removal of the calcium, due to the adhesions. In time, shoulder motion will return. We have never observed a recurrence of the calcium in the same shoulder if it has been completely removed at surgery.

Summary

Calcific deposits in the tendinous cuff of the shoulder joint may be silent and asymptomatic, or chronically disturbing with subacromial impingement. Occasionally, they may become acutely reactive and extremely painful. Prompt, specific, and relieving treatment is greatly appreciated by the patient. The surgeon, however, should always keep in mind other conditions that may cause calcific deposits in and around joints.

REFERENCES

1. Bateman JE: The Neck and Shoulder, WB Saunders, Philadelphia, 1978
2. Bosley RC: Report on thirty total acromionectomies. Personal communication, Boulder, Colorado
3. Bosworth BM: Calcium deposits in the shoulder and subacromial bursitis. A survey of 12, 122 shoulders. JAMA 116:2477, 1941
4. Codman EA: The Shoulder. RE Kreiger, Malabar, Florida, 1984
5. Codman EA: The anatomy of the subdeltoid bursa and its clinical importance. Boston Med Surg J May: 613, 1906
6. DePalma AF: Surgery of the Shoulder. JB Lippincott, Philadelphia, 1973
7. Gerber C, Terrier F, Ganz R: The role of the coracoid process in the chronic impingement syndrome. J Bone Joint Surg 67B:703, 1945
8. Hammond G: Complete acromionectomy. J Bone Joint Surg 53A:173, 1971
9. Kessel L: Clinical Disorders of the Shoulder. Churchill Livingstone, London, 1982
10. McCarty, DJ, Gatter RA: Recurrent anterior inflammation associated with focal apatite crystal deposition. Arthritis Rheum 9:804, 1966
11. Moseley HF: Surgery of the Shoulder Region. Surg Clin North Am 43:1521, 1963
12. Moseley HF: Shoulder Lesions. E & S Livingstone, Edinburgh and London, 1969
13. Neer CS, Marberry TA: The disadvantages of radial acromionectomy. J Bone Joint Surg 63A:416, 1981
14. Neer CS: Anterior acromioplasty for chronic impingement syndrome in the shoulder. A preliminary report. J Bone Joint Surg 54A:41, 1972
15. Neer CS, Bigliani LU, Hawkins RJ: Rupture of the long head of biceps related to subacromial impingement. Orthop Trans 1:111, 1977
16. Resnick CS, Resnick D: Crystal deposition disease. Semin Arthritis Rheum 2(4):39B, 1983
17. Uhthoff HK, Sakar K, Hammond DI: The subacromial bursa: a clinicopathological study. p. 121. In Bateman, Walsh (eds): Surgery of the Shoulder. CV Mosby, Toronto, 1984
18. Warren RE, Diner DM, Inglis AE, Pavlos H: The carocoid impingement syndrome. Read at Second Meeting of the American Shoulder and Elbow Surgeons, American Academy of Orthopaedic Surgeons, New Orleans, Feb. 19–20, 1986

Tendon Ruptures

Robert D. Leffert
Carter R. Rowe

RUPTURES OF THE ROTATOR CUFF

History

Although Monro[29] in 1788 is credited with calling attention to ruptures of the rotator cuff, and Smith[45] observed them in cadavers in 1834, it was Codman[8–12] who convinced the medical profession that rotator cuff lesions constituted one of the primary causes of shoulder disability. At the beginning of this chapter, we should keep in perspective Codman's reflection: "In fact, in aged people, it is hard to obtain a perfectly normal shoulder joint, just as it is to find a perfectly normal aorta."

Pathologic Findings

There are many factors involved in the process of weakening and ultimate rupture of the rotator cuff. The natural history of rotator cuff lesions is one of attritional changes and eventual deterioration that expose the glenohumeral joint to varying degrees of arthrosis.

The anatomical arrangement of the rotator cuff causes the tendinous attachment to wear and ultimately tear beneath the acromial arch. Every upward motion of the extremity extracts a price from its longevity. Were it not for the protective mechanism of scapular rotation, the rotator cuff would be short-lived. This may be seen in the increase in rotator cuff pathology seen in those who use weight machines for their deltoids in commercial health clubs. The position of resisted horizontal adduction and abduction at 90° of elevation while in the seated position fixes the scapula and allows the rotator cuff to be ground under the acromial arch, which inflicts great trauma to the critical zone of the tendon. Furthermore, patients with trapezius palsy or even marked weakness of the trapezius from disuse may develop secondary subacromial impingement for a similar reason.

The arterial blood supply has been shown to be quite tenuous at the attachment of the supraspinatus to the rotator cuff.[8,39,41] Also, the dependent position of the arm tends to wring out the vessels by traction, thus further reducing the already scant blood supply. The tendon is exposed to direct and indirect trauma, especially in contact sports. Age takes it toll on the tensile strength of the tendon. DePalma[14] found that approximately one in every four subjects from the fifth decade on can be found to have a rupture of the rotator cuff of varying degree. Men were more frequently affected than women, manual laborers more frequently than sedentary workers, and the dominant arm more frequently than the nondominant. The majority of ruptures occur after age 45 due to these mechanical and attritional factors. Yet ruptures can occur in active, young, healthy athletes. We have had to repair ruptured rotator cuffs in professional hockey players in their late 20s and early 30s. Ruptures may also result from systemic diseases such as rheumatoid arthritis, gout, and neurotrophic joints. The ruptures may be iatrogenic, as in the case of repeated steroid injections into the rotator cuff, which cause degenerative changes in the tissue collagen with resultant tendon necrosis and subsequent rupture.

Developmental defects, such as nonunion or lack of fusion of one of the three epiphyseal centers of the acromion may predispose to impingement and thus rupture of the rotator cuff, as pointed out by Neer[31] and Mudge.[30]

Glenohumeral instability with anterior subluxation may cause subacromial impingement. Often the clinical picture may be difficult to define. If only the impingement is recognized and treated, the patient continues to be symptomatic because of the instability. Finally, in the patients whom Rowe and Zarins described with anterior subluxation (so-called dead arm syndrome), there was a surprisingly high incidence of enlargement of the seam between the supraspinatus and subscapularis out over the humeral head accompanying the glenohumeral instability. This combination can be a factor in the difficult anatomic problem involved in restoration of the stability of the joint.

Classification

Although rotator cuff ruptures may be grouped as complete and incomplete, acute or chronic, degenerative or traumatic, their patterns are quite consistent.

GRADE IA: TRANSVERSE OR HORIZONTAL TEARS

These occur horizontally across the insertion of the tendon to the tuberosity (Fig. 6-21A). Usually the supraspinatus ruptures first, although the tears may extend either anteriorly or posteriorly into the subsca-

pularis or infraspinatus. At surgery, tendon-to-tendon closure is usually successful.

GRADE II: LONGITUDINAL TEARS

The rupture extends in line with the tendon and muscle fibers from 1 cm to 3 or 4 cm in length and at times to the extent that the humeral head may actually protrude up through the ruptured tendon (Fig. 6-21B). These tend to be more in posttraumatic situations or with instability. When reduced, the tendons can be closed anatomically and tendon-to-tendon repair is usually satisfactory.

Interstitial tears of the rotator cuff are painful and identified only by a smooth, soft depression of the tendon. These are usually missed by arthroscopy or arthrography. In this situation, ultrasonography, nuclear magnetic resonance,[46] and bursography may help to clarify the picture. Similar incomplete ruptures may occur in the patellar tendon and the tendo Achilles. Tami and Ogawa[47] reported an interesting case of this type in 1985.

GRADE II (COMBINATION OF I AND II)

The combination of the transverse longitudinal rupture is commonly seen with varying degrees of retraction from the tendon (Fig. 6-21C). This produces a stellate type of tear.

GRADE III: MASSIVE AVULSION OF THE CUFF

At surgery, the humeral head resembles a billiard ball due to complete retraction of the tendon (Fig. 6-21D). Usually the supraspinatus and infraspinatus are involved, and in some patients parts of the subscapularis or teres minor may also be torn. Usually there is eburnation of the bone and degenerative change within the articular cartilage at this point.

Diagnosis

Diagnosis will depend on the type of rupture, the mode and mechanism, pathologic condition, and age of the patient. The process may occur slowly over time with attrition, or acutely with trauma.

The rotator cuff rupture that occurs slowly on an attritional basis may not be diagnosed until impinge-

ROTATOR CUFF TEARS

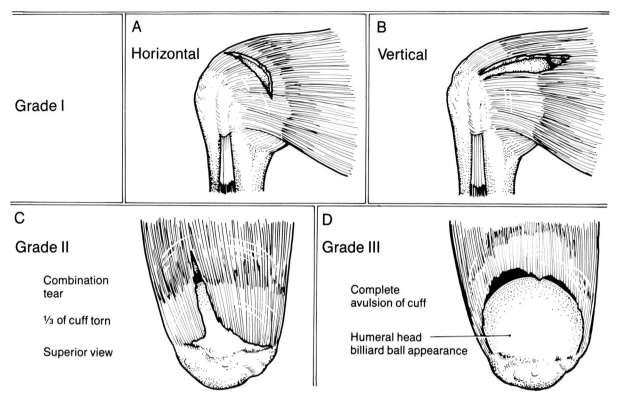

Fig. 6-21. Types of rotator cuff tears. Grade I. (**A**) The transverse or horizontal tears. (**B**) The vertical tear. Grade II. (**C**) Combination of **A** and **B**. Grade III. (**D**) Complete avulsion of the rotator cuff: the "billiard" ball tear.

ment of the hypertrophic tendon edges and subacromial bursa beneath the coracoacromial ligament causes symptoms. The discomfort of a rotator cuff rupture is usually more disturbing at night than during the day, perhaps due to muscle spasm after the shoulder muscles have relaxed. Weakness of abduction will then develop in many cases. The defect of the rotator cuff may actually be palpable through the skin over the humeral head. Usually passive range of motion is maintained in most of these cases, while active range and strength are diminished, particularly in the midrange. There will be a disturbance of scapular rhythm and a positive drop-arm and impingement sign. Radiographs will show a cephalad migration of the humeral head with a break of the smooth inferior line between the medial neck of the humerus and the inferior glenoid. There will be varying degrees

of degenerative change of the joint margins, head, and subacromial surfaces (Fig. 6-22).

The type of rupture that occurs suddenly in a more active person is characterized by acute pain and weakness of abduction. A specific traumatic episode is usually identified. The degree of weakness and pain will depend on the size of the rupture and the degree of mechanical decompensation. In some patients, abduction cannot be initiated. In others, abduction is possible to 90° but cannot be maintained against downward pressure on the arm. One must differentiate between limited motion due to pain, and limited motion due to rotator cuff weakness. This can be clarified by (1) observing whether an injection of local anesthetic into the subacromial space eliminates the pain and restores abduction; (2) double-constrast arthrography and arthrotomography or a subacromial bur-

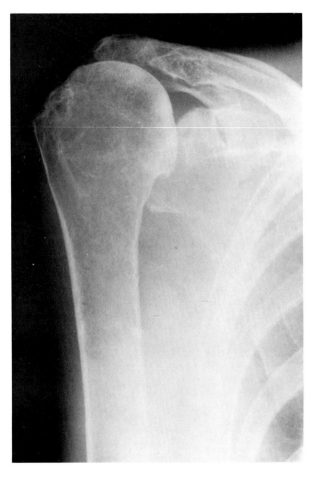

Fig. 6-22. A high-riding humeral head is characteristic of rupture of the rotator cuff.

sagram to outline the rupture; (3) arthroscopy of the glenohumeral joint into the subacromial space, although it is possible to miss tears by this method. Recent advances in ultrasonography[24] and magnetic resonance imaging[46] have been shown to be helpful in diagnosing rotator cuff rupture.

Treatment

Because of differences in experience and teaching among surgeons, a number of different schools of thought have evolved regarding the management of the ruptured rotator cuff. Opinions vary, with one maintaining that the shoulder should be operated upon as soon as possible after the diagnosis has been made and the tendon repaired while fresh and before adhesions have had a chance to develop.[1–3,12,17,18,22,33] Another advises that the patient should be observed for a period of 6 weeks to 3 months following acute onset of symptoms before a decision to operate is made, since many patients heal sufficiently to become asymptomatic during this time and ultimately will do as well as those who have had surgery.[21,24,41–43] After a period of observation, if weakness and pain persist, surgical repair can be carried out without prejudice to the ultimate result. Harrison McLaughlin was an advocate of early operation on rotator cuff ruptures for many years. Later in his career, he operated on fewer of them because he became convinced that many would recover without surgery.

In the preoperative evaluation of a patient with an old rupture of the rotator cuff it is most important to define precisely why the patient is now seeking surgery. Is it because of pain, or weakness of the shoulder, or both? If the patient's chief complaint is pain, the shoulder must be carefully examined for adhesions that cause restricted range of motion. Mild and moderate periarticular fibrosis can be eliminated at the time of surgery, although chronic adhesions that are firm usually cannot, and even if the rotator cuff is successfully repaired, the painful restriction of motion will persist. In some cases, it may even be made worse by the surgery. Some of these patients will ultimately require arthrodesis of the shoulder if their painful restriction continues.

In the interest of providing the best care for the rotator cuff tear, the surgeon should carefully consider the patient's circumstances and requirements, which will require an eclectic philosophy drawing from all schools of thought. In high-performance athletes, there is a greater pressure for early diagnosis and treatment. Older patients, not under pressure for top performance, have more liberal time constraints. Some older patients can be helped considerably by instructing them in the proper use of the arm to avoid stress and impingement on the rotator cuff. By achieving elevation and lateral rotation with the forearm supinated, they enlist the aid of the short head of the biceps and coracobrachialis in a supplementary maneuver. Some of these patients may be so satisfied with this adjustment that surgery is not necessary (Fig. 6-23). Several patients are illustrative of this therapeutic approach. One was a 45-year-old man,

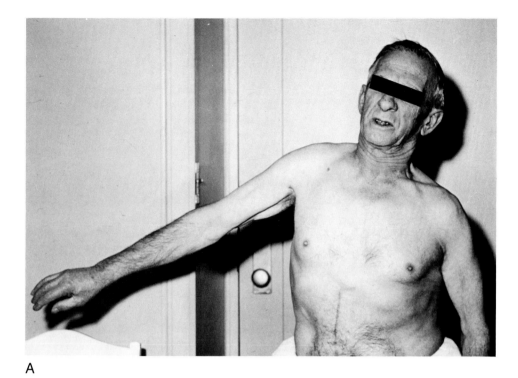

A

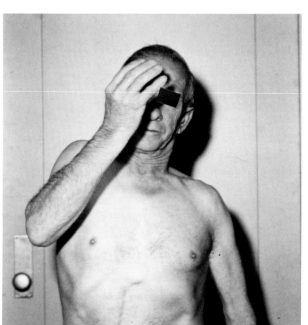

B

Fig. 6-23. Much can be gained by using the short head of biceps and coracobrachialis to elevate the arm in supination, instead of attempting to elevate the arm in abduction. Both patients had rotator cuff ruptures demonstrated on arthrograms. Their presenting complaints were "inability to raise my arm." (**A**) Patient referred to us for repair of ruptured rotator cuff. (**B**) He was satisfied when instructed to use his short head of biceps and coracobrachialis by forward flexion in supination instead of his nonfunctioning abductors, to reach his face and head. (*Figure continues.*)

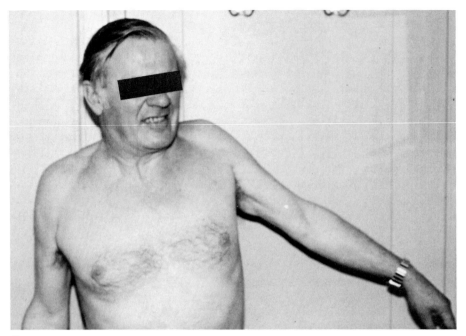

C

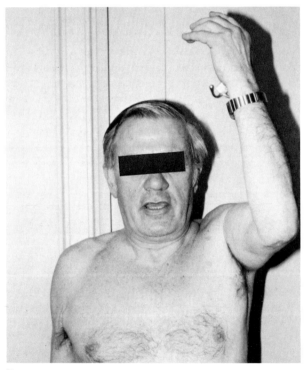

D

Fig. 6-23 (*Continued*). (**C**) This patient was also referred for surgical repair of his ruptured rotator cuff. (**D**) As he had had previous major abdominal surgery, he was very happy to use his flexors, instead of his abductors, and avoid surgery.

who worked with produce, carrying heavy crates. He came to the office because he had heard that we "did not operate on all rotator cuff ruptures." His examination revealed no power of abduction with a normal deltoid muscle. He had no pain; weakness was his limiting factor. He was instructed to return to work and to elevate the arm in forward flexion and lateral rotation and to avoid abduction. Three weeks later he felt better and at 3 months could initiate abduction which, although weak, was useful. At 6 months, he had regained strong abduction and forward flexion and was working full-time doing heavy work.

Another interesting observation was of a patient who was admitted to the service of Dr. Cave many years ago for a Bankart procedure because of recurrent anterior dislocations of his shoulder. He was examined the night before surgery by one of us and his abduction was strong. He had full range of motion. During the night, the patient unfortunately died of a coronary occlusion. At postmortem examination the next day, his shoulder was explored and found to have a massive rotator cuff rupture with a completely bald humeral head. The lesion was obviously chronic, yet clinically he had excellent abduction. The clinical experience of Rockwood,[40] Hawkins[17] and our own patients has demonstrated that in selected cases at surgery, when a massive cuff rupture is found and repair is impossible by means of mobilization, good results have been obtained by thorough decompression. This consists of acromioclavicular arthroplasty, resection of the coracoacromial ligament, and anterior acromioplasty.

In an unpublished follow-up study of rotator cuff repair we carried out at the Massachusetts General Hospital, seven severe unrepaired rotator cuff tears in which only the "decompression operation" was performed were compared to 24 repaired rotator cuffs for pain, motion, strength, and function. The patients whose rotator cuffs were not repaired did as well as those whose were, with a surprisingly slightly better score in motion and strength in the former. Evidently, relief of pain and return of function had occurred merely from eliminating the impingement. DePalma's experience[14] has shown that with complete avulsion of the cuff, the size of the lesion or tear is not always a factor that determines the degree of dysfunction. He stated "I believe that the degree of impairment of function is directly related to the loss of muscle balance." He maintained that "As long as the

remaining portion of the cuff is capable of balancing the pull of the deltoid, no loss of abduction ensues." Consequently, the pull of the subscapularis, teres minor and long head of the biceps may compensate for the loss of the supraspinatus and infraspinatus function. The two patients illustrated in Figure 6-24 had complete absence of the rotator cuff at surgery except for a small portion of the subscapularis and teres minor. It was impossible to mobilize the cuff in either patient. In neither of these was an attempt made to repair the cuff, and decompression was carried out consisting of resection of the coracoacromial ligament with debridement of the chronically thickened subacromial bursa and soft tissue, with complete relief of pain and good function.

Thus, a reasonable approach to the management of rotator cuff ruptures would be one of selectivity. The surgeon who routinely operates on all torn cuffs will operate on some patients who would recover spontaneously. Some may be made worse by surgery. Nevertheless, the surgeon who is fearful of repairing the rotator cuff will leave many shoulders painful and disabled.

For most patients who are not high-performance athletes, a waiting period of 3 to 6 weeks following the acute onset of symptoms will allow the surgeon to determine whether healing is taking place. If surgery is then chosen, in our experience the cuff will not have undergone significant additional deterioration or so much retraction as to make repair impossible. For the elderly patient in whom a severe cuff tear that cannot be repaired by ordinary means is found at surgery, decompression with early motion may prove most successful.

The most definite indication for early surgery is the professional athlete in his or her late 20s or early 30s with a proven rotator cuff tear. Early surgical repair rather than procrastination would be indicated. In these patients, the tissues are better in terms of their blood supply and capacity to heal. Over the years, we have had a number of professional football players and hockey players whose acutely ruptured rotator cuffs were repaired with minimal loss in terms of ultimate results.

The patient in Figure 6-25 represents a good indication for surgical repair in an active, somewhat older professional. He is a 45-year-old policeman, a pistol instructor at the Police Academy, who was disabled by chronic pain and weakness of the right shoulder

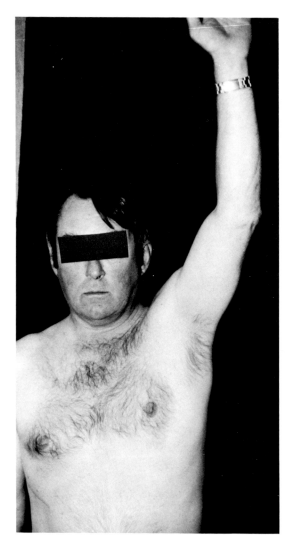

A

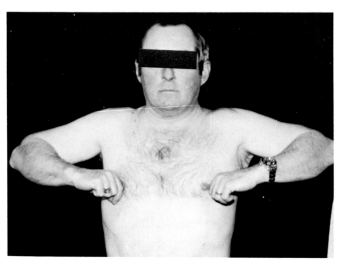

B

Fig. 6-24. Examples of "decompression" of the subacromial space for complete unrepaired rotator cuff ruptures. The ruptures were not repaired. (**A,B,C**) At surgery, patient was found to have a severe rupture of the left rotator cuff. We were unable to identify his rotator cuff to repair it. Resection of the coracoacromial ligament and debridement of the subacromial space without any attempt to repair the tendon was carried out. Six months later, the patient has no pain and complete range of motion, and an excellent functioning shoulder. My secretary, who is quite strong, was unable to depress his arm. At 3 years follow-up, his shoulder remains strong with no degenerative changes by radiographs. (*Figure continues.*)

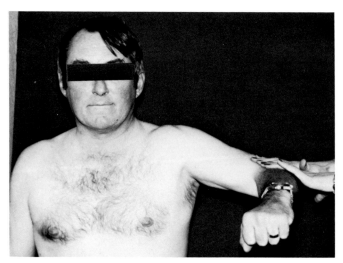

C

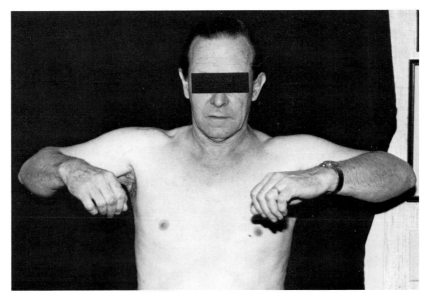

Fig. 6-24 (*Continued*). (**D,E,F**) Patient at surgery had a complete "billiard ball" rupture of his right shoulder. There was no rotator cuff to repair except a remnant of subscapularis and teres minor. Surgery consisted only of resection of the coracoacromial ligament and debridement of the subacromial space. Six months after surgery the patient had no pain, excellent range of motion, and a good functioning arm. At 2 years follow-up, his condition remains the same.

D

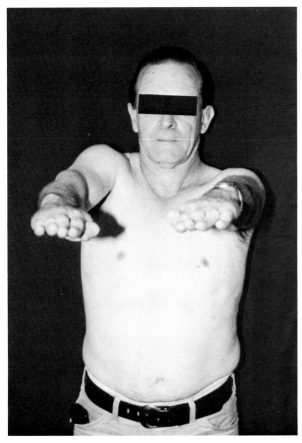

E

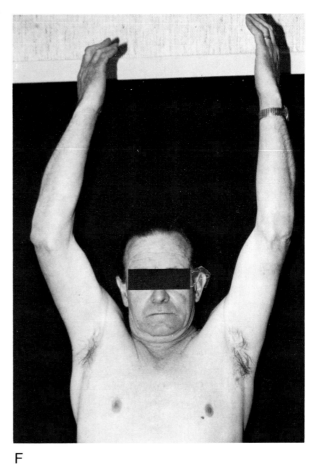

F

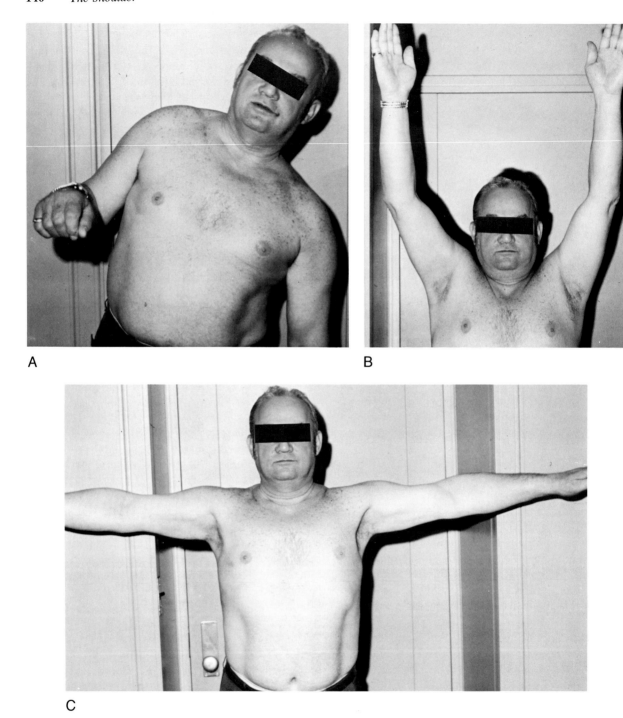

A

B

C

Fig. 6-25. Repair of massive rotator cuff tear with a "trench" in the humeral head and fascia lata reinforcement. (**A**) Patient was disabled as a pistol instructor in the Police Academy because of a weak painful right shoulder and inability to abduct. (**B,C**) Six months after surgery, he has complete range of motion, a strong shoulder, and is back with full duties as a pistol instructor.

to the point where he was unable to perform his duties. After a discussion of the options of treatment, he chose surgery. On exploration, a massive tear was found which fortunately could be mobilized and secured to a bony trough, with a strip of fascia lata. His result was excellent with complete range of function and painless motion. After surgery he returned to full duty.

SURGICAL APPROACHES AND OPERATIVE TECHNIQUES

Limited Anterior Deltoid-Splitting Approach

This is particularly applicable in younger patients, especially for athletes in whom minimal disturbance of the anatomy is desired so that they may return to contact sports. Several professional hockey players have responded to this limited technique with little loss of time from the ice. In using this approach it is mandatory to confine it to that area above the level of the axillary nerve, which ordinarily runs 5 cm below the acromion.

Enlarged Exposures

DELTOPECTORAL GROOVE INCISION

This utility incision has a number of advantages in allowing for visualization of the subacromial arch in relation to the underlying rotator cuff and permitting operative repair and decompression. If the anterior deltoid is not detached during the exposure, there is no risk of postoperative detachment and retraction—a complication that can be extremely disabling. The incision begins over the acromioclavicular joint and goes anteriorly and inferiorly to bisect the coracoid process. If the arm is adducted, the skin folds will indicate just where the incision should end above the anterior axilla. A slightly curved vertical line directed medially into one of these folds rather than laterally out to the arm will lie in Langer's lines and will heal with absence of the hypertrophic scarring so often seen. The arm is then abducted on an armboard or a padded stand for easy identification of the

deltopectoral groove and the cephalic vein. The use of self-retaining retractors in the skin obviates the need to clamp most of the subcutaneous bleeders and the cephalic vein can be mobilized laterally with the deltoid and preserved in most cases. It is easier to identify the deltopectoral groove if one begins inferiorly, since there is more fat there. Since the tip of the coracoid process underlies the interval between the muscles, it is a readily palpable landmark. Particularly in heavily muscled individuals, adequate relaxation must be provided by the anesthetist, or it will not be possible to repair extensive cuff tears without detaching part of the anterior deltoid.

When hemostasis has been obtained, the coracoacromial ligament is easily defined and an incision is made parallel to its inferior surface from the coracoid to the acromial attachment. An elevator may then be introduced posterior to the ligament so that when the ligament is detached from the coracoid, the underlying rotator cuff is protected. The cutting cautery is useful in this maneuver because a rather constant branch of the thoracoacromial artery will be divided at the most superior point of attachment of the ligament and bleeding can be troublesome if the vessel is not coagulated. The ligament can then be grasped and sharply removed in its entirety, along with any osteophytes present at its acromial attachment. The degree of compression of the cuff by these osteophytes and the anterior-inferior edge of the acromion can be very accurately assessed by means of this approach. If traction is applied on the arm, one can inspect the entire coracoacromial arch, including the undersurface of the acromioclavicular joint. Often there will be an osteophyte on the inferior aspect, usually stemming from the lateral clavicle. If it is present, the lateral end of the clavicle may be removed either from above or from below; take care to protect and spare the coracoclavicular ligaments.

The soft tissues on the undersurface of the anterior acromion are removed and then one decides how much bone must be resected to allow for clearance of the repaired cuff. Although originally we used osteotomes for this purpose, an air drill and burr provide an easily controlled means of accomplishing this part of the procedure. Since the bone that is removed is not the deltoid origin, but anterior and inferior to it, there is no fear of later detachment of the muscle. Furthermore, a uniform thickness of bone need not be removed, but only those areas actually or poten-

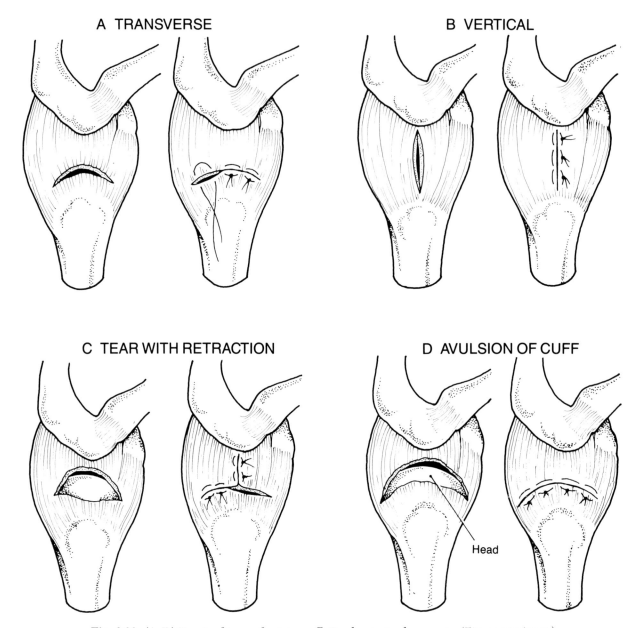

Fig. 6-26. (A–D) Repair of tears of rotator cuff. Tendon-to-tendon repair. (*Figure continues.*)

tially impinging on the cuff. When the decompression has been completed, there will be adequate space in which to assess the cuff and its potential for repair. In those patients in whom significant delay has resulted in retraction of the tissues, gentle traction combined with blunt dissection both inside and outside the torn cuff will allow a surprising degree of mobilization, and in many cases an edge-to-edge repair after the surfaces have been freshened. By varying the position of the arm, different parts of the humeral head and cuff can be presented in the wound so that repair can be effected.

The exposure demonstrated in the previous section for tendinitis and impingement is also a very satisfactory anterior exposure for rotator cuff tears, and is favored by Dr. Rowe.

E MASSIVE AVULSION AT INSERTION

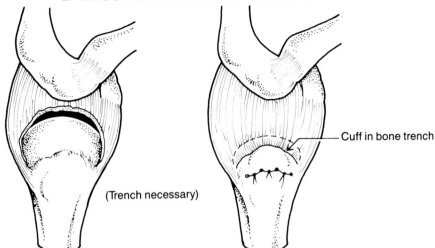

(Trench necessary)

Cuff in bone trench

Fig. 6-26 (*Continued*). (**E–G**) Massive tears repaired into a bony trench made along the articulate surface of the humeral head. (*Figure continues.*)

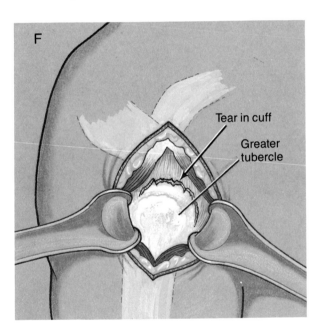

Tear in cuff

Greater tubercle

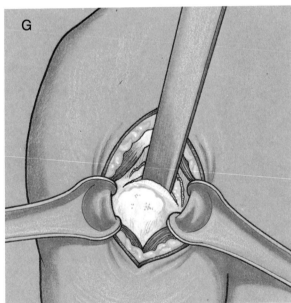

SUPERIOR INCISIONS

These can provide greater exposure to the posterior cuff, including the infraspinatus and teres minor. Kessel,[20] Gschwend,[16] Debeyre,[13] Ozaki et al.,[34] and Mikasa[27] have described their use of different transacromial approaches with satisfactory result. Closure of the acromial osteotomy is secured by suture of the osteoperiosteal flaps. We have not used these approaches, which are said to provide significant advantage in exposure of the rotator cuff.

Operative Cuff Repair

Whenever possible, we prefer direct suture of tendon to tendon, such as with longitudinal and horizontal tears (Fig. 6-26A–E). However, with very large tears in which the tendon has retracted from the tuberosities, a bony trough at the border of the articular surface of the humeral head may be necessary for implantation of the freshened tendon (Fig. 6-26F,G). This encourages improved healing and strength of the repair. It is important to ensure that the superior

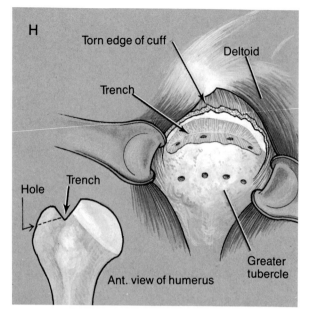

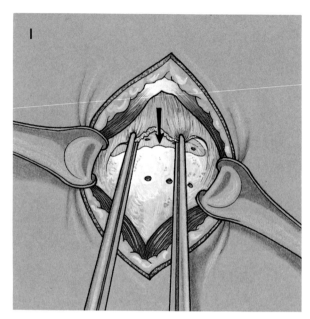

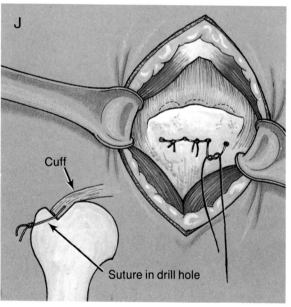

Fig. 6-26 (*Continued*). (**H–J**) Drill holes are then made through the greater tuberosity. The freshened rotator cuff is drawn into the trench and secured with cotton or synthetic sutures. A strip of fascia lata may be used when indicated.

edge of the trough is smooth, to eliminate the shearing action on the tendon. Drill holes are made through the greater tuberosity to secure the repair. (Fig. 6-26H–J). Fascia lata may be used to reinforce the repair if necessary, although we have tended to use it very rarely recently. If there is a large space at the site of repair that cannot be closed, a graft may be used to cover the defect as recommended by Wolfgang,[48] Neviaser,[33] and Post.[36] Debeyre[13] recommends that chronic tears with retraction of the cuff be treated by mobilization of the supraspinatus from its fossa, so that it may be advanced laterally and reattached with little tension. The results are reported as favorable. However, this is a technically

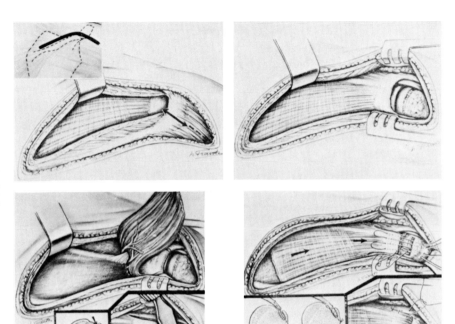

Fig. 6-27. The Debeyre technique of advancing the supraspinatus distally to the humeral head.

difficult operation with the possibility of both devascularization and denervation of the supraspinatus if the mobilization is excessive (Fig. 6-27).

Another method used to cover the humeral head is by transferring the subscapularis and teres minor muscles superiorly[4,6,33] or by shifting the course of the long head of the biceps over the greater curvature of the humeral head into a new channel.[6,36] With chronic ruptures of the rotator cuff, the function of the biceps tendon increases and is often found to be hypertrophied, since it is compensating for the loss of the rotator cuff.[6] Its increased size indicates increased function (Fig. 6-28). Consequently, we would not recommend removing this important tendon to tenodese it to the bicipital groove or coracoid.

If the acromion has an unfused epiphysis, it should be resected if it is a small piece, or grafted if it is large.[30,31]

Complications

The use of isolated inert tissues, such as freeze-dried fascia, autogenous fascia lata, coracoacromial ligament, or the resected biceps tendon adds avascular tissue to an area of poor blood supply. Conse-quently, the incidences of rejection, infection, or scarring may be increased, despite the fact that there are limited indications for their use. We do not believe that nonbiological materials have been shown to have any place in the repair of defects of the rotator cuff and prefer to perform a generous decompression in those cases in which repair cannot be done.

Postoperative adhesions should be minimized as much as possible. Early gentle passive gliding motion of the arm, as can be obtained with pendulum exercises, will minimize adhesion formation as well as stimulate circulation.

Postoperative infection is the surgeon's nightmare. Careful preoperative skin care and inspection of the skin immediately before surgery are most important. Opinions differ as to the indications for antibiotic therapy. Dr. Rowe uses them for 48 hours postsurgery, although Dr. Leffert does not. In our experience, there has been one deep infection in the past 30 years of rotator cuff repairs. That occurred when a strip of fascia lata from the thigh was used to secure the cuff.

The postoperative detachment of the deltoid that accrues from excessive mobilization of the muscle or from failure to reattach and protect it properly is a significant cause of disability. If an acromionectomy is done rather than an acromioplasty as described,

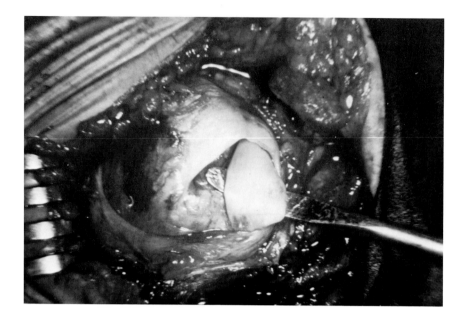

Fig. 6-28. In chronic rotator cuff ruptures, the biceps tendon hypertrophies as it compensates for the missing rotator cuff.

the length–tension relationships of the deltoid will be changed significantly. Because the complexity of the muscle includes limited tolerance for that, function will be severely aversely affected. Although it has been possible in a few cases to restore function in patients who have had late detachment of the deltoid, it is a technically very difficult operation, and one the patient must realize cannot be considered as having a certain result. Postoperatively, patients should be splinted in abduction for 6 weeks and then begin gentle graded exercises.

Postoperative Care

For small and medium tears, which are securely repaired, we allow the arm to rest at the side of the body in a sling and begin gentle pendulum motion within the first week postoperatively. For larger tears, we tend to begin these motions at about 2 weeks to stimulate healing and minimize the formation of adhesions. The sling is used during this period but the patient should be instructed in how to protect the wound with plastic drape so that showers may be taken.

During the 1950s and 1960s, the airplane splint was routinely used in the postoperative management of rotator cuff repairs. Today we seldom use it and

have encountered no difficulty. Patients' comfort has been significantly enhanced and we believe that there is less adhesion formation and more stimulation to healing. If the repair at surgery is secure only in an abducted position, the likelihood of disruption when the arm is returned to the anatomical position is very great. Both Bateman[3] and Mode[28] have commented on the use of the brace in the postoperative rehabilitation of the shoulder.

Whether patients are sent to physical therapy in the postoperative period varies with the surgeon and the circumstances. Dr. Rowe prefers to instruct the patient personally in the exercises. Although Dr. Leffert does instruct the patients in the pendulum exercises in the hospital, at the 2-week office visit (when the subcuticular suture is removed) patients are routinely referred for instructions in physical therapy as outpatients. The therapists are provided with a copy of the operative note so that they understand the procedure, as well as the precautions, and are encouraged to communicate with the surgeon if there are any questions. The patient is asked to demonstrate the pendulum exercises to the therapist and it is stressed that these are not active exercises. The patient bends from the waist, keeping the feet apart with the knees slightly bent, and lets the arm go limp. The analogy of comparing the arm to an elephant's trunk is used to promote a gentle swinging of the arm as the weight is shifted from one foot to the other. It is explained that making big circles with the dependent arm is an active exercise, mostly involving the movement of the scapula on the thorax.

The patients are instructed that at 2 weeks they may begin to discard the sling so that by 3 weeks they have been weaned out of it. Some find that sleeping in the sling at this time is uncomfortable, and they are taught how to place pillows behind their back so as to not roll over onto their arm.

At 3 weeks, the patients return to the physical therapist to receive instruction in supine, active-assisted range-of-motion exercises. The humerus is flexed with the forearm supinated or the elbow may be flexed and the arm cradled in the other arm. Side-lying exercises are taught for scapular motion. Internal and external rotation of the arm is done with a pillow behind the arm to flex the humerus slightly and take the stress off the cuff. Diagonal exercises and horizontal rocking of the arm into abduction using the sound arm are taught. The usual program of exercises is to begin with each of these done for 3 or 4 minutes at a time, twice a day, increasing to 6 or 7 minutes after a week. This will ultimately involve 1 hour of exercise per day. Exercises are added one at a time so that those that are provocative or painful can be isolated and discarded. The patients receive an explanation of what was done at surgery. They are encouraged to do gentle pendulum exercises, as well as exercise using a large, inflatable beachball placed on a table around which they may push it every hour or so.

At 5 weeks, supine diagonal exercises are begun. At the 6-week visit, the patient is instructed in standing, active-assisted exercises. The nature of the movement of the scapula on the ribcage and the contribution to total shoulder girdle movement are stressed and patients are encouraged to watch the movement of the scapulae in the mirror. They begin exercises against gravity for elevation and receive guidance in activities of daily living, such as the use of the arm in bathing or holding a newspaper, as well as use of table utensils. However, they are cautioned against activities such as holding a blow-dryer or attempting to lift heavy weights.

During the first 6 months following repair, we believe very strongly that no attempt should be made to "strengthen" the shoulder with resisted exercises or by lifting weights. This is the period to regain

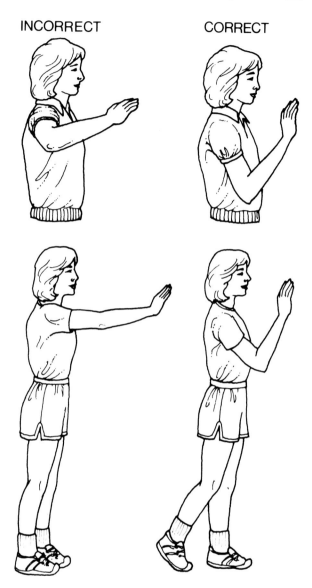

Fig. 6-29. Elimination of strain to the shoulder and repair. **(A)** Avoid the "flying elbow" and extend arm, as it adds strain to the repair. **(B)** To avoid strain, flex the elbow and take a step forward to reach for an object.

motion and to heal the torn cuff. In our experience, one of the most common causes for poor results or the failure of rotator cuff repair is aggressive physical therapy, particularly with weights, or forceful passive exercises before the cuff repair has healed sufficiently.

Although tendon-to-bone healing may eventually occur, we are never certain of the degree of healing or the time element. We doubt very much if the healing is ever as strong as normal in patients 50 years or older. In the patient's attempt to rehabilitate the shoulder, it is most important that the body move with the shoulder (Fig. 6-29). Resistive horizontal motions in the sitting position in 90° of abduction, in which the position of the scapula is fixed and the rotator cuff repeatedly forced under the acromial arch, must be avoided. This is an abnormal shoulder position in which scapulothoracic rhythm is eliminated. Unfortunately, these positions are too frequently used routinely in many so-called health centers and exercise areas. Push-ups from the floor will also overtax the rotator cuff, as the scapula is fixed. Resumption of normal activities with the arm must be tailored to the individual and the lesion repaired. Usually by about 6 months, most activities can be tolerated. Those patients in contact sports should be cautioned to keep the arm close to the body in contact and to move their body with every shoulder motion. This advice will go far in protecting this vulnerable area.

RUPTURES OF THE BICEPS TENDON

The long head of the biceps tendon may rupture proximally either from the supraglenoid tubercle of the scapula, at the entrance to the bicipital groove proximally, or at the exit of the tunnel at the musculotendinous junction (Fig. 6-30). The muscle mass moves distally in such cases, producing the typical "Popeye" appearance of the arm. The rupture of the biceps tendon distally involves both heads and the muscle mass migrates proximally.

Pathologic Findings

As pointed out by DePalma,[14] "After the fourth decade, degenerative changes in the form of thickening, widening and shredding of the biceps tendon occur."

Sometimes patients can describe the incident of rupture with a forceful flexion of the arm. However, at times rupture may occur from a minor incident or even spontaneously. The pathologic process within the tendon can be compared to that of the tendo Achilles: microtears render it vulnerable to forceful rupture. A sudden sharp pain is experienced with dehiscence of the tendon. The degree of ecchymosis will depend on the site of the tear; it is less in the avascular portions and quite noticeable at the musculotendinous junction.

Diagnosis of the rupture of the proximal long head of the biceps tendon is evident on the basis of the distal retraction of the muscle mass. Partial ruptures may also occur and are characterized by local pain and weakness with only slight muscular deformity. Rupture of both heads of the biceps distally is not as obvious cosmetically. Impairment of function also differs between the proximal and distal tendon ruptures. Rupture of the proximal tendon may show little if any weakness in flexion of the forearm since this function is carried out primarily by the brachialis, and short head of the biceps. However, there may be weakness of supination of the forearm with rupture of the long head. This would be particularly bothersome in someone such as a carpenter, who must use a screwdriver. With rupture of the distal biceps tendon, there is not only weakness of supination of the forearm but also marked weakness of elbow flexion.

Treatment

RUPTURE OF THE PROXIMAL BICEPS TENDON

When this occurs in the active, younger person (which is infrequent), surgical repair is usually indicated. When rupture occurs in middle-aged or older persons, there is less indication for surgical repair. The majority of patients will accept the cosmetic deformity and would be perfectly satisfied with the strength of flexion. They seldomly complain of the lessened power of supination. Dr. Edwin Cave ruptured the long head of his biceps tendon when jumping his horse and continued for 10 years without pain during a busy orthopaedic surgical practice, as well as continuing to ride and curl. His only complaint was "a little weakness when tightening a difficult screw."

Open surgical repair produces a long scar and usually cannot completely restore the underlying anatomy. The technical steps are outlined in Figure 6-31. The coiled up distal end of the tendon is usually

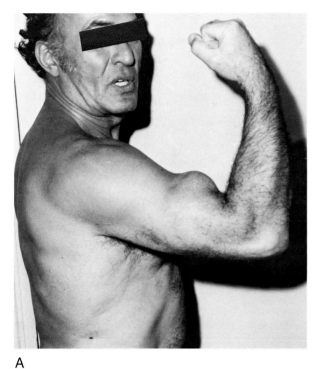

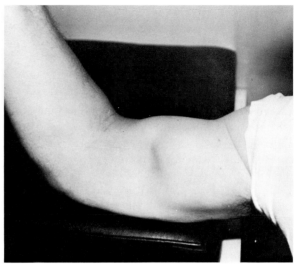

B

Fig. 6-30. (**A**) When the proximal long head of the biceps ruptures, the muscle mass moves distally. (**B**) When the distal head of the biceps ruptures, the muscle mass moves proximally.

A

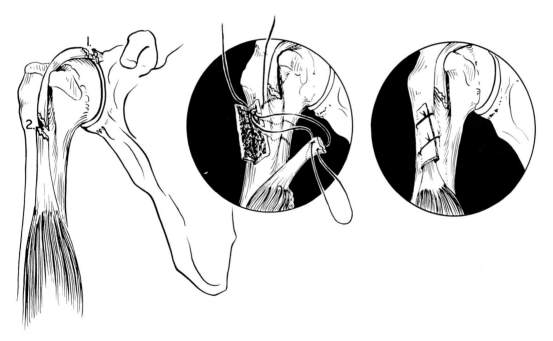

Fig. 6-31. Technique of repairing long head of biceps rupture. When end-to-end repair is not possible, the intraarticular tendon should be resected and the distal tendon fixed in a trap door of the humerus. (Reproduced with permission from Cave EF, Boyd RJ: Injuries to major tendons. p. 961. In Cave EF, Burke JF, Boyd RJ (eds): Trauma Management. Copyright © 1974 by Year Book Medical Publishers Inc., Chicago.)

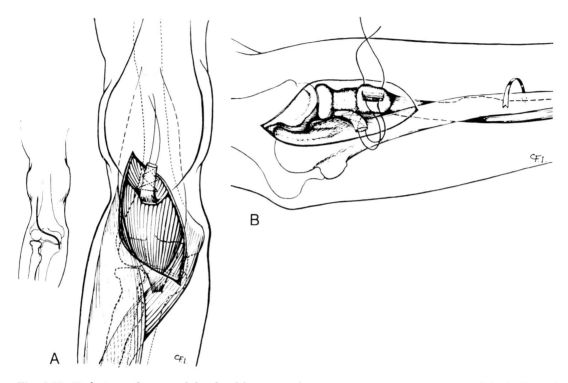

Fig. 6-32. Technique of repair of the distal biceps tendon. Two exposures are necessary. **(A)** The line of the anterior skin incision. In the larger drawing, the retracted biceps tendon is seen in the upper portion of the incision with a silk suture in place. By retracting the distal end of the incision, the canal of the biceps tendon is located between the brachialis and the pronator teres on the medial side and the brachioradialis on the lateral side. **(B)** The radial tuberosity as seen through the posterior approach. Note the full pronation of the radius. The suture is in place, preparatory to insertion of the end of the tendon into the trap door.

found beneath the attachment of the pectoralis major to the humerus. If not, it can be picked up with a separate incision. If the distal end of the tendon cannot be reattached strongly to the proximal end, the intraarticular portion of the biceps tendon should be resected and the distal stump attached to the coracoid process, the conjoined tendon, or to a trap door in the humerus (Fig. 6-31). The surgical exposure should remain lateral to the conjoined tendon. The musculocutaneous nerve may be injured as it enters the conjoined tendon. The entrance of the nerve into the muscles may vary from 3 cm below the coracoid process to as far down as 6 cm. Neer has drawn attention to the correlation between proximal biceps ruptures and tear of the rotator cuff in middle-aged and older patients. After rupture, if symptoms of weakness continue, exploration of the rotator cuff is indicated.[31] Figure 6-32 shows the technique of repair of a chronic midbiceps rupture using strips of fascia lata.

RUPTURE OF THE DISTAL BICEPS TENDON

Surgical repair of the distal biceps tendon ruptures is recommended regardless of age, due to the functional loss of forearm flexion. Before Boyd and Anderson[5] reported their method of exposure in 1961, the anterior approach for reinsertion of the biceps tendon was used and carried a risk of injury to the radial nerve. Attaching the tendon to the brachialis muscle was less effective. Meherin and Kilgore[26] reported six patients in whom the tendon was reattached anteriorly to the radial tuberosity, with two

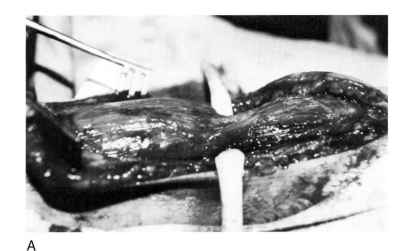

A

Fig. 6-33. (A) Operative photo of the torn biceps of a 21-year-old mechanic who fell 10 feet down an elevator shaft and struck his arm on a steel bar when he landed. Although there was no break in the skin, the biceps was ruptured, as seen here, 5 months past injury. There was nothing but scar at the isthmus over the rubber drain, and the distal stump of muscle was totally denervated as shown by EMG. He had marked weakness of supination. (B) Repair was done using multiple laces of autogenous fascia lata. (C) Postoperative result: he has essentially normal function, including strong supination.

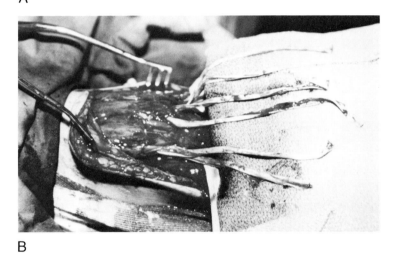

B

C

permanent partially damaged radial nerves and one complete nerve injury. Dobbie[15] also reported two radial nerve injuries from this procedure.

The approach recommended by Boyd and Anderson has proved to be safe and effective (Fig. 6-32).

To locate the end of the tendon, a curvilinear incision is made over the anterior aspect of the elbow joint. The tendon is usually found curled up 5 to 6 cm above the joint. Care must be taken to protect the lateral antebrachial cutaneous nerve. A suture is placed in the distal tendon and the interval between the radius and ulna through which the tendon originally passed is identified. No further dissection is carried out anteriorly. A second incision is made over the posterolateral aspect of the elbow joint, similarly to the approach used by Boyd for the radial head and proximal ulna.[5] Elevation of the muscle origins from the lateral surface of the ulna is carried out along the plane of the interosseous membrane, exposing the head and neck of the radius by retracting the supinator muscle laterally. The radial nerve is protected during this maneuver. The forearm is then fully supinated, exposing the radial tuberosity. A trap door is made in the tuberosity with small, sharp osteotomes and two drill holes are placed through the cortex of the radius. Then the end of the tendon is passed from the anterior incision through the interval by means of a curved hemostat or a small tendon passer, out through the posterior incision between the radial neck and ulna. The elbow is flexed and the sutures are passed through the drill holes in the bony canal. Thus, the tendon is resutured to its original insertion. Reinforcing sutures are placed along the tendon in the soft tissues and interosseous membrane. A cast is applied with the elbow flexed 45 to 60° and the forearm in neutral position. Immobilization is discontinued at 6 weeks and graduated exercises begun in supination, pronation, flexion, and extension.

RUPTURE OF THE BICEPS WITHIN ITS SUBSTANCE

Rupture of the biceps is a very unusual lesion that usually results from a combination of forced flexion and direct pressure on the muscle. A case of this unusual injury is presented in Figure 6-33.

RUPTURE OF THE TRICEPS TENDON

The triceps tendon has been likened in function to the quadriceps tendon by Cave.[7] Whereas rupture of the quadriceps is not uncommon, rupture of the triceps is. It is mostly likely associated with systemic disease, such as hyperparathyroidism,[37] Paget's disease, or rheumatoid arthritis. The tendon inserts not only directly into the olecranon, but beyond it into the forearm fascia, much as the quadriceps does with the patella. Complete rupture of the tendon can be repaired by direct suture or, if it has torn from the olecranon process, directly to the bone by drill holes to ensure the repair. Turning down a flap of the superficial tendon, as with the quadriceps, adds to the strength of the repair.

Serfoss et al.[44] found only two cases of triceps rupture in the literature and added one of their own. This was a 44-year-old man with hyperparathyroidism who had experienced a grand mal seizure and was unable to extend his right elbow afterwards. The rupture had occurred just proximal to the olecranon. Direct repair to the olecranon was successful. The author emphasized the association of tendon avulsion and primary hyperparathyroidism.

RUPTURE OF THE PECTORALIS MAJOR TENDON

Although also an unusual injury, rupture of the pectoralis major tendon is more common than that of the triceps (Fig. 6-34). Kawashima et al.[19] reported two cases and cited the first recorded rupture of the pectoralis major in 1822; 32 cases have been reported in the world literature during the past 150 years. A traumatic rupture can be mistaken for congenital absence of the pectoralis major. The traumatic rupture is usually produced by sudden, unexpected muscle contraction during pulling or lifting. The patient experiences sudden pain and develops local ecchymosis and swelling. As the swelling subsides, a sulcus and deformity are visible. Subsequently, the patient notes weakness of the arm in adduction and internal rotation.

Marmor[23] and Park and Espinella[35] questioned the essential function of the pectoralis major muscle. Marmor indicated that in normal shoulder function it is not essential, but it is necessary for athletic performance. Park and Espinella[35] reviewed 10 ruptures of the pectoralis major treated surgically, with 8 excellent and 1 good result (1 case was not further detailed). Of 12 ruptures treated conservatively, 2 resulted in excellent and 7 in fair recovery. One patient died and was lost to follow-up. Purlasky and Martin[38] also commented on conservative treatment and stated that although spontaneous function may return with

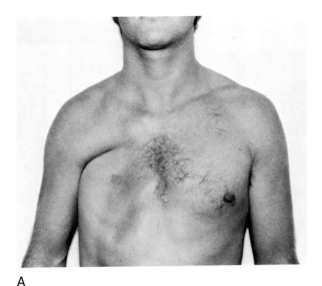
A

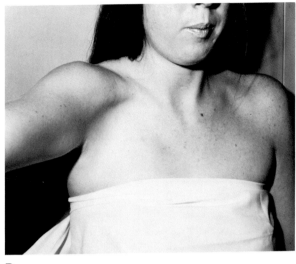
B

Fig. 6-34. Ruptures of the pectoralis major muscle. (**A**) Congenital rupture of the sternal portion of the right pectoralis major muscle. (**B**) Rupture of both heads of the right pectoralis major muscle.

nonoperative treatment, recovery is slow and "full power never restored." This is in contrast to patients with congenital absence of the pectoralis major who complain little of weakness and usually are bothered only by the cosmetic appearance (Fig. 6-34).

REFERENCES

1. Bakalim B, Pasila M: Surgical treatment of rupture of the rotator cuff tendon. Acta Orthop Scand 46:751, 1975
2. Bassett RW, Cofield RH: Acute tears of the rotator cuff. Clin Orthop Rel Res 176:18, 1983
3. Bateman JE: The diagnosis and treatment of tears of the rotator cuff. Surg Clin North Am 43:1523, 1963
4. Bateman JE: The Shoulder and Neck, 2nd ed. WB Saunders, Philadelphia, 1978
5. Boyd HB, Anderson LD: A method of reinsertion of the distal biceps brachii tendon. J Bone Joint Surg 43A:1041, 1961
6. Bush LF: The torn shoulder capsule. J Bone Joint Surg 57A:256, 1975
7. Cave EF: Twins (extra) ordinary—the knee and elbow. Sir Robert Jones Lecture. Bull Hosp Joint Dis 26:127, 1965
8. Codman EA: Ruptures of the supraspinatus—1834 to 1934. J Bone Surg 19:643, 1937
9. Codman EA: Complete rupture of the supraspinatus tendon. Operative treatment with report of two successful cases. Boston Med Surg J May:708, 1911
10. Codman EA: Obscure lesions of the shoulder—rupture of the supraspinatus tendon. Boston Med Surg J V. 6, 1927
11. Codman EA: The Shoulder. RE Kreiger, Malabar, Florida, 1984
12. Cofield RH: Acute tears of the rotator cuff. Can Orthop Rev 175:18, 1983
13. Debeyre J, Patte O, Elmclik E: Repair of ruptures of the rotator cuff of the shoulder. J Bone Joint Surg 47B:36, 1965
14. DePalma AF: Surgery of the Shoulder, 3rd Ed., JB Lippincott, Philadelphia, 1983
15. Dobbie RP: Avulsion of the lower biceps brachii tendon. Analysis of 51 previously unreported cases. Am J Surg 51:662, 1941
16. Gschwend N: A surgical approach to rotator cuff tears. p. 202. Bateman, Welch (eds): Surgery of the Shoulder. BC Decker, Philadelphia, 1984
17. Hawkins RJ, Hoberka P, Misamore GW: Surgery for full thickness rotator cuff tears. Presented at the Annual Meeting, American Academy of Orthopaedic Surgeons, Atlanta, Georgia, February, 1984
18. Heikel HVA: Rupture of the rotator cuff of the shoulder. Experiences of surgical treatment. Acta Orthop Scand 39:477, 1968
19. Kawashima M, Sato M, Forisi F et al: Rupture of the pectoralis major. Two cases. Clin Orthop Rel Res 109:115, 1975

20. Kessel L: Clinical Disorders of the Shoulder. Churchill Livingstone, London, 1982

21. Lundbloom K: On pathogenesis of rupture of the tendon aponeurosis of the shoulder joint. Acta Radiol 20:563577, 1939

22. Lundberg BJ: The correlation of clinical evaluation with operative findings and prognosis in rotator cuff rupture. In Bayley I, Kessel L (eds): Shoulder Surgery. Springer-Verlag, Berlin, 1982

23. Marmor L, Recktal C, Hall CB: Pectoralis major muscle. Function of the sternal portion and mechanism of rupture of normal rupture. J Bone Joint Surg 43A:81, 1961

24. Matsen FA, Mack LA, Kilcoyne RF: Sonographic evaluation of the rotator cuff; delivered to the 3rd meeting of American Shoulder and Elbow Surgeons, Boston, November 1, 1984

25. McLaughlin HL: Repair of major cuff ruptures. Surg Clin North Am 43:1535, 1963

26. Meherin J, and Kilgore ES: The treatment of ruptures of the distal biceps brachii tendon. Am J Surg 99:636, 1960

27. Mikasa M: Trapezius transfer for globar tear of the rotator cuff. In Bateman, Welsh (eds): Surgery of the Shoulder. BC Decker, Philadelphia, 1984

28. Mode M: Shoulder rehabilitation after rotator cuff surgery. In Bateman, Welsh (eds): Surgery of the Shoulder. BC Decker, Philadelphia, 1984

29. Monro A: A Description of all the Bursaw Mucosae of the Human Body. Elliott, Edinburgh, 1788

30. Mudge K, Wood VE, Frykman GK: Rotator cuff tears associated with os acromiale. J Bone Joint Surg 66A:427, 1984

31. Neer C, Bigliani L, Norris T, Fisberg: The relationship between the unfused acromial epiphysis and subacromial impingement lesions. Orthop Trans 7:138, 1983

32. Neer CS, Craig EV, Fukuda H: Cuff tear arthropathy. Orthop Trans 5:447, 1981

33. Neviaser RJ, Neviaser TJ: Reconstruction of chronic tears of rotator cuff. In Bateman, Welsh (eds): Surgery of the Shoulder. BC Decker, Philadelphia, 1984

34. Ozaki J, Fugimoto S, Masuhara K: Repair of rotator cuff tears with synthetic fabrics. In Bateman, Welsh (eds): Surgery of the Shoulder. BC Decker, Philadelphia, 1984

35. Park JY, Esppiniella JL: Rupture of the left pectoralis major muscle. Report of a case. Surgery 25:110, 1949

36. Post M: The Shoulder, Surgical and Non-surgical Management. Lea & Febiger, Philadelphia, 1978

37. Preston ET: Avulsion of both quadriceps tendons in hyperparathyroidism. JAMA 221:406, 1972

38. Pulaski EJ, Martin GW: Rupture of the left pectoralis major muscle. Report of a case. Surgery 25:40, 1949

39. Rathbun JB, MacNab: The microvascular pattern of the rotator cuff. J Bone Joint Surg 52B:540, 1970

40. Rockwood CA: Shoulder function following decompression and irreparable cuff lesions. Presented at the Second Annual Meeting of the American Shoulder and Elbow Surgeons, Rochester, Minnesota, 1983

41. Rothman RM, Parke WW: The vascular anatomy of the rotator cuff. Clin Orthop 41:176, 1965

42. Rowe CR: Ruptures of the rotator cuff. Selection of cases for conservative treatment. Surg Clin North Am 43:176, 1976

43. Samilson RL, Binder WF: Symptomatic full thickness tears of the rotator cuff. Orthop Clin North Am 6:449, 1975

44. Serfoss R, Tripi J, Bowers W: Triceps brachii rupture. J Trauma 16:244, 1976

45. Smith JG: Pathological appearances of seven cases of injury of the shoulder joint with remarks. London Med Gazette, 14:280, 1834; reported in Am J Med Sci 16:219, 1834

46. Steiner RE: Nuclear magnetic resonance—its clinical application. J Bone Joint Surg 65B:533, 1983

47. Tamai K, Ogawa K: Intratendinous tear of supraspinatus tendon exhibiting winging of the scapula. Clin Orthop Rel Res 194:159, 1985

48. Wolfgang BL: Surgical repair of tears of the rotator cuff of the shoulder. J Bone Joint Surg 56A:14, 1974

Idiopathic Chronic Adhesive Capsulitis ("Frozen Shoulder")

Carter R. Rowe
Robert D. Leffert

Perhaps the least understood of the shoulder's many problems is chronic adhesive capsulitis, which is referred to under a number of descriptive terms, such as periarthritis, pericapsulitis, bursitis, tendinitis, and adhesive capsulitis. There are a number of unusual aspects of this syndrome:

1. Its cause is unknown.
2. It does not occur in other joints or parts of the body.
3. It is usually a self-limited syndrome, when untreated, passing through three distinct phases of 3 to 4 months each (Fig. 6-35):
   The *freezing* phase
   The *frozen* phase
   The *thawing* phase
4. In most cases, the shoulder and its tissues recover completely with time, although Simmons in 1949[36] reported that there may still be significant residual restriction after 3 years. Some forms of treatment may upset or prolong nature's schedule.
5. It may involve the opposite shoulder, but rarely recurs in the same shoulder. This was confirmed by Codman[9] and also by Lundberg.[22] We have seen only one patient who appeared to have a recurrence 2 years after successful treatment and resolution of the problem. She had an underlying seizure disorder, which ultimately was found to be caused by a contralateral intracranial meningioma.
6. In our series,[3] 70 percent of the patients were women. These findings were in agreement with those of DePalma,[11] Bateman,[4] and Lundberg.[22] The nondominant limb is more commonly affected than the dominant.
7. It occurs between 40 and 60 years of age (the menopausal period).
8. It is not associated with calcific deposits in rotator cuff, rupture, or attritional changes of the cuff.
9. Radiograms are consistently normal.
10. Frozen shoulder is not associated with arthritis or malignancies. A number of systemic diseases have been linked with the condition, including thyroid disorders, diabetes, and autoimmune diseases.[5,6,38] Although several reports have indicated a higher incidence of the first two by retrospective studies of patients with stiff shoulders, further analyses have generally failed to establish positive statistical correlations. The initial impression of increased levels of HLA-B27 and decreased IgA in the serum of frozen shoulder pa-

155

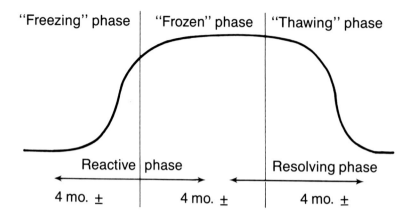

"Freezing" phase   "Frozen" phase   "Thawing" phase

Reactive | phase   Resolving phase

4 mo. ±   4 mo. ±   4 mo. ±

Fig. 6-35. Natural history of idiopathic adhesive capsulitis (frozen shoulder). When untreated, the syndrome consists of three distinct stages: freezing, frozen, and thawing. Each phase usually lasts 4 months, but may vary.

tients has not only not been confirmed by subsequent studies by the same workers, but has also not been found by others.[7,22,35] Hence the autoimmune theory is still unproven.

PATHOLOGIC BASIS

In 1896, Duplay[12] described the syndrome as *periarthritis scapulo-humerale* and Putnam[32] as painful periarthritis. Codman[9] first used the term *frozen shoulder* and remarked "This is a class of cases that I find difficult to define, difficult to treat and difficult to explain from the point of view of pathology." Neviaser[27–29] in 1945 described the problem as "adhesive capsulitis." Pasteur[30] in 1932, Lippmann[19] in 1943 and DePalma[10] in 1952 associated tenosynovitis of the long head of the biceps with frozen shoulder, and believed it to be the initiating pathologic change. Today the tendinitis is considered merely an extension of the reactive capsule of the joint into the bicipital sheath. Neviaser[27] observed at surgical exploration that the capsule was adherent to the humeral head in 9 of 10 explored shoulders. With the advent of the arthroscope, Johnson[17] has not observed adhesions of the capsule to the humeral head, but "a reactive synovitis of the non-rheumatoid type." Wiley et al.[40] also agrees with Johnson ". . . in no patients in the preliminary studies on frozen shoulders were we able to see obliteration of the infraglenoid recess, indeed in no patient were there any intra-articular adhesions whatsoever." These are interesting obser-

vations. Perhaps the manipulation and traction in the shoulder necessary to suspend the arm and perform shoulder arthroscopy eliminated the soft adhesions to the humeral head observed by Neviaser. The conflicting observations of investigators may also be due to the specific stage of the frozen shoulder. If the shoulder is arthroscoped during the freezing phase, a reactive synovitis and no adhesions would be expected. However, if the shoulder is arthroscoped in the frozen or thawing phase, the capsule may well be contracted and adherent to the humeral head, as we have seen and as reported by Neviaser and Lundberg. We have also observed adhesions between the rotator cuff and the undersurface of the acromial arch, eliminating its gliding surfaces, as noted by Codman and by Rowe.[3]

The pathologic sections of the bursa and capsule in the late stages we obtained revealed only a mild lymphocytic reaction. We found no evidence of infection or leukocytic reaction. Cultures of the tissue showed no growth. Observations made by Lundberg[22] in 1969 are significant: electron microscopy ". . . in a few cases, did not reveal any obvious changes in the ultrastructure of the collagen of the joint capsule." Also "analysis of the glycosaminoglycans in joint capsules from frozen shoulders, revealed an increase in the amount of hexosamines. The increase was confined to the glycosaminoglycans, heparin sulfate and chondroitin sulfates, whereas hyaluronic acid is decreased." The syndrome, with its three separate phases and its total recovery (if the tissues are not traumatized by treatment), remains a mystery. We are unable to explain why no other joints of the body are similarly involved. It is clear that more investigative study is needed.

CLINICAL PICTURE

Idiopathic adhesive capsulitis should not be confused with other conditions that create adhesions and/or painful restriction of shoulder motion, such as

1. Arthritides
2. Neglected dislocations, particularly posterior
3. Calcific tendinitis
4. Local tumors
5. Stroke shoulder
6. Cerebral and pulmonary lesions
7. Referred pain (cervical or abdominal)
8. Rotator cuff tears
9. Immobilization of shoulder following fracture

Specific reference is made to the rotator cuff tear since ordinarily patients even with major tears do not have significant restriction of motion, although they do have pain and weakness. However, a rotator cuff derangement including a tear can, with time, produce restricted motion and be confused with idiopathic frozen shoulder. In addition to taking a general and local history and performing physical examination as well as radiographs of the shoulder, the arthrogram is particularly valuable as a diagnostic and, in some cases, therapeutic tool. In addition to what can be observed in a contrast study, the normal shoulder will usually accommodate 20 to 35 ml of fluid, and as little as 5 to 10 ml in a patient with adhesive capsulitis. Some rough estimate of the degree of contracture may be gained from the amount that can be introduced under digital pressure. As stated, rotator cuff tears, which usually do not have significant restriction of passive motion, may sometimes be responsible for the stiff and painful shoulder, and can be identified by arthrography.

True, idiopathic "frozen shoulder" usually comes on silently during the middle decades of life and is ordinarily not associated with a specific cause. Immobilization is probably an important factor, however, particularly when there has been stress, such as surgery or long confinement to bed. Other factors that may initiate immobilization of the shoulder are periods of abnormal emotional tension, such as caused by a death in the family, or periods of intense mental concentration and lack of normal function of the arm. There often is initial pain, present even at rest, and

which may prevent sleep. Within a few weeks, this gives way to discomfort only with attempted motion. The loss of motion is progressive, the pain is constant, and eventually quite debilitating (Fig. 6-36). It is often worse at night, when the patient is unable to find a comfortable position for the arm. If the patient continues to immobilize the limb, glenohumeral motion may be totally lost and a substitution pattern of scapulothoracic motion will prevail. Some patients will then assume that they are actually improving, since the joint is no longer as painful. They subconsciously alter their pattern of use to accommodate the restriction. Most patients, however, retain enough glenohumeral motion to prevent comfortable function. When the limited ranges of motion of the shoulder are exceeded, pain may radiate down the arm over the C6 dermatome and proximally up the trapezius to the neck. There may be numbness or tingling down the arm to the hand, all of which may mimic discogenic radiculopathy at C6. When the pain is severe, the biceps reflex may be observed to be depressed, adding further confusion with the cervical disc. However, in the frozen shoulder the pain is not reproduced or made worse by motions of the cervical spine, but by attempts to move the glenohumeral joint. Radiation of the pain to the hand involves the dorsum and all the fingers, rather than specifically the radial side of the hand or to the base of the thumb. True motor weakness is absent.

TREATMENT

Therapy should be based on the stage of the disease. In the acute, or "freezing" stage, the shoulder responds poorly to all the usual forms of treatment, including manipulations, injections, anti-inflammatory medications, heat, rest, liniments, ultrasound, diathermy, acupuncture, and sometimes physical therapy. Patients may become emotionally depressed and exhausted. They are often accused of "not working hard enough" at physical therapy but find that the harder they work, the tighter their shoulder becomes. They are driven by their doctors, their therapists, their spouses, and their employers to "work harder and not let the shoulder freeze." These pa-

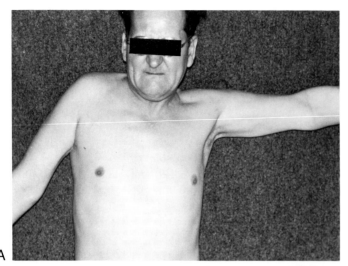

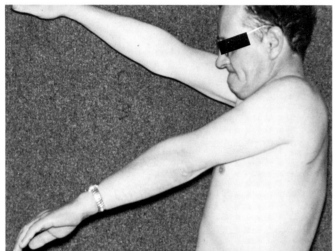

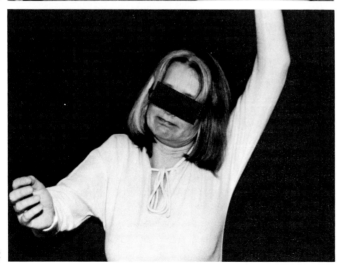

Fig. 6-36. (**A** and **B**) A 45-year-old man in the "freezing" phase of his right shoulder. Note the distress and discouragement in his face. (**C**) A 40-year-old woman in the "frozen" phase of her right shoulder. Again, note the expression of fatigue and pain.

tients may develop a true "guilt complex." They do not understand why they are not improving and wonder whether they will ever get well. Some of them even suspect that they may have cancer.

Many of these patients, when they are first seen and have had an opportunity to talk for a while, break down completely. They express hopelessness because they feel that no one understands, and they can no longer bear the burden. In most cases, no one has calmly explained to them the cause and nature of their problem or its natural history and what to expect. Once the patient has had a reassuring explanation and assurances that the shoulder will improve with time, they are able to bear the pain and begin to relax. It is also most important to convey that they have an inherent capacity to improve with time and their own efforts, and can begin to assume responsibility for the healing process rather than being subjected to treatments dictated by other people. This change of attitude is striking.

Some years ago when Dr. Rowe was in charge of the Shoulder Clinic at the Massachusetts General Hospital, routine treatment was manipulation and forceful physical therapy. The aim was to "keep the shoulder from freezing." Over the years, it became apparent that this form of treatment did not seem to shorten the course of the syndrome, and often seemed to make the patient worse. As we were not helping these patients, it was obvious that we did not understand the natural history of adhesive capsulitis. Some unanswered questions came to mind: "How long would the syndrome last if we did nothing?" "Since forceful exercises and manipulation were painful, were they necessary?"

For answers, we selected a number of patients and observed them *without* any form of treatment, except for pain medication as needed and a sedative at night, so that they would get adequate rest. They were, however, encouraged to use the arm as normally as possible. To our surprise, these patients fared better than those we were treating and trying to keep their shoulders from "freezing."[3] On the basis of these patients, we realized that the natural history of frozen shoulder consisted of three distinct phases: the freezing phase: $+/-$ 4 months; the frozen phase: $+/-$ 4 months; and, the thawing phase: $+/-$ 4 months.

Although, in general, these patients took approximately a year to go through the cycle, they all recovered completely. They were helped greatly during this time by *knowing* they would get better and that there was medication to help them.

Freezing Phase

Treatment must be highly individualized and based on the stage of the disease. The freezing phase is a reactive phase. For the patient with an acutely and globally painful shoulder, physical therapy in the form of exercise will only cause additional discomfort. There may be little to do but provide comfort by means of a sling for a limited time along with appropriate analgesics. Because sleep is disturbed, a selected sedative is useful as well. The transcutaneous nerve stimulator may be of use in this phase and later stages of treatment.[34] There is no proof that systemic steroids are more effective than nonsteroidal anti-inflammatory agents, which may have a place in therapy here with the additional benefit that they have an analgesic effect. Shoulders in our clinic that were manipulated in the freezing phase were apt to freeze again with prolongation of the syndrome and, in some instances, permanent damage. We have seen several patients in whom repeated manipulations had been carried out in the reactive phase, and their shoulders became permanently stiff, one with a cowl of myositis ossificans completely encircling the glenohumeral joint.

The technique of arthroscopy in the early or freezing phase as recommended by Johnson,[17] with "simple lavage followed by intraarticular injection of cortisone without manipulation" is encouraging.

Frozen Phase

In the frozen phase, although the shoulder becomes tighter, the pain becomes less and the patient is more comfortable. If patients are seen for the first time during this phase, having received their treatment elsewhere, it is most important to be certain that the diagnosis is correct. As stated, other conditions may mimic frozen shoulder; unrecognized chronic posterior dislocation and even neoplasm may occasionally be discovered. The value of the arthrogram has already been commented upon.[28]

The patient should be seen regularly, once a month, and encouraged to use the arm within the limit of range of comfort. If the limb is neglected or overprotected, the patient risks developing all of the clinical features of "shoulder–hand syndrome."[13] Not all patients with frozen shoulders develop dystrophic hands, although some do. There appears to be a significant overlap between these two entities and reflex sympathetic dystrophy, which may complicate and considerably prolong the recovery from frozen shoulder. These patients may be considerably benefitted by treatment with stellate ganglion blocks. The technique of continuous blockade has proved to be extremely effective in reversing this part of the clinical complex, although the insertion of the catheter requires hospitalization for approximately 1 week. During this time, intensive, supervised, and active rather than passive exercise is performed. The recent experience has been summarized by Linson and coworkers.[18]

Thawing Phase

During this phase, patients report that the motion of the shoulder gradually returns. They are optimistic and confident of recovery. The pain is no longer disturbing. They are carefully instructed to carry out gentle pendulum exercises and stretching on a regular basis during the day. They are encouraged to take their arms through a range of motion that they can tolerate, without force. This is emphasized also by Post[31] and Lundberg.[22] It is important that forceful exercise be avoided. Patients are encouraged and reassured that the condition is self-limited and that they *will* get well. (Fig. 6-37) They are encouraged to continue with their jobs and to use the extremity, even though motion is limited. Not all patients require formal physical therapy, although some do. Much of the thrust of the therapist's activities is educational and directed at correcting abnormal shoulder girdle mechanics. Because of the often long period of glenohumeral restriction of motion, the substitution of scapulothoracic motion becomes a difficult pattern to discard. The therapist can be very helpful in this regard, and patients can be taught to appreciate when their scapulae are moving abnormally. Patients are extremely relieved when they understand the nature of their problem. They do not become depressed or discouraged nearly as easily. In general, the less aggressive the physical therapy, and the more naturally the patient uses the arm within the range of comfort,

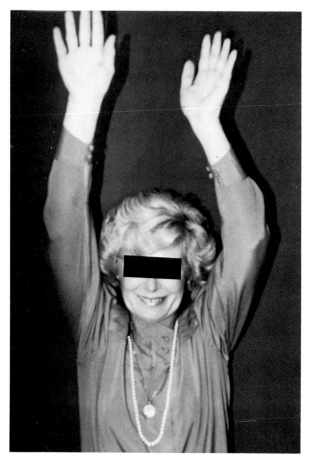

Fig. 6-37. The "thawing" or recovery phase. This patient did not receive manipulations, physical therapy, or injections: only gentle stretching and use of her shoulder as tolerated, which she carried on at home. "You told me in a year I would be perfectly all right. I am!"

the shorter the period of pain and limited motion.

In an attempt to assess the efficacy of the various conservative means of management of frozen shoulder, a prospective study is presently being conducted in the Physical Therapy Department of the Massachusetts General Hospital. This is comparing the results of treatment with formal and regular physical therapy and a home program of "as natural use as possible" by patients with range of motion exercises as tolerated.

There is wide variation in the management of frozen shoulder.[37] Grey[14] evaluated 21 patients with 25 frozen shoulders. Treatment was limited to reassurance and occasional analgesics. No attempts were made to keep the shoulder from freezing. Forceful physical therapy or manipulation was not used. Twenty-four of the 25 shoulders returned to normal within 2 years of the onset of symptoms. Both DePalma[10] and Post[31] managed their frozen shoulders in a similar manner. A careful study of their treatment is recommended.

Of all the considerations of treatment of the patient with a frozen shoulder, closed manipulation is undoubtedly the most controversial. Even among those who are committed to manipulation, there is disagreement as to whether it is most effective if done within the first 6 months or second 6 months following the onset of symptoms. Haines and Hargadon[15] reported in 1982 on 78 cases of frozen shoulder treated by primary manipulation and steroid injection and concluded that the method was safe, satisfactory, and effective. Eighty-three percent of patients so treated had a full range of pain-free movement during 8 weeks of the manipulation. Charnley[8] in 1959 stated "While I have not been able to prove my own belief that early manipulation of the shoulder speeds up the process of rehabilitation, I consider that I have established that the bad reputation of early manipulation is without foundation." Lloyd-Roberts and French[21] in 1959 reported encouraging results, as did Neviaser[27] and Reeves.[33] Lloyd-Roberts and French compared two groups, one receiving manipulation, and the other not. At 6 months, 44 percent of the nonmanipulated group had good results, whereas 67 percent of those with manipulation had good results. Reeves reported that 66 percent of patients following manipulation had good results at 6 months. However, Hazelman[16] reported no difference in a prospective study comparing steroid injections, physical therapy, and manipulation. Murnayhan[26] believed that manipulative treatment shortened the time "during which the shoulder range of motion is extremely decreased. It does not, however, appear to shorten the overall course of the disease." Lundberg's experience[22] was similar.

The mechanism by which manipulation produces release of the contracted structures has been documented by Neviaser,[27] McLaughlin,[24,25] as well as Lundberg.[22] The snapping that one hears during manipulation is not, as one might assume, usually "adhesions being torn," but often the contracted inferior capsule of the glenohumeral joint rupturing in those cases that regain motion. In some, the subscapularis

as well as other structures may tear. Neviaser has performed delayed arthrograms to show reconstitution and normalization of the capsule in patients who regain their motion following manipulative rupture.[28] The potential and reported complications of manipulation under anesthesia include fractures and dislocations of the humerus, ruptures of the rotator cuff, increased inflammation and scarring, and even radial palsy. If manipulation is done, it must be carefully performed with particular attention to avoid dislocation. No attempt should be made to increase medial rotation, since the supra- and infraspinatus would be at risk of rupture.

The decision for manipulation should, we believe, be made in the late frozen or early thawing phase. We have not, however, used this modality within the last 13 years. DePalma[10] in 1952 stated "Manipulation of frozen shoulders is a dangerous and futile procedure," and both he and McLaughlin[25] independently recommended open release of contracted structures that did not respond to conservative therapy. MacNab,[23] reporting on the then "Current Status of the Frozen Shoulder" to the 1982 Meeting of the American Shoulder and Elbow Surgeons, advised initial conservative treatment but "If despite a well-supervised physiotherapy program it is impossible to restore useful range of movement to the shoulder, then a more aggressive approach may have to be employed, including hydraulic distention, manipulation under general anesthesia, or surgical release of the contracted structures." If one does choose open release, a number of structures may require incision, including a hypertrophied coracohumeral ligament, a portion of the subscapularis, and capsule. It is essential that patients follow an active mobilization program immediately following the surgery lest the gains in range of motion be lost.

The remaining mode of treatment, that of hydraulic distention, is a serendipitous consequence of diagnostic arthrography, and may actually increase motion by stretching or even rupturing the capsule if sufficient volume and pressure are applied.[1,2,20] This may explain Johnson's encouraging results of rapid mobilization following early "simple lavage" (by arthroscopy) followed by intraarticular injection of cortisone without manipulation or physical therapy.[17]

Although this is usually a "self-limited" disease, it is by no means benign. We have defined the natural course of the disease and the three definite stages of freezing, frozen, and thawing (Fig. 6-35). We caution against too aggressive therapy, which in some instances may prove worse than the disease. Several patients we have seen, who "did not respond" to manipulation (sometimes repeated), and long sessions of physical therapy, were finally found to have unrecognized a chronic (unreduced) posterior dislocations of the shoulder. This can very easily mimic "frozen" shoulder, as AP views are usually interpreted as normal. A good rule is that if the patient does not improve, take a true axillary view of the shoulder.

REFERENCES

1. Andren L, Lundberg BJ: Treatment of rigid shoulders by joint distention during arthrography. Acta Orthop Scand 36:45, 1965
2. Annexton M: Arthrography can help free frozen shoulder. JAMA 241:9, 1979
3. Aufranc OE, Barr JS, Rowe CR: The upper extremity. In The American Academy of Orthopaedic Surgeons, Instructional Course Lectures. 14:118–119, J.W. Edwards, Ann Arbor, Michigan, 1957
4. Bateman JE: The Shoulder and Neck, 2nd ed. WB Saunders, Philadelphia, 1978
5. Bridgeman JF: Periarthritis of the shoulder and diabetes mellitus. Ann Rheum Dis 31:69, 1972
6. Bulgen DY, Hazelman B, Ward M, McCallem M: Immunological studies in frozen shoulder. Ann Rheum Dis 37:135, 1978
7. Bulgen DY, Hazelman B, Ward M, McCallem M: Immunological studies in frozen shoulder. J Rheum 91:883, 1982
8. Charnley J: Periarthritis of the shoulder. Postgrad Med J 35:384, 1959
9. Codman EA: The Shoulder. R.E. Kreiger, Malabar, Florida, 1984
10. DePalma AF: Loss of scapulohumeral motion (frozen shoulder). Ann Surg 135:193, 1952
11. DePalma AF: Surgery of the Shoulder, 3rd edition. JB Lippincott, Philadelphia, 1983
12. Duplay S: De la periarthrite scapulo-humerale. Rev Prat Trav Med 53:226–227, 1896
13. Edeiken J, Wolferth CC: Persistent pain in the shoulder region following myocardial infarction. Am J Med Sci 191:201, 1936
14. Grey RG: Frozen shoulder. J Bone Joint Surg 60A:564, 1978
15. Haines JF, Hargadon EJ: Manipulation as the primary treatment of the frozen shoulder. JR Coll Surg Edinb 27:5, 1982
16. Hazelman BL: The painful stiff shoulder. Rheum Phys Med 11:413, 1972
17. Johnson LL: Arthroscopy of the shoulder. Orthop Clin North Am (2):197, 1980
18. Linson M, Leffert RD, Todd D: The treatment of upper extremity reflex sympathetic dystrophy with prolonged continuous stellate ganglion blockade. J Hand Surg 8:153, 1983
19. Lippmann RK: Frozen shoulder, periarthritis, bicipital tenosynovitis. Arch Surg 47:283, 1943
20. Lloyd GJ, McIntyre JL, Older MWJ: The treatment of shoulder stiffness by hydrostatic manipulation. J Bone Joint Surg 60A:564, 1978
21. Lloyd-Roberts GC, French PR: Periarthritis of the shoulder. Br Med J 20:1569, 1959
22. Lundberg BJ: The frozen shoulder—clinical and radiographical observation. The effect of manipulation under general anesthesia. Structure and glucosaminoglycan content of the joint capsule. Acta Orthop Scand Suppl 119:1, 1969
23. MacNab I: Frozen shoulder—current status. Orthop Trans 7:137, 1983
24. McLaughlin HL: On the "frozen shoulder." Bull Hosp Joint Dis 12:383, 1951
25. McLaughlin HL: The "frozen shoulder." Clin Orthop 20:126, 1961
26. Murnayhan JP: Adhesive capsulitis of the shoulder. p. 154. In Surgery of the Shoulder. BC Decker, Philadelphia, 1984
27. Neviaser JS: Adhesive capsulitis of the shoulder. A study of the pathological findings in periarthritis of the shoulder. J Bone Joint Surg 27:211, 1945
28. Neviaser JS: Arthrography of the Shoulder. Charles C. Thomas, Springfield, Il, 1975
29. Neviaser JS: Adhesive capsulitis and the stiff and painful shoulder. Orthop Clin North Am 11:327, 1980
30. Pasteur F: Les algies de lepaule et la physiotherapie de la teno-bursites bicipitale. J Radiol Electrol 16:419, 1932
31. Post M: The Shoulder—Surgical and Nonsurgical Management. Lea & Febiger, Philadelphia, 1978
32. Putnam JJ: The treatment of a form of painful periarthritis of the shoulder. Boston Med Surg J 107:536, 1882
33. Reeves B: Arthrographic changes in frozen and post traumatic stiff shoulders. Proc R Soc Med 59:827, 1966
34. Rizk TE, Christopher RP, Pinals RS et al: Adhesive capsulitis (frozen shoulder): a new approach to its management. Arch Phys Med Rehabil 64 (1):29, 1983
35. Seignalet J, Sany J, Caillens JP, Lapinski H: Lack of association between HLA-B27 and frozen shoulder. Tissue Antigens 18:364, 1981

36. Simmons, FA: Shoulder pain with particular reference to the frozen shoulder. J Bone Joint Surg 31B:462, 1949

37. Stein I: Managing frozen shoulder syndrome. Orthop Rev 5:92, 1976

38. Van der Korst JK, Colenbrander H, Cats A: Phenobarbital and the shoulder-hand syndrome. Ann Rheum Dis 25:553, 1966

39. Wiley AM, Older WJ: Shoulder arthroscopy. Am J Sports Med 8:31, 1980

Dislocations of the Shoulder

7

Carter R. Rowe

More progress has been made in the evaluation and treatment of instabilities of the shoulder since the mid-1960s than in any previous time in history.

Prior to this time, except in a few exceptions, all dislocations were considered the same, their pathologic basis was assumed to be the same, and their treatment was, unfortunately, the same. In the 1960s, variations from the usual types of dislocation were being identified:

In 1969, the author reported on the "atraumatic" dislocation and subluxation, to differentiate it from the common traumatic dislocation.[118] Previously, Gallie[50] had referred to a small group of patients whose recurrent dislocation occurred "without traumatism," and Platt had been concerned with the absence of the Bankart lesion at surgery occasionally seen as pointed out by Osmond-Clarke.[104]

In 1969, Blazina and Satzman published their experience with recurrent transient subluxation as a distinct type of shoulder instability in athletes.[14] Since then a number of authors have confirmed their findings[11,97,110,113] and added variations of the transient syndrome.[124]

In 1973, the author, with Pierce and Clark, published an in-depth study of the voluntary dislocation syndrome, in which it was demonstrated that patients were able to subluxate their shoulders with voluntary muscle control.[122] Although voluntary dislocations had been referred to in the past (see below, Dislocations), no thorough study had been made of the syndrome in relation to the combination of the voluntary muscle force–couples control responsible for the shoulder disorder. Another significant finding in this study was that a small but significant number of these patients suffered from personality and psychiatric problems, which markedly influenced their response to treatment.

In 1980, Neer and Foster[97] drew our attention to another variant of shoulder instability: patients with ligament laxity of the shoulders of the atraumatic, or of the voluntary, group whose shoulders became unstable from repeated subluxations or dislocations. Frequently, they were unstable in more than one direction, or "multidirectional." Neer has referred to this group as "involuntary" dislocators, to differentiate them from the voluntary group.

Thus, at the present time, there are five distinct types of shoulder instability, rather than a single type (Table 7-1).

In addition to the different types of dislocations,

Table 7-1. The Five Categories of Shoulder Instabilities

I. Traumatic
    Traumatic injury
	IV. Transient subluxation
	    ("Dead arm" syndrome)
	    Forceful overextension of arm in elevation

II. Atraumatic Functional incidence	

III. Voluntary
    Patient's muscle control
	V. Involuntary subluxation
	    Instability due to chronic laxity of capsule
	    Multidirectional±

Table 7-2. Instabilities of the Shoulder

Five Categories	Six Causative Lesions
1. Traumatic	Capsule
2. Atraumatic	1. Avulsion from rim (Bankart lesion)
3. Transient	2. Excessive Laxity
4. Voluntary	Bone
5. Involuntary	3. Hill-Sachs lesion
	4. Fracture glenoid rim
	5. Variations in glenoid tilt
	Muscle
	6. Rupture

Note: there is no one "essential" lesion.

six different causative factors or "essential" lesions associated with instability of the shoulder have been identified (Table 7-2).

HISTORICAL REVIEW

Dislocation of the shoulder is one of our earliest injuries. The wall paintings of Egyptian tombs from as early as 3,000 B.C. attest to this, with accurate drawings of manipulations to reduce the dislocated shoulder. These appear similar to the present Kocher method.[64] It is interesting to read the accounts of Brockbrank and Griffith[24] of the various and ingenious methods used in the past to reduce the dislocated shoulder, some of which, unfortunately, resulted in major injury to the arm, and, at times, to the entire person.

With the beginning of Olympic games in 776 B.C., more attention must have been given to the vulnerable shoulder joint. Hippocrates[61] in the 4th century B.C. records some of the problems of instability of the shoulder and devised methods of closed reduction using either the fist or heel in the axilla as a fulcrum to reduce the dislocation. He is credited also with the first surgical procedure to correct recurrent anterior dislocations. Red hot irons, "which are not too thick, nor much rounded," are inserted into the anterior inferior structures of the shoulder (he must have had hardy patients), eliminating recurrence by means of scar tissue, or cicatrix. Although he did not record the complications, he did warn against injury to "the glands of the axilla, for this would be attended with great danger, as they are adjacent to the most important nerves." Hippocrates' technique must have been superb. It is interesting that he not only recognized the usual traumatic dislocation but also indicated that some patients could "dislocate their joints without pain, and reduce them in like manner." Perhaps these were voluntary dislocators. We must also credit Hippocrates with recognition of the chronic "unreduced" dislocation of the shoulder: "when attempts to reduce a dislocated shoulder have failed—whatever acts are performed or by carrying the arm around by their side."

Little attention was given to the shoulder, or, in fact, to the patient, during the Dark Ages. It was not until the 18th and 19th centuries that easier and less traumatic methods were devised to reduce shoulder dislocations. White[4] in 1764 and Cooper[31] in 1824 found that the shoulder could be reduced with the arm in abduction and elevation. Cooper also recognized posterior as well as anterior dislocations. The Kocher[68] method introduced in 1870 proved to be effective but required more muscular relaxation to reduce the shoulder than suspension or elevation procedures as demonstrated by Stimpson in 1907[134] and by Milch[86] in 1938.

Broca and Hartman[23] in 1890 and Ricard in 1894[112] were the first surgeons since Hippocrates to attempt capsulorrhaphy or a surgical repair for recurrent dislocations of the shoulder. With the advent of sterile surgical technique and anesthesia, numerous operative procedures were reported. The evolution of pathology and treatment of recurrent dislocations of the shoulder is interesting. Flower[46] in 1861 described the humeral head defect, which was reported 79 years

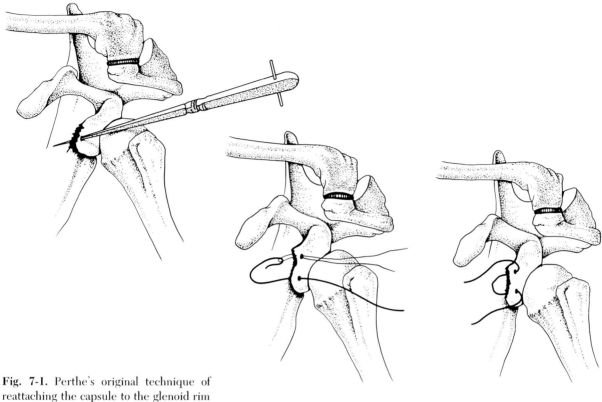

Fig. 7-1. Perthe's original technique of reattaching the capsule to the glenoid rim (1906). (Moseley HF: Shoulder Lesions. ES Livingstone, Edinburgh, 1969.)

later by Hill and Sachs.[58] Caird in 1887 also described the humeral head defect as well as the detached labrum and capsule.[25] Broca and Hartman in 1890 confirmed the findings of detachment of the anterior labrum and capsule from the glenoid rim, and first suggested that recurrent dislocations were intracapsular. They also described the bony defect of the humeral head. Although we give Bankart credit for the "Bankart repair," Perthes in 1906 was the first to suggest that the separated labrum and capsule should be reattached to the glenoid rim.[108] He demonstrated his technique using drill holes through the rim of the glenoid (Fig. 7-1). Bankart, in 1923[9] and in 1938,[10] popularized Perthes' technique and stressed the importance of corrrecting the "essential lesion" by reattaching the avulsed capsule back along the glenoid rim to rebuild support (Fig. 7-2). Many "essential lesions" and surgical techniques have developed since 1923 (see section on pathology below).

FACTS AND FIGURES

Prognosis

A number of investigators have reported interesting findings that have added to our knowledge of the natural history of the incidence of recurrent shoulder dislocations.

OVERALL INCIDENCE

Hovelius reported a 1.7 percent incidence of shoulder dislocations in the Swedish population, and a 7 percent incidence of shoulder dislocations in Swedish hockey players.[62] Simonet et al.[132] reported an incidence of 8.2 percent per 100,000 of initial traumatic shoulder dislocations in Olmsted County residents of Minnesota. Both Hovelius and Simonet reported an incidence of twice as many male as female patients.

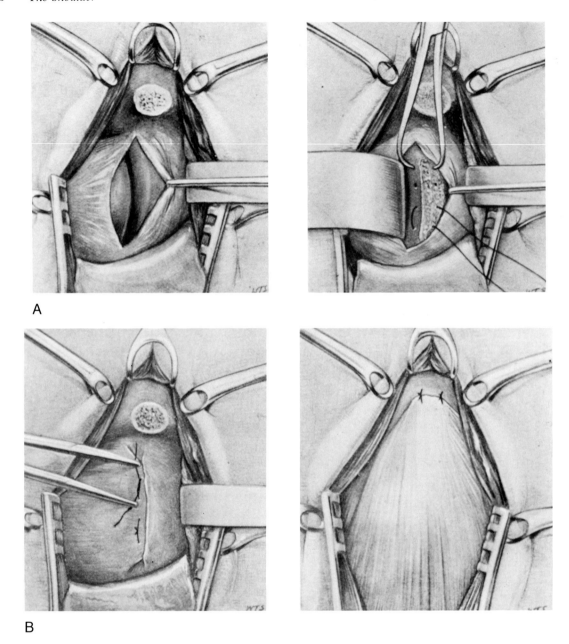

A

B

Fig. 7-2. Bankart's original repair of the capsule to the rim (1923). (Bankart ASB: Recurrent or habitual dislocation of the shoulder. Br Med J 2:1132, 1923.)

The author[117] analyzed 1603 shoulder injuries in patients admitted to the Emergency Ward of the Massachusetts General Hospital, in 1956. Five hundred (31 percent) were dislocations of the shoulder. Ninety-eight percent were anterior dislocations and 2 percent were posterior. There were 251 initial or primary dislocations in patients under 45 years of age,

and 249 initial dislocations after age 45, which are interesting figures.

Kazar and Relovszky[69] in 1969, reported an overall incidence of 27 percent recurrent shoulder dislocations following initial dislocation. Simonet's further study of 116 patients reported an overall incidence of recurrence of 66 percent, in patients under the age of 20 years. However, they found an 82 percent recurrence rate among athletes, and only 30 percent among nonathletes. In 1961, the author reported an overall incidence of shoulder recurrence of 42 percent. Our figures[123] closely parallel those of McLaughlin.[83] In our study, the recurrence rate was 94 percent under the age of 20, 72 percent between the ages of 20 and 40, and only 14 percent after the age of 40 (Table 7-3). Twenty-eight percent of these were occasional "recurrers" and 72 percent were "frequent recurrers." Seventy percent recurred within the first 2 years, 19 percent from 2 to 5 years, 6 percent from 5 to 10 years, and 5 percent from 10 to 20 years. Ninety-seven percent were anterior dislocations and 3 percent were posterior dislocations. Of all patients, 5.4 percent had suffered nerve injuries of the brachial plexus.

Throughout our study on the prognosis of primary dislocations of the shoulder, regardless of the many associated factors of recurrence, *the age of the patient was the most significant factor determining the incidence of recurrence* (Table 7-3). Other investigators[140,143,148] found that recurrence depended on the length of initial immobilization of the shoulder. Aronen[5] reported a lowering of the recurrence rate with a controlled rehabilitation program. This was a factor in our study, yet the age differential remained the determining factor. Henry's studies[56] are of interest. Among 121 acute traumatic dislocations of the shoulder in young athletes in his series

Of 62 immobilized shoulders, 56 (90 percent) recurred.
Of 59 not immobilized, 50 (85 percent) recurred.

He concluded that immobilization in the young athlete had little if any effect on the incidence of recurrence. An associated fracture of the greater tuberosity definitely lowered the incidence of dislocation in our series to 4.5 percent, yet those with fractures of the tuberosity had an average age of 60 years, and the expected recurrence rate in this age group was only 14 percent. The degree of initial trauma was another factor that lowered the incidence of recurrence. However, when the age of the patient was analyzed, there was a differential of 20 to 30 years between the recurrers and nonrecurrers.

There were also interesting preoperative findings in a sample of 162 initial recurrent anterior dislocations in our series.[112]

88 percent were complete anterior dislocations. Of these
86 percent were traumatic recurrent dislocators.
14 percent were atraumatic recurrent dislocators (there has been an increase of this category in recent years).
12 percent were transient anterior subluxations (this category is also on the increase).
27 percent gave a positive family history of shoulder dislocations.
12 percent were bilateral shoulder dislocations (an incidence comparable to Moseley and Overgaard's figure of 10 percent)[87]
85 percent were right-handed and 13 percent left-handed.
2 percent were ambidextrous.

Table 7-3. Age of Patient at the Time of Primary Dislocation in Relation to the Incidence of Recurrence

Age of Patient (yrs)	Number of Primary Dislocations	Number of Recurrences	Incidence of Recurrences (%)
1–10	4	4	100
11–20	49	46	94
21–30	64	51	79
31–40	16	8	50
41–50	33	8	24
51–60	63	9	14
61–70	50	8	16
71–80	32	2	6
81–90	10	0	0
	321	136	42
Total shoulders (3 bilateral cases)	324		
Under 20 years			94
20–40 years			74
Over 40 years			14

(Rowe CR, Sakellarides HT: Factors related to recurrences of anterior dislocation of the shoulder. Clin Orthop 20, 1961.)

CLASSIFICATION (TABLE 7-1)

Traumatic Dislocation

This is the most common type, and is usually the result of a direct or indirect traumatic injury. A high incidence of traumatic lesions are present consisting of avulsion of capsule and labrum from the glenoid rim (Bankart lesion), trauma to the glenoid rim, Hill-Sachs lesions of the humeral head, and secondary laxity of the joint capsule.

This category has a predictable response to surgical repair and a less predictable response to resistive exercises.

SUBGROUPS

1. Traumatic chronic unreduced dislocation. Dislocation that has been unreduced for 3 or more weeks.
2. Luxatio erecta (inferior dislocation)

Atraumatic Dislocation or Subluxation

The causative factor is a functional shoulder motion, or stress, of the arm as in excessive throwing, pitching, swimming, or serving in tennis.

There is a lower incidence of traumatic lesions in this group.

There is a higher incidence of generalized laxity of capsule and joint.

Good response to a program of resistive exercises is seen. This should be tried before deciding on surgery.

Voluntary Dislocation or Subluxation

This is produced by voluntary suppression of selected motor-couples of the shoulder and activation of others. There are two categories of voluntary subluxators.

SUBTYPE I

These patients have "normal" personalities and are helpful and cooperative in their treatment. They have an excellent response to a program of specific resitive exercises, and explanation of the syndrome to the patient and family. Some of the group who have ceased actively dislocating their shoulder but have experienced secondary laxity of the joint capsule and muscle may be considered "involuntary" subluxators (see below).

SUBTYPE II

These patients have emotional or psychiatric disturbances and use their ability to subluxate or dislocate their shoulders at will for gainful purposes. These patients have an extremely poor response to surgical procedures.

Traumatic Recurrent Transient Subluxation

This is the result of forceful hyperextension of arm, a direct blow to the elevated shoulder, or excessive repetitive elevation and external rotation of the arm as in serving in tennis or pitching. The patient may be aware, or unaware, of the subluxation. It is commonly referred to as the *dead arm* syndrome.

Patients have a fair response to exercises and a predictable response to surgical repair.

Involuntary Dislocation or Subluxation

The capsule and ligament of the shoulder in some voluntary and atraumatic dislocations will become overstretched and lax from repeated subluxations, or dislocations will occur merely from the position of the arm, without voluntary action of the muscles. This is termed *involuntary* instability. These may be multidirectional (unstable anterior, posterior, or inferior)

This group of patients has a good response to specific resistive exercises, and a good response to specific surgical procedures when indicated.

SUBGROUP I

Paralytic subluxation may be considered under the *involuntary* group, as it results from intrinsic passive laxity of the supporting structures.

All of the five groups may be *acute* or *recurrent, anterior,* or *posterior.*

EXAMINATION

History

Specific information should be obtained on the following:

1. The mechanism of initial injury (traumatic, atraumatic, voluntary).

2. The position of the dislocated arm (locked in external rotation or in internal rotation).
3. The ease or difficulty of reduction.
4. The mechanism of recurrence (the activity and position of the arm prior to recurrence).
5. The length and type of immobilization of the shoulder following the initial dislocation.
6. Signs and symptoms of nerve injury.
7. The extent of the patient's physical limitations. Is the patient satisfied to leave the shoulder as it is?

Physical Examination

One should note the following:

1. The general laxity of the patient's joints, including the fingers (Fig. 7-3), elbows, and knees.
2. A concise check of the motor and sensory deficits, areas of atrophy, weakness, or numbness.
3. Circulation of the arm (radial pulse) in positions of neutral, in elevation, and external rotation.
4. The patient should demonstrate the positions they avoid or in which they are apprehensive.
5. Testing positions for instability (discussed below).

ANTERIOR INSTABILITY

Standing

The patient avoids, or is apprehensive, when the arm is elevated and externally rotated, such as the position of throwing, serving in tennis, or swimming overhand (Fig. 7-4A). The examiner should raise the patient's arm in complete elevation, extension, and some external rotation. At the same time, pressure is applied posteriorly to the humeral head (Fig. 7-4B,C). With anterior instability of the shoulder, the patient registers apprehension and may quickly drop the shoulder. In marked instability, the patient may refuse to put the arm in this position for fear that the shoulder might dislocate. This is known as the "apprehension" test.

POSTERIOR INSTABILITY

The arm is placed in forward flexion of 90° in internal rotation and some adduction (Fig. 7-5). The arm is directed posteriorly. Adducting the arm may increase posterior instability.

Standing

With the patient standing in forward flexion of 45° with the arms relaxed, pointing toward the floor, the

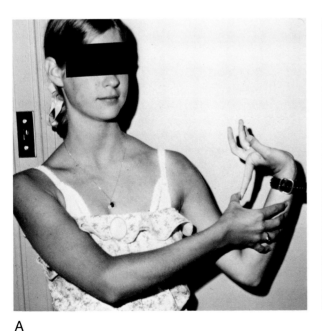

A

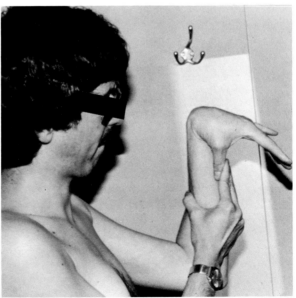

B

Fig. 7-3. Hyperextension of the fingers is a good indicator of generalized ligament laxity. (**A**) Moderate laxity. (**B**) Severe laxity.

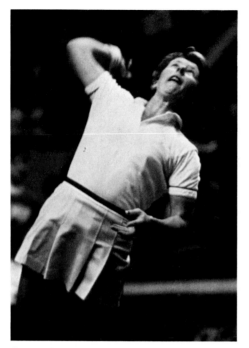

A

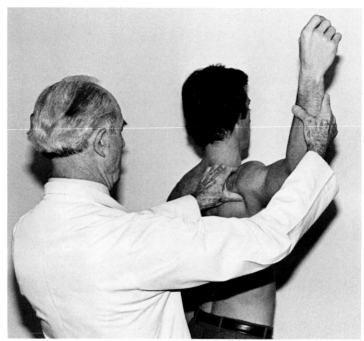

B

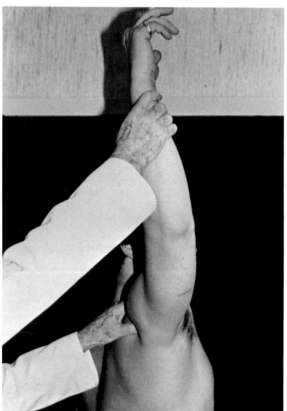

C

Fig. 7-4. The apprenhension test for *anterior* instability. (**A**) This represents the position in which the patient states "my arm goes dead" when serving in tennis or throwing. (**B**) The arm is elevated in external rotation with pressure applied posteriorly to the humeral head. (**C**) The arm may be slightly extended in this position.

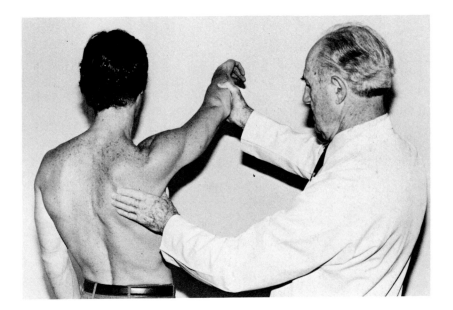

Fig. 7-5. For posterior shoulder instability, the arm is raised in forward flexion and pronation and some adduction.

arm is pulled down slightly. Pressure is applied posteriorly to the humeral head with some extension of the arm for anterior instability (Fig. 7-6A), for posterior instability (Fig. 7-6B), pressure is anteriorly to the humeral head in slight flexion or directly down for inferior instability (Fig. 7-6C). This a very sensitive test: tł.e patient is able to completely relax the shoulder, bending forward with hands pointing to the floor, which we find is far more effective than in the sitting position.

Supine

It is helpful to have the patient near the edge of the examining table, with the examiner supporting the patient's arm under his or her own arm. This leaves both hands free to manipulate the shoulder anteriorly, posteriorly, or inferiorly. This can easily be accomplished by grasping the shoulder with one hand to stabilize it. The other hand can put posterior or anterior pressure on the humeral head (Fig. 7-7A, B). Pulling down gently on the arm aids in producing instability. A third maneuver is to have the patient place one hand behind the head, as one would relax at night, and apply pressure posteriorly to the humeral head, while extending the arm slightly (Fig. 7-7C).

Prone

Have the patient face down near the edge of the examining table, allowing the arm to "hang" over the edge of the table. In this position, anterior, posterior, or downward pressure can be applied to the arm. Gerber and Ganz[52] illustrate very clearly their method of examining the shoulder for instability.

PATHOLOGIC BASIS FOR RECURRENT DISLOCATIONS

It is evident that much of the confusion and controversy over the specific pathologic basis of recurrent dislocations of the shoulder, and the "causative factors," are due to the lack of careful layer-by-layer dissection of the tissues of the shoulder *at the time of surgical repair.* Theories on the pathologic basis of instability must be based on living, functioning tissue. Dissection of tissue at autopsy, or fixed tissues of a cadaver, will *not* reveal the laxity of the capsule, muscle trauma, or labral instability of fresh tissue. When careful dissection is carried out at surgery, the

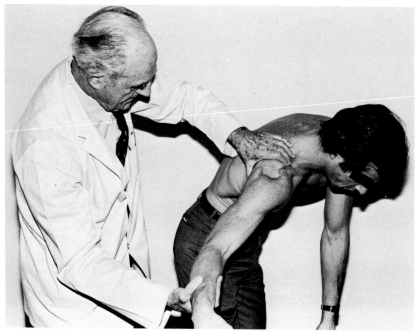

A

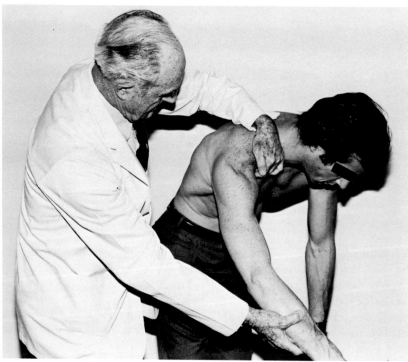

B

Fig. 7-6. Anterior, posterior, and inferior instabilities can also be effectively tested by having the patient lean forward with arms pointing to the floor. (A) For anterior instability. (B) For posterior instability. (*Figure continues.*)

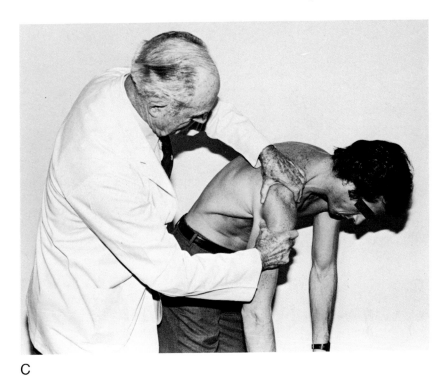

Fig. 7-6 (*Continued*). (**C**) For inferior instability.

C

surgeon will note *more than one "essential"* lesion, related to shoulder instability. Each pathologic lesion should be recognized and steps taken to correct all of them, to restore the important "balance" to the coordinated muscular action of the shoulder.

For instance, the surgeon who transplants the subscapularis muscle and leaves unrecognized and uncorrected a large Bankart lesion along the rim of the glenoid, has left a major defect unrepaired. The surgeon who corrects a Bankart lesion, yet leaves unrecognized and unrepaired a redundant overstretched capsule or rupture of the capsule from the neck of the humerus, has not returned maximum stability to the shoulder. The surgeon who recognizes neither of these lesions, and cuts through muscle and capsule, relying on scar tissue and limited motion of the shoulder to provide stability, falls short in restoring stability to the shoulder. Transplanting muscles through muscle, may upset the delicate functional balance of the shoulder.

The various pathologic lesions may be categorized into three areas (Fig. 7-8):

1. Capsular lesions
2. Muscular lesions (not in figure)
3. Bony lesions

Capsular Lesions

There are three lesions of the capsule:

1. Rupture of the capsule and labrum from the rim of the glenoid (the Bankart Lesion)
2. Rupture of capsule from the humeral neck
3. Excessive laxity of capsule secondary to repeated injury

THE BANKART LESION

The majority of investigators agree that the most common lesion accounting for recurrent dislocation and subluxations of the shoulder is loss of stability along the rim of the glenoid, due to avulsion of the capsule and labrum from the rim, better known as

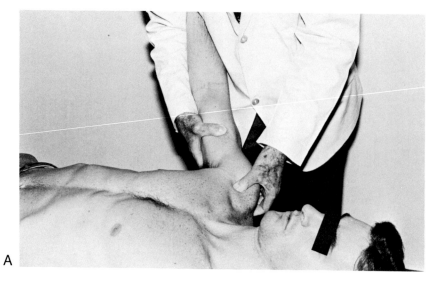

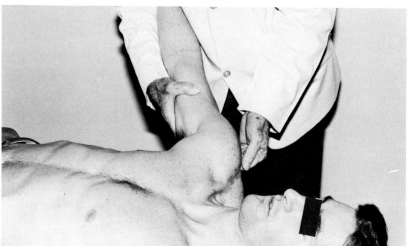

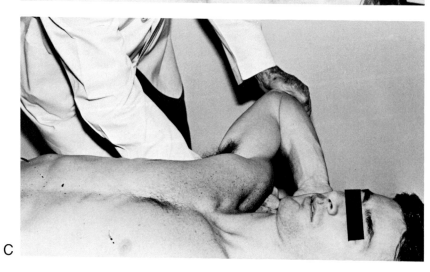

Fig. 7-7. With the patient supine supporting the arm, near the edge of the examining table. (**A**) Apply gentle pull to the arm and downward pressure to the humeral head for posterior instability. (**B**) Posterior upward pressure is applied for anterior instability. (**C**) Extending the arm over the clenched fist will also indicate anterior instability.

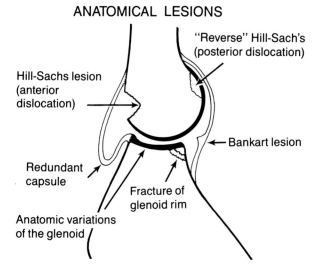

ANATOMICAL LESIONS

"Reverse" Hill-Sach's (posterior dislocation)

Hill-Sachs lesion (anterior dislocation)

Bankart lesion

Redundant capsule

Fracture of glenoid rim

Anatomic variations of the glenoid

Fig. 7-8. Outline of the anatomic lesions producing instability of the shoulder. The muscular lesions are not shown.

"the Bankart lesion"[18] (Fig. 7-9A). Bankart considered avulsion of the capsule and labrum to be the "essential" lesion. Rather than the "essential" lesion, we suggest that the Bankart lesion be considered the "most common" causative lesion of recurrent dislocations of the shoulder. Avulsion of the capsule from the glenoid rim was noted early by Caird[25] in 1887, then by Broca and Hartman[23] in 1890, and Perthes[108] in 1906. It was later popularized by Bankart[9] in 1923. We have classified the Bankart lesion into four types (Fig. 7-10).

The incidence of the Bankart lesion in our follow-up series was 85 percent in traumatic recurrent dislocations,[121] 64 percent in recurrent transient subluxations,[124] and 84 percent in patients reoperated upon for previous failed surgical procedures.[126] The lesion was *absent* in voluntary dislocators and in the majority of "atraumatic" and "involuntary" recurrent dislocations. Magnuson[76] thought that the capsule had little to do with holding the humeral head onto the glenoid. However, the large majority of investigators recognize the avulsed capsule and labrum as the most common and most important cause of shoulder instability.

EXCESSIVE LAXITY OF THE CAPSULE

An abnormal redundancy was present in 28 percent of our traumatic recurrences, in 26 percent of transient subluxations, and in 86 percent of failed surgical procedures. It was present in all of the voluntary subluxators in our series.[122] The degree of redundancy is determined at surgery with the shoulder in complete external rotation (Fig. 7-10). If the capsule can be elevated 0.5 cm, it is considered mildly lax; if it can be lifted 1 cm, it is considered moderately lax; and if it can be lifted beyond 1 cm, it is severely lax. We consider capsular laxity one of the essential lesions, or causative factors, in shoulder instability.

Rupture through the capsule was present in 3 percent of the traumatic dislocations. In 14 percent, the labrum was displaced into the joint, as a bucket handle split (Fig. 7-9B,C).

Muscle Lesions

Although some investigators consider a pathologic condition of the subscapularis muscle as the primary cause of shoulder instability,[37,79,137] we found a rather low incidence of injury to the subscapularis muscle per se, as did Adams.[1] In our series of 158 shoulders operated on for recurrent anterior dislocation, the subscapularis muscle was considered normal in 83 percent.[121] The muscle was "attenuated" or "inadequate" in 10 percent, and ruptured in 7 percent (Fig. 7-12A).

In the past year, we have observed two unusual muscle lesions associated with recurrent anterior dislocations. Both were avulsions of the insertion of the capsule and subscapularis tendon from its attachment along the lesser tuberosity of the humerus. In one the entire attachment was ruptured off the lesser tuberosity and infolded under the body of the subscapularis muscle into the joint (Fig. 7-12B). In the other, the attachment of the subscapularis and capsule was ruptured off the lesser tuberosity and neck of the humerus with the long head of biceps tendon displaced into the joint (Fig. 7-12C). Nicola[100] in 1942 and Fahey and DeCosola[45] in 1942 reported instances in which the capsule was noted to be avulsed from the neck of the humerus and considered it one of the causative factors of instability. In both of our cases the attachment of the subscapularis and capsule was repaired back to the lesser tuberosity and neck, following which a standard Bankart procedure was carried out, repairing two large Bankart lesions. We emphasize again the importance of thorough exposure of the subscapularis muscle and capsule and its proxi-

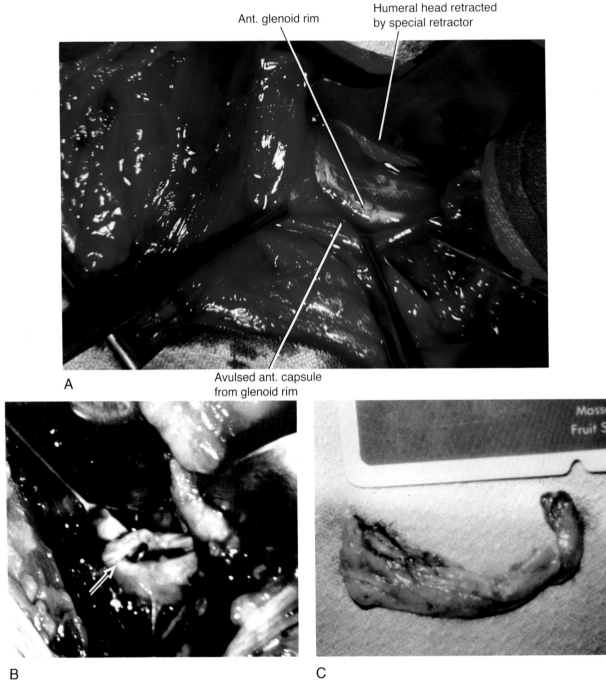

Ant. glenoid rim

Humeral head retracted
by special retractor

A

Avulsed ant. capsule
from glenoid rim

B

C

Fig. 7-9. (**A**) Labeled Bankart lesion shows avulsion of capsule and labrum from anterior glenoid rim of a left shoulder. The labrum is usually worn and not distinguished from the capsule. (**B**) A bucket handle split of the labrum. (**C**) The removed labrum has hypertrophied, resembling a knee meniscus. (Fig. A from Rowe CR, Patel D, Southmayd WW: The Bankart procedure. A long-term end-result study. J Bone Joint Surg 60A:1, 1978.)

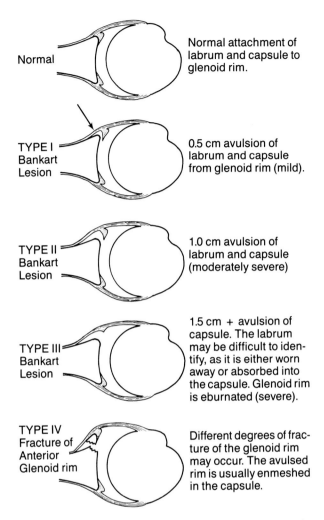

Normal	Normal attachment of labrum and capsule to glenoid rim.
TYPE I Bankart Lesion	0.5 cm avulsion of labrum and capsule from glenoid rim (mild).
TYPE II Bankart Lesion	1.0 cm avulsion of labrum and capsule (moderately severe)
TYPE III Bankart Lesion	1.5 cm + avulsion of capsule. The labrum may be difficult to identify, as it is either worn away or absorbed into the capsule. Glenoid rim is eburnated (severe).
TYPE IV Fracture of Anterior Glenoid rim	Different degrees of fracture of the glenoid rim may occur. The avulsed rim is usually enmeshed in the capsule.

Fig. 7-10. Classification of the Bankart lesion (four types).

mal humeral attachments, as well as its glenoid rim attachment. The investigative contributions of Turkel et al.[141] to the pathomechanics of the articular capsule concluded that, in the lower range of abduction, the subscapularis muscles, the superior capsular ligament of the capsule, and the coracohumeral ligament stabilize the joint to a large extent. From 0 to 45° abduction, the joint is protected by the subscapularis, the middle glenohumeral ligament, and superior fibers of the inferior capsular ligament. At 90° of abduction, the inferior capsular ligaments are the main restraint to anterior instability of the joint.

We consider the attenuated and ruptured muscles as definite "causative factors" for instability of the shoulder. Another muscle lesion noted in our series in 1984 was the enlargement of the normal seam between the subscapularis and supraspinatus tendons (Fig. 7-13A,B). *The seam is considered pathologic when it enlarges out over the humeral head to the lesser and greater tuberosity.* This occurred in 20 of 37 shoulders operated on for recurrent transient anterior subluxations of the shoulder.[124] This lesion would also appear to be a factor in instability of the shoulder. We were reassured when we found that Codman[28] had also commented on this finding in two operated cases in 1906.

The greatest degree of iatrogenic injury to the subscapularis muscle was in the series of shoulders in which initial surgery for recurrent dislocation had failed.[102,126,149,107] The Bristow procedure produced the greatest degree of scarring and trauma to the subscapularis muscle, followed by the duToit procedure. Next was the Putti-Platt procedure and, to a lesser degree, the Bankart procedure. As one would

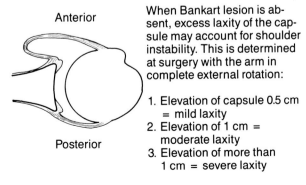

Anterior

Posterior

When Bankart lesion is absent, excess laxity of the capsule may account for shoulder instability. This is determined at surgery with the arm in complete external rotation:

1. Elevation of capsule 0.5 cm = mild laxity
2. Elevation of 1 cm = moderate laxity
3. Elevation of more than 1 cm = severe laxity

Fig. 7-11. Classification of the laxity of the joint capsule.

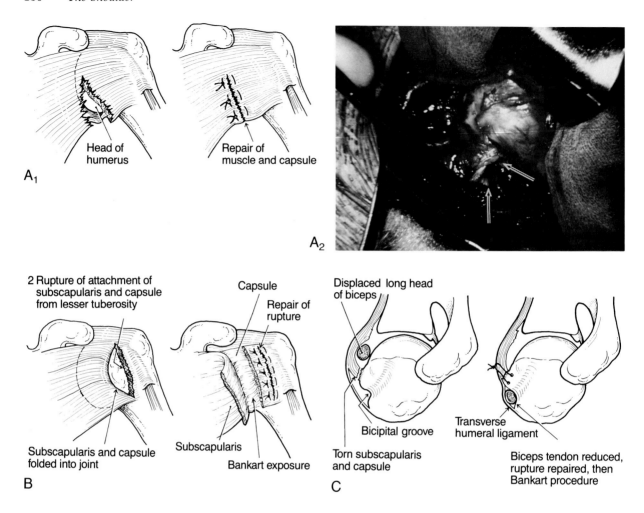

Fig. 7-12. Types of rupture of the subscapularis muscle associated with recurrent anterior dislocation. (**A1**) Direct rupture through the body of the subscapularis muscle and capsule. (**A2**) Traumatic rupture of inferior subscapularis muscle. (**B**) Avulsion of the attachment of the subscapularis from its attachment to the lesser tuberosity, with curling under into the joint. This was repaired, following which a Bankart procedure was carried out. (**C**) Avulsion of the subscapularis from the lesser tuberosity with dislocation of the long head of biceps tendon into the joint. This was repaired and a Bankart procedure then performed. (Fig. A2 from Rowe CR, Patel D, Southmayd WW: The Bankart procedure. A long-term end-result study. J Bone Joint Surg 60A:7, 1978.)

expect, the Nicola and Magnuson procedures produced the least scarring of the subscapularis muscle, as the muscle was left intact.

Bone Lesions

Palmer and Widen[106] considered the Hill-Sachs lesion of the humeral head to be the "essential lesion" of recurrent anterior dislocations. Again, we suggest that the Hill-Sachs lesion be considered *one* of the causative lesions of recurrent anterior dislocation, rather than the "essential" lesion. In our follow-up study[121] in 1978, we found Hill-Sachs lesions of the humeral head in 77 percent of 142 traumatic dislocations, in 40 percent of transient subluxators,[124] and in 76 percent of failed surgical repairs.[126] They were absent in voluntary dislocations.[122]

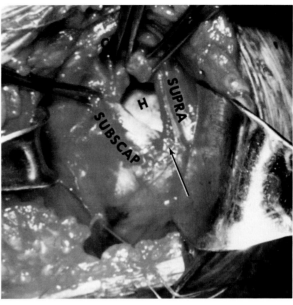

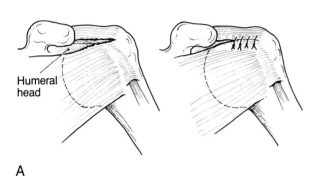

Humeral head

A   B

Fig. 7-13. (**A**) Enlargement of the seam between the subscapularis and the supraspinatus over the head of the humerus to the greater tuberosity. Repair should be limited to the dome of the head, otherwise elevation may be limited. (**B**) Traumatic enlargement of the seam between the subscapularis and supraspinatus tendons over head of humerus in a left shoulder (arrow points to greater tuberosity). The seam was closed over the curvature of the humeral head. *Supra,* supraspinatus tendon; *H,* humeral head; *Subscap,* subscapularis tendon; *C,* coracoid process. (Fig. B from Rowe CR, Zarins B: Recurrent transient subluxation of the shoulder. J Bone Joint Surg 63A:863, 1981.)

CLASSIFICATION OF HILL-SACHS LESIONS

Hill-Sachs lesions of the humeral head are produced by the recoil impaction of the head against the rim of the glenoid at the time of dislocation (Fig. 7-14A). The lesion is an impacted compression fracture of the head (Fig. 7-14B). We have classified Hill-Sachs lesions into three groups (Fig. 7-15):

1. A *mild* lesion (Fig. 7-15A)
2. A *moderately* severe lesion (Fig. 7-15B)
3. A *severe* lesion (Fig. 7-15C)

FRACTURES OF THE GLENOID RIM

The glenoid rim was damaged in 73 percent of our traumatic dislocations. In 44 percent the rim was fractured by the impact of the humeral head. We consider this another causative factor in recurrent dislocation. Fractures can be defined as

1. Mild chip fracture (Fig. 7-16A)
2. Moderately severe fracture (an eighth to a quarter of the width of the fossa) (Fig. 7-16B).
3. Severe fracture (larger than a quarter of the fossa) (Fig. 7-16C).

At surgery, the fractured rim of the glenoid is usually enveloped in the avulsed capsule. Forty-five percent of the glenoid rims were damaged in the transient subluxators. No glenoid rim trauma or degenerative changes were noted in the voluntary dislocators.

Mechanism of Injuries in Primary Dislocations

A review of injuries producing the dislocations in our studies revealed that a forceful extension or abduction of the arm was found in 30 percent, forceful

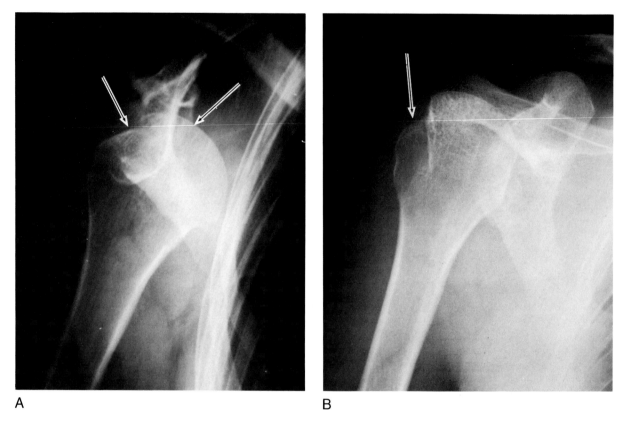

A   B

Fig. 7-14. (**A**) Origin of a Hill-Sachs lesion (due to recoil impaction of the dislocated head against the rim of the glenoid) (see arrows). (**B**) Severe Hill-Sachs lesion of the superior lateral aspect of the humeral head after reduction (see arrow).

elevation and external rotation of the arm in 24 percent, a direct blow to the shoulder in 29 percent, and a fall on the outstretched hand or arm in 17 percent.

Our findings do not substantiate Bankart's theory of the mechanism of injury, since 30 percent of the recurrent dislocations in our series were caused initially by a forceful abduction or extension of the arm, a dislocation that Bankart claims never recurred.[9] Also, only 29 percent of the recurrent dislocations were caused initially by a direct blow to the shoulder or elbow, an injury that Bankart thought was the sole cause of recurrent dislocations. It is our opinion that both the so-called "ordinary" or "nonrecurrent" and the "recurrent" dislocations, as noted by Bankart, may produce the same lesion.

CLOSED REDUCTION

The usual methods of closed reduction using the Kocher method, and "the heel or fist" in the axilla, result in a pulling contest against the shoulder muscles in spasm. This can produce a very difficult contest, often requiring intravenous administration of diazepam (Valium) or meperidine (Demerol), or a light general anesthesia (Fig. 7-17).

Sir Astley Cooper[31] in 1828 observed that when the arm was in full elevation, the controlling muscles of the shoulder joint were relaxed, and reduction could be more easily accomplished in this position than by pulling on the arm with the muscles in spasm. I quote from his book *A Treatise on Dislocations and*

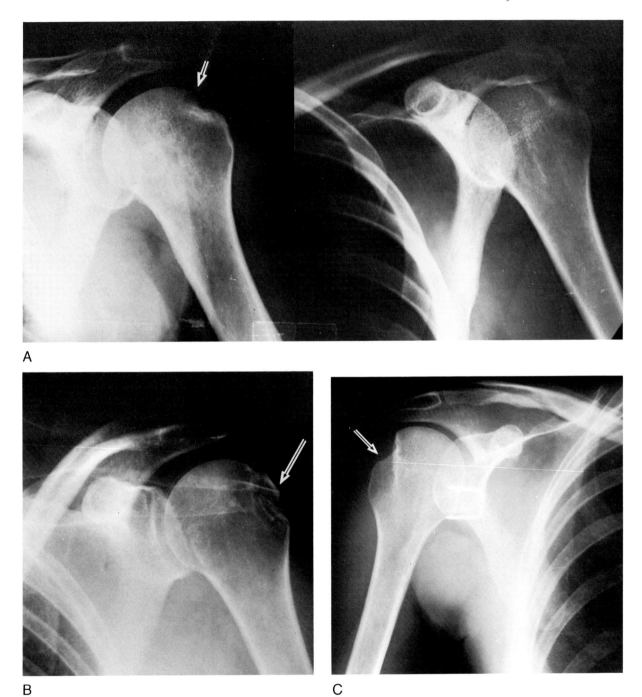

Fig. 7-15. Classification of Hill-Sachs lesions. (**A**) Mild lesion (arrow) (compression of ⅙ of circumference of humeral head). (**B**) Moderate severe lesion (arrow) (compression from ⅙ to ¼ of circumference). (**C**) Severe lesion (arrow) (compression of greater than ¼ of circumference).

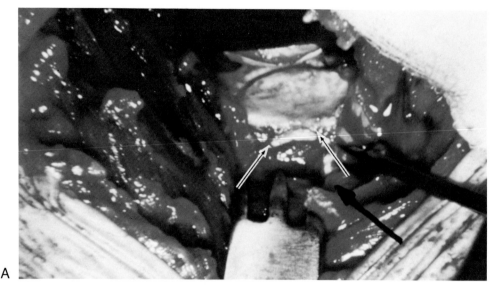

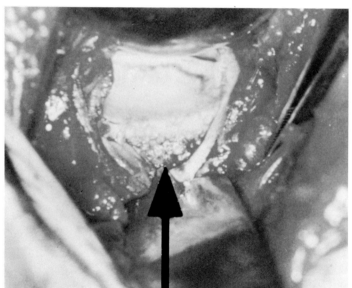

Fig. 7-16. Classification of fractures of the glenoid rim due to impaction of the humeral head. (A) Mild (or chip) fracture (arrows). (B) Moderately severe fracture (⅛ to ¼ of the width of the fossa). (C) Severe fracture (larger than ¼ of the width of the fossa).

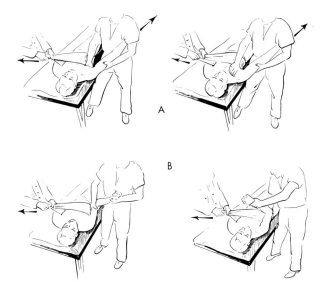

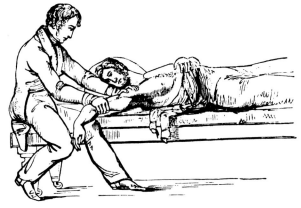

Fig. 7-17. Many methods of reduction pull against muscles in spasm. Pulling on the arm with the fist or foot in the axilla or in the Kocher position results in pulling against muscles in spasm. (Reproduced with permission from Rowe CR, Marble AC: Shoulder girdle injuries. p. 254. In Cave EF (ed): Fractures and Other Injuries. Copyright © 1958 by Year Book Medical Publishers, Inc., Chicago.)

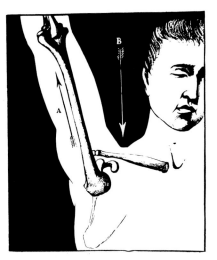

Fig. 7-18. Was White telling us in 1764 to reduce the shoulder in elevation? (Moseley HF: Shoulder Lesions. E & S Livingstone, Edinburgh 1969.)

Fractures of the Joints (p. 304): ". . . the dissection explains the reason that the arm is sometimes easily reduced soon after the dislocation, by raising it suddenly above the horizontal line, and placing the fingers under the head of the bone, so as to raise it toward the glenoid cavity, which every tyro knows will sometimes reduce it, *because in this position, the muscles of opposition are relaxed so as to oppose no resistance to reduction.*" This good advice remained dormant until E.A. Codman,[27] in explaining the pivotal paradox of shoulder motion, pointed out that combined internal and external rotation of the shoulder decreases from the position at the side of the body to complete elevation where it "is practically nil, *for the humerus cannot be further rotated externally or internally.*" In other words, the rotating muscles in full elevation become inactive, and relaxed. Therefore, muscle spasm present with the arm in the anatomical position at the side of the body is neutralized to a great extent in elevation and reduction in the elevated position can more easily be accomplished. This explains Sir Astley Cooper's observation in 1825. Evidently, White[4] was telling us that the shoulder should be reduced with the arm in elevation in 1764 (Fig. 7-18).

In 1955, a patient arrived at the emergency ward at the Massachusetts General Hospital with a luxatio erecta dislocation (Fig. 7-19). I found that the patient's shoulder could be easily reduced by applying traction to the arm in elevation; by placing my thumb under the humeral head, it could be easily lifted back into the glenoid. Another case of luxatio erecta is shown being reduced on the x-ray table in Figure 7-20. Since this time, we have routinely reduced anterior dislocations by gently and *slowly* elevating the arm to full elevation in the luxatio erecta position, in which position the muscles relax. The humeral head can then

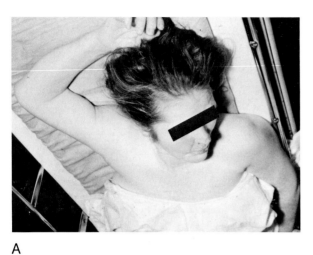

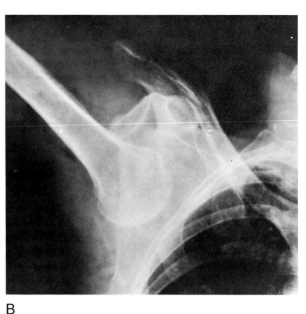

A   B

Fig. 7-19. (A) The arm of a luxatioerecta dislocation can be easily reduced by adding gentle traction to the elevated arm and placing one's thumb under the head, assisting it back into the glenoid. This taught us the technique of reducing an anterior dislocation. **(B)** Gently bring the arm into elevation, in which position it can be reduced, usually without the need of relaxants.

be replaced with little difficulty (Fig. 7-21). Usually no medication is necessary. This reduction can be done on the x-ray table after the prereduction films are taken.

In 1949, Milch[86] also observed that dislocation of the shoulder was more effectively carried out with the arm in elevation. The Stimson technique[134] (Fig. 7-22), with the patient prone and the arm relaxed at

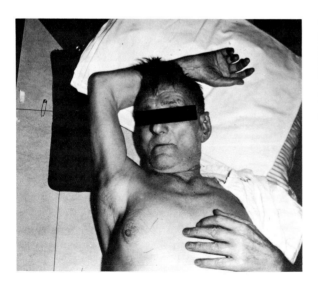

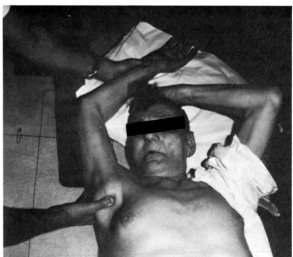

Fig. 7-20. Another luxatioerecta dislocation that was reduced on the x-ray table.

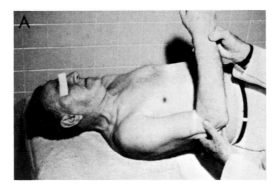

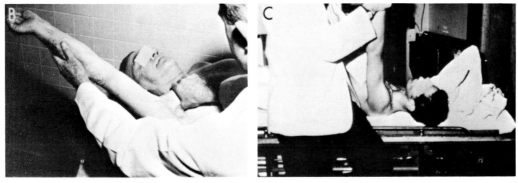

Fig. 7-21. Technique of reducing shoulder by placing arm in elevation (this can be performed usually without medication). **(A)** The arm is gently supported, and *slowly* raised into elevation. **(B)** Then with gentle traction upward and outward, the thumb is placed under the humeral head reducing it onto the glenoid. **(C)** Reduction of left anterior dislocation without pain medication of a jockey who had been thrown from his horse. (Reprinted with permission from Rowe CR, Cave EF: Shoulder Girdle Injuries. p. 266. In Cave EF (ed): Fractures and Other Injuries. Copyright © 1958 by Year Book Medical Publishers, Inc., Chicago.)

90° of flexion over the side of the table, uses the same principle of elevation, traction, and relaxation. Bosley,[17] in 1979, introduced an addition to the Stimson procedure with the "scapula maneuver." With the patient in the prone position and a weight applied to the arm (Fig. 7-23), the scapula is rotated with the heel of the hand, to position the glenoid fossa medially toward the humeral head, thus assisting in its reduction. This is a safe and very effective method of reduction.[3]

Another method that has gone unnoticed in most textbooks is a gentle modification of the Kocher method, recommended by Leidelmeyer[75] in 1977, by Mirick[88] in 1979, and by Danzl et al.[21,34] in 1985, referred to as the "external rotation method." The patient is supine. The elbow is flexed to 90° and slowly adducted to the patient's side. The arm is then slowly externally rotated, stopping "every few degrees until spasm and resistance abate." By the time external rotation is complete, reduction occurs. The authors claim that the majority of patients were reduced within 5 minutes. Danzl et al. claimed success in 78 of 100 dislocations. Some patients may need more relaxation of their muscles, particularly those whose shoulders have been dislocated for a longer period of time. The usual relaxant is diazepam (Valium) 5 mg intravenously. One should remember that patients have variable reactions to drugs. It is safe to have an intravenous line ready in case of drug reaction or overdose.

The reader should also be cautioned about nerve injuries in closed reductions of the shoulder.[15]

An occasional learning experience for residents covering the emergency ward, is seeing a patient whose

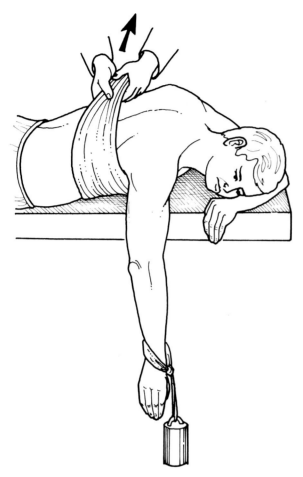

Fig. 7-22. The Stimson method employs the same principles of relaxation of the muscles in flexion. (Redrawn with permission from Cave EF, Rowe CR: p. 422. In Cave EF, Burke JF, Boyd RD (ed): Trauma Management. Copyright © 1974 by Year Book Medical Publishers, Inc., Chicago.)

shoulder they have been unable to reduce, even with light anesthesia to learn, to their embarrassment, that the patient's shoulder has been unreduced for several years. This usually occurs when there is a communication problem between the physician and the patient.

Immobilization

For the young adult, our studies indicate that a period of immobilization of 3 weeks in internal rotation and adduction was associated with the lowest recurrence rate.[117] Some investigators,[140,143,148] how-

ever, advise longer periods of immobilization. Yoneda and associates found a low rate of recurrence in a follow-up study of 100 athletes whose shoulders had been immobilized for 6 weeks. Aronen[5] stresses the need for rigid adherence to a rehabilitation program. This program was carried out at the U.S. Naval Academy. During a follow-up period of 35.8 months, his recurrence rate was only 25 percent. Emphasis was on restriction of activities until the goals of the rehabilitation program were reached.

For the patient 45 years or older, shorter periods of immobilization are indicated since the recurrence rate after age 45 is only 12 percent. We immobilize the shoulder in patients in this age group, for comfort only, with early mobilization as tolerated, to avoid limited motion of the shoulder and formation of adhesions.

Exercise

With the young adult, gradual resistive exercises are begun at 3 weeks, in internal rotation and adduction to avoid pull on the healing anterior capsule, yet allow benefit from the stimulation of early motion. This is increased to external rotation and abduction at the fourth to sixth week. Return to competitive athletics is delayed until the patient has regained *full motion, good strength,* and has no *apprehension* with his or her arm in elevation. This may take from 6 to 8 weeks or longer. A shoulder restraint may be used at first when the patient returns to competitive contact sports. It is a good rule, however, to caution the athlete to keep the hands and arm *in front of the body* as much as possible, and avoid extending the arm beyond the coronal plane of the body. The patient should be cautioned also that when the arm is moved *the body should be moved in the same direction,* at the same time. In so doing, strain is removed from the shoulder and absorbed in the body motion. Leverage of the extended arm is eliminated. Also, the motion is more fluid and coordinated, improving one's tennis, golf, fencing, throwing (pitching), and many other sports. As we have pointed out previously (Chapter 6), shoulder exercises taken with the patient strapped in a *sitting* position grinds the rotator cuff under a *fixed* scapula (acromial arch), straining the capsule of the shoulder, creating overuse tendinitis of the rotator cuff, chronic bursitis, and, at times,

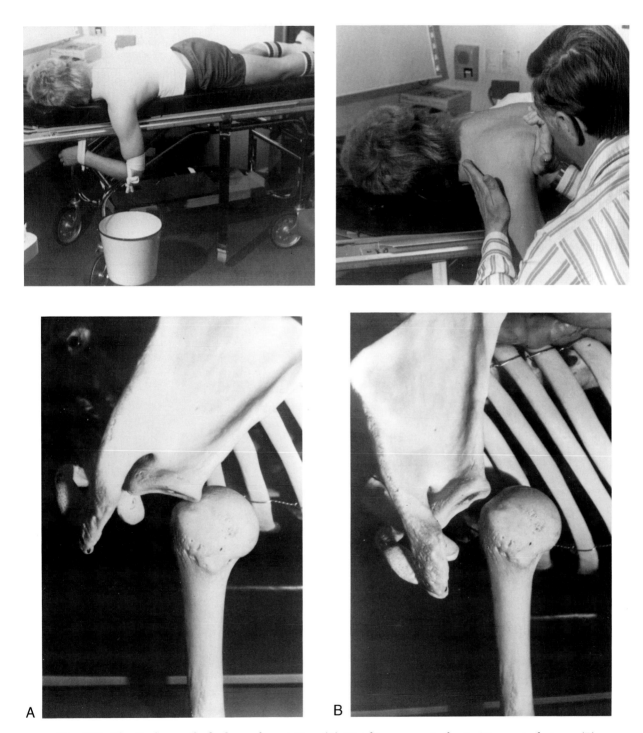

Fig. 7-23. The Bosley method of scapular rotation. (**A**) Weight on arm similar to Stimson technique. (**B**) Pressure on the spine of the scapula rotates the glenoid toward the humeral head. (*Figure continues.*)

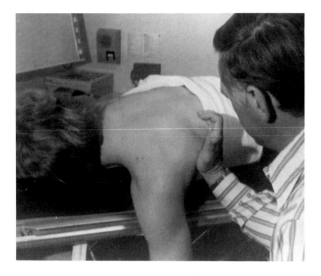

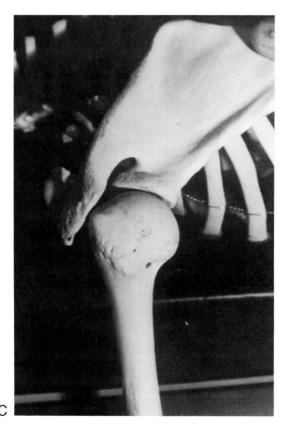

C

Fig. 7-23 *(Continued)*. **(C)** Reduction by pushing upward and anterior on the head. (Courtesy of Rex C. Bosley, December 1985.)

subluxation of the shoulder. We stress again, that it is far more physiological, and less traumatic to the rotator cuff, to move the body when performing shoulder exercises, and avoid the 90° position of abduction. Use of wall weights with the body moving is easier and causes less strain on the shoulder than in the sitting position. Rowing, swimming, golf, and cutting wood are effective and safe exercises for the shoulder.

SURGICAL PROCEDURES FOR RECURRENT DISLOCATION AND SUBLUXATION

We will consider only those operative procedures more commonly used today. Table 7-4 outlines the chronological order of procedures for repair of shoulder instabilities. These will be discussed in the following order:

Repair of capsule and labrum back to the glenoid rim
 Bankart procedure
 duToit procedure
 Viek procedure
 Eyre-Brook procedure
 Moseley procedure
Muscle and capsule plication
 Putti-Platt procedure
 The Symeonides procedure
Muscle and tendon sling procedures
 Magnuson-Stack procedure
 Bristow-Helfet-Latarjet procedure
  Modifications
 The Boytchev procedure
 Nicola procedure
 Gallie-LeMesurier procedure
 Boyd transfer of long head of biceps (for posterior dislocation)
Bone block
 Eden-Hybbinette procedure
 DeAnquin procedure (through a superior approach to the shoulder)
Osteotomies
 Weber (humeral neck)
 Saha (humeral shaft)

Table 7-4. Chronology of Surgical Procedures for Recurrent Dislocations

4TH Century B.C.	Hippocrates
1890	Broca and Hartman
1894	Ricard
1906	Perthes
1920	Eden
1923	Bankart
1923	Putti (credits Codivilla)
1925	Platt
1932	Hybbinette
1934	Nicola
1942	Rowe and Cave (modification of Bankart)
1943	Magnuson-Stack
1947	Moseley
1948	Gallie-LeMesurier
1948	Eyre-Brook
1954	Latarjet
1956	Saha
1956	duToit (credits Fouche and Allen 1937)
1958	Rowe (capsulorrhaphy; double breasting along rim of glenoid)
1958	Bristow-Helfet
1959	Viek (credits Luckey 1949)
1965	DeAnquin
1966	Kretzler
1967	Scott
1972	Symeonides
1972	Connolly (infraspinatus transfer)
1974	Boytchev (reported by Conforti)
1980	Neer (capsular shift)
1980	Protzman (capsular shift)
1984	Weber (osteotomy of proximal humerus)

Scott and Kretzler osteotomy of scapular neck (for posterior dislocations)

Bestard osteotomy of scapular neck (for anterior and posterior dislocations)

Muscle transplant to humeral head

The Connolly procedure (transplantation of infraspinatus muscle into the Hill-Sachs lesion for anterior dislocation)

McLaughlin procedure (transplantation of subscapularis into the medial humeral head defect for posterior dislocation)

Saha transplants to the humeral shaft

Capsulorrhaphies

Neer anterior–inferior and posterior capsular shifts

Protzman capsular shift

Rowe glenoid capsulorrhaphy

The Bankart Procedure

This is the author's choice when a Bankart lesion is present. When the lesion is absent, we use the capsulorraphy technique described below.

AIM

The Bankart procedure involves a detailed layer-by-layer dissection, identification of the causative pathology, correction of the pathology, and return of the muscles to their original attachments for complete range of motion, stability, and strength. By returning all muscles to their original attachments, the important *muscle balance* of the shoulder is maintained. By avoiding the transfer of tissues, and eliminating the use of metal screws, staples, or pins, complications are minimal.

STEPS

Step 1. Careful layer-by-layer dissection of muscles and capsule down to the rim of the glenoid; avoid cutting across muscle layers.

Step 2. Recognition and repair of pathologic lesions; there is often more than one lesion.

Step 3. When a Bankart lesion is present, the capsule is repaired back to glenoid rim by direct suture through bone (no metal screws, staples, or spikes are used).

Step 4. When the capsule is *not* avulsed, the modified capsulorrhaphy is carried out. It is important to check the capsular attachment to the humeral neck, as well as along the glenoid rim.

Step 5. No postoperative immobilization is used. Early motion of the extremity has proved beneficial to healing, and a relief to the patient.

SUGGESTIONS FOR AN EASIER AND STRONGER PROCEDURE

1. A relaxant anesthesia is essential: it affords relaxation of the deep muscles, better exposure, and improved surgical technique.

2. The patient is placed supine on the operating ta-

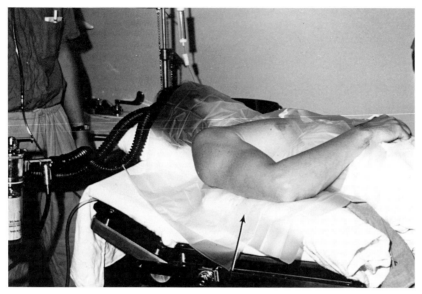

A

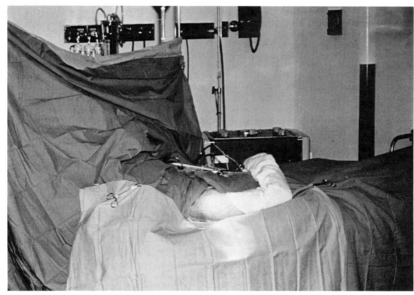

B

Fig. 7-24. (A) The patient is placed supine, with a folded blanket under the arm, allowing the head to displace posteriorly, away from the rim of the glenoid. A sandbag is *not* placed behind the shoulder. **(B)** The anesthetist is placed on the opposite side of the table, giving room for an assistant at the top of the table. (*Figure continues.*)

ble, moved slightly to the opposite side of the table to allow resting space for the arm (Fig. 7-24). We do not recommend the semisitting position, or suspending or placing the arm in abduction on an arm board, since this displaces vital structures laterally toward the incision.

3. A sand bag is *not* placed behind the shoulder.

This will displace the humeral head forward, making it more difficult to expose the rim of the glenoid.

4. Instead, a folded blanket or half-sheets are placed under the arm to elevate the elbow. This displaces the humeral head posteriorly, improving the exposure of the glenoid rim (Fig. 7-24A).

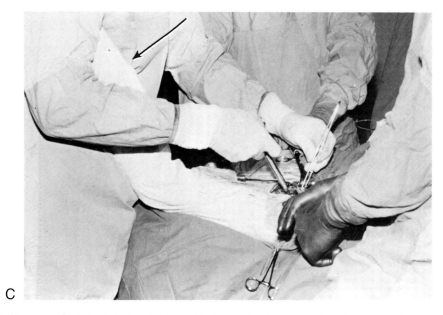

Fig. 7-24 (*Continued*). (**C**) It is helpful to hold the patient's arm under the surgeon's arm; freeing the assistant's hands to help the surgeon. This can be a great help.

5. The anesthetist is placed on the opposite side of the table. This frees the head of the table for an assistant (Fig. 7-24B).
6. It is helpful for the surgeon to hold the patient's arm under his or her arm (Fig. 7-24C): under the inner arm for internal rotation and under the outer arm for external rotation. This frees the hands of your assistant. By lowering the table, the surgical exposure is improved.
7. Proper instruments are necessary. Information on the instruments used by the author, can be obtained on request (Kirwan Surgical Products, 81 Island Creek Road, Duxbury, MA 02332).

INSTRUMENTS

1. Specially designed humeral head retractors are necessary (Fig. 7-25A).
2. Single- or triple-pronged capsule retractors (gently driven into the scapula neck to retract the medial flap of capsule). The fourth instrument is a blunt retractor, used as indicated for muscle retraction (Fig. 7-25B).
3. Reading from left to right (Fig. 7-25C), the straight scaphoid gouge is used to initiate the hole through the cortex of the neck of the glenoid. This allows the curved glenoid punch to pass through the bone more easily and safely. The cortex of the bone is usually quite dense due to repeated trauma. We do not use a drill, although this can be used. The curved glenoid punch creates the hole. The three-sided clamp and awls complete the holes. By using the above instruments, the holes can be kept small. We have fractured the glenoid rim only once in 40 years.
4. Suture Passing Instruments (Fig. 7-25D).
   a. On the left is the #5 Mayo ½ taper needle, which is strong and has the correct curve to pass through the hole. If necessary, the curve of the needle can be changed with two needle holders.
   b. On the right is the hooked suture passer that can be used when the curved needle fails. All of the above instruments have essentially the same radius of curve

TECHNICAL STEPS

Step 1. A slightly curved incision is made from the coracoid process down to the axillary fold (Fig. 7-26). A shorter incision can be used in female patients. The incision should not

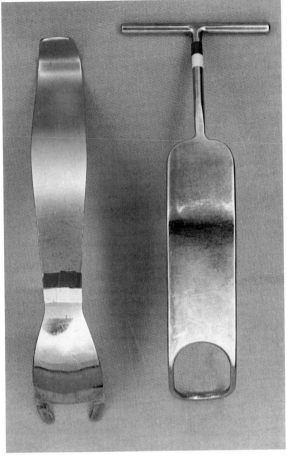

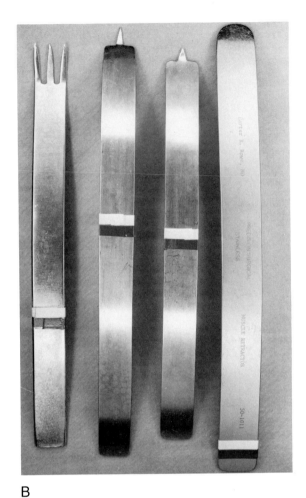

A

B

Fig. 7-25. Instruments for Bankart procedure: **(A)** Humeral head retractors: Left, designed by the author; right, designed by Professor Fukuda of Japan. **(B)** Single or triple pronged capsule retractors: on extreme left, a deep blunt retractor for the coracoid muscles on the right. (*Figure continues.*)

be carried lateral to the axillary fold or onto the arm, because the scar will spread. We have not found it necessary to release the deltoid muscle from the clavicle. A fatty seam usually identifies the interval between the pectoralis major and the deltoid muscle. Developing the seam by blunt dissection will expose the cephalic vein, which may lie superficial or deep. At times it may be absent. The cephalic vein is not ligated but is retracted laterally with the deltoid muscle. Be careful to free the vein up over the coracoid process.

Step 2. Osteotomy of the coracoid process is optional (Fig. 7-27). We prefer to do it especially in muscular individuals, since it gives better exposure of the subscapularis and the superior aspect of the shoulder, eliminates traction on the common tendon of the short head of biceps and coracobrachialis, and thus protects the musculocutaneous nerve. (By following this technique we have never injured or compromised the musculocutaneous nerve or had a nonunion after resuturing the coracoid).

Step 3. The arm is then completely externally ro-

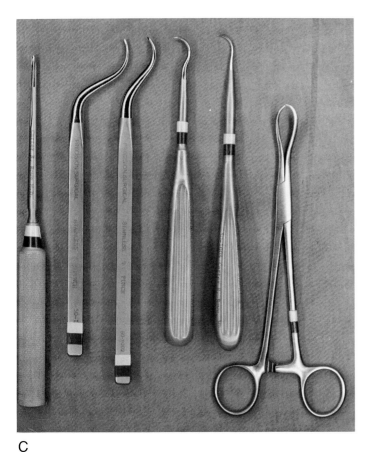

C

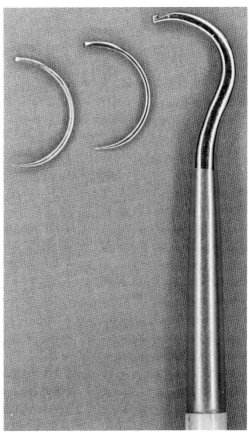

D

Fig. 7-25 (*Continued*). (**C**) From left to right: the straight scaphoid gouge (to initiate the hole in the glenoid neck); the curved spikes or punch (to direct the hole); the awls (to develop the hole); the three-sided clamp (sharp on three sides, completes the hole). (**D**) Suture-passing instruments. Left, #5 Mayo ½ taper needle; right, hooked suture passer (if the needle is not successful).

tated, giving full exposure to the entire sub-scapularis muscle and tendon attachment (Fig. 7-28). Ligation of the anterior circum-flex vessels that course along the inferior border of the subscapularis muscle is also optional. We prefer to do this because it gives better exposure of the inferior capsular ligament and the axillary capsular fold at 6 o'clock, where strong overlapping repair is needed. We have had no ill effects from ligation of the vessels, or injury to the nerve. However, the circumflex vessels can be pre-served. Rockwood[116] leaves attached a small strip of inferior subscapularis to protect the circumflex vessels and axillary nerve.

Step 4. Many surgeons have difficulty removing the subscapularis muscle and tendon from the anterior capsule. This important step can be accomplished quite *easily and effectively*. We offer a few helpful suggestions (Fig. 7-29):

   a. First, place the arm in complete external rotation.

   b. Then begin the dissection of the tendon of the subscapularis muscle halfway be-tween the bicipital groove and the mus-

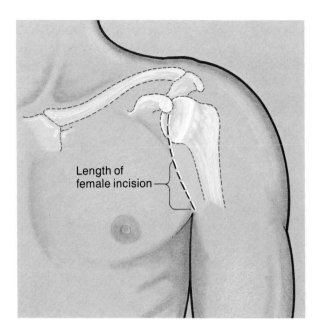

Fig. 7-26. Skin incision.

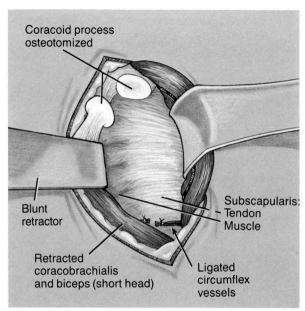

Fig. 7-28. External rotation of the arm exposes the subscapularis. Ligation of circumflex vessels is also optional. We prefer to do so for better exposure of the inferior capsular fold.

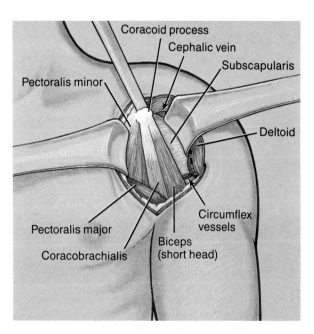

Fig. 7-27. Osteotomy of coracoid is optional. We use it for better exposure of the subscapularis muscle.

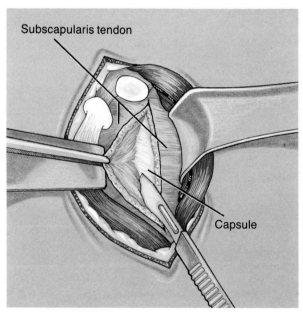

Fig. 7-29. Dissection of subscapularis tendon and muscle from the anterior capsule—a most important step. By turning the subscapularis muscle back, the axillary nerve is protected.

cle portion of subscapularis, thus leaving adequate tendon for strong reattachment. Since the capsule and tendon are one in this area, the knife blade should be held almost horizontal, *thus leaving some tendon attached to the capsule, to avoid entering the joint.* If the capsule is nicked, repair it and continue your dissection.

c. When the dissection approaches the muscle of the subscapularis, the capsule becomes evident. The muscle can then be easily removed either with serrated scissors or a winged tip periosteal elevator down to the glenoid rim, thus exposing the entire capsule. If the subscapularis muscle is turned back intact, rather than splitting it or transecting it, the axillary nerve is protected (as evidenced by no injury to the axillary nerve in our series). It is here that the capsule should be carefully examined, first for its attachment to the lesser tuberosity and humeral neck, then for general laxity. This is determined *by completely externally rotating the shoulder,* in which position the capsule should normally stretch tightly across the humeral head. The degree of laxity is illustrated in Figure 7-11. If the capsule can be lifted more than 2 cm in external rotation, it is considered abnormally lax and constitutes a factor in the shoulder's instability. If the capsule is abnormally lax, determine whether the laxity is due to avulsion from the neck of the humerus, or lesser tuberosity, or from the anterior glenoid rim. If there is avulsion, it should be repaired. Then continue opening the capsule along the anterior glenoid rim (see Fig. 7-12).

Step 5. With the anterior capsule completely exposed, the degree of laxity of the capsule is then determined. *This is an important step.* With the arm in neutral zero position, normally the capsule can be lifted up 1 cm or more. With the arm in complete external rotation, the capsule should stretch tightly across the anterior humeral head. If, as stated in Step 4, the capsule can be lifted up 1 to 2 cm in complete external rotation, it is considered abnormally lax and constitutes a factor in the shoulder's instability.

Step 6. The capsule should be opened 0.5 cm lateral to the glenoid rim (Fig. 7-30A). This must be done with *the arm in complete external rotation.* This is another very important step. If the capsule is opened with the shoulder in neutral position, the arm will be limited in external rotation postoperatively. When it is opened with the arm in complete external rotation, the patient will gain external rotation more easily. The capsule is then opened vertically by placing one Allis forceps directly over the rim of the glenoid and a second forceps 0.5 cm lateral to the rim (Fig. 30B). The vertical opening of the joint along the glenoid rim is essential for exposure of the rim as well as the entire interior of the joint, and the posterior capsule.

Step 7. This will give an adequate mesial flap, to double breast over the lateral flap in closure. The Bankart lesion, if present, is exposed (avulsion of the capsule and labrum from the glenoid rim) (Fig. 7-31). If a capsular lesion *is* present, a Bankart procedure is carried out. If a lesion is *not* present, a capsulorrhaphy is performed (see below). This is done with no change in the surgical approach.

Step 8. The humeral head retractor is then inserted into the joint (Fig. 7-32A). This should allow complete exposure of the glenoid rim and the joint, not only anteriorly but posteriorly as well. When a well-developed Bankart lesion is present, the medial flap is held back with a single- or triple-pronged spike driven into the scapular neck, to give excellent exposure of the rim. The rim and neck of the scapula are then freshened with a small osteotome or curette (Fig. 7-32B). This is most important to ensure strong healing of the capsule back to bone. Next, the scaphoid gouge is used to perforate the cortex of the scapular neck and initiate the holes (Fig. 7-32A). This makes it much easier and much safer for the curved spike to pass through

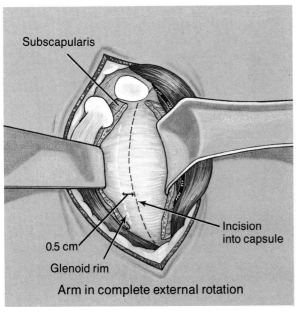

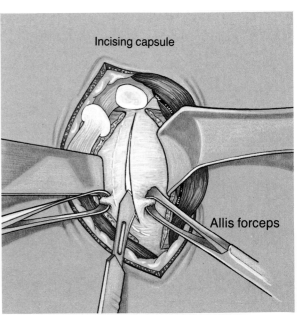

A

B

Fig. 7-30. (**A**) The arm is completely externally rotated and the laxity of the capsule tested. (**B**) The capsule is then opened vertically 0.5 cm lateral to the glenoid rim. The arm must be in external rotation when you enter the capsule.

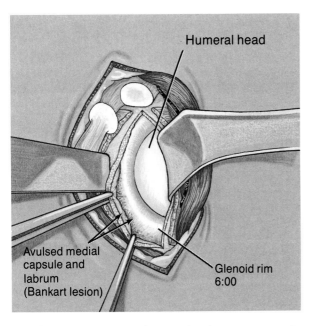

Fig. 7-31. Upon opening the capsule, the presence or absence of a Bankart lesion is identified. If present, a Bankart procedure is performed. If not, a capsulorrhaphy is performed. No change in incision or approach is necessary.

the rim without injury to the bone. Since the glenoid rim may be dense from repeated dislocations, the use of the scaphoid gouge is a definite help. Drill holes may be made, but the scaphoid gouge is safer. With a well-developed Bankart lesion, the labrum is usually nonexistent, having been worn away or retracted in the avulsed capsule. Severe fractures of the rim may include a fifth, a quarter, or even a third of the glenoid fossa (Fig. 7-16). The fractured portion of the rim is usually enmeshed in the capsule.

We have never found it necessary to use a bone graft to compensate for the fractured glenoid rim, regardless of the size of the fracture. Routine repair of the capsule to the remaining rim has proved successful. Although a bone graft has been considered at times, it could not be fitted smoothly enough, in our opinion, to avoid secondary arthrosis. In fact, our follow-up studies show that with fractures of the glenoid rim the recurrence rate using the standard Bankart

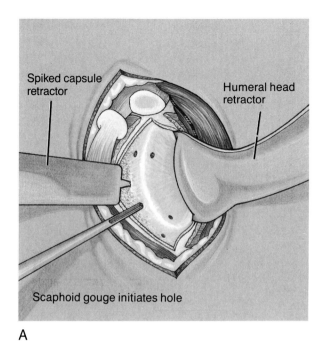

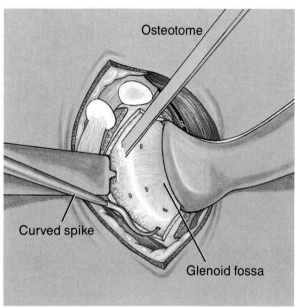

Fig. 7-32. (A) The humeral head retractor is inserted. The medial capsule is retracted by a single or triple pronged retractor driven into the neck. A scaphoid gouge is next used to initiate the holes in the neck of the glenoid, making it much easier for the curved spike to pass through. **(B)** The rim and neck are then decorticated or freshened with a small osteotome to promote healing when reattached. The holes are developed by the curved spike; introduce it first from the neck side, then the joint side.

technique was only 2 percent, which was surprisingly lower than our overall recurrence rate of 3.5 percent.

Step 9. Three holes are then made through the rim of the glenoid after the neck has been freshened with a small osteotome. For a left shoulder, the holes should be made at 2 o'clock, 4 o'clock, and 6 o'clock. We stress again that *the 6 o'clock hole is the most important fixation point*, as this is the area of greatest strain to the capsule when the arm is in full elevation, such as in throwing, serving in tennis, a basketball lay-up, and in forceful contact sports. In many other types of repairs, postoperative subluxation may occur because of lack of stability of the axillary fold of the capsule and the inferior capsular ligament at 6 o'clock. With stability restored at 2, 4, and 6 o'clock, the shoulder is secure in all positions; superior, mid, and inferior. One-point fixation alone will leave the other two areas unprotected either above or below the fixation. For adequate exposure of the glenoid neck, the medial capsule is retracted by inserting either the single- or triple-pronged retractor into the neck, depending on the degree of separation of the capsule. The curved spike is then tapped (after the hole is begun with the scaphoid gouge), first from the neck side, then from the articular side. This instrument should be carefully introduced in each direction until you can feel that the entrances meet.

Step 10. The three-sided clamp is then introduced to give the holes correct curvature (Fig. 7-33). The small awls are used to complete the holes. The holes should not be made very large, and should be placed 3 to 4 mm from the rim. As noted, we have had only one rim fracture in the past 40 years using this technique.

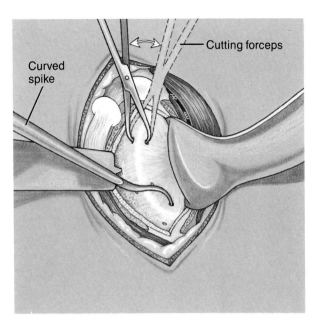

Fig. 7-33. The hole is then enlarged by the three-sided cutting clamp. Small awls are used to complete the holes.

Step 11. We prefer cotton sutures in our shoulder surgery because of cotton's low reaction to the tissues, its strength, and secure knot formation. Two strands of #0 cotton are passed through each hole, either with the #5 Mayo ½ taper needle (we prefer the Richard's needle (Richard's Medical Co., Memphis, Tennessee) because of its strength and exact curve) (Fig. 7-34A), or with the barbed suture retriever (Fig. 7-34B).

Step 13. After the sutures have been passed through the glenoid holes, the humeral head retractor is removed and the arm brought into neutral position. The sutures are passed through the lateral flap of capsule, securely tying it to the glenoid rim with the arm in 35° of external rotation. This will allow the beginning of adequate external rotation postoperatively. The capsule can be accurately taken up according to the degree of redundancy present. After tying the suture, they are left long (Fig. 7-35A). One strand

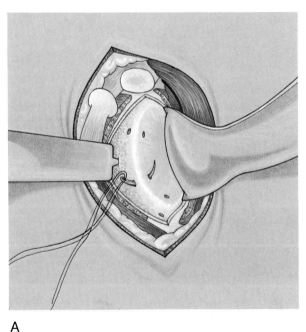

A

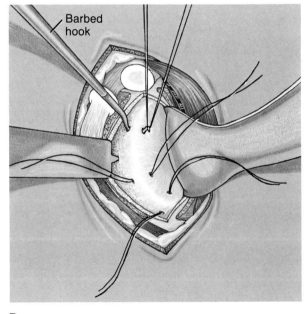

B

Fig. 7-34. The sutures are passed through the holes either with (**A**) a #5 Mayo ½ taper needle, or (**B**) the barbed suture retriever. We prefer double strands of 0 cotton sutures, although single synthetic sutures may be used.

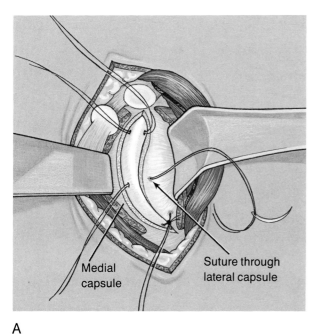

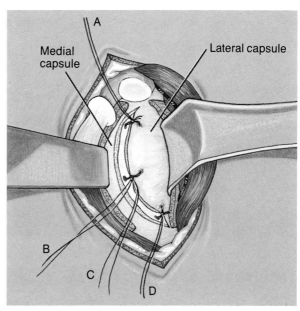

A   B

Fig. 7-35. (A) After passing the sutures through the rim, the head retractor is removed and the arm brought to the neutral position. The sutures are then passed through the lateral flap of capsule and tied to the glenoid rim, its original location. (B) One strand at *A* and *D* is cut. The strands at *B* and *C* are not cut.

at A and D is cut (Fig. 7-35B). Both strands at B and C are left long.

Step 14. Next, the sutures are passed through the medial capsule, to double-breast the medial capsule over the lateral capsule. One of the strands of sutures is cut at A and at C. Both strands are passed through at B (Fig. 7-36).

Step 15. Strand A is then tied to B, and strand C tied to strand D (Fig. 7-37). This technique securely overlaps and double breasts the repair along the entire glenoid rim. It is important that suture D be passed deep through the axillary fold and the inferior capsular ligament at 6 o'clock, to ensure *strong support of the capsule when the arm is in full elevation*. The free edge of the medial capsule is then stitched to the capsule. No other repair gives the support of *double breasting the capsule along the entire glenoid rim*. This improves on nature's single layer of capsule and takes the place of the worn or absent labrum, giving depth and security to the glenoid fossa.

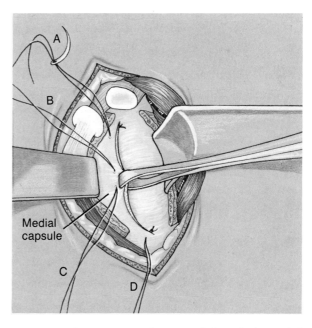

Fig. 7-36. The sutures are then passed through the medial capsule, single strands of suture at *A* and *D*, and both strands at *B*.

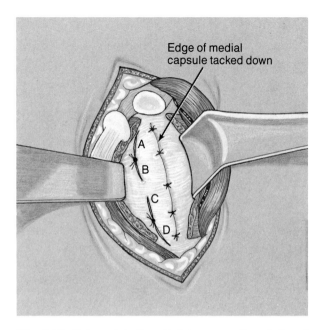

Fig. 7-37. Suture *A* is then tied to suture *B*, and *C* and *D*, thus securely double-breasting the capsular repair along the entire glenoid rim. The free edge of the medial flap is stitched to the capsule.

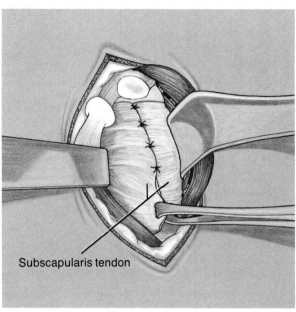

Fig. 7-38. In closure, all muscle layers are returned to their original attachments. The subscapularis is sewn back to its original attachment intact.

We have *found no evidence of degenerative changes* due to the holes in the rim of the glenoid in our follow-up studies ranging from 2 to 30 years. This is because all bone irregularities and holes along the rim are covered by the smooth capsule, leaving a soft surface for the humeral head to function against, instead of bone grafts, staples, or screws, which may cause degenerative changes.

Step 16. In closure, *all tissues are returned to their original attachments* (Fig. 7-38). The subscapularis muscle is identified and reattached to its origin along the lesser tuberosity with double strands of #20 cotton. The muscle is *not* shortened. If, however, the lower attachment of the subscapularis muscle is found to be abnormally thin or ruptured, this can be reinforced by lowering its attachment. Start the resuturing superiorly, so that the muscle attachment is smooth under the coracoid. If there has been an abnormal opening of the seam be-

tween the subscapularis and the supraspinatus tendons, it is closed over the surface of the head, but not back to the coracoid because this would limit elevation. With careful anatomical exposure and repair, and replacement of tissue to its normal attachments, we have not had an incidence of injury to the axillary nerve or to the musculocutaneous nerve.

Step 17. We prefer to reattach the coracoid by direct suture through the bone, rather than with a screw. A hole is made through the osteotomized fragment of coracoid with the scaphoid gouge, and then a hole is made through the base of the coracoid process (Fig. 7-39A). The handle of the scaphoid gouge should be depressed into the axilla, so that the hole comes out on top of the base of the coracoid. Two strands of #0 cotton are passed through the holes with the #5 ½ taper needle. A second suture is then passed through the tendinous attachment of the coracoacromial ligament and the edge

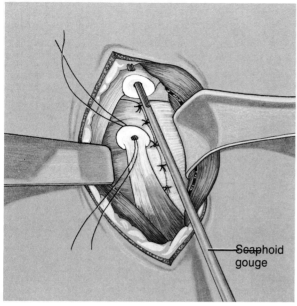

A

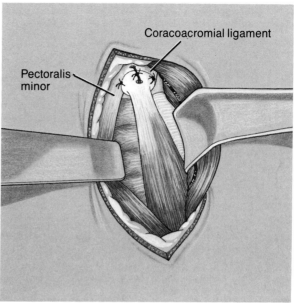

B

Fig. 7-39. (**A**) The coracoid is reattached by making a hole through the osteotomized coracoid fragment with a scaphoid gouge, and then a hole through the coracoid base. Double strands of 0 cotton are passed through the holes, plus sutures through the border of the coracoacromial ligament and base of coracoid. A third suture may be passed through the pectoralis minor attachment if needed. (**B**) These are securely tied giving excellent fixation.

of the common tendon of the coracoid. A third suture may be passed through the pectoralis minor attachment if necessary.

Step 18. The three sutures are then securely tied (Fig. 7-39B). As evidence of its strength, we have not had an incidence of nonunion or avulsion of the coracoid in our follow-up radiographs, despite early motion of the shoulder and later exposure of the arm to every type of contact sport, heavy labor, or to full combat duty in the armed forces. The wound is next checked for small bleeding points. The skin is then closed without drainage. It has never been necessary to use a Hemovac (although the use of one is optional), nor have we used a blood transfusion for this operation. Blood loss has been minimal. An antibiotic is given intravenously during surgery and for 48 hours afterwards.

Step 19. The vertical sketch illustrates the double-breasting strength along the rim (Fig. 7-40). Again, there are no bone grafts that may not unite, nor any screws or staples that may break, loosen, or erode the head.

Step 20. A wrap-around sling is optional for 1 or 2 days (Fig. 7-41). Active gentle pendulum exercises and the use of the arm and hand are begun as tolerated. We have not found it necessary to send the patient to physical therapy following surgical repair. Patients are instructed in the use of the arm and appropriate exercises, which they carry out themselves. The shoulder heals on its own schedule.

WHEN A BANKART LESION IS NOT PRESENT

Another advantage of the Bankart technique is that the exposure is the same whether there is a Bankart lesion or not. One technique shifts easily into the other (for capsulorrhaphy technique, see below).

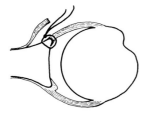

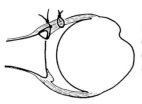

BANKART REPAIR

Reattaches lateral capsular flap to glenoid rim

Plus, added strength from double breasting the medial capsule, reinforcing the entire glenoid rim from 2:00 to 6:00.

Fig. 7-40. The vertical sketch illustrates the double breasting strength of the repair, along the glenoid rim and the smooth capsular surface for the humeral head. This explains the absence of degenerative changes secondary to the repair.

POSTOPERATIVE CARE

Since no muscles have been transected or transplanted, and no bone transplanted in the technique described above, long periods of immobilization and support to the shoulder are not necessary. This is a great relief to the patient. The arm is completely free in 1 to 2 days, when gentle pendulum exercises can begin. Patients can shower on the fourth day, using soap and water on the incision (Fig. 7-42). When

discharged, the patient is fully dressed with no slings or casts (Fig. 7-43). The patients are happy that they do not have to spend hours attending physical therapy. The necessary therapy is carried out during the day by the patient. Our routine is as follows:

Step 1. *Early Motion.* If a sling is applied at surgery, it is usually discarded on the second postoperative day. The arm is free, and gentle pendulum exercises are begun which stimulate healing and aid in regaining motion. By the third day, the patient should be able to reach the face, and to begin progressive function of the extremity. On the fourth or fifth postoperative day, the sutures are removed, and the patient leaves the hospital, to be seen in the office in 3 weeks.

Step 2. Because as the patient does not have to attend physical therapy to regain motion and function of the arm, valuable time is saved. Patients accomplish this on their own with our instructions. They may return to school or work in 10 days or 2 weeks, and are encouraged to use their extremity to write and function within the range of tolerance. They are cautioned to avoid straining their shoulder with lifting or pushing. They are seen for an office check-up once every 3 weeks for 3 months, then once every 3 months for a year.

Step 3. By the third week, they begin gentle pro-

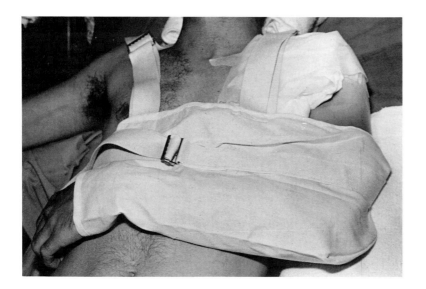

Fig. 7-41. A wraparound sling is applied to protect the arm during recovery from anesthesia.

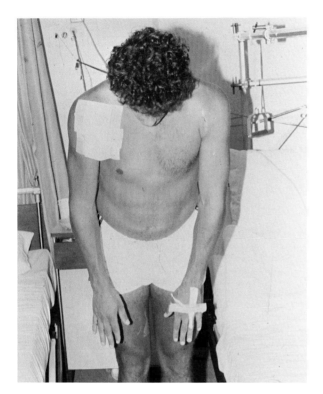

Fig. 7-42. On the second postoperative day, the sling is discarded and the patient may begin gentle elbow flexion and pendulum exercises.

gressive exercises in inward and outward rotation of the arm, abduction to 45°, and increasing forward flexion by gentle stretching. This is "healing time," and should not be abused.

Step 4. From the eighth to tenth week, progressive resistive exercises are increased with the aid of rubber bands (Thera-bands), elastic belts, or springs (Fig. 7-44). Normal functional activities are encouraged such as use of wall-weights, swimming, light rowing, squash, or golf. Wall-weights coordinate shoulder and body motion. This is carried out gradually and not forced, so that normal healing processes are not disturbed but stimulated. I was interested in a patient on whose right shoulder I had performed a Bankart procedure a year previously. He had gone to England after surgery and I had not seen him for a year. I asked him if he had seen a doctor.

"No." Had he received physical therapy? "No, I did what you told me to do, that is to let my shoulder recover on its own schedule." He had complete range of motion and full function of his shoulder. Perhaps he is telling us something!

Step 5. At 6 months, patients should have regained 90 to 100 percent of motion, good strength, and have no apprehension of their shoulder in elevation and rotation. Contact sports, hockey, football, heavy labor, and combat duty are allowed. Patients are advised, however, to keep their arms and hands in front of them, and avoid forceful action on the extended or abducted extremity when possible. Also, they should take *a good body turn* in the use of the arm, in throwing sports, such as football, serving in tennis, or throwing a baseball. This relieves strain on the shoulder and produces a smoother and more effective function.

In summary, the aim of the Bankart procedure is to restore stability to the shoulder safely without interrupting the important balance of the shoulder muscles. This is accomplished by careful layer-by-layer exposure of the shoulder, identifying the causative factors producing the joint instability, and correcting them. All muscles are returned to their original anatomical attachments. In this way, the normal coordinated rhythmic balance of shoulder function is restored. Metal screws, staples, or pins are not used. Muscle layers are not transected or transplanted to unnatural sites. Early motion with the absence of slings or supports is well received by the patient.

RESULTS

Follow-up evaluation was scored by a 100 unit rating sheet, which included stability (50 units), motion (20 units) and function (30 units) (Table 7-5). Seventy-four percent (103 shoulders) were rated excellent, 22.5 percent (33 shoulders) good, and 3 percent (4 shoulders) poor results. Thus, 96.5 percent were graded good to excellent results. The recurrence rate was 3.5 percent, which has remained the same in our follow-up studies to date. It is important to note that *our "recurrence rate" includes both postoperative subluxations and dislocations.* We do not evaluate

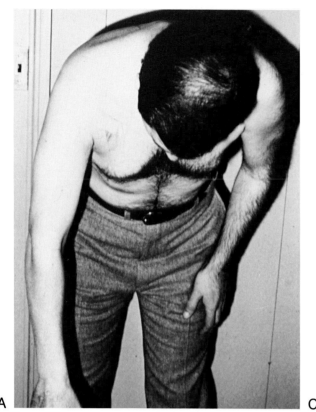

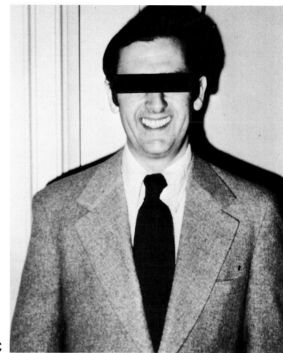

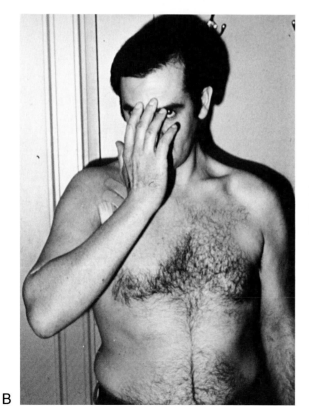

Fig. 7-43. The patient leaves the hospital on the fourth or fifth postoperative day. (**A**) With pendulum exercises. (**B**) Patient can touch his face. (**C**) Fully dressed. May return to office.

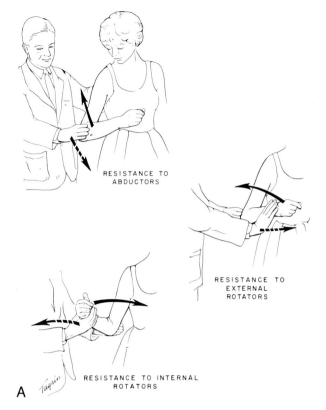

RESISTANCE TO
ABDUCTORS

RESISTANCE TO
EXTERNAL
ROTATORS

RESISTANCE TO INTERNAL
ROTATORS

A

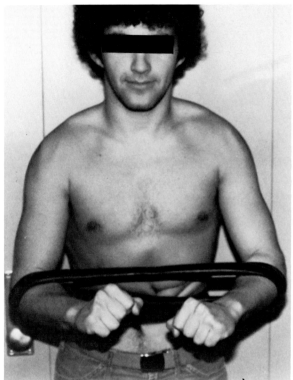

B₁

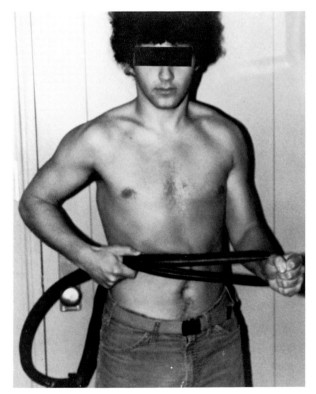

B₂

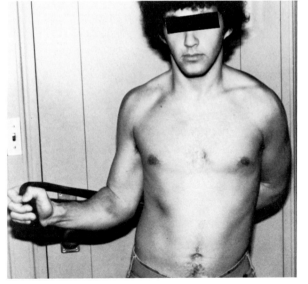

B₃

Fig. 7-44. Specific resistive exercises in abduction (to 45°), internal rotation, and external rotation can be carried out by the patient at intervals during the day. (**A**) With help of friends or family. (**B**) Using elastic belt or Thera-bands. (1) Abduction to 45°. (2) External rotation. (3) Internal rotation. (*Figure continues.*)

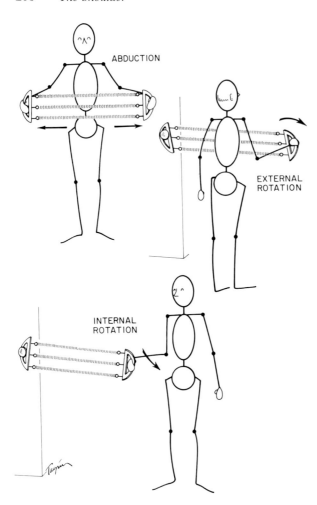

ABDUCTION

EXTERNAL ROTATION

INTERNAL ROTATION

Fig. 7-44 (*Continued*). (**C**) We emphasize again that shoulder strengthening exercises should have body motion with shoulder motion, when possible.

them separately. We consider a postoperative recurrent subluxation just as disabling as a postoperative recurrent dislocation. All follow-up examinations were seen personally by the author.

EVALUATION OF POOR RESULTS

In our follow-up study in 1978,[121] there were 5 recurrences in 145 patients. Excess laxity of the supporting tissues was present in two loose-jointed patients. This was early in our study and today we would have put more time into specific resistive exercises. The other three patients experienced severe postop-

erative trauma (roping a steer at a rodeo, an epileptic fit, and a violent fight soon after surgery).

In one instance, recurrent subluxation occurred as the result of reparative surgery on a Bristow procedure referred to us. Another was a patient with a severe Hill-Sachs lesion. A Connolly procedure eliminated the patient's instability. Our further experience with the Connolly procedure is reviewed in the next few pages. Much can be learned from the following specific questions.

SPECIFIC QUESTIONS

1. *What Has been the Experience Using the Bankart Procedure with Severe Hill-Sachs Lesions?*
We have follow-up information on 110 shoulders with Hill-Sachs head lesions.

Thirty shoulders seen initially with a mild Hill-Sachs lesion experienced no recurrence, 32 were excellent, and 8 were good results. Sixty-four repairs had moderately severe head lesions, with a recurrence rate of 4.7 percent. Sixteen shoulders had severe head lesions, with a recurrence rate of 6 percent. Thus, of the 80 shoulders with moderate to severe Hill-Sachs lesions, 5 percent recurred. This is an acceptable result for *initial* surgical repair and only 1.5 percent higher than our overall recurrence rate of 3.5 percent. What additional steps can be taken for *failed* initial surgery complicated by severe Hill-Sachs lesions?

Since our publication in 1978, we have used the Connolly procedure (transfer of the infraspinatus muscle into the severe Hill-Sachs lesion) on four occasions. Three had been failed procedures referred to us. Two incisions are used: an anterior one to repair the Bankart lesion (which each had), and a second superior incision for transfer of the infraspinatus muscle. There have been no recurrences of dislocation to date using this combination. However, because of two previous unsuccessful surgical procedures and advanced traumatic joint changes, one patient's shoulder may require either a joint replacement or arthrodesis. We have not used the Weber osteotomy, but appreciate its principle. Weber reports a 6 percent recurrence rate and a 1 percent subluxation rate, or 7 percent instability rate.

2. *What Has been the Experience with Using the Bankart Procedure for Recurrent Dislocations Complicated by Fractures of the Glenoid Rim?*

Table 7-5. Rating Sheet for Bankart Repair

Scoring System	Units	Excellent	Good	Fair	Poor
Stability					
No recurrence, subluxation, or apprehension	50	No recurrences	No recurrences	No recurrences	Recurrence of dislocation
Apprehension when placing arm in certain positions	30	No apprehension when placing arm in complete elevation and external rotation	Mild apprehension when placing arm in elevation and external rotation	Moderate apprehension during elevation and external rotation	Marked apprehension during elevation or extension
Subluxation (not requiring reduction)	10	No subluxations	No subluxations	No subluxations	
Recurrent dislocation	0				
Motion					
100% of normal external rotation, internal rotation, and elevation	20	100% of normal external rotation; complete elevation and internal rotation	75% of normal external rotation; complete elevation and internal rotation	50% of normal external rotation; 75% of elevation and internal rotation	No external rotation 50% of elevation (can get hand only to face) and 50% of internal rotation
75% of normal external rotation, and normal elevation and internal rotation	15				
50% of normal external rotation and 75% of normal elevation and internal rotation	10				
50% of normal elevation and internal rotation; no external rotation	5				
Function					
No limitation in work or sports; little or no discomfort	30	Performs all work and sports; no limitation in overhead activities; shoulder strong in lifting, swimming, tennis, throwing, no discomfort	Mild limitation in work and sports; shoulder strong; minimum discomfort	Moderate limitation doing overhead work and heavy lifting; unable to throw, serve hard in tennis, or swim; moderate disabling pain	Marked limitation unable to perform overhead work and lifting; cannot throw, play tennis, or swim; chronic discomfort
Mild limitation and minimum discomfort	25				
Moderate limitation and discomfort	10				
Marked limitation and pain	0				
Total units possible	100				

(Rowe CR, Patel D, Southmayd WW: Method of results evaluation for Bankart repair of recurrent anterior dislocation of the shoulder. Reprinted from J Bone Joint Surg 60A (1), 1978.)

To our surprise, the recurrence rate in this group was only 2 percent, which is lower than our overall rate of 3.5 percent.[121] Eighteen shoulders had one-sixth of the glenoid fossa fractured as the result of recurrent dislocations, with no recurrence (10 were graded excellent, 5 good, and 3 were lost to follow-up). Twenty-six had one-quarter of the fossa fractured off, with 1 recurrence (15 had excellent results, 8 were good, and 2 were lost to follow-up). Seven shoulders had one-third of the glenoid fossa fractured off (five were graded excellent, two were lost to follow-

up). Of the 44 shoulders with rim fractures that were evaluated, 98 percent were rated good to excellent, with only one recurrence. *In these shoulders, no bone grafts or muscle transplants were used to reinforce the rim.* The fractured fragments were not replaced, since they could not be secured without irregularity along the rim. Routine Bankart repairs were carried out, regardless of the size of the rim defect. Our incidence of 31 percent of patients with fractures of the glenoid rim compares with D'Angelo's[33] 31.5 percent rate. Other investigators report lower incidence of glenoid rim fractures. Palmer and Widen[106] reported 20 percent, Symeonides[137] 18 percent, and DePalma[38] 11 percent. It has been stated that unless the fractured glenoid fossa is built up by a bone graft it "may be virtually impossible to restore muscle balance."[38] With direct repair of the capsule back to the fractured glenoid rim by the Bankart technique, we are happy to have a different experience.

3. *Does the Return of Complete External Rotation Weaken the Bankart Procedure?*

Some investigators[65,79] have stated that return of complete external rotation following surgical repair was associated with an increased incidence of recurrence or subluxation. In our experience, the opposite has been true. Only 2 percent of our 86 patients with return of complete external rotation experienced recurrence; none of the 30 patients with return of 75 percent of normal external rotation had recurrences. Conversely, in our eight patients whose external rotation was limited to less than 50 percent of normal, two experienced recurrence.

Therefore, from our follow-up studies, *the return of maximum external rotation was associated with a definite decrease in the incidence of recurrence, rather than an increase.* This is understandable, because, with limited external rotation, a force will expend itself against the repair and, if great enough, will disrupt the repair. On the other hand, with complete external rotation, the force is not obstructed and tearing would be very difficult.

Return of stable and complete external rotation has been greatly appreciated by patients who are baseball players, pitchers, tennis players, football quarterbacks, basketball players, and swimmers. Patient D.B. (Fig. 7-45) played 4 years of football at a large university after a Bankart procedure on his dominant shoulder with no recurrences. He has been stable for over 15 years. Patient S.H. (Fig. 7-46) demonstrates complete range of motion 6 years following a Bankart procedure on his right shoulder. He is a good athlete and takes part in all sports. There are no degenerative joint changes in his shoulder. Seventy-five percent of the 375 patients undergoing Bankart procedures had return of 100 percent of motion, 20 percent had return of 75 percent of motion, and 5 percent had less than 75 percent of motion.

4. *How Has the Bankart Procedure Stood up for the Athlete?*

In our 1978 report, 67 of 161 patients were involved in athletics prior to their shoulder injury. Only two patients failed to return to their previous sport. There were 46 *dominant* arms and 31 *nondominant* arms involved. Of the 46 dominant arms, only one patient failed to return to his original sports activity. Thirty were engaged in throwing sports. Of these, 10 (33 percent) were able to throw or pitch a baseball as hard as they had prior to injury. They were able to throw a football as hard as they had prior to injury, and to serve as hard in tennis, swim as powerfully, or "spike" a volleyball as forcefully as prior to injury. The remaining 20 patients in throwing sports (67 percent) could throw a football or softball or serve as hard in tennis, but could not throw a baseball as hard as formerly. A number of the 46 patients whose dominant arms were involved became superior athletes after their shoulder repair, including two college pitchers, two college catchers, one triple letter athlete, three professional hockey players, one professional basketball player, one college tennis champion, seven college (see Figs. 45-46) and two professional football players, and one backstroke swimming champion at the U.S. Naval Academy.

Of the 31 patients in whom the *nondominant* shoulder was repaired, only *one* was not able to return to sports activities in which he had participated before his injury. The other 30 had no limitations and in many instances were superior athletes, including 10 college and 1 professional football players, 8 three letter athletes, 5 competitive swimmers, 1 hammer thrower who placed third in the Olympic tryouts in the east, an All-New England basketball center, a member of the U.S. Olympic Ski Team, a college hockey goal tender, and 2 college weight lifters. These results certainly speak for themselves. Again, we point out that a recurrent subluxation is recorded the same as a recurrent dislocation in our follow-up rating.

5. *Does the Bankart Procedure Cause Late Degenerative Changes along the Glenoid Rim?*

This was a concern to us when we began to use the Bankart procedure in World War II. Would the holes in the rim of the glenoid and articular surface result in spur formation, or late degenerative changes along the rim? As we began to have follow-up studies, we did not see late joint changes, which was encouraging to us. The answer came in our 1978 report on 124 patients evaluated for up to 30 years (an average of 6-year follow-up), with no late degenerative

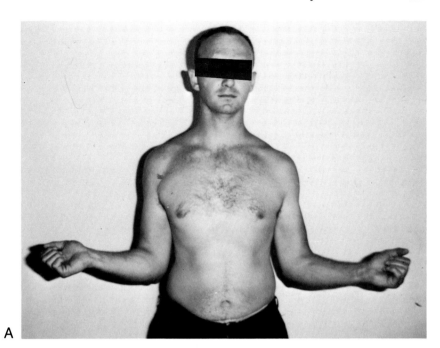

Fig. 7-45. Patient after Bankart repair of his right shoulder (dominant arm). He played 4 years of football at a large university. He continues with a strong shoulder and no recurrences (15 years). Note complete range of external rotation. (**A** and **B**).

A

B

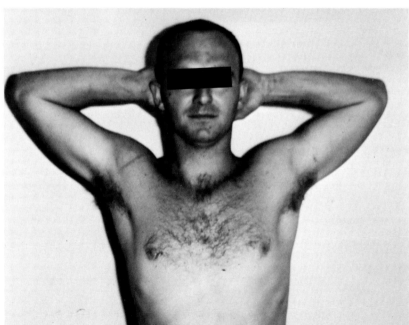

changes that were not present preoperatively. Again, this was a very pleasant surprise to us. The reason for this, we assume, was that the holes in the articular surface of the glenoid are covered by the capsule, leaving a smooth articular surface. Also, we are careful to keep the holes in the glenoid rim small. It is most important that the rim not be traumatized when one is reattaching the capsule and making the holes. Special instruments are necessary for this.

Figure 7-46 shows a film of S.H.'s right shoulder

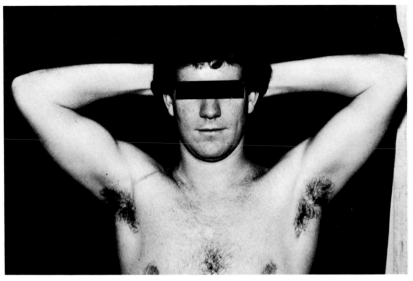

A

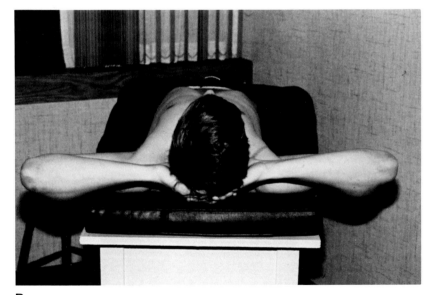

B

Fig. 7-46. Patient has complete range of motion. (**A**) and (**B**) External rotation. (*Figure continues.*)

6 years after his Bankart procedure with a smooth untraumatized rim. Figure 7-47 (patient J.B.) shows a right shoulder 15 years after a Bankart procedure. There are no degenerative changes. One year after surgery, J.B. joined the Marines and had active combat duty in Korea; he has full range of motion and no recurrences. In Figure 7-48, the patient's left shoulder, 26 years after a left Bankart procedure, shows no degenerative changes. He has complete range of motion, no recurrences, and a strong shoulder. When this procedure is compared to the changes present following other procedures, the time and effort in performing a Bankart procedure seem worthwhile.

6. *Has Early Motion Affected Your Results?*

Early motion has affected our results in a very *beneficial* way. With our Bankart and capsulorrhaphy technique, the repair is strong enough for the patient to

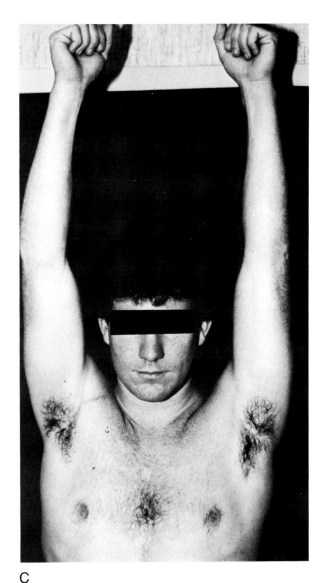

C

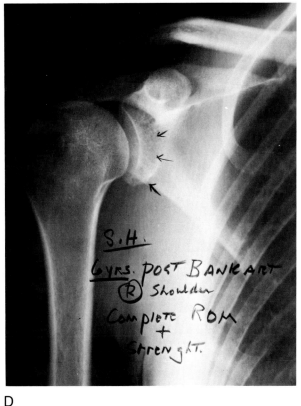

D

Fig. 7-46 (*Continued*). (**C**) Elevation. (**D**) Illustrates lack of traumatic or degenerative changes after 6 years as a three-letter man in college.

begin motion on the first or second postoperative day. Since no screws or staples are used, and no healing of bone to bone with transplants is required, motion could be started in the recovery room if necessary. We look forward to a safe method of immediate passive motion for our Bankart repairs, since we feel the repair is strong enough to tolerate this.

We have found that early motion stimulates healing, reduces edema and adhesion formation, and improves the status of the extremity, as well as the comfort and satisfaction of the patient in having a free extremity to be used as tolerated to dress, shower, and wet the incision on the third or fourth postoperative day.

We have used early passive and active motion on the second to third day in all of our Bankart repairs over the past 20 years. Patients carry out their own physical therapy immediately after surgery. We have had no complications from this routine, only the good effects of early function.

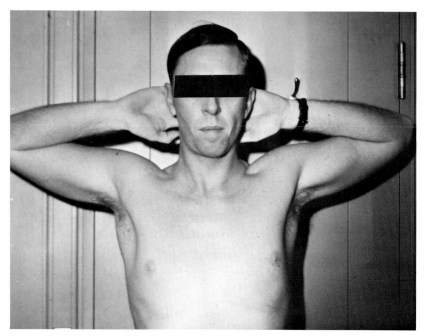

A

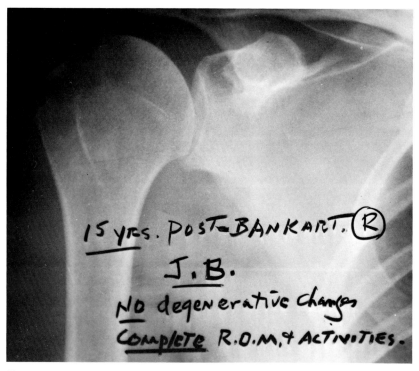

B

Fig. 7-47. **(A)** Patient 15 years after Bankart procedure of his right shoulder, followed by full combat duty with Marines in Korea. **(B)** No dislocations or degenerative changes of the joint.

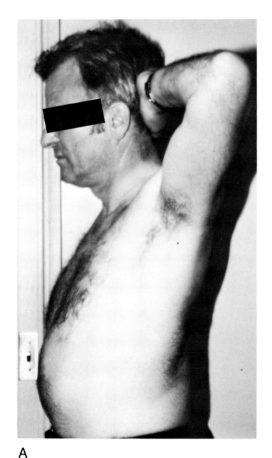

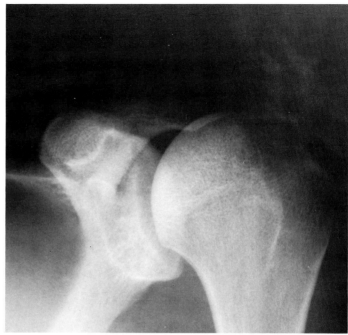

B

Fig. 7-48. (A,B) Patient's left shoulder shows no degenerative changes 26 years after Bankart procedure. He had full function in sailing, golf, and work with no recurrences.

A

COMPLICATIONS

Since 1946, 475 Bankart procedures have been evaluated with one infection, an incidence of 0.002 percent. The infection was not evident until a year after surgery. Fortunately, it did not involve the joint. Following local debridement, the shoulder has been normal. We point out that our surgery has not been performed under ultraviolet light or in the greenhouse. One patient in 1953 extruded two strands of silk sutures which were removed and the small sinuses spontaneously closed, with no evidence of infection. Since then, we have routinely used cotton sutures and have had no suture reaction. One patient had a postoperative hematoma that required evacuation and closure. His wound healed uneventfully (four other patients had mild postoperative hematomas, all of which absorbed before discharge). Two patients experienced a thrombophlebitis of the cephalic vein, which cleared up when treated with warm com-

presses. These occurred during the period when we ligated the cephalic vein. None have occurred since we have omitted ligation of the vein (1975). There has been no injury to the musculotendinous nerves. We credit this to osteotomizing the coracoid process, which eliminates traction on the common tendon. Only one patient experienced temporary deltoid weakness postoperatively. However, electromyograms confirmed that the axillary nerve was intact and his muscle strength returned. There have been no nonunions of the osteotomized coracoid process after repair by direct suture. There were no late degenerative changes or arthrosis of the shoulder joint or the glenoid rim, during a 30 year follow-up. Mild changes in one shoulder were present preoperatively and did not increase following surgery. This is good testimony to the lack of trauma with the Bankart repair.

Samilson records arthropathy of the shoulder following recurrent anterior dislocations, to which the reader is referred.[128,129]

Modifications of the Bankart Procedure

THE DUTOIT PROCEDURE

In 1956, G.T. duToit and D. Roux[40] reported on a modification of the Bankart procedure in a 24 year study of what they termed "the Johannesburg procedure," which they credit to F.P. Fouche and A.L. Allen in 1937. Instead of reattaching the lateral capsule directly to the rim of the glenoid by holes through the rim, they attached the capsule to the scapular neck using one or two staples. Boyd and Hunt[19] of the Campbell Clinic in 1965 modified the procedure by using barbed staples, and by exposing the joint by splitting the subscapularis muscle and capsule in

line of its muscle fibers, without removing the subscapularis from the capsule (Fig. 7-49). The staples could be inserted within or outside the joint capsule. The capsule was then closed horizontally. This became a very popular technique due to its simplicity; however, disturbing loosening of the staples, even though barbed, can occur from sudden heavy lifting, or in contact sports. Another disturbing complication was degenerative changes along the glenoid rim and, at times, intraarticular migration of the staples.[102,116,126,149]

THE VIEK TECHNIQUE

The Viek[142] procedure was published in 1959. Viek credits the idea of pull-out wires for securing the anterior capsule to the scapular neck to Luckey.[77] Although no follow-up report was given, the surgical approach seems sound and the technique worthy of study.

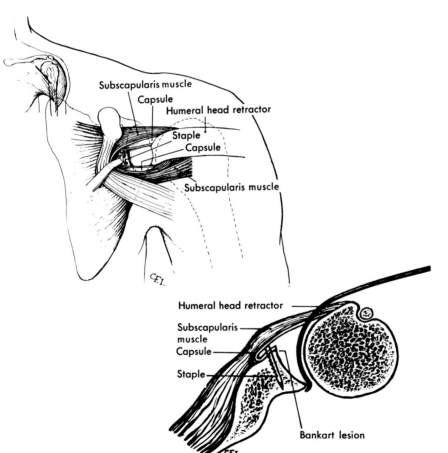

Fig. 7-49. The duToit procedure (Boyd modification). The avulsed capsule is reattached to the neck of the scapula by one or two barbed staples rather than to the glenoid rim. (Boyd HB, Hunt HO: Recurrent dislocations of the shoulder. The staple capsulorrhaphy. J Bone Joint Surg 47A:1514, 1965.)

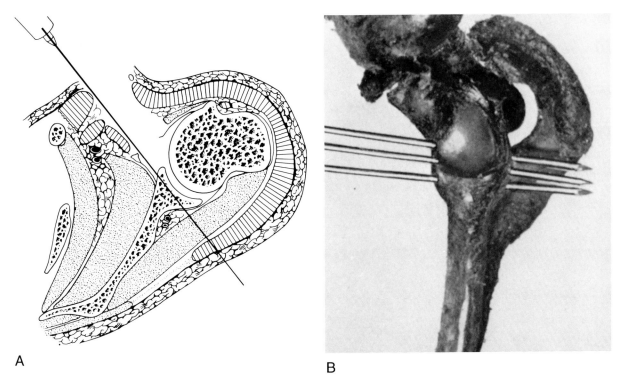

Fig. 7-50. The Viek technique. (**A**) Wire through the scapular neck. (**B**) Three ⅛″ Steinmann pins (end of pullout sutures are threaded through the eye of the pins) (Viek P, Bill BT: The Bankart shoulder reconstruction—the use of pullout wires and other practical details. J Bone Joint Surg 41A:236, 1959.)

The patient is placed on the side. The anterior glenoid rim is approached through the deltopectoral space, the subscapularis muscle is separated from the anterior capsule, which is opened, and a humeral head retractor is used to expose the glenoid fossa (Fig. 7-50). Braided wire (00) sutures are placed through the detached capsule, with pull-out wires that exit anteriorly. Wire sutures are then passed through the scapular neck, by means of three ⅛″ Steinmann pins (the ends of the sutures are threaded through eyes in the Steinmann pins), out through the skin of the scapula, and tied. The wires are removed 3 to 4 weeks postoperatively. This is an ingenious technique.

We have two comments. First, one of the reasons it was devised was the fear of trauma to the rim of the glenoid by the Bankart technique. This is a very good reason, if the Bankart procedure is not correctly performed. However, we have had no traumatic changes along the rim of the glenoid in our follow-up studies from 2 to 30 years. The reason for this is

that the holes are covered by the soft capsule. We emphasize use of proper instruments and small holes.

Second, for extra strength, we recommend double breasting the lateral and medial capsule folds along the glenoid rim, from 2 to 6 o'clock, especially at 6 o'clock where the greatest strain to the shoulder is exerted when the arm is elevated. Although the Viek technique inserts three pins, it would seem difficult to place one as inferiorly as 6 o'clock. However, this is an excellent technique and worthy of study.

THE EYRE-BROOK PROCEDURE

The Eyre-Brook[44] procedure (Fig. 7-51) was presented in 1948. Rather than repairing the capsule directly to the glenoid rim by holes through the rim, Eyre-Brook proposed, as did Viek, reattaching the capsule to horizontal holes made in the neck of the scapula, just off the rim. This is an excellent alternative to the Bankart procedure, especially when the rim has been badly damaged. Arthur Eyre-Brook,

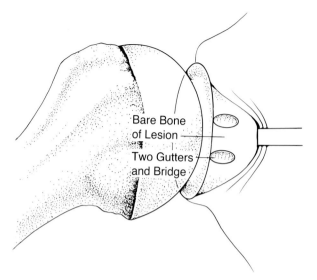

Fig. 7-51. The Eyre-Brook procedure. The capsule is reattached to the neck of the glenoid, rather than through the rim. (Eyre-Brook AL: Recurrent dislocation of the shoulder. Lesions discovered in seventeen cases, surgery employed, and immediate report of results. J Bone Joint Surg 30B:39, 1948.)

who assisted Bankart during his training, credits this modification to him. Thus, Bankart must have varied his technique in this procedure. Perhaps an additional hole should be made at 5 or 6 o'clock for strength

along the inferior capsular ligament to protect the arm in full elevation.

THE MOSELEY PROCEDURE

Moseley[91,92] introduced an unusual modification in 1947, by inserting a vitallium rim along the glenoid neck as a base for suturing and double breasting the capsular repair (Fig. 7-52). Although this procedure has not had popular acceptance, it is indicated as an alternative in large fractures of the glenoid rim and fossa.

In 1986, Ellison[42] reported his inside-out procedure at the meeting of the American Orthopaedic Association. The subscapularis muscle is not separated from the anterior capsule, but is "turned back," from its attachment to the lesser tuberosity. With a ³⁄₁₀″ drill, holes are made in the rim of the glenoid neck as in the Bankart procedure. The holes (usually six) are completed with a special punch. Sutures are placed through the holes, then through the capsule from "inside out," and sutured to the glenoid rim.

Matsen[79a] uses a somewhat similar technique, turning down the subscapularis and capsule from its attachment to the lesser tuberosity. The lateral capsule is then reattached to the glenoid rim.

Cofield[28a] approaches the anterior rim of the glenoid according to our technique with three holes in

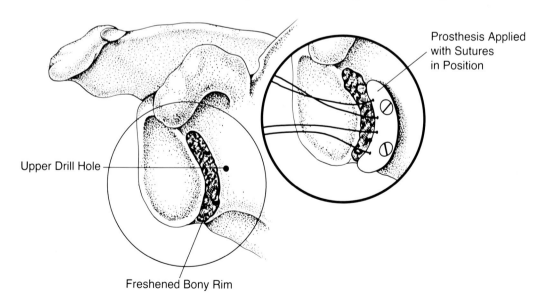

Fig. 7-52. The Moseley procedure. Insertion of vitallium rim along the glenoid neck as a base for the capsular repair. (Moseley HF: Shoulder Lesions. E & S Livingstone, Edinburgh, 1969.)

the glenoid rim. The lateral capsule is then split horizontally, and reattached to the glenoid rim by the capsular shift technique.

Other Procedures

MUSCLE AND CAPSULE PLICATION

The Putti-Platt Procedure

Sir Harry Platt became disturbed by the absence of Bankart's *"essential"* lesion at surgery in some recurrent anterior dislocations of the shoulder. He therefore devised a simpler procedure of shortening and double breasting the subscapularis muscle and capsule. He first performed this procedure at the Ancoats Hospital, in Manchester, England, on November 13, 1925. However, he was not aware that Victorio Putti of Italy had devised a similar procedure in 1923, crediting the idea to his former teacher Codivilla at the University of Bologna. It remained for Osmond-Clarke to report the procedure in 1948, giving it the eponymous title, the "Putti-Platt" procedure[104] (Fig. 7-53).

Technique. This is a strong procedure, and is easier to perform than the Bankart. It became very popular in Britain during World War II. The arm is rotated laterally, bringing the subscapularis muscle and tendon into full view. The subscapularis muscle and capsule are sharply divided 2.5 cm medial to the insertion to the lesser tuberosity down through the capsule. The joint is inspected. When no Bankart lesion is present, the lateral flap of subscapularis muscle and capsule are sewn to the "soft tissue" along the rim

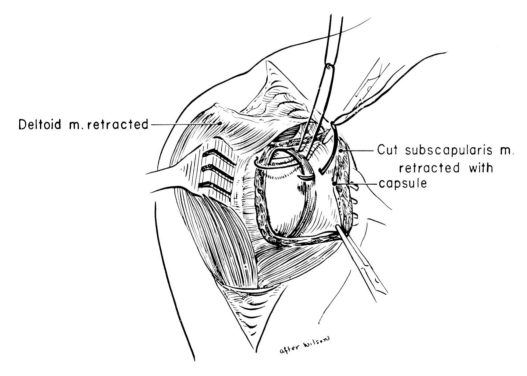

Fig. 7-53. The Putti-Platt procedure. The subscapularis muscle and capsule are sharply divided 2.5 cm medial to the lesser tuberosity. When no Bankart lesion is present, the lateral flap of capsule and muscle is sewn to the "soft tissues" along the rim of the glenoid. The medial flap is then double breasted over the lateral flap. When a Bankart lesion is present, the glenoid neck is "freshened" and the lateral flap sutured "to the deep surface of the medial capsule on the undersurface of the medial flap." (Reprinted with permission from Rowe CR, Marble AC: Shoulder girdle injuries. p. 254. In Cave EF (ed): Fractures and Other Injuries. Copyright © by Year Book Medical Publishers, Inc., Chicago, 1958.)

of the glenoid under the medial flap of muscle. The medial flap is then double breasted over the lateral flap. If a Bankart lesion is found (avulsion of the labrum and capsule from the rim of the glenoid), the bone is freshened and the lateral flap is then sutured to the deep surface of the medial capsule on the undersurface of the medial flap. The capsule is not reattached directly to the bone of the glenoid rim. The medial flap is then double breasted over the lateral flap.

Comments. Although this is a strong procedure, it has the disadvantage of limiting external rotation, which is a definite concern to the dominant arm of many athletes, such as tennis players, baseball, and basketball players, and to anyone who needs a complete, smooth, rhythmic overhead motion of the arm and shoulder. However, some patients have return of normal external rotation. Another concern is that if full range of motion is obtained, it may be at the expense of stretching and weakening of the shortened subscapularis muscle. Perhaps, if the lateral flap were lengthened beyond 2.5 cm, freer motion would be obtained. I agree with Rockwood[116] and Symeonides[137] that if only 2.5 cm of lateral subscapularis and capsule are used, and "attached" to the soft tissues of the raw bone on the underside of the mesial flap, if the patient regains complete external rotation beyond the neutral zero position, it may be at the expense of disruption of the repair from the glenoid rim and overstretching of the double breasted tissues, and thus loss of stability.

We have found, however, with patients we have reoperated on for failed Putti-Platt procedures, that the subscapularis muscle is not scarred to the point that it could not be removed from the anterior joint capsule, which is an advantage for the reoperating surgeon. Some patients are not disturbed by limited external rotation (if it is not severe) and are perfectly satisfied with the strength of the Putti-Platt procedure, and its limited motion.

The Symeonides Procedure

Technique. The same principles of the Putti-Platt procedure apply to the Symeonides[137] procedure, which the author describes as a "simplified" Putti-Platt procedure. The medial flap or stump of the divided subscapularis and capsule is sewn over the lateral flap (the lateral flap is not sewn to the rim). The simpler procedure was preferred because suturing the lateral part of the cut subscapularis and capsule to the anterior aspect of the neck of the scapula was, in many cases, difficult and unsatisfactory due to the lack of sufficient soft tissue elements. It seemed likely that this part would be detached or weakened as soon as the first movements of the shoulder were begun.

Comments. Symeonides considers the shortening of the subscapularis muscle to be the source of the strength of his repair. On the other hand, in our Bankart repairs the subscapularis muscle is reattached back precisely to its original insertion, without any degree of shortening of the muscle, and yet our long-term recurrence rate is only 3.5 percent. The strength of the Symeonides technique is perhaps due as much to shortening of the capsule as to the shortening of the subscapularis muscle.

MUSCLE AND TENDON SLING TRANSFER PROCEDURES

A number of "sling" procedures that have been designed to stabilize the shoulder are discussed here.

The Magnuson-Stack Procedure

Technique. In 1943, Magnuson and Stack[79] proposed detaching the insertion of the subscapularis muscle from the lesser tuberosity and transferring it laterally across the bicipital groove to the shaft of the humerus with the arm in internal rotation to function, not only as a sling, but also to limit external rotation (Fig. 7-54). Although Magnuson performed "only a few of these procedures" (personal communication), it was popularized chiefly by his associate, J.K. Stack. A number of modifications have been made by DePalma in 1963,[38] Badgley and O'Connor[7] in 1965, Bailey[8] in 1967, Compere in 1980 (personal communication, 1982), and Rockwood[116] in 1984. These modifications are helpful and indicated. Rockwood and Compere recommend opening the joint and repairing the capsule back to the glenoid rim, if it is avulsed. DePalma leaves the inferior margin of the subscapularis muscle intact to avoid injury to the anterior circumflex vessels and axillary nerve.

Comments. This is a comparatively easy procedure. The design, however, is to restrict external rotation of the arm as well as to have the sling effect of the subscapularis muscle across the front of the joint.

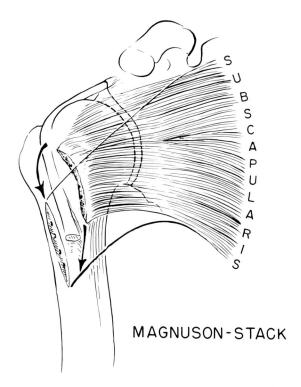

S
U
B
S
C
A
P
U
L
A
R
I
S

MAGNUSON-STACK

Fig. 7-54. The Magnuson procedure. The insertion of the subscapularis is detached from its insertion to the lesser tuberosity, the arm is internally rotated, and the muscle transplanted to the shaft of the humerus. (Reprinted with permission from Rowe CR, Marble AC: Shoulder girdle injuries. p. 254. In Cave EF (ed): Fractures and other injuries. Copyright © by Year Book Medical Publishers, Inc. Chicago, 1958.)

Unfortunately, limiting external rotation eliminates the coordinated rhythmic motion of the shoulder, especially when the dominant arm is involved, which is so important in above-the-shoulder function especially in sports. Its indication, it would seem, would be in the older age group, rather than in young active athlete. The technique of implantation of the subscapularis tendon into the humeral shaft by different surgeons varies. When the tendon is secured only by staples or screws into the shaft, the transplant may pull off, as has occurred in a number of unsuccessful Magnusons we have seen (see below). A more secure technique would be to countersink the tendon into a bony trough in the humeral shaft, securing the tendon through drill holes, as recommended by

DePalma and Rockwood. The wise surgeon, however, warns his or her patient preoperatively that external rotation of the shoulder will be limited. Rockwood advises checking the transplant at surgery to be certain the arm can be externally rotated to neutral zero position before securing the tendon. One of the advantages of the procedure is, however, that if it fails and reoperation is necessary, the subscapularis muscle and capsule are in excellent condition for a Bankart repair, or some other reconstructive procedure.

The Bristow-Latarjet-Helfet Procedure

Technique. This involves transplantation of the coracoid process with its tendon attachments through the subscapularis muscle to the neck of the glenoid. In 1958, Helfet[55] proposed a combination of bone block and sling procedure to give anterior stability to the humeral head. He states that the idea was suggested to him by his chief, Rowley Bristow, during his training in England. Although Bristow is reported not to have performed the procedure, Helfet popularized the idea over the past 15 years. As with the Putti-Platt procedure, the concept of transplanting the coracoid process had previously been proposed. Latarjet[72] reported a similar procedure in 1954, actually 4 years prior to Helfet's report. Consequently, the procedure should now be referred to as the Bristow-Latarjet-Helfet technique. Originally Helfet merely inserted the osteotomized coracoid process (with the attached short head of biceps and coracobrachialis) "through a vertical slip, an inch or an inch and a quarter long, in the middle two-thirds of the musculo-fibrous junction of the muscle [subscapularis muscle]." The joint is opened and the neck of the scapula "rawed," after which the coracoid process is placed on this surface *without* metal fixation (Fig. 7-55). The coracoid tip was merely sutured to the edges of the subscapularis muscle. Postoperatively, the arm is supported in a collar cuff sling for 6 weeks. Helfet reports two recurrences in 30 patients evaluated: an incidence of 7 percent. MacKenzie[78] also favors the Bristow technique.

Modifications

1. McMurray[84] in 1958, and Mead and Sweeney[85,136] in 1964 split the subscapularis muscle and tendon in line with its fibers, opened the joint, and se-

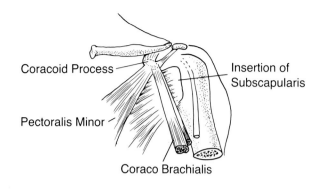

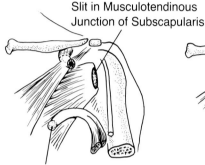
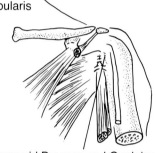

Tip of Coracoid Process
and Conjoined Tendon

Coracoid Process and Conjoined Tendon
Passed Through this Slit to
Neck of Scapula and Held by
Sutures to Margins of Subscapularis

Fig. 7-55. The Bristow-Helfet-Latarjet procedure. The coracoid process with the attached short head of biceps and coracobrachialis muscle is transplanted through the subscapularis muscle to the neck of the scapula. Helfet did not use metal fixation. (Helfet AJ: Coracoid transplantation for rewiring dislocation of the shoulder. The Rowley Bristow operation. J Bone Joint Surg 40B:198, 1958.)

cured the coracoid process to the anterior glenoid neck with a screw.

2. In 1969, Bonin[16] did not split the subscapularis muscle but separated it from the capsule and attached the coracoid to the glenoid neck with a screw.

3. In 1970, May[80] divided the subscapularis muscle from the lesser tuberosity, split it, explored the joint, and fixed the coracoid to the neck of the glenoid with a screw. The subscapularis was then double breasted over the conjoined tendon with half of the muscle above and half below the tendon (Fig. 7-56).

4. In 1985, Braly and Tullos (Fig. 7-57) emphasized that the Bankart lesion, when present, should be corrected and that external rotation should not purposely be restricted.[22] In their procedure, the subscapularis muscle is "incised transversely to its fibers approximately 1 cm medial to its insertion." It is tagged and *then separated from the anterior capsule and turned back.* The capsule is incised vertically along the rim in a "T" shape, to expose the joint. The glenoid neck is then decorticated, the coracoid is secured to the glenoid neck with a malleolar screw to "ablate the pseudo-pouch lying on the anterior aspect of the glenoid," and the capsule repaired. Tullos states that since using the AO cancellous screw they have not had any problem with loosening of the screw. The subscapularis tendon is then resutured to its insertion, thus eliminating the sling effect of the Bristow procedure "and the tangle of anatomy." Braly and Tullos use good principles and technique in their modification.

5. Rockwood[116] uses the Latarjet procedure only when a large portion of the glenoid rim has been avulsed. The entire coracoid process is filleted out and screwed onto the neck by "laying it flat" onto the neck of the scapula using two screws instead of one, which gives a larger base for the coracoid transplant.

Mead[85] points out that the effectiveness of the Bristow procedure was due to the transplanted coracoid

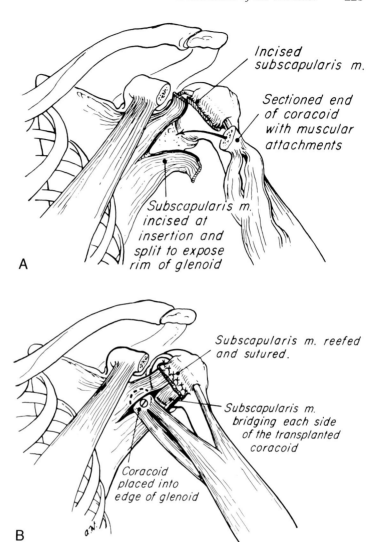

Incised
subscapularis m.

Sectioned end
of coracoid
with muscular
attachments

Subscapularis m.
incised at
insertion and
split to expose
rim of glenoid

A

Subscapularis m. reefed
and sutured.

Subscapularis m.
bridging each side
of the transplanted
coracoid

Coracoid
placed into
edge of glenoid

B

Fig. 7-56. The May modification of the Bristow procedure. (**A**) The subscapularis muscle is divided and the joint is explored. (**B**) The coracoid process is fixed to the neck of the scapula with a screw. The subscapularis muscle is then double breasted over the conjoined tendon, with half of the tendon above and half below. (May VR: A modified Bristow operation for anterior recurrent dislocation of the shoulder. J Bone Joint Surg 52A:1010, 1970.)

tendon, preventing the subscapularis muscle from displacing upward in elevation of the arm. The bone-blocking effect of the coracoid is questionable: if it is close enough to the joint to function as a bone block, it may cause traumatic arthrosis; if placed down on the glenoid neck, its bone-blocking function is minimal.

Comments. A number of points of discussion regarding the Bristow-Latarjet-Helfet procedure have arisen. The primary concern is the disruption of the muscle balance in shoulder function by the damage inflicted on the subscapularis muscle (tying it down and transforming it in various degrees of scar tissue)

with elimination of the plane between the subscapularis and the capsule. In patients with failed Bristow procedure who have come to us and others for reoperation the damage to the subscapularis is appreciable in all cases. In a recent patient, the scar tissue was so dense that we were unable to dissect through it to the joint for fear of injuring the musculotendinous or axillary nerves. This has been observed by other surgeons.[48,59,97,102,116,149] This is one of the greatest drawbacks of the procedure. In reoperating on patients with Bankart, Putti-Platt, Magnuson, Nicola, and duToit procedures, the damage to the subscapularis muscle tissue has been far less than we find in patients who have had Bristow procedures.

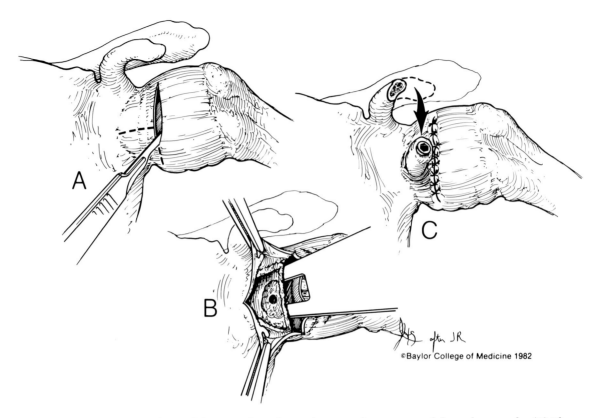

Fig. 7-57. The Braly-Tullos modification. The subscapularis muscle is separated from the capsule. (**A**) The capsule is incised in a T-shape. (**B**) The coracoid is secured to the scapular necks with a cortical screw. (**C**) The capsule is repaired and the subscapularis resutured to its original insertion. (Braly WG, Tullos HS: A modification of the Bristow procedure for recurrent anterior shoulder dislocations and subluxations. Am J Sports Med 13:81, 1985.)

Another disturbing problem is loosening or breakage of the screws and nonunion of the transplant.[6,101] Zuckerman and Matsen[149] in 1984 reported 37 patients with failed Bristow procedures. Twenty-four had loose screws and three had fracture of the transplant. Forty-one percent had "significant injury to the articular surface of the glenohumeral joint."

Norris has recently reported on 20 failed Bristow procedures.[102] Of these, 18 had symptomatic nonunion and loosening of the screw of the coracoid transplant, 15 subluxated beneath the implant, and 8 had unrepaired labral detachments.

Hovelius[62] of Sweden also reported in 1982 that only 52 percent of the transferred coracoids healed, 28 percent had fibrous healing, and in 16 percent the screw had migrated. However, as with many orthopaedic procedures, the technique of the Bristow procedure is perfected by some surgeons who report few complications and good results.[2,76,80] We would encourage those who are interested in this procedure to learn the secret of those who report successes.

The Boytchev Procedure

Technique. Conforti, in 1974 and 1980, summarized his experience with the Boytchev procedure and his modifications. The coracoid tip with its three attached muscles is routed deep to the subscapularis muscle and then back to its original attachments. In a very well illustrated article,[29] Conforti reports on 17 patients who had no recurrence.

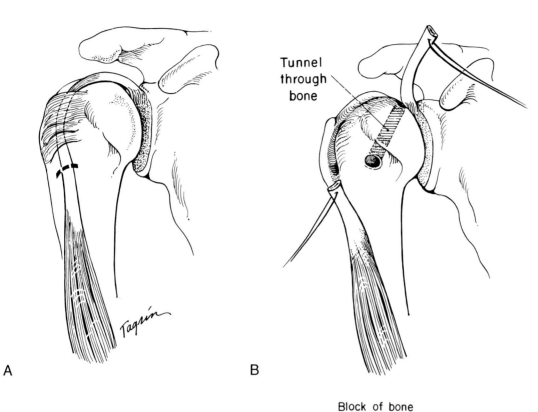

A

B

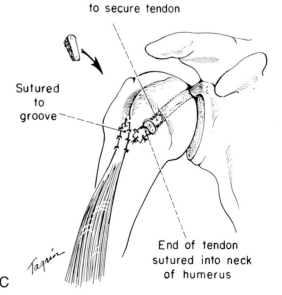

C

Fig. 7-58. The Thompson modification of the Nicola procedure. The transplanted long head of biceps tendon is used as a ligamentum teres. (**A**) Divison of the tendon. (**B**) Transplantation through the humeral head. (**C**) Fixation of the biceps tendon with a plug of bone. The distal biceps tendon is implanted into the biceps canal.

Comments.   One should be concerned, however, with complications to the musculocutaneous and axillary nerves and, the instability of unrepaired Bankart lesions, excessive capsule laxity, or severe Hill-Sachs lesions that are left unrepaired. Further follow-up study is indicated.

Long Head of Biceps Transplant: Nicola Procedure

Toufick Nicola[99] in 1934 transplanted the long head of biceps tendon through the humeral head to function as a ligamentum teres. It was a very popular procedure during the 1930s; however, during World War II it proved not to be strong enough for combat duty and was discontinued in favor of the Bankart and Putti-Platt procedures. In a follow-up study at the Massachusetts General Hospital in 1956,[117] the recurrence rate of the Nicola procedure in civilians was 53 percent. Adams[1] in 1948 reported an incidence

of 36 percent and Lange[71] in 1951 reported a 33 percent recurrence rate.

A modification of the Nicola procedure was presented by Thompson[138] in 1965, in which the transplanted biceps tendon was used specifically as a ligamentum teres, which greatly increased the stability of the joint (Fig. 7-58). The tendon is secured in the bony canal with a plug of iliac bone. The distal biceps tendon is then transplanted into the bicipital groove or to the coracoid process. We have used Thompson's modification in the past as an adjunctive procedure in paralytic shoulders and selected voluntary dislocations with satisfactory results.

The Gallie-LeMesurier Procedure

In 1948, Gallie and LeMesurier proposed a technique for inserting "a new ligament" taken from the iliotibial band across the anterior inferior aspect of the capsule and glenoid rim[50] (Fig. 7-59). This tech-

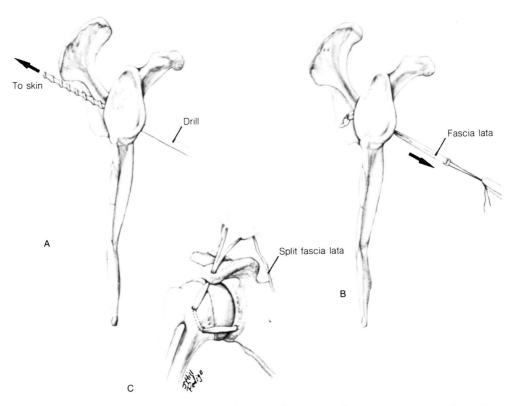

Fig. 7-59. The Gallie-LeMesurier procedure. The aim of this procedure was to create a "new ligament" for shoulder stability from the iliotibial band. This procedure is effective also for multidirectional instabilities. (Post M: The Shoulder. Lea & Febiger, Philadelphia, 1978.)

nique stabilizes posterior instability as well as anterior instability of the shoulder. The procedure has been used extensively by Bateman of Toronto, and is well described in his book.[11]

The principle of stabilizing the shoulder via the scapula led also to the Viek procedure[142] as well as recent modifications by Caspari,[26] using a strip of fascia from the thigh to reinforce the anterior inferior capsule.

Although the Gallie procedure is an unusual technique, it has the advantage of creating little interference with the muscle balance of the shoulder. Early motion is advised, and a very good range of postoperative motion is expected. Also, the procedure is applicable for multidirectional instabilities because it controls anterior, inferior, and posterior instabilities. This technique has been little appreciated by surgeons interested in the shoulder and deserves further study and experience with its advantages.

BONE BLOCK PROCEDURES

Although the Bristow-Latarjet-Helfet technique may be considered a bone block procedure, it is listed under sling procedures.

The Eden[41] and Hybbinette[65] Procedures

This procedure was designed as a buttress to the Hill-Sachs lesion of the humeral head, thus preventing the Hill-Sachs lesion from slipping over the anterior glenoid rim (Fig. 7-60). The procedure has been used extensively by Palmer and Widen of Sweden.[106] The bone block is removed from the iliac crest, and shaped to fit over the bony defect of the glenoid rim. The use of fixation screws is optional. Although we have not found it necessary to use this technique, it has its indications for large fractures of the glenoid rim and severe Hill-Sachs lesions of the humeral head. In the past, we have considered using this technique for large fracture of the glenoid rim, but in each instance we were not satisfied with the accurate and smooth placement of the graft along the glenoid rim and were concerned with the possibility of late traumatic changes to the joint. In each case, we used the standard Bankart procedure with success. Hindmarsh and Lindberg[60] in 1967 reported an increased risk of postoperative arthrosis of the joint in a long term follow-up study using the Hybbinette-Eden technique. Also, Oster[105] reported a recurrent dislo-

cation rate of 18 percent. Palmer and Widen[106] report a recurrence rate of 7 percent.

The DeAnquin Procedure

DeAnquin[35,36] uses a unique superior shoulder approach to the anterior glenoid neck and securely places a bone graft into the Bankart defect. This is secured by sutures through the glenoid rim and bone graft plus the medial flap of the capsule. DeAnquin states very clearly that the bone graft is used *not to block the humeral head but only to extend the width of the glenoid surface.* In instances of a large Hill-Sachs lesion, DeAnquin fills in the head lesion with bone graft and, at times, with the infraspinatus muscle. His recurrence rate of 0.7 percent is a justification of his procedure. We have not used his bone graft procedure but appreciate its unusual approach. We also agree with his experience that with severe Hill-Sachs lesions consideration must be given to filling the head defect, preferably with the infraspinatus transfer or a bone graft.

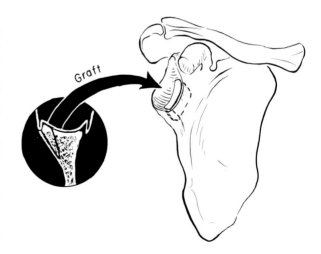

Fig. 7-60. The Hybbinette-Eden procedure. The aim is to extend the glenoid fossa, thus creating a buttress to prevent the Hill-Sachs lesion from slipping on the rim. The graft is obtained from the iliac crest. Fixation is optional. (Reprinted with permission from Rowe CR, Cave EF: p. 275. In Cave EF (ed): Fractures and Other Injuries. Copyright © 1958 by Year Book Medical Publishers, Inc., Chicago.)

OSTEOTOMIES

Osteotomy of the Glenoid Neck

For recurrent anterior dislocation a number of surgeons have reported performing an anterior osteotomy of the glenoid neck. Saha[127] reviews the technique of removing a wedge from the posterior neck of the scapula in those cases showing an anterior tilt (Fig. 7-61). Bestard[13] reports 49 anterior glenoplasties in which a 0.5 cm wedge of bone was inserted anteriorly to correct anterior tilt of the glenoid (Fig. 7-61B) with only a 2 percent recurrence rate. He also reports 12 posterior wedged glenoplasties for recurrent posterior dislocation using the Scott-Kretzler technique.

The Scott-Kretzler procedure is discussed below.

Rotational Osteotomies of the Surgical Neck of the Humerus

Weber[144] in 1969 devised another optional procedure, a rotational osteotomy of the proximal humeral neck, for patients with severe Hill-Sachs lesions of the humeral head. The osteotomy rotates the humeral head medially, thus displacing the head defect away from the glenoid rim and making available more head surface when the arm is in elevation and external rotation, which is a very ingenious concept (Fig. 7-62). In doing this procedure, the subscapularis muscle should be shortened. Weber's results are very commendable. On a 100 unit evaluation scale, his follow-up (average 8 years) results were 71 percent excellent, 19 percent good, 3 percent fair, and 7 percent poor. His recurrence rate was 6 percent plus 1 percent subluxation or 7 percent instability rate, which is very good considering that his patients had large Hill-Sachs lesions. Our results using the Bankart procedure with moderately severe Hill-Sachs were 5 percent recurrence and only 6 percent with severe lesions. This included recurrent dislocations and subluxations.

Humeral Shaft (The Saha Procedure)

Saha[127] used a rotational osteotomy at the junction of the upper and mid-thirds of the humeral shaft to improve the stability of the shoulder, as did Debevoise[37] in 1971. Saha also describes techniques by Meyer-Burgdorff[94] in which the tilt of the glenoid

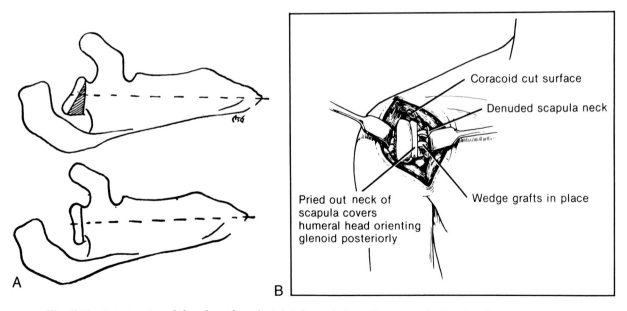

Fig. 7-61. Osteotomies of the glenoid neck. **(A)** Saha technique for removal of wedge from posterior neck for recurrent anterior dislocation. **(B)** Bestard technique of anterior wedge osteotomy for recurrent anterior dislocation. (Fig. A from Saha AK: Recurrent Anterior Dislocation of the Shoulder: A New Concept. Academic Publishers, Calcutta, India, 1969; Fig. B from Bestard EA, Schoene HR, Bestard EH: Glenoplasty in management of recurrent shoulder dislocations. Contemp Orthop 12(3):50, 1986.)

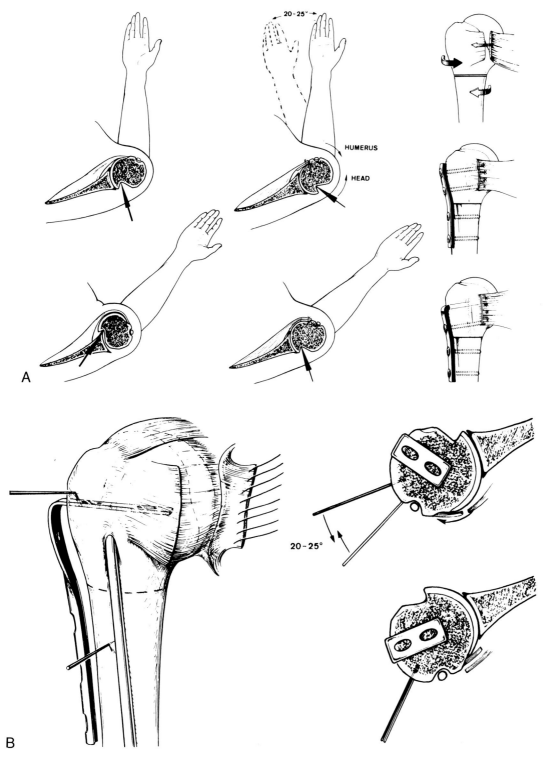

Fig. 7-62. Weber osteotomy. (**A** and **B**) The humeral head is rotated inward or medially, thus displacing the head defect away from the rim of the glenoid. (*Figure continues.*)

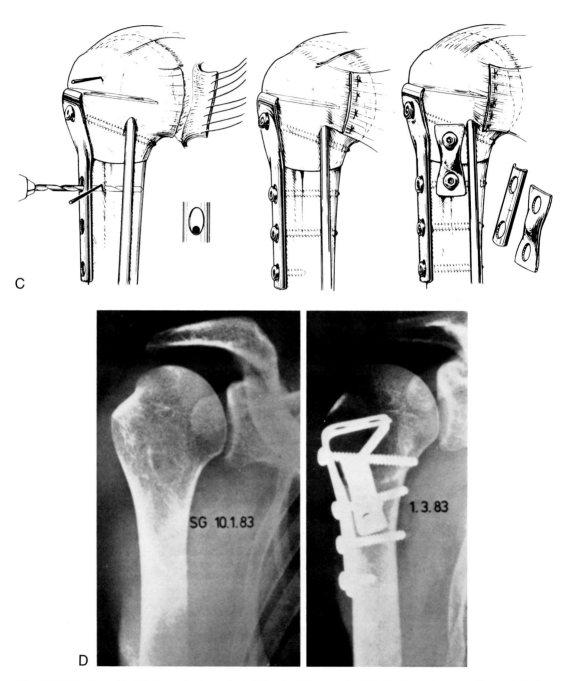

Fig. 7-62 (*Continued*). (**C**) The osteotomy is stabilized with an angled blade plate plus a small, semitubular, two-hole plate. The subcapularis tendon and capsule are overlapped. (**D**) A patient after surgery. (Weber BG, Simpson A, Hardegger F: Rotational Osteotomy for recurrent anterior dislocation of the shoulder associated with large Hill-Sachs lesions. J Bone Joint Surg 66A:1443, 1984.)

fossa in recurrent anterior dislocations is corrected by removing a posterior wedge of the glenoid neck (usually 5 mm in width). This was the forerunner of the Scott and Kretzler neck osteotomies for recurrent posterior dislocations.

MUSCLE TRANSPLANTATION

The Connolly Procedure

Indications. The primary purpose for the Connolly procedure is to fill the defect of the humeral head with the infraspinatus muscle, thus eliminating the chance of the defect slipping over the rim of the glenoid. In 1972 Connolly reported 90 shoulders operated on for recurrent anterior dislocation of the shoulder,[30] 10 of which had severe Hill-Sachs lesions in which he transplanted the infraspinatus muscle. He emphasized, however, that *repair of the Bankart lesion should be carried out also.* To date, Connolly has not reported a follow-up study of the patients on whom he has used this procedure. However, Willis et al. report a follow-up study of 53 patients on whom this technique was used.[146]

Technique (Fig. 7-63). The patient is placed on his or her side, with the involved shoulder up. Two incisions are used: a posterior one for the infraspinatus

muscle transplantation, and an anterior one for anterior repair of the shoulder. The infraspinatus insertion is released and the defect in the humeral head, which is located just under the infraspinatus insertion, is freshened to bleeding bone. Three or four holes are made through the base of the greater tuberosity. The infraspinatus tendon is shortened 1 cm so that the transplant will be under proper tension. The infraspinatus tendon with its attached capsule is transplanted snugly into the defect with sutures through the holes. Thus, an intraarticular lesion is changed to an extraarticular lesion by this procedure. The shoulder is protected for a period of 3 weeks, after which graduated passive and active exercises are begun.

We have used a superior approach along the anterior acromion, instead of a posterior approach, as used by Connolly (see Chap. 3). By internally rotating the arm, the infraspinatus tendon and Hill-Sachs lesion come into full view. I have found this a more direct and less extensive exposure than the routine posterior shoulder approach. With a very large Hill-Sachs lesion, the cavity may be filled by taking more bone from the greater tuberosity with the infraspinatus tendon transplant. I strongly support Connolly's suggestion that the shoulder also be exposed anteriorly and the Bankart lesion repaired, if present.

I have not used the Connolly procedure alone for

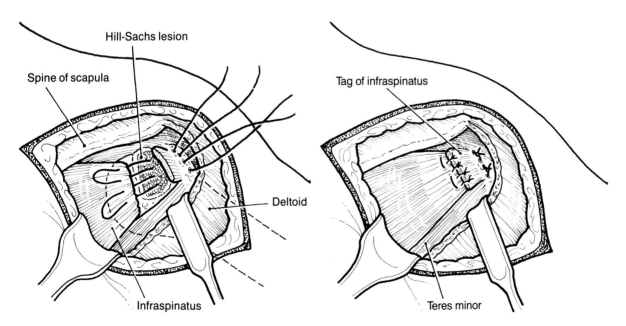

Fig. 7-63. The Connolly procedure. Transplantation of the infraspinatus muscle into the Hill-Sachs lesion.

primary repair. I have used it only in patients with failed repairs, in combination with a Bankart repair, who have a severe Hill-Sachs lesion. Willis et al.[146] in 1981 reported a series of 53 shoulder repairs using only the Connolly technique. Of 37 primary or initial repairs, there was a 6 percent recurrence dislocation rate, but also a 6 percent subluxation or a 12 percent instability rate for the procedure. Eight of the patients with failed primary repairs, however, had no recurrence following secondary surgery. This procedure would seem to have its primary indication in previously failed procedures. None of our second surgical procedures, with severe Hill-Sachs lesions plus Bankart lesions, have failed when we used the combination of a Bankart and a Connolly procedure.

The Saha Procedure

Saha[127] in 1969 reported his experience from 1956 to 1965 with 45 consecutive cases of recurrent anterior dislocations treated with transplantation of the latissimus dorsi muscle posteriorly from its insertion to the lowest posterior limit of the greater tuberosity and the lower insertion of the infraspinatus tendon. His theory is that when the arm is in abduction the adductor power of the latissimus dorsi is transferred to reinforce the subscapularis and short posterior steering muscles, holding the humeral head back and lessening its anterior advance or dislocation. The results of this procedure in Professor Saha's hands have been most encouraging, with no recurrences. However, I would be concerned with the patient who may have a large Bankart lesion and redundant capsule anteriorly. The transplant, however, may be effective with patients with large Hill-Sachs lesions, since the transplant is close to the lower border of the head defect and may fill some part of the defect.

The McLaughlin Procedure

See section on posterior dislocation, below, for discussion of this procedure.

CAPSULORRHAPHIES

The causative pathology of instability of the shoulder, when a Bankart lesion or severe Hill-Sachs lesion is *not* present, in the majority of cases, is excessive laxity or redundancy of the anterior capsule, particularly the inferior ligament and axillary capsular fold.

One must remember also that laxity of the capsule may be due not only to laxity along the glenoid rim but also from avulsion along the neck of the humerus. Associated with the lax capsule may be deficiencies of the subscapularis or minor degrees of avulsion of the capsule, associated with unidirectional or multidirectional instabilities of the shoulder. As pointed out by Neer, there seems to be an increase in the involuntary category of capsular instability. At least they are being more frequently identified and carefully studied. Under the rubric of capsular laxity we should include also laxity of the supporting tissues due to paralysis of different types.

Three commonly used capsulorrhaphies have been devised to restore stability to the shoulder in these instances:

1. The Neer Inferior Capsular Shift[97]
2. The Protzman anterior capsular procedure[110]
3. The Rowe capsulorrhaphy[124]

The Neer Capsular Shift Procedure

Indications. As a rule, Neer excludes patients with Bankart lesions and patients with voluntary dislocations. However, if a Bankart lesion is encountered the capsule is repaired by the Bankart technique with holes in the rim of the glenoid. The procedure can be carried out both anteriorly and posteriorly by separate approaches for multidirectional instabilities.

Neer states that the principle of the capsular shift procedure is "to detach the capsule from the neck of the humerus and shift it to the opposite side of the calcar not only to obliterate the inferior pouch and capsular redundancy on the side of the surgical approach, but also to reduce laxity on the opposite side." This is a very logical concept, which is receiving wide acceptance.

Technique. The procedure is performed through one or two surgical approaches, either anterior or posterior. The subscapularis muscle is partially removed from the anterior capsule (Fig. 7-64A1). The anterior capsular incision is T-shaped (Fig. 7-64A2) and repair is obtained by double breasting the anterior capsular flaps. The posterior approach and repair are illustrated in Figure 7-64B1. The infraspinous muscle is separated from the posterior capsule. A similar T-incision is made, overlapping the superior flap with the inferior flap (Fig. 7-64B2). The double

Fig. 7-64. The Neer capsular shift. (**A**) The anterior capsular shift. (**1**) The subscapularis tendon and muscle are partially removed from the anterior capsule. (**2**) The capsular incision is T-shaped, its stem is on the glenoid rim, and the top across the neck of the neck of the humerus. The repair is obtained by double breasting the inferior flap over the superior flap. (*Figure continues.*)

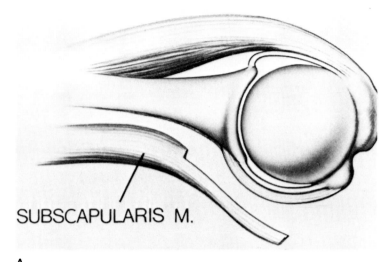

SUBSCAPULARIS M.

A₁

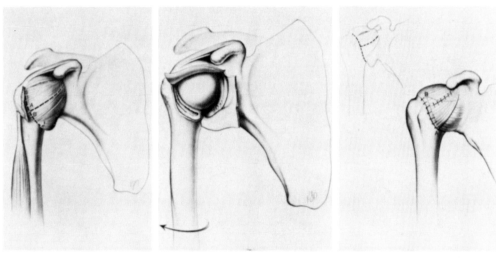

A₂

breasting of the capsular flaps is an excellent step in adding strength to the repair.

Postoperative immobilization is continued in a cast (or splint) for 5 to 6 weeks. Progressive resistive exercises are begun at the twelfth week, but the patient is cautioned against swimming, heavy lifting, or participating in sports for 1 year. Although Neer's report is a "preliminary" one, only 1 patient of 49 received an unsatisfactory rating. He rightly cautions against performing surgical procedures on the voluntary dislocator with personality or emotional problems. We agree with Neer that instability of the shoulder producing unidirectional and multidirectional instability present clinical problems that call for further study and research.

The Protzman Capsulorrhaphy

The Protzman technique is a combination of the capsular overlapping shift and a modified Putti-Platt procedure. It is used for all types of shoulder instabilities.

An anterior approach is used (Fig. 7-65). The subscapularis muscle is removed from the anterior capsule so that the capsule can be assessed as to its looseness. This determines where the vertical cut is to

INFRASPINATUS M.

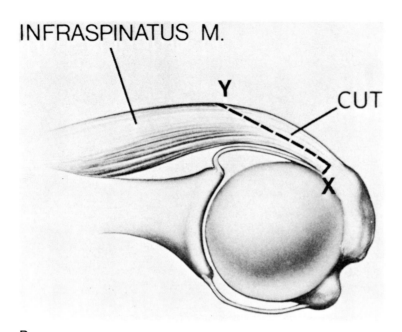

Y

CUT

X

Fig. 7-64 (*Continued*). (**B**) The posterior capsular shift. (**1**) The infraspinatus muscle is removed from the posterior capsule. (**2**) A T incision is made, overlapping the superior flap with the inferior flap. (Neer CS, Foster CR: Inferior capsular shift for involuntary inferior and multidirectional instability of the shoulder. A preliminary report. J Bone Joint Surg 62A:897, 1980.)

B₁

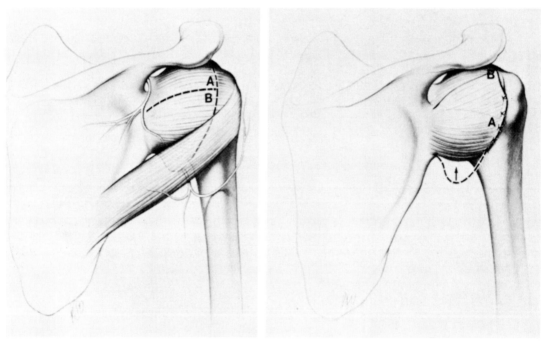

B₂

be made. Protzman stressed this part of his technique: "after the vertical cut is made, I stick a finger or look into the capsule. The "T" portion of the cut is then made so that the glenoid side of the "T" inter-sects the glenoid at the point of maximum Bankart defect." Thus, the capsulorrhaphy is "tailored" to the direction of instability. The "tailoring" is a very good point, as the repair on the glenoid should be strong

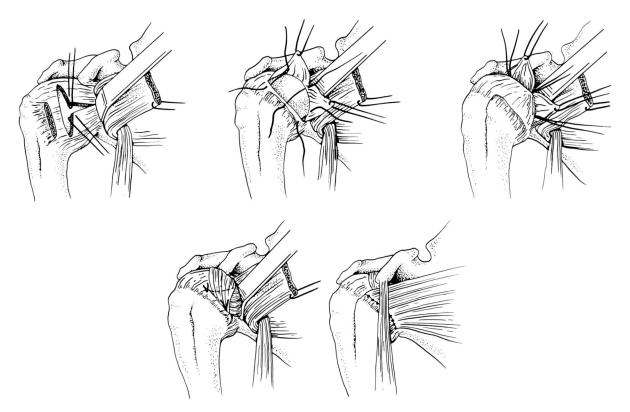

Fig. 7-65. The Protzman technique. The subscapularis muscle is removed from the anterior capsule. The joint is opened with a T incision. The lateral capsular flap is sewn to the "soft tissue" of the glenoid rim. The superior and inferior flaps are then double-breasted. (Protzman RR: Anterior instability of the shoulder. J Bone Joint Surg 62A:909, 1980.)

over the extent of the Bankart lesion. Protzman also emphasizes reattaching the capsule to the glenoid rim by sewing the lateral stump to the soft tissues of the glenoid rim, similarly to the Putti-Platt procedure. The superior and inferior flaps are then double breasted over it. This is a combination of strong techniques. Protzman's rate of recurrence of subluxation or dislocation as of 1980 was 5.6 percent.

Rowe Capsulorrhaphy

The surgical approach for our capsulorrhaphy is the same as the approach used for the standard Bankart procedure (Fig. 7-66). The capsule is opened vertically 0.5 cm lateral to the glenoid rim. The advantage of this approach is that regardless of whether a Bankart lesion is present, both the Bankart procedure and the capsulorrhaphy repair can be used with the same capsule opening. No alteration of the incision is necessary. The laxity of the capsule is taken up as necessary and double breasted along the rim of the glenoid where support is most needed. The degree of tightening of the capsule is determined by external rotation of the arm prior to suturing. This must be carefully carried out, as tightening of the anterior capsule too much in multidirectional subluxations, may, as Neer points out in the capsular shift, subluxate the head posteriorly. With complete removal of the subscapularis muscle from the capsule and exposure of the entire anterior and inferior capsule and, to some extent, the posterior capsule, a *balanced* repair can be performed.

Technique. To double breast the anterior capsule along the glenoid rim, the suture is first passed under the medial attachment of the labrum into the joint,

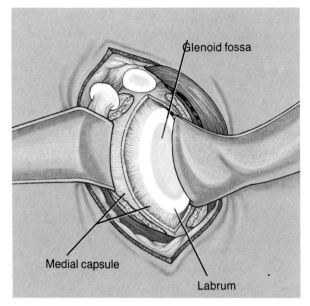

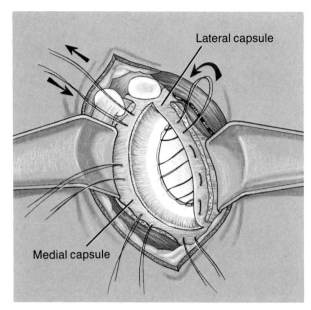

A

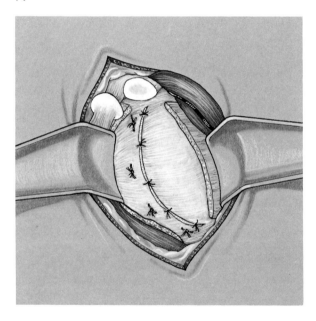

Fig. 7-66. The Rowe capsulorrhaphy (left shoulder). **(A)** The approach is the same as for the Bankart procedure. the suture is begun through the medial flap of capsule under the labrum, out through the lateral flap of capsule, then back through the capsule, and under the labrum and mesial capsule. This is repeated along the rim of the glenoid down to 6 o'clock. If there is multilocular instability, the capsular repair can be carried posteriorly from the anterior incision, and the posterior capsule can be taken up as needed to eliminate the redundancy. The sutures pull the lateral capsule onto the labrum. The mesial flap of capsule is then double breasted over the repair, adding extra-strength to the repair, along the rim of the glenoid, where reinforced repair is needed. (*Figure continues.*)

then passed out and back in the lateral capsule, and back under the labrum (Fig. 7-66). With anterior instability usually four or five sutures are usually used, at 1, 2, 4, and 6 o'clock (for a left shoulder). Care is taken to eliminate the excessive laxity of the axillary fold of capsule and strengthen the repair along the inferior border of the glenoid. The degree of tightening of the anterior capsule is tested before the sutures

are tied. Usually 30° of external rotation is satisfactory. Tightening the sutures pulls the lateral capsule under the labrum. The sutures are then tied, double breasting the medial flap over the lateral flap to give maximum strength along the rim of the glenoid, where it is needed most. With *multidirectional* instability, sutures can be inserted through the posterior capsule, at 6 and 7 o'clock (to strengthen the posterior capsule).

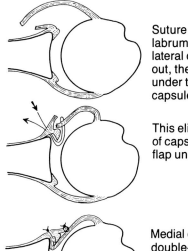

Suture passes under the labrum, is carried through lateral capsule from inside out, then outside in, back under the labrum and lateral capsule.

This eliminates redundancy of capsule and attaches the flap under labrum.

Medial capsular flap is double-breasted over lateral capsule for extra strength, leaving a soft, strong repair along the glenoid rim.

Fig. 7-66 *(Figure Continued)*. **(B)** A vertical view of the capsulorrhaphy demonstrating the capsular buttress along the rim of the glenoid, which is smooth, nonirritating, and strong. The laxity of the capsule is taken up.

B

To date, this has worked successfully. We have had to expose the shoulder posteriorly on only one occasion in the past 20 years, for a multidirectional dislocation.

The incision is closed in layers. Postoperative care is similar to that for the Bankart routine. No sling or other support is used after the first 3 days; from then on the arm is free. This is followed by gradual increasing motion and use of the arm as tolerated. It has not been necessary to send patients to physical therapy or to immobilize the arm. They can do their exercises at home, at school, or at work. Resistive exercises with rubber bands are started 10 to 12 weeks postoperatively. The shoulder should be ready for contact sports 6 months postoperatively. At that time, the patient should have full or near full range of motion, good strength of the shoulder, and no apprehension on elevation of the arm. When primary instability of a multidirectional instability is inferior, this technique eliminates the inferior capsular laxity and returns stability to the shoulder in positions of elevation of the arm. When the primary instability is posterior and not multidirectional, one must decide whether to use a capsular repair or the Scott glenoplasty. Unfortunately, the posterior capsule is not as strong (with reinforced capsular ligaments) as it is anteriorly. For this reason, we have favored the Scott osteotomy over capsular repair for specific posterior instability.

THE PARALYTIC SHOULDER

All three of the techniques for capsulorrhaphies as described may be considered for the paralytic shoulder. However, in many instances the paralytic shoulder may need additional support. We have found the Thompson modification of the Nicola technique an excellent procedure for inferior subluxation of the humeral head (see Fig. 7-58). It serves as a strong ligamentum teres.

RECURRENT TRANSIENT ANTERIOR SUBLUXATION (DEAD ARM SYNDROME)

A perplexing and frustrating shoulder syndrome, the "dead arm" syndrome was a puzzle to orthopaedic surgeons for many years. The patient, usually a good athlete, presents with a history of being unable to throw, serve forcefully in tennis, swim free style, "spike" a volleyball, or use their arm forcefully overhead because of a sudden sharp "paralyzing" pain in their shoulder after an overthrust of the arm in elevation and external rotation, or hyperextension. I recall such patients in the 1950s. The usual diagnoses were "tendinitis" or biceps tendon instability. Patients are frustrated and discouraged. No form of treatment has helped them and no specific diagnosis of their shoulder problem has been made.

In 1969 Blazina and Satzman[14] were the first to publish their findings with this syndrome. They reported on the transient shoulder subluxation in which the patient was aware of arm slipping out and back in. Later, other investigators recorded their experience with the same clinical problem.[11,73,90,97,113,124]

In 1981 we published our experience with recurrent transient subluxation of 58 patients and 60 shoulders, and added another dimension to the syndrome:[124] those patients who were *not* aware of their shoulder subluxating, but only of a sudden pain.

In our study, two groups were identified. In group I (27 shoulders), patients were *aware* of the sensation of their shoulders "slipping out and back in" on forceful elevation and external rotation of the arm. In group II (33 shoulders), patients were *not aware* of their shoulders subluxating; their only complaint was a sudden sharp "paralyzing" pain in the action of throwing, or sudden use of the arm in elevation and external rotation. This group proved to be difficult to identify and were frequently misdiagnosed and incorrectly treated.

It was interesting that both groups had similar mechanisms of injury, the same complaints and physical findings, comparable pathologic lesions at surgery, and similar results after similar surgical treatment. Group II had not previously been identified in the literature. Again, we find that Codman had observed a somewhat similar syndrome in baseball pitchers, which he termed "a glass arm," due to pain and loss of power.[28]

My first introduction to the dead arm syndrome in patients who were *not* aware of their shoulder subluxating was with a jockey in 1962, who, after having been thrown from his horse, was later no longer able to reach back and whip his horse when racing. He had been seen by a number of orthopaedic surgeons, as he was an exceptional jockey. His shoulder had not responded to the usual forms of treatment. All investigative studies, radiographs, and other tests were negative.

His complaint was direct: "Doctor, I am not paid to ride, I am paid to win. Will you look into my shoulder? If you don't find anything, I'm no worse

off. If you find something, fix it, and maybe I'll be able to ride again."

This was certainly an open challenge. Although he was sincere and motivated, we were somewhat reluctant to explore his shoulder with so little to go on, since at that time arthroscopy had not been developed and arthrograms were not helpful. To our surprise, at surgery we found a well-developed Bankart lesion. After it was repaired the jockey returned to full competition with a painless, strong shoulder.

This explained to us the complaints of a number of college athletes we had seen in the 1950s, who, after an overpull of their arm in elevation and extension, had complained of a "dead arm" that never returned to full function in spite of rest, exercising, and investigation. Some had been labeled as experiencing "loss of heart," being "no longer motivated or aggressive," or it was thought that it was in their head."

Mechanism of Injury

Thirty-five of the sixty shoulders (58 percent) had experienced forceful external rotation in positions of elevation or abduction. Seventeen (28 percent) had experienced a direct blow to the shoulder. Eight shoulders (13 percent) had produced their subluxation by excessive throwing or hard serving in tennis. This is a very interesting group; these were frequently diagnosed and treated as "tendinitis."

Eighty-five percent occurred in sports such as football, baseball, basketball, hockey, tennis, skiing, boxing, and karate, while 15 percent occurred when the patient fell from a height or sustained a direct blow at work.

Physical Examination

All 60 shoulders showed a positive "apprehension test." This test is best carried out with the patient standing and relaxed. The arm is taken into maximum elevation and external rotation, and forward pressure is applied to the posterior aspect of the humeral head (Fig. 7-4). In this position, the patient suddenly becomes apprehensive and the pain and weakness in the shoulder are reproduced. The patient frequently will demonstrate the position of the arm in throwing or serving in tennis. This test can also be carried out with the patient supine (Fig. 7-7A), with the arm in abduction or elevation; posterior pressure is applied to the humeral head. The diagnosis of transient subluxation is not dependent on the actual demonstration of subluxation, during the physical examination, or even with fluoroscopy. In fact, the shoulder could not be anteriorly subluxated in some instances even when the patient is under anesthesia, although the problem may be due to hyperlaxity of the anterior capsule. A number of patients in our series were sent to us because their doctor was *not* able to demonstrate subluxation of the shoulder, although a positive apprehension test, a positive history, and at surgery, explanation of the shoulder's instability, were available.

Differential Diagnosis

A number of conditions should be considered and carefully excluded:

1. Thoracic outlet syndrome, or partial vascular occlusion
2. Injury or stretching of the brachial plexus
3. Cervical disc disease
4. Subacromial or coracoid impingement syndromes of the shoulder, with or without rotator cuff tear
5. Lesions of the long head of biceps tendon (rare in our experience)
6. Injury to the acromioclavicular joint
7. The patient, who usually has work-related injury, suddenly sprains his shoulder in heavy lifting or in sudden overpull of his shoulder

The specific points in diagnosis are an active athletic individual, whose arm has been forcefully hyperextended or elevated, whose arm subsequently fails in overhead functions, and who has a positive apprehension test. *In the absence of a strongly positive apprehension test and a consistent history, one should suspect conditions other than transient subluxation.* The "industrial shoulder," overpulled at work, must be carefully differentiated. The history and physical findings are not as consistent nor is their response to treatment as predictable.

Radiographic Findings

Hill-Sachs lesions of the humeral head were present in 24 (40 percent) of the 60 shoulders; these were mild in 19, moderate in 3, and severe in 2. Traumatic changes of the anterior or inferior glenoid rim as illustrated with axillary views were present in 27 shoulders (45 percent). More recently, we have found arthroscopy or arthrotomography of the shoulder to be helpful when there is a question of the diagnosis. Although demonstration of instability by fluoroscopy could be helpful, we have not found that this was necessary.

Previous Diagnoses

Thirty-three shoulders (55 percent) had been diagnosed as having some condition other than subluxation when they were first seen by us. Eight of the 33 shoulders were in group I (those who were aware of their shoulder slipping), and 25 in group II (those who were *not* aware of their shoulder slipping). A diagnosis of a "pinched nerve" was made in nine patients, bursitis or tendinitis of the biceps tendon in four, subluxation of the long head of biceps tendon in three, a rupture of the cervical disc in three, and a thoracic outlet syndrome in two shoulders. A neurologic diagnosis had been made in 12 patients (20 percent), cervical myelography had been carried out in two, and electromyograms in three patients. The frequency of incorrect diagnosis in group II reflects the difficulty in making the diagnosis when the patient is *not* aware of any displacement of the humeral head during activity.

Previous Treatment

Previous nonoperative treatment consisted mainly of injections of the subacromial bursa, systematic anti-inflammatory drugs, physical therapy, ultrasound, diathermy, and, in five patients, "manipulative" treatment. Previous incorrect surgical procedures had been performed in seven patients. These included "decompression" of the shoulder for impingement syndrome in three patients (all in group II) and tenodesis of the long head of biceps tendon in three patients (two were in group II).

Treatment

Nonoperative

We routinely treated transient subluxations conservatively at first with a program of specific resistive exercises in internal rotation, external rotation, and abduction of the arm to strengthen the stabilizing muscles of the rotator cuff, and with instructions to avoid positions of overextension or elevation of the arm in sports. These exercises can be carried out by manual resistance or by the use of elastic bands or belts (see Fig. 7-44). This program should be continued for 2 months. Pain and disability of the shoulder were decreased in 8 of 60 shoulders (13 percent), eliminating the need for surgery.

Surgical

In our 1981 series, 50 shoulders were operated on. In the 32 shoulders with typical Bankart lesions, a standard Bankart procedures was performed. The 18 shoulders with excessive laxity of the capsule, rather than a Bankart lesion, were treated with our capsulorrhaphy, which eliminates the redundant capsule, and double breasts the capsule along the glenoid rim.

Since 1981, 30 more patients have been operated on for recurrent anterior transient subluxation. Our experience correlates accurately with the 60 patients reported in 1981. We emphasize again the importance of layer-by-layer exposure of the shoulder down to the glenoid rim, to identify the various pathologic factors responsible for the shoulder's instability and to correct them.

The postoperative management is also similar to that used for routine Bankart procedures. A sling is used for 2 to 3 days, after which the arm is free. Pendulum exercises are begun a few days after surgery. Many of the patients returned to light work within 4 to 6 weeks, and by 3 months swimming, rowing, and taking part in light sports was permitted. By 6 months, a complete range of motion is expected and participation in contact sports and heavy labor is permitted.

Surgical Pathology

Bankart lesions were found in 32 (64 percent) of the 50 operated shoulders. Of these, 17 cases were mild, 10 were moderate, and 5 were severe. Excess laxity of the anterior capsule was present in 26 percent of the operated patients, and excess opening of the seam between the subscapularis and supraspinatus tendons over the humeral head was present in 20 shoulders. When the opening extends out over the head of the humerus, that part over the head is closed. Other pathologic lesions were loose bodies in one shoulder. In another, an abnormal insertion of the pectoralis minor tendon was noted extending over the coracoid process into the coracohumeral ligament and greater tuberosity. The tendon was released and reattached to the coracoid, where it belonged. In two shoulders the glenoid labrum was split longitudinally as a bucket-handle tear of the meniscus in the knee (Fig. 7-9B, C). In none of the 50 shoulders was there any evidence of instability or subluxation of the long head of the biceps tendon, although the intertubercular ligament was thinner in patients with excess generalized ligament laxity.

Results

In our grading system, 50 units were given for function, 10 for pain, 30 for stability, and 10 for motion. Our postoperative results were 70 percent excellent, 24 percent good, and 6 percent fair results. Of interest were the five shoulders with severe fractures of the glenoid rim treated with a routine Bankart repair; all had excellent results. The presence of a Hill-Sachs lesion did not affect the results adversely in this group. The two shoulders with severe Hill-Sachs lesions, and three with moderately severe lesions, had excellent results. There were 33 dominant shoulders. Of these, 21 (64 percent) were able to return to forceful throwing and were able to participate in sports and work.

Two patients were professional tennis instructors who returned to play. One professional National Hockey League player continues to play 3 years after surgery. Of the fifteen nondominant shoulders, 87 percent had no limitations in sports or work and returned to all activities that they had participated in before injury. Of eight patients operated on whose injury was produced by hard pitching, four were graded excellent; they could pitch hard and throw hard. Four were graded as good results. These four patients could throw a football as far as they could prior to injury, and serve hard in tennis, but were unable to pitch forcefully. The left shoulder of the young lady in Figure 7-67 had been painful and use-

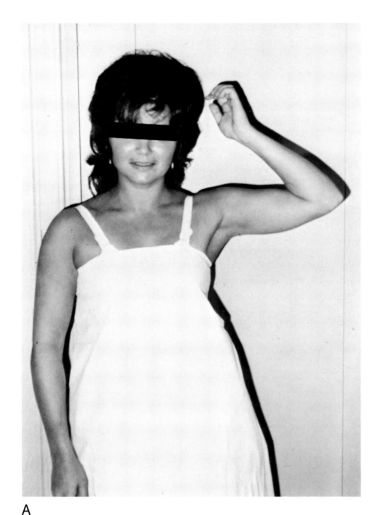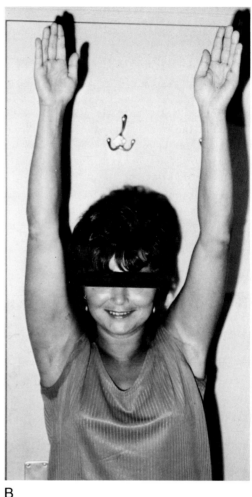

A   B

Fig. 7-67. **(A)** This young lady's left arm had been useless ("I couldn't swat a fly") because of sudden pain in her arm since she had fallen down stairs and checked her fall with her outstretched left arm. **(B)** At surgery, an avulsed labrum and excess laxity of the capsule were found. Following repair of her labrum and capsulorrhaphy, her shoulder has been excellent. "Now I can swat flies and throw again."

less after she had fallen down her cellar stairs and checked the fall with her outstretched left arm. At surgery a separated labrum and excessive laxity of the capsule were found. The labrum was reattached to the glenoid rim and excessive laxity of the capsule eliminated. Her result has been excellent.

The college hockey player in Figure 7-68 had disabling subluxation of both shoulders resulting from "boarding." He had undergone bilateral tenodesis of the long head of biceps in both shoulders, which had proved unsuccessful. At surgery, a severe Bankart lesion was found in the right shoulder and severe

laxity of the capsule was found 8 months later in the left shoulder. He returned to college hockey postoperatively and then was accepted at the Air Force Academy. His result was excellent.

The young man in Figure 7-69 presented an interesting problem. He was a two letter athlete in basketball and a baseball pitcher at a large state university. His right arm had been "dead" for 2 years following excessive pitching, and it was unresponsive to all forms of conservative treatment and rest. At surgery, excessive laxity of the anterior capsule was found and corrected by our routine capsulorrhaphy. Eight

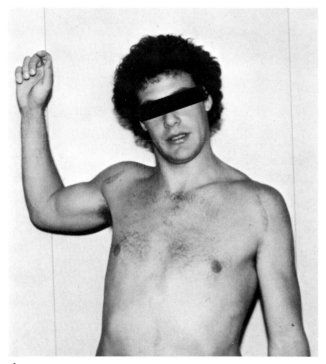

A

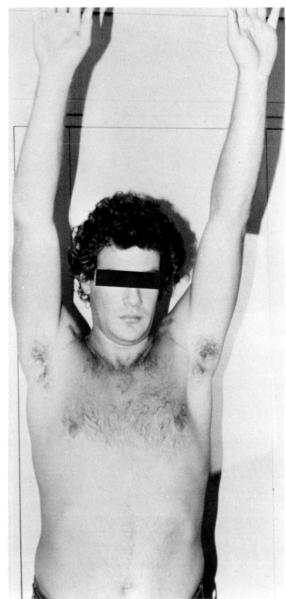

B

Fig. 7-68. (A) This college hockey player had had previous unsuccessful tenodesis of the long head of biceps of both shoulders, without relief to his "dead arm." he could not tolerate the position of throwing. **(B)** At surgery, a severe Bankart lesion was found in his right shoulder and, 6 months later, excessive laxity of the capsule in the left shoulder. After a Bankart on the right shoulder, and capsulorrhaphy in the left shoulder, he returned to hockey and was then accepted to the Air Force Academy.

months later, he pitched his senior year and was on the basketball team.

Analysis of Fair Results. Of five patients studied, two with fair results were treated with exercises with little improvement. Of the three patients treated surgically, two had work-related injuries. At surgery, one had a type I Bankart lesion; however, the patient continued to have discomfort and postoperative adhe-

sions with a 25 percent loss of abduction and external rotation and limited use of the arm in above-shoulder activities.

The fourth patient with generalized ligament laxity had a good result for 2 years, and then reproduced his shoulder difficulties by heavy lifting. The fifth patient also did very well for a year, when he was thrown against a tree, after an automobile accident and sustained a new injury to his shoulder.

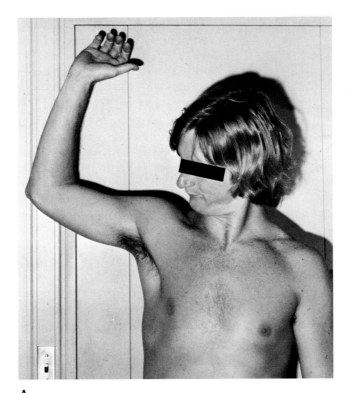

A

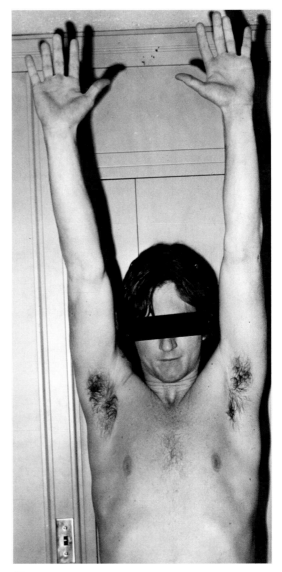

B

Fig. 7-69. (**A**) This college athlete's right shoulder had been "dead" (no strength) and painful for 2 years after excessive pitching. His arm was "no good" in this position. (**B**) At surgery, excessive laxity of the capsule was present for which a capsulorrhaphy was performed. Eight months following surgery, he returned to varsity pitching and, in his senior year, played basketball.

Complications. There were no infections or serious complications in this series. In one shoulder, a postoperative hematoma developed that closed secondarily after evacuation. One patient developed a thrombophlebitis of the cephalic vein that resolved uneventfully in 10 days. There were no nonunions of the coracoid process.

After a successful anterior capsular repair one patient developed posterior subluxations two years later. Although the condition has not been completely relieved, he has been helped with specific resistive exercises to strengthen his infraspinour and teres minor muscles. The patient did not have a Bankart lesion, only a redundant capsule. Neer and Rockwood, with good reason, caution that with capsulorrhaphy the shoulder may become unstable in the opposite direction in patients with ligament laxity or in whom the repair has been too restrictive anteriorly.

Radiographic Follow-Up

There were no late degenerative or traumatic joint changes on follow-up radiograms except for one, in which mild joint changes were present on the preoperative films. These had not increased at the patient's 5 year follow-up examination.

Comments

We emphasize again the importance of a detailed history and careful physical examination in an active athlete or person who has experienced a forceful overextension of their shoulder, followed by a "dead arm." Although some patients with work-related injuries may seem to be in this category, usually they are not. This group usually includes only the active athlete. It is significant that 11 percent of 60 shoulders in our series had undergone previous unsuccessful surgical procedures, such as acromioclavicular arthroplasties or tenodesis of the long head of biceps tendon. Fifty-five percent had been diagnosed as having some condition other than subluxation, when first seen by us. Although transient subluxations may occur posteriorly, they are much less common in athletes. These will be considered in the discussion of posterior instability.

In the differential diagnosis, thoracic outlet syndrome, brachial plexus injuries, tears of the rotator cuff, and impingement syndromes should be carefully ruled out.

Identification of recurrent anterior transient subluxations of the shoulder has been a step forward in relieving many good athletes and workers of a disability that, in the past, has been poorly defined and treated.

CHRONIC (UNREDUCED) DISLOCATIONS

Chronic dislocations of the shoulder have been known to the medical professional since the writings of White[145] in 1741 and Cooper[31] in 1825. However, in the past, there has been no standard or accepted definition of *when an unreduced shoulder becomes "chronic."* Bennett[12] and Cubbins[32] refer to unre-

duced shoulder dislocations merely as "early" and "older" without a specific time reference. Other investigators[11,39,81,91,115,130,147] have merely used the terms *acute* and *chronic*. Souchen (1891) did offer a definition: "we will call recent, all dislocations no older than a month, this is somewhat arbitrary, but adopted to fix a limit."[133] The only other authors to offer a definition were Schulz et al.[130] (1969) who considered a dislocation not recognized within 24 hours to be chronic. Unless an accepted definition for chronic dislocations is adapted, it will be difficult to compare one contributor's results with those of another. After analyzing reports by other orthopaedic surgeons, we suggest that *3 weeks* be an acceptable period to define chronic dislocations.

Incidence

This section is based on our study of 24 shoulders in 1982, plus two since then, for a total of 26 shoulders, whose dislocations had been unreduced from 3 weeks to 33 years.[126] There were 8 anterior, 16 posterior, 1 superior, and 1 inferior dislocation. There was only one bilateral posterior chronic dislocation, which was due to a seizure.

To determine how often the average orthopaedic surgeon sees a chronic dislocation of the shoulder, we canvassed 208 orthopaedic surgeons in New England.[126] As would be expected, the incidence was directly related to the length of time the surgeon had been in practice. Thirty-three percent of orthopaedic surgeons who had been in practice from 1 to 5 years had treated one or more chronic dislocations, 51 percent of orthopaedic surgeons in practice from 5 to 10 years, 70 percent in practice from 10 to 20 years, and 90 percent in practice for 20 years plus. It was interesting that 65 percent of the reported chronic dislocations were anterior and 35 percent posterior.

History

The patient's complaint in relation to the time of injury and subsequent disability may be confusing and quite inadequate, especially if the dislocation occurred during a seizure. The usual complaint is loss of motion and pain in the shoulder.

Diagnosis

Of the 24 patients with chronic dislocations of the shoulder reported by us in 1982, the mechanism of injury was as follows:

A fall	11
Motor vehicle	6
Seizure	4
Assault	1
Manipulation of shoulder	1
"Since youth"	1
Unknown	2
Total	26

Of these, 20 (77 percent) were not recognized by the patient or doctor and 6 were. Of the eight anterior dislocations, three were diagnosed before admissions and five were not. Two had been treated for sprain and one for rotator cuff tear. Of the 16 posterior dislocations, only 2 had been diagnosed prior to examination, and 14 had not (86 percent). Three had been treated for "frozen shoulder," two for bursitis, one for a "cracked glenoid," and one as a "spastic." The one superior dislocation was unrecognized and the single inferior dislocation was recognized.

Physical Examination

The chronic anterior dislocation is easier to recognize clinically than a posterior dislocation, as radiographs of the anterior dislocation are positive, whereas with a posterior dislocation they may be interpreted as normal. In the chronic anterior dislocation the deformity of the shoulder is also more pronounced, with its prominent acromion and absence of shoulder contour. Also, the shoulder is fixed in external rotation and the patient is unable to reach across the body anteriorly or posteriorly (Fig. 7-70).

As pointed out in the section on posterior dislocations a number of clinical signs will aid in diagnosing a posterior dislocation. If the patient is asked to flex elbows to 90°, it will be noted that the shoulder and arm are locked in internal rotation on the injured side (Fig. 7-71A). An additional characteristic sign is the inability of the patient to turn the palm of the extended arm upward; although the forearm is in complete supination, the arm is fixed in complete internal

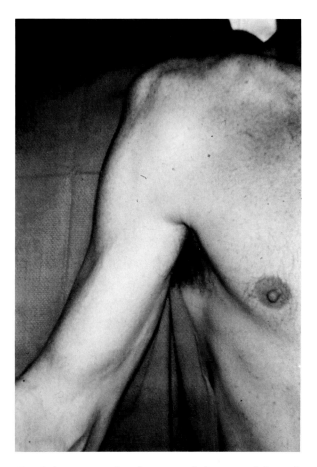

Fig. 7-70. An unreduced anterior dislocation of the right shoulder. Note that the arm is locked in external rotation.

rotation (see Fig. 7-85B). The patient with an unreduced posterior dislocation can easily confuse the examiner; he or she will demonstrate motions across the body anteriorly and posteriorly and will be able to elevate the extremity well above the head with the aid of scapular rotation. The examiner may also miss the abnormal prominence of the shoulder, as this is posterior. This can be picked up best by observing the shoulders from above (see Fig. 7-86). A chronic superior dislocation can be clearly diagnosed by an AP radiogram (Fig. 7-72).

There are two steps one should take when seeing a patient who has had a shoulder injury, but who has *not* responded to physical therapy and continues to have limited motion (not always painful) of the shoulder:

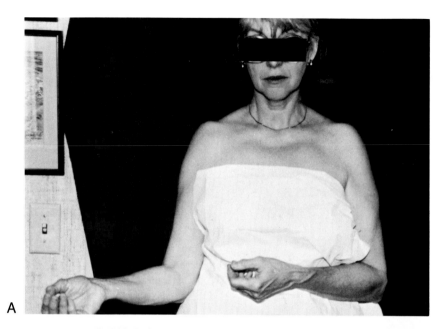

A

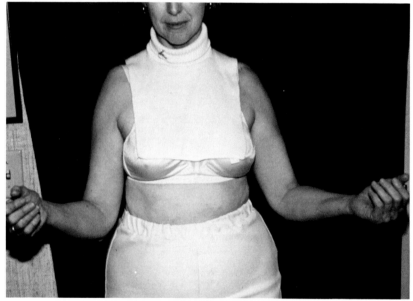

B

Fig. 7-71. **(A)** An unreduced posterior dislocation of the left shoulder. The arm is locked in internal rotation. **(B)** After open reduction. The shoulder has regained external rotation. She is no longer depressed and has gained weight.

1. With the patient standing, grasp the lower angle of the scapula. As the arm is moved upward in a chronic dislocation the scapula will move immediately. The head of a posterior dislocation will be more firmly fixed to the scapula than the anterior dislocation.
2. When in doubt, *take a true axillary view* or a Y-lateral view (we do not consider the transthoracic view accurate enough to be satisfactory). This will establish the diagnosis (Fig. 7-73). A safe rule is: to never manipulate a *frozen shoulder* without taking an axillary view.

Treatment

Treatment may be considered in the five categories discussed here.

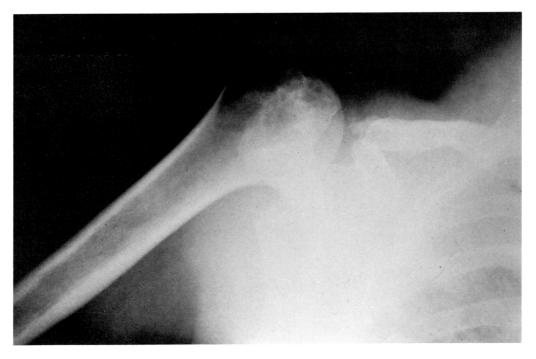

Fig. 7-72. The arm is an unreduced superior dislocation is in neutral rotation.

NO TREATMENT

Eight patients received no treatment and preferred to leave the shoulder dislocated. One result was good, four were fair, and three were poor. It is interesting that the untreated posterior dislocation scored higher (average 65 units) than the untreated anterior dislocation (average 49 units). This is understandable, since the arm in the unreduced posterior dislocation is in a more functional position than in an anterior dislocation. The arm rests at the side of the body in internal rotation. In this position, the patient is able to reach across the body anteriorly and posteriorly, the face, and above the head. With the arm close to the body, the extremity is under the lifting fulcrum of the shoulder. The arm of an unreduced anterior dislocation is abducted from the body and in external rotation and away from the fulcrum of the shoulder and, therefore, is not in a strong position. Thus, it is in a weaker position for lifting, as well as for reaching the midline of the body anteriorly or posteriorly, or the face or back.

MANIPULATION

Only two patients in our series underwent manipulative reduction. One was reduced 3 weeks after injury, the other at 4 weeks. We agree with DePalma,[39] Rockwood and Green,[115] and Schulz[130] that manipulative reduction should *not* be undertaken before careful consideration is given to the patient's age, degree of osteoporosis of the humerus, status of the vascular system, and period of time the shoulder has been dislocated. Forceful manipulation may result in fracture of the humerus, and nerve or vascular damage. The surgeon should visualize exactly what is to be accomplished. In chronic dislocation, the head is firmly wedged over the rim of the glenoid. It is necessary to free the head gradually with traction and gentle flexion and extension. If the head is adequately mobilized, with continued traction it may be possible to lift it back into the glenoid. If, however, one is unable to mobilize the humeral head, the wisest approach is either to offer no further treatment or to discuss open reduction with the patient later.

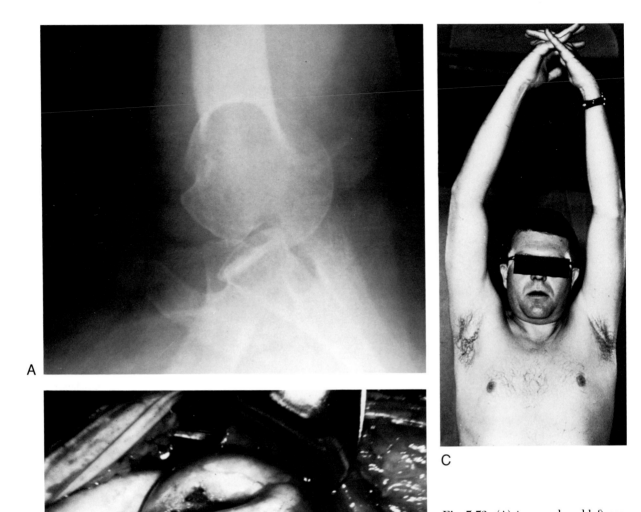

Fig. 7-73. (**A**) An unreduced left posterior dislocation of 3 months' duration. (**B**) Deep cleft in humeral head at surgery. The head was not resected. (**C**) The patient 15 years after open reduction with complete range of motion and function. (Figs. B and C from Rowe CR, Zarins B: Chronic unreduced dislocations of the shoulder. J Bone Joint Surg 64A:500, 1982.)

OPEN REDUCTION WITH PRESERVATION OF THE HUMERAL HEAD

Indications

With careful analysis and an atraumatic surgical approach, this category of treatment gave the best results. An anterior approach was adequate for the anterior dislocations. Obtaining adequate exposure of the chronic posterior dislocation was more difficult. Several points should be considered.

If the dislocation has been unreduced for 3 or 4 months, the humeral head will be osteoporotic and may be easily injured in freeing it up, if exposure is not adequate. To avoid injury to the vunerable head, one should have anterior, lateral, as well as posterior exposure. In 2 of our 12 posterior dislocations the subscapularis muscle and anterior capsule were drawn so tightly across the glenoid fossa that resection of the subscapularis attachment and capsule was necessary to reduce the humeral head.

Nerves and blood vessels in the scar tissue could be injured with inadequate exposure. For these reasons, we have used the "utility" or deltoid turn-down approach for posterior dislocations present for 3 or 4 months or longer. In deciding whether the humeral head should be sacrificed, remember that the shoulder is not a weight-bearing joint, and will function with much more damage to the head than the hip, knee, or ankle would tolerate. When in doubt, give nature a chance before discarding the humeral head.

Figure 7-73A shows an unreduced posterior dislocation (axillary view) of 3 months duration. Figure 7-73B illustrates the deep cleft in the head at surgery. A weight-bearing joint would not tolerate the degree of damage this head had received. We did not remove the head, and the patient has had no pain and a stable shoulder with excellent motion for 15 years (Fig. 7-73C). In another chronic posterior dislocation, the cartilaginous cap had a "ping-pong" in-and-out defect. At the 5-year follow-up, the head had survived and was functional.

Postoperative Care

Because of the fear of redislocating the shoulder postoperatively, many surgeons have used transarticular fixation with screws (Fig. 7-74A), Steinmann pins (Fig. 7-74B), or with pins from the acromion to the head. (Fig. 7-74C). Plaster casts or braces are also commonly used (Fig. 7-74D). Although fixation devices have been used to ensure reduction, they unfortunately eliminate needed early motion to the cartilage of the humeral head and add trauma to an already traumatized head.

We have *not* found it necessary to use any of the above methods. We find that early, safe postoperative motion is possible, without redislocation, by these simple rules:

1. If the arm remains posterior to the coronal plane of the body, we have not experienced a posterior dislocation regardless of the rotation of the arm
2. If the arm remains supported anterior to the coronal plane of the body, we have not experienced an anterior dislocation.

As demonstrated in Figure 7-75, this can be accomplished simply and comfortably with an elastoplast strapping to the humerus for a posterior dislocation, which allows early motion of the shoulder in backward extension and flexion of the elbow to reach the mouth. For an anterior dislocation, the Rowe sling (Fig. 7-76) allows motion from zero to forward flexion and adduction. These supports to the arm are put on at surgery and remain on for 3 weeks, at which time they are changed to removable supports to be worn at night for 3 weeks. We emphasize again that we have *not* experienced a dislocation or subluxation of an acute or a chronic dislocation after reduction using the above simple technique during the postreduction period. The patients are happy, comfortable, and safe. Early motion of the shoulder is possible.

Results

NO TREATMENT

Of the eight patients who had no treatment, one result was good, four were fair, and three were poor (see Table 7-6 for evaluation criteria). It was of interest to note that the three untreated posterior dislocations (average 65 units) scored higher than the four untreated anterior dislocations (average 49 units). This is understandable, since the arm is in a more functional position with an unreduced posterior dislocation (no abduction, arm at side of body, and in internal rotation) than the unreduced anterior dislocation (with the arm in abduction and external rotation).

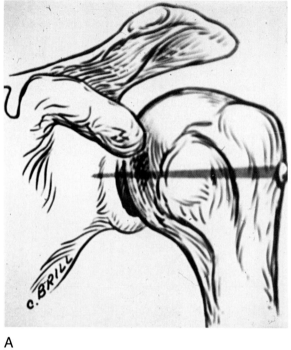

A

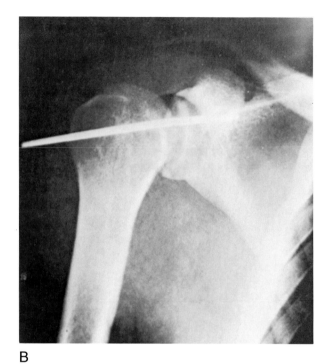

B

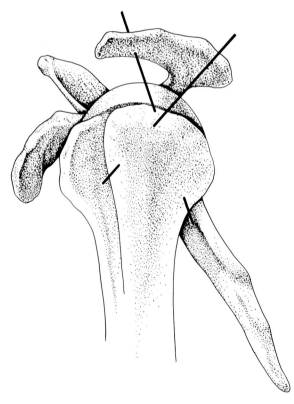

C

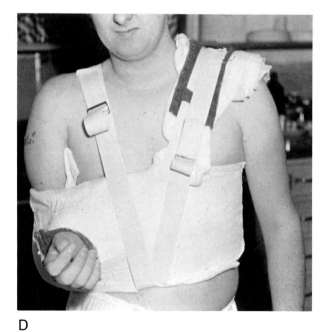

D

Fig. 7-74. Methods of transarticular fixation frequently used postreduction. (**A**) Screws. (**B,C**) Pins. (**D**) Plaster casts used for a recurrent posterior dislocation. The above techniques eliminate needed early safe motion of the shoulder. (DePalma AF: Surgery of the Shoulder. 3rd Ed. JB Lippincott, Philadelphia, 1983, p. 493.)

MANIPULATION

Unfortunately, we were unable to reach the two patients whose shoulders were reduced by manipulation.

OPEN REDUCTION WITH PRESERVATION OF THE HUMARAL HEAD

Nine shoulders (35 percent) had open reduction with preservation of the humeral head. This category scored higher than all other categories. In reviewing the literature, there is, in general, a pessimistic prognosis for open reduction of the chronic unreduced shoulder. The *very encouraging results* with open reduction in this study have been due, we believe, to adequate exposure of the humeral head at the time of surgery (thus reducing trauma to the head when reduced) and to the simple and effective postoperative support to the shoulder, allowing early motion of the join that's so important for nourishment of the articular cartilage and ligaments. This was accomplished by *not* transfixing the humeral head with screws or

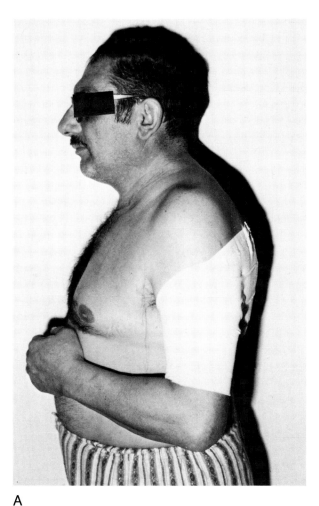
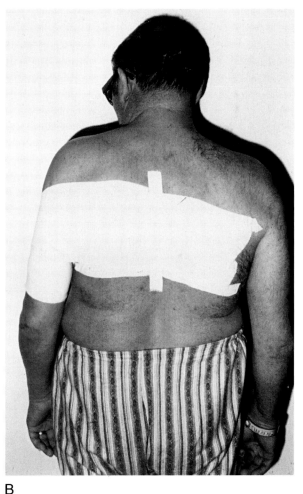

A   B

Fig. 7-75. A simpler, safer, and more comfortable method of maintaining reductions is recommended. **(A,B)** For a posterior dislocation, an elastoplasty strap is applied around the arm onto the back, which eliminates forward flexion but allows flexion of the elbow and backward extension of the arm. As long as the arm does not go anterior to the coronal plane, the shoulder has not dislocated posteriorly. This simple method has been comfortable and most effective, and can be applied at the time of surgery. (*Figure continues.*)

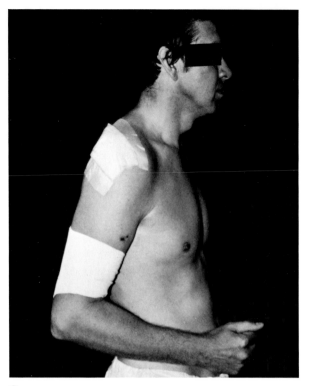

C

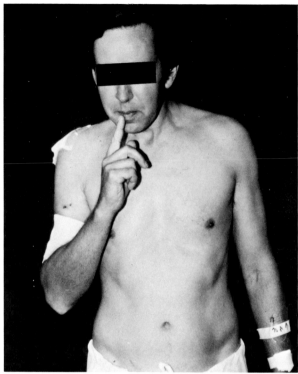

D

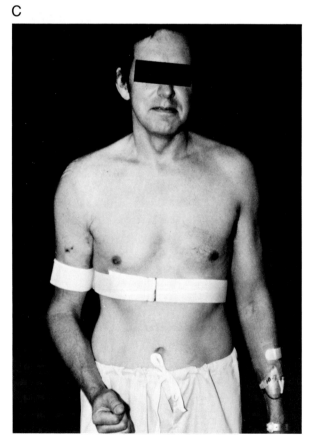

E

Fig. 7-75 (*Continued*). **(C,D)** Illustrated motion posteriorly and ability to reach the mouth. Patient 3 days after open reduction of posterior dislocation. **(E)** After 3 weeks, a removable belt may be worn at night for a week.

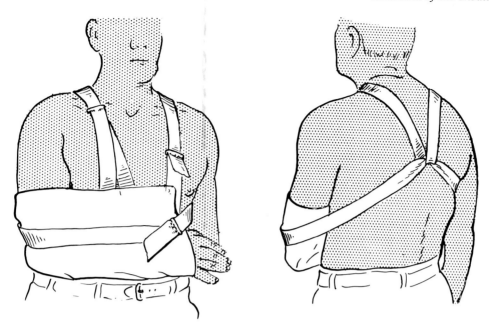

Fig. 7-76. Sling for an anterior dislocation. As long as the arm remains supported anterior to the coronal plane, the shoulder has not dislocated anteriorly. (Rowe CR, Marble AC: Shoulder girdle injuries. p. 254. In Cave EF (ed): Fractures and Other Injuries, Yearbook Medical Publishers, Chicago, 1958.)

pins, or immobilizing the shoulder after reduction in a plaster spica or splints. Of the nine open reductions, there were two excellent results (average 95 units), four good results (average 80 units), and three fair results (average 55 units). The overall average was 77 units (good).

REPLACEMENT OF THE HUMERAL HEAD (NEER PROSTHESIS)

Of the three patients, one had an excellent result (90 units), one a good result (70 units), and one a fair result (55 units), an average of 72 units (good). The fair result was a very intriging patient in whom the shoulder had been posteriorly dislocated for 33 years. He was happy to get his arm away from his body with external rotation, and was very satisfied with his result. Chronic adhesions kept him from having a good result. The good result was a patient whose posterior dislocation went unrecognized for two years. Chronic adhesions had developed that did not disappear after a satisfactory Neer replacement and kept her from having an excellent result.

RESECTION OF THE HUMERAL HEAD (JONES PROCEDURE)

It was necessary to remove the humeral head in seven patients and reattach the rotator cuff to the shaft of the humerus (Fig. 7-77). This was a very challenging group as they did not qualify for a shoulder replacement. The functional results of the Jones procedure were a surprise to us, with one good result and three fair results (an average of 65 units) (Table 7-6). We should keep this procedure in mind since there will be instances in which it may be needed, such as a failed septic case.

Summary

The eight untreated shoulders averaged 56 units (fair), the nine shoulders with open reduction and preservation of the humeral head averaged 77 units (good), the three Neer procedures averaged 72 units (good), and the four shoulders with the Jones procedure averaged 65 units (fair). Thus, the average rating for all surgical procedures was 71 units (good), which

Table 7-6. Results: Evaluation for Chronic Unreduced Dislocation

	Rating Units (100)	Excellent (90–100)	Good (70–89)	Fair (50–69)	Poor (Less than 50)
Pain					
No pain	30	No pain	Mild discomfort; no medication	Moderate disabling pain (occasional medication)	Constant disabling pain (constant medication)
Mild	25				
Moderate	20				
Severe	0				
Motion					
100% of normal elevation external & internal rotation	40	100% shoulder motion	75% of elevation, internal or external rotation	50% of elevation, lacking internal or external rotation	Can barely reach face; no rotation
75% of normal elevation external & internal rotation	30				
50% of elevation and lack of internal or external rotation	20				
25% or less of elevation, and lack of internal and external rotation	0				
Function (Strength & stability)					
Normal strength, activities, and stability of shoulder	30	Performs usual work and sports. Adequate strength in lifting, pushing, throwing. No instability.	Mild to moderate limitation in work and sports. No instability.	Moderate limitation in overhead work & lifting. Unable to throw. Mild to moderate apprehension of arm in extended position.	Unable to use arm in gainful activities. Recurrent subluxation or dislocation.
Mild limitation of activities and strength. No instability	25				
Moderate limitation of activities and strength; apprehension of shoulder in certain positions.	15				
Severe loss of strength, activities, and recurrent subluxation or dislocation.	0				
Possible total	100				

is a much more favorable prognosis for this condition than had previously been reported in the orthopaedic literature.

We emphasize the following points:

1. *All* chronic dislocations of the shoulder do not have to be reduced. The patient may be happy to remain as he or she is.
2. Before attempting a closed reduction, the surgeon should be certain of the length of time the shoulder has been dislocated, the age of the patient, and the physical condition of the humeral shaft.
3. Improved surgical results can be obtained:
   a. *Adequate* surgical exposure should be used to avoid injury to the already injured humeral head.
   b. Use gentleness in reduction, whether closed or open.
   c. *Early*, safe, active and passive postreduction motion can be obtained, thus eliminating transfixation of the joint with pins or screws, or immobilization of the shoulder with a plaster cast, by a simple strapping of the arm (for posterior dislocation) or a sling (for anterior dislocation).

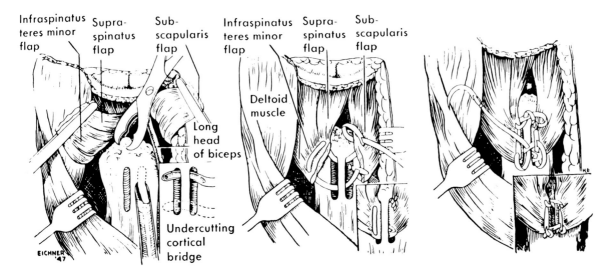

Fig. 7-77. The Jones procedure. The humeral head is resected; the bony attachments of the rotator cuff removed and the tendons of the rotator cuff are attached to the prepared humeral shaft. It is important to snug up the shaft into the glenoid. (Jones L: The shoulder joint—observations in the anatomy and physiology. Surg Gyn Obstet 75:443, 1942. Reprinted by permission from Surgery, Gynecology and Obstetrics.)

VOLUNTARY DISLOCATION AND SUBLUXATION[*]

Although voluntary dislocation of the glenohumeral joint was described by Portal[51] in 1722, little subsequent attention was given to this unusual and interesting syndrome for many years. The literature has consisted largely of single case reports or small series of three, four, or five patients.[33,49,53,89,111] Although some of these were successfully treated surgically, more often initial surgery was followed by multiple recurrences and further unsuccessful operative procedures.

Shoulder instability in these patients develops either spontaneously or after insignificant trauma. Although they are numerically uncommon, their management remains a difficult problem. Many voluntary dislocators begin to dislocate in childhood or adolescence following trivial trauma or none at all. In some cases, they voluntarily dislocate their shoulders many times each day. Some may use this maneuver to amuse or annoy those around them, to attract attention, or to relieve emotional tension.[63,67,134,135,138]

Others may try to abandon the maneuver, only to find that certain activities or assumption of a particular position will invariably produce a dislocation. Some of these patients never dislocate as a habit. In some, their luxations can be voluntarily produced despite the fact that they never occur in the course of everyday activities (Fig. 7-78). What characterizes all of the patients in this category, termed voluntary, is that their dislocations follow little or no trauma and are usually painless or minimally painful. Reduction does not require the assistance of another person, being effected by muscular activity or a series of stereotypic gyrations of the humerus and scapula (Fig. 7-79). Secondary traumatic changes of the joint usually do not occur in these patients, although some have been reported.

History and Physical Examination

As a rule, the voluntary dislocator will give very little, if any, history of significant trauma or injury. Many of them state that they found out they were able to slip their shoulder in or out of its socket without injury, whereas others had a minor incident to

[*] Robert D. Leffert co-authored this section.

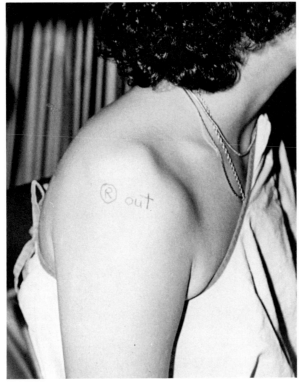

A

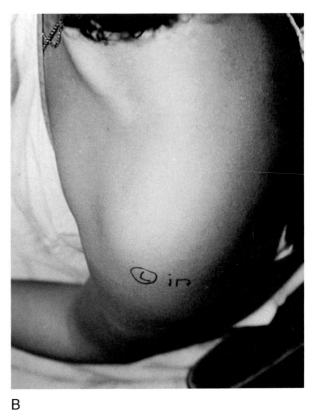

B

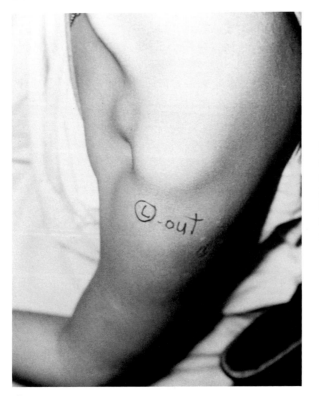

C

Fig. 7-78. An 18-year-old woman showing ability to subluxate both shoulders voluntarily despite not experiencing instability with functional activities. **(A)** The right shoulder anteriorly and inferiorly subluxated. **(B)** The left shoulder in normal position with the muscles relaxed. **(C)** The left shoulder inferiorly subluxated with asymmetrical muscle contraction.

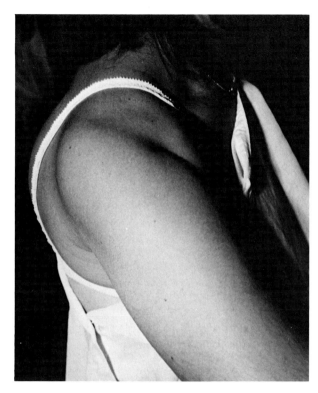

Fig. 7-79. This 16-year-old girl voluntarily produces posterior subluxation of the right glenohumeral joint accompanied by winging of her scapula.

the shoulder. The involuntary or atraumatic dislocator will give an account of a single or repeated injury or overuse of their arm, following which the shoulders were unstable.

The largest group of these patients was reported in 1973 by Rowe et al.,[122] who describe clinical, roentgenographic, electromyographic, and psychiatric findings in 26 patients with voluntary dislocation in one or both shoulders. In this study of 40 shoulders, eight (31 percent) had emotional or character problems (category I), whereas 18 (69 percent) had no psychological or emotional problems (category II). On the basis of the clinical and electromyographic analysis, it was believed that redislocation was produced by suppression of an element or one of the muscle forces responsible for normal shoulder motion. The displacement was unidirectional in 20 patients (posterior in 12, anterior in 4, and inferior in 4). In the other 20 shoulders, dislocations were in more than one direction (anterior, posterior, and inferior in

eight; anterior and posterior in six; inferior and posterior in six). The majority of patients were between the ages of 12 and 19. Thirty-five percent had bilateral involvement. Forty-two percent reported that the onset was spontaneous; they demonstrated their shoulder instability "as a trick." The remainder reported a mild injury with the onset, such as a fall, lifting, or taking part in an athletic event. Sixty-five percent had moderate to marked laxity of other joints, while the remainder did not have hyperlaxity. No patient had the characteristic findings of Ehlers-Danlos syndrome.

In May, 1976, Leffert and co-workers began a video-electromyographic prospective study of 23 additional patients who exhibited voluntary dislocation of one or both shoulders.[74] There were 11 male and nine female patients. Their ages ranged from 14 to 31 years, with an average of 18.5 years. Of 19 patients in whom the duration of the shoulder dislocation was known, 6 had the problem for a year or less, 3 between 2 and 3 years, 5 greater than 5 years, and 5 "for as long as I can remember."

Eight patients had no history of trauma, realized that they could voluntarily dislocate one or both shoulders, but did not do it as a habit. Three additional ones dated the onset to strenuous activity (one while dancing and two while competitively swimming) and then were in the same category. Eight patients began to dislocate "as a habit" or "to relieve tension": one after playing tennis without obvious injury and one after strenuously throwing a ball. One tripped over a wire and, although he had no shoulder pain, found that he could voluntarily dislocate his shoulder. Of the same group of 20 patients, 15 characterized their shoulders as being painless or having minimal discomfort with their dislocations. Three had mild pain, one had moderate pain and one, a physician's daughter, claimed severe pain, for which she periodically received intramuscular Demerol.

The physical build of the voluntary and involuntary dislocators may show little differences. In fact, those with involuntary subluxations or dislocations may have more generalized ligamentous laxity than the voluntary dislocators. The 1976 study showed that half of the patients had no evidence of generalized laxity, while six had moderate laxity without a family history. No patient in either the 1973 or the 1976 study had Ehlers-Danlos syndrome.

With careful observation, one may notice subtle

differences in facial expression and attitude between the voluntary and involuntary groups of dislocators. The voluntary dislocator is quite willing to demonstrate his or her "trick" and shows a facial expression that seems to say "Now you try and figure this out!" The involuntary dislocator is not so eager to demonstrate the instability of the shoulder, and the facial expression says "I hope you can help me."

As a rule, the diagnosis is not difficult to make. However, at times it may be difficult. Take as an example the patient who states that each time he abducts his arm to 90° in internal rotation the shoulder "pops out." Is this due to voluntary muscle control or involuntary instability of the shoulder? We have observed that the voluntary dislocator usually tightens or "sets" as abduction and internal rotation are initiated. The scapula may begin to wing at the same time. The involuntary dislocator does not exhibit this preliminary maneuver. This subtle differential finding has been of value in our assessment of these patients. Of the 26 shoulders in the 1976 study, 17 dislocated only posteriorly, 3 inferiorly, and 1 anteriorly. Three were multidirectional posterior and inferior, while two were multidirectional posterior and anterior. Hence, of the unidirectional pure dislocators, 17 of 26 (65 percent) were posterior, and of those with multidirectional dislocation, 5 of 26 (19 percent) had posterior dislocations as a major feature.

Radiographic Findings

None of the patients we have observed in either of the series, no matter how often they had dislocated or subluxated their shoulders, showed any radiographic evidence of trauma to the glenohumeral joint or a Hill-Sachs lesion. Only those patients who had previously had unsuccessful operative procedures showed degenerative changes. Of the 26 involved shoulders in the second series, 3 were judged abnormal because of slight to moderate flattening of the glenoids. No measurements of humeral version or glenoidal inclination were obtained in these patients.

Electromyographic Studies

In the original 1973 study,[122] the force-couple control of the shoulder mechanism was investigated in detail. Normal control of shoulder motion depends on the rhythmic function of muscle force-couples that rotate and elevate the humerus and scapula. For instance, the humerus is rotated and elevated by the coordinated action of the deltoid pulling upward and the subscapularis, infraspinatus, and teres major pulling inward against the glenoid fossa, aided by upward and oblique pull of the supraspinatus. Simultaneous muscle action by suppression of one-half of a force-couple and activation of another force-couple may produce voluntary anterior, posterior, or inferior displacement of the humeral head. Also we found that displacement of the humeral head can be accomplished by varying positions of the arm and by various muscle combinations (Fig. 7-80). These combinations are worthy of careful study.

In the 1976 study,[74] 20 patients underwent video EMG analysis of their shoulder motion both in the reduced position and while voluntarily dislocating and reducing their shoulders. In most cases both shoulders were examined, even when one was uninvolved. The flexible wire technique of Basmajian and Stack was employed with percutaneous insertion of fine nylon-coated flexible Karma wire through a #25 needle, which was then withdrawn (Fig. 7-81A). The following muscles were examined routinely: deltoid, supraspinatus, infraspinatus, subscapularis, latissimus dorsi, and pectoralis major. Other muscles examined, when indicated, included biceps, triceps, serratus anterior, and rhomboids. All needle insertions were verified for accuracy of placement by stimulation prior to the connection to the EMG preamplifier. Spring clips designed in our laboratory provided motion-free electrode connections to avoid artifacts in the integrated EMGs.

The recording apparatus was arranged so that four channels of EMG signals from four different muscles could be obtained simultaneously (Fig. 7-81A), although the EMG was constantly monitored to detect possible artifacts. The signals were rectified and filtered and then put into a bar graft generator, so that the four channels of running integrated EMG could be studied. By means of a video mixer, they were then displayed on the screen of a monitor, the other half of which showed the simultaneous picture of the moving shoulder (Fig. 7-81B).

Stop action and 7:1 slow motion made detailed analysis of motion and muscle activity possible. Since only four channels could be used at any one time, the process had to be repeated several times to study all the pertinent muscles. Although there was no abso-

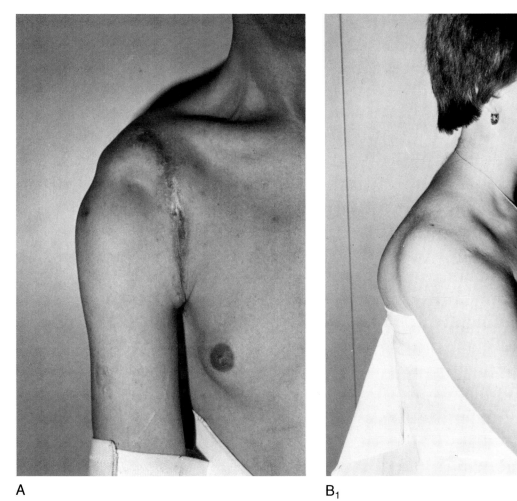

A

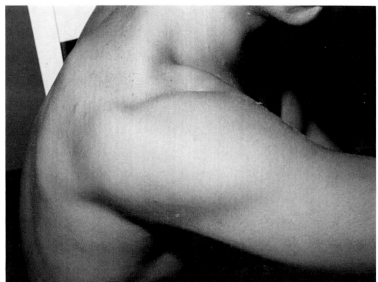

B$_1$

B$_2$

Fig. 7-80. Displacement of the humeral head can be accomplished with various positions of the arm or differing muscle combinations. (**A**) Inferior displacement is usually with the arm at side of body. (Patient's surgical repair had been unsuccessful.) (**B**) Posterior displacement (1) With the arm slightly flexed. (2) Arm in forward flexion. (*Figure continues.*)

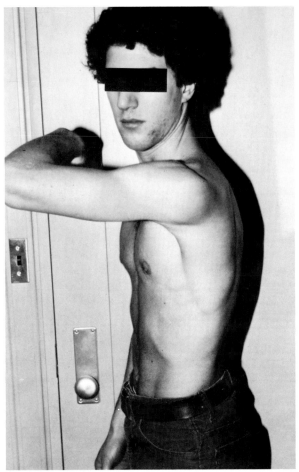

B₃

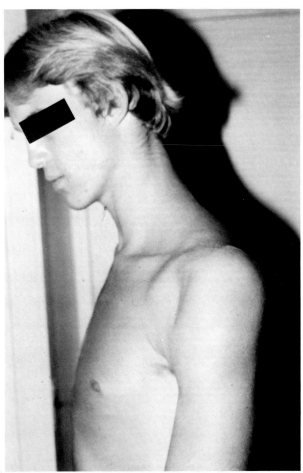

B₅

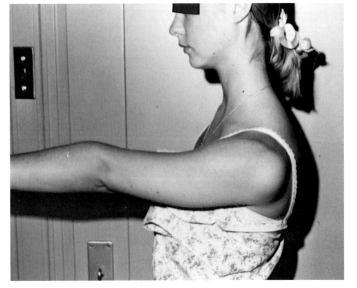

B₄

Fig. 7-80 (*Continued*). (3) Arm in forward flexion and 90° internal rotation. (4) Arm in forward flexion 90° and in neutral rotation. (5) With the arm in neutral at side of body. (*Figure continues.*)

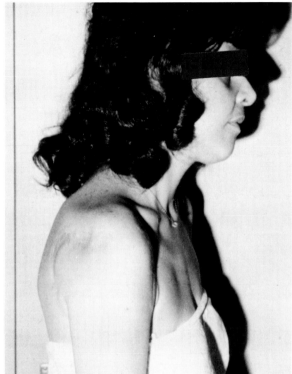

C₁

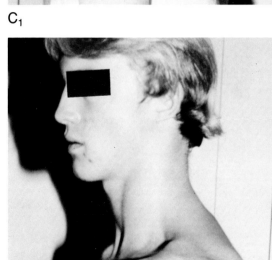

C₃

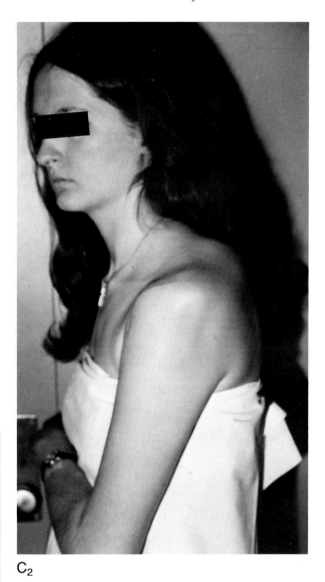

C₂

Fig. 7-80 (*Continued*). (**C**) Anterior displacement. (1) With arm in neutral at side of body. (2) With arm in forward flexion and internal rotation. (3) With arm in backward extension.

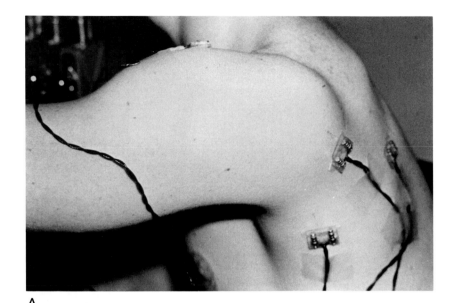

A

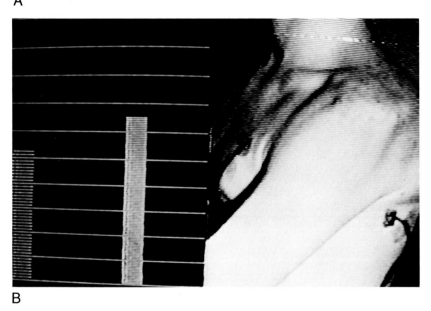

B

Fig. 7-81. (A) This patient has had wire electrodes inserted into the anterior and posterior deltoid muscles, as well as latissimus dorsi and infraspinatus. (B) Photograph taken from the split video screen during testing of the inferior dislocation in which latissimus dorsi (left histogram) and pectoralis major (right histogram) are active in producing the dislocation.

lutely uniform pattern of muscular activity seen, in all cases a number of important observations were made.

In 7 of the 17 pure posterior dislocations, no abnormal motor activity was necessary to produce the dislocations; the patient merely had to forward flex the humerus, adduct slightly, and then allow the forearm to drop so that the humerus was medially rotated. An immediate, painless, posterior dislocation resulted. This could be considered an involuntary type. Lateral rotation or extension of the arm reduced the

dislocation. Two of these seven also winged their scapulae by suppressing serratus activity at the time of their dislocation, as did one additional patient in whom it appeared to be the mechanism of dislocation without additional muscular hyperactivity (Figs. 7-79, 7-82). Another simultaneously exerted overactivity of the latissimus dorsi to produce his dislocation while he winged his scapula. In the majority of the remaining posterior dislocators it was possible to demonstrate overactivity of the latissimus dorsi in the production of posterior dislocation in patients who could

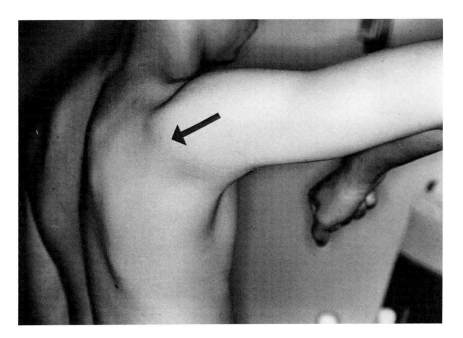

Fig. 7-82. An example of winging of the scapula at the time of posterior dislocation.

not be passively dislocated. In several patients, there was simultaneous activity of the posterior deltoid. In three patients with inferior dislocation, the pectoralis major was conspicuously hyperactive, with one of these also requiring the activity of the latissimus dorsi to depress the humeral head. One patient (the only one who had significant complaints of pain and who had had an unsuccessful Bankart procedure) had tetanic contraction of the latissimus and chronic but episodic inferior dislocation of the humerus. Although considered primarily to be an inferior dislocator, on one occasion an axillary view had shown her to be completely dislocated posteriorly.

All patients tolerated the examination with multiple electrode insertions without difficulty. The patients did not experience significant pain. Since one video monitor was turned so that they could watch it, they usually became actively absorbed and interested in the proceedings. The wires were gently removed at the end of the sessions, which generally took 1.5 hours. There have been no adverse aftereffects of wire electrode insertion.

Treatment

The evolution of treatment of voluntary dislocation of the shoulder has been fascinating. In the 1960s, our attention was first focused on this syndrome be-

cause of a number of patients admitted to the Massachusetts General Hospital after unsuccessful surgery for this condition. As we studied these patients and identified how they produced their dislocations, we realized that this was not a surgical problem. Since the report in 1973, we have resorted to surgery in only three patients for this problem. All other patients have responded to conservative treatment. This has also been the experience of others.

CONSERVATIVE

Once the differentiation between voluntary and involuntary instability is made, the next important step is to establish whether the patient has any emotional problems that will directly effect the response to treatment. It may take one or two interviews before this can be clearly identified. We have found it most helpful to have a family member present during the examination. Frequently, the family is perplexed by conflicting medical opinions that they have gotten about diagnosis and treatment. A clear explanation should be made to the family and to the patient, detailing how the dislocation is produced by abnormal muscle activity. With a clear explanation, the mystery of the patient's performance is dispelled and a treatment plan can then be outlined.

First, the patient is instructed to cease performing "the trick." A program of exercises is outlined that must be specific for the patient rather than generalized. Exercising the wrong muscles, or activating those that cause the dislocation, can not only perpetuate the problem but even make it worse.

Therefore, for those patients in whom the pattern of muscular activity was difficult to define clinically, a video EMG analysis was done. The activity patterns and positions were explored and, once the pattern of instability was known, the specific exercise program was designed with the physical therapist to increase stability by strengthening the antagonists of the muscles responsible for the dislocation. With exposure to additional patients, we very infrequently now use EMG analysis because we have become more adroit at defining clinically the responsible force-couples.

For all patients, the initial exercise program was designed to avoid any pattern in which the patient felt unstable. In most cases, a home exercise program consisting of three or four key exercises performed two or three times per day was prescribed. Elastic webbing was often used for resistance, and the patient was instructed on how to use a door jamb to secure one end of the elastic. Hand-held weights were often used in the same positions. Although biofeedback was used early in the series in an attempt to "inhibit the overactive muscles," this modality was not found to be of great benefit: although a patient might be able to relax a specific muscle in certain static positions while using biofeedback, it proved almost impossible to eliminate that muscle's activity from functional patterns during daily activities that required proximal stability (cocontraction) for distal limb function.

In addition to specific exercises, patterns of use of the arm were reviewed with each patient, who was urged to avoid positions that caused dislocation. Sometimes a simple modification of the manner in which the arm was used was enough to reduce the frequency of dislocation markedly. For example, teaching a patient with posterior dislocations to forward flex the arm in lateral rotation would immediately reduce the number of dislocations. Patients who dislocated as a "tension reliever" were admonished against the practice and urged to employ other means. Usually the "tension" was relieved after muscle tone had been regained by exercises. All patients were provided with written instructions during the initial sessions. In some cases, the patients returned for several outpatient refresher sessions. It is *most important* to make sure that these patients do not become independently involved in commercial weight machine gymnasiums, because of the very real possibility of developing the wrong muscles to excess and thereby vitiating the entire therapeutic exercise program.

It is important also that the patient carry out the exercises three times daily at home or at school and that they be checked once a month for 3 or 4 months to monitor progress (See Fig. 7-44). During this period, the patient will demonstrate whether she has been cooperative and interested in helping herself, or whether she is uncooperative and having emotional difficulties, using the ability to subluxate or dislocate the shoulders to gain attention, relief from responsibilities, or, in some instances, to obtain medication.

Occasionally, psychiatric consultation is necessary. This may present a problem, since the patient and the family may be reluctant to undergo a psychiatric interview. In addition, the psychiatrist must be familiar with the syndrome and the problems it entails. A clear explanation is helpful to the patient and family, emphasizing that the key to successful treatment is a careful understanding of all factors involved in the problem. Both the patient and family usually accept the suggestion, although not invariably. It is important that at subsequent interviews all findings and recommendations are openly discussed with all concerned. In the past 10 years, the incidence of these patients with significant psychiatric difficulties has shown a marked drop—to about 15 percent. Perhaps a clearer understanding of the entity and a more responsible approach to the patient's problems have become factors in the lessening of the chances of patients taking advantage of their "trick." An understanding doctor may prove an excellent psychiatrist.

SURGICAL

Although the unwary surgeon would see no contraindication to surgical attempts to stabilize the patient's shoulder and eliminate the subluxation or dislocation in an *uncooperative* patient, it has been our experience; and that of others, that such surgery is doomed to failure. We have had the opportunity to see many patients operated upon without success in the category I patient (those with significant psychiatric problems). Surgery in these instances will not only help but often also may prove harmful to the patient, by exacerbating dependence and psychiatric problems.

A few typical patients with unresolved emotional problems will serve to illustrate.

Case 1

P.McG., a 19-year-old man, twisted his left shoulder and was seen in the emergency ward because of anterior and posterior dislocations of his left shoulder and anterior, posterior, and inferior dislocations of his right shoulder. The following surgical procedures were performed during periods of unrecognized psychiatric disturbances:

Left shoulder (at another hospital)
1956: anterior Putti-Platt (temporarily successful)
1956: posterior Bankart (unsuccessful)
1958: posterior Bankart, repeated (unsuccessful)
1958: posterior bone block (unsuccessful)
1961: shoulder arthrodesis

Right shoulder (performed at Massachusetts General Hospital)
1959: posterior osteotomy, neck of glenoid (unsuccessful)
1960: anterior Bankart (unsuccessful)
1960: posterior Eden-Hybbinette (unsuccessful)
1960: shoulder arthrodesis

Fortunately, the shoulders were fused in a functional position that has allowed him to work successfully as a bartender for the past 15 years with only minor complaints of left shoulder pain during periods of emotional stress (see Chap. 16).

Case 2

P.S. was a young woman seen early in our series because of her ability to dislocate both shoulders.

Left shoulder (performed at another hospital)
1950: posterior capsulorrhaphy (unsuccessful)
1960: (performed at Massachusetts General Hospital) posterior bone block and Bankart (successful)

Right shoulder
1963: (Massachusetts General Hospital) posterior bone block and capsular reefing (unsuccessful)
1963: We recognized her psychiatric difficulties and advised against further surgery, although she requested it

During the next 20 years of follow-up, she continued to dislocate her right shoulder during periods of emotional stress.

In contrast, during the period of the study, three patients in category II (normal psychiatric profiles) with voluntary dislocation of their shoulders were operated on because of secondary laxity of the shoulders from repeated "involuntary dislocations." All have had good results. Figure 7-83 shows a good response to surgery. Figure 7-84 shows a typical category II patient who responded to specific resistive exercises with excellent results.

Another patient, who was not included in the EMG analysis group, was unable to keep the humeral head from going posteriorly no matter what she did. She had rather flat glenoids bilaterally even though dislocation was present only on the right side. She underwent a glenoidal osteotomy using Scott's technique.[131] Her osteotomy consolidated readily and she was free of dislocations for 3 months, when she reported a feeling of instability without frank dislocation; none could be produced by either the patient or surgeon. She was started on a program of strengthening exercises for her lateral rotators, with marked improvement in their bulk and tone and complete relief of her symptoms. Eleven months postoperatively, having not done her prescribed exercises for 5 months, she reported a spontaneous dislocation and reduction. She was restarted on her exercises with relief of her symptoms. She was last seen at 1 year following surgery. Whether she will have to continue the exercises indefinitely is unknown, but it is clear that without surgical intervention she would have been unable to do them at all because of a total lack of joint stability. It cannot be overemphasized that for the patient with *severe psychiatric problems* that preclude cooperation in the physical therapy program, emotional difficulties must be resolved before the shoulder can be successfully treated. Surgery is contraindicated in such circumstances, as has been well documented.

Results

In the 1973 study, of the 15 patients with emotional and psychiatric problems (category I) who are not cooperative, 14 continued to subluxate and dislocate their shoulders to gain attention, avoid responsibilities, or obtain drugs. The alarming story of this group

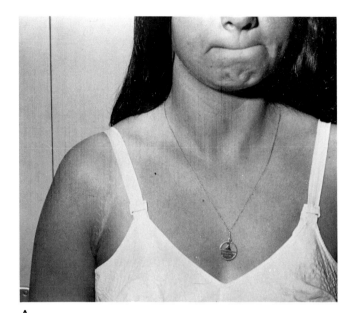

A

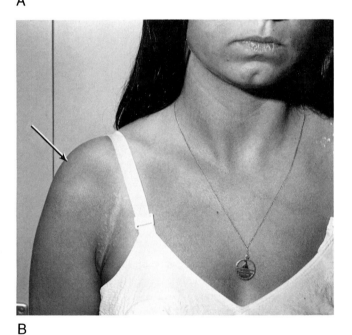

B

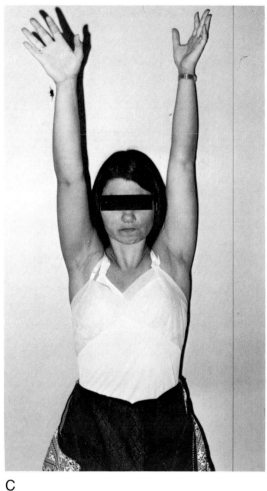

C

Fig. 7-83. (A) A 19-year-old woman who continued to dislocate her right shoulder inferiorly after unsuccessful surgery. **(B)** She was cooperative but her shoulder continued to "slip out" (arrow indicates inferior subluxation). She responded to a capsulorrhaphy plus a Thompson modification of a Nicola procedure. She has been a successful physical therapist for 10 years. Her good result was due to lack of emotional problems and cooperation.

is that a total of 35 operations had been performed on these patients by qualified orthopaedic surgeons, with only one successful result. Today, however, we are much more alert to the recognition and treatment of voluntary dislocators. Of the 31 cooperative patients in the 1973 study, in the absence of psychologi-

cal disorders, 28 responded to conservative treatment with good and excellent results and 3 with fair results. This last group had voluntarily ceased dislocating their shoulders, but instability persisted on a nonvoluntary basis, necessitating surgical reconstruction. The results were excellent in all three, as stability

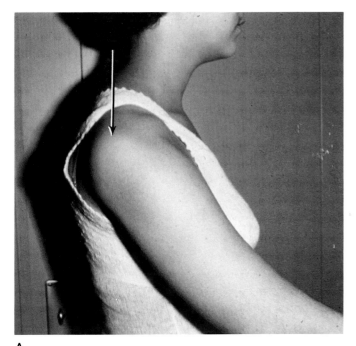
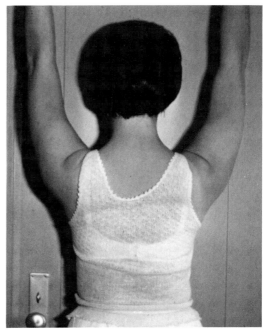

A   B

Fig. 7-84. (**A**) A typical patient in category II (with normal personality) who was seen because her shoulder "slipped out" during archery, or even when she was carrying books (arrow indicates posterior subluxation). (**B**) After 3 months of specific resistive exercises, she returned to archery and could lift a chair without instability of her shoulder.

was restored, and the patients did not voluntarily attempt to break down their repairs.

Of the 20 patients in the 1976 series, all in category II, 13 reported that they had completely stopped dislocating under all circumstances. Two experienced marked improvement and rarely dislocated. Five were still dislocating when last seen or contacted. Two had experienced significant lessening of their dislocations while doing their exercises, but had become bored with them and ultimately reverted to their original status. One of these went to a commercial exercise program to strengthen his muscles and lost the initial benefit of his medically prescribed exercises. One patient did her exercises sporadically and reported that although her frequency of dislocations did not change, the moderate discomfort she had with them was completely alleviated.

One patient, a lax-jointed and multidirectional dislocator, could not do the exercises because her shoulder would dislocate in any position. An additional patient (category I) had severe psychiatric problems

and continued to dislocate inferiorly and posteriorly on an episodic basis. She is currently receiving psychotherapy.

There was no correlation of results with age, duration of symptoms, bilaterality, radiographic changes, sex, or joint laxity. Even though there was no correlation in the unidirectional dislocators, of the 5 failures of treatment, 2 were multidirectional, although only 5 of the 26 affected shoulders were multidirectional.

The pathologic basis of posttraumatic dislocations is well recognized, although which of the reported anatomical lesions is most important is still occasionally debated. There are no such predictable lesions in the voluntary dislocator. In the few cases that have been described at operation, the findings have usually been a patulous capsule and rather stretched and inadequate musculature. Rarely does one find labral detachments or head defects. Evidence of arthrosis in the joint is not usually seen unless there has been previous surgery. We believe that the dynamic dysfunction of the force-couples of the musculature produces the voluntary type of dislocation, although joint laxity may contribute to the problem. That the majority of voluntary dislocations are posterior in direction is more easily understandable in this context when one considers the position needed to produce this type: forward flexion and medial rotation. This position is assumed for a great many activities of daily living. It puts the lateral rotators at a great disadvantage mechanically, since they are unable to contract strongly and press against the posterior capsule, thus keeping the humeral head from going posteriorly. If an overpulling medial rotator and head depressor such as latissimus dorsi or pectoralis major is superimposed on the already barely compensated muscular–capsular apparatus, dislocation results.

Case Reports

T.R. was a 14-year old, left-handed white girl who was examined because of bilateral voluntary posterior shoulder dislocations that began at age 12. There was no history of trauma and no pain, but she had severe functional limitations because forward flexion of her arms to the horizontal would invariably produce posterior dislocations. Although she could reduce the dislocations without difficulty and never dislocated as a habit, she was incapacitated by them. She exerted moderate, generalized joint laxity and had snapping hips, but was otherwise normal and asymptomatic. The pertinent family history was negative.

Radiographs of her shoulders were negative. A video EMG analysis of her shoulders during dislocation revealed that her latissimus dorsi and, to a lesser constant degree, posterior deltoids were hyperactive during the production of her dislocations. Both sides were identical.

On the basis of her analysis, an exercise program was prescribed to strengthen the lateral rotators with the arms 30° flexed and abducted. This position was shown on EMG to inactivate the latissimus in this patient and so was judged correct for her. Using this routine, she stopped dislocating and has remained asymptomatic for the 30 months she was evaluated. She participates in strenuous activity without difficulty.

M.M.T., a 16-year-old girl, had had difficulty with both shoulders "as long as I can remember." There was no history of trauma and she had no functional limitations, although she would often be awakened by dislocations, anteriorly on the right and inferiorly on the left. She had bilateral subluxating patellae and a family history of hyperlaxity.

Clinical examination showed her to be able to dislocate voluntarily her right shoulder anteriorly and the left inferiorly by contraction of the pectoralis major in both cases, which was verified by EMG. Reduction occurred spontaneously with relaxation of the muscles. Other than generalized joint hyperlaxity, there were no abnormalities. A program of strengthening exercises was prescribed for the lateral rotators of the humerus without eliciting contraction of the pectorals. She did her exercises faithfully and, at 28 months, was totally asymptomatic.

R.Z. was a 20-year-old white man who was evaluated for a 1-year history of posterior dislocations of his nondominant shoulder. There was no history of trauma, but he did admit to "cracking it to relieve tension." In addition, forward flexion, adduction, and medial rotation of the humerus would produce posterior dislocations, which made it impossible for him to participate in athletics. There was no pain and he had had no therapy. There was slight hyperlaxity of the upper extremity joints and a negative family history.

His examination revealed that passive positioning of the shoulder as described would produce posterior dislocation and, although he could dislocate actively using the latissimus, muscular activity was not necessary. Radiographs of his shoulder were normal.

He was advised to stop cracking the shoulder to relieve tension and, after video EMG studies, was given a program of lateral rotator-strengthening exercises. With 2 months, the frequency of dislocation had dropped to once a week. Then, hoping to accelerate the recovery process and build up his muscles, he began to attend a commercial exercise gymnasium regularly. When contacted at 1 year, he had reverted to his pretreatment status.

Summary

As is shown by the results of these two series, it is possible to treat successfully even long-duration voluntary dislocators by nonoperative exercise techniques. Not all patients can be so treated, even if one excluded those who will not cooperate in the exercise program. The category I patient who is emotionally disturbed requires psychiatric, not surgical, intervention. However, excellent results can be obtained with conservative treatment in the cooperative patient after a careful and thorough examination and an explanation of how the subluxation or dislocation is produced, followed by a guided exercise program to rehabilitate the supporting muscles of the shoulder.

POSTERIOR DISLOCATION

Incidence

In our review of 500 shoulder dislocations in 1956, we found the incidence of posterior dislocations to be 2 percent.[117] McLaughlin, in his series of 581 shoulder dislocations, reported an incidence of 3.8 percent.[82] In 1949, Wilson and McKeever[147] reported a 1.5 percent incidence. Because posterior dislocations are being recognized more frequently today, the overall incidence is perhaps higher than has been reported in the past.

Diagnosis

It is well to review again the clinical characteristics of a posterior dislocation so that one may be more alert to its presence and more accurate in diagnosis.

With a posterior dislocation, the arm is locked in *internal rotation* (whereas in an anterior dislocation the arm is locked in external rotation). This is easily picked up by asking the patient to flex both elbows to 90° (Fig. 7-85). The fixed position of internal rotation of the dislocated shoulder will be evident. Also, if the patient is asked to extend both arms, he or she will be unable to turn the palm of the dislocated arm upward. Even though the arm is in complete supination, it is locked in internal rotation. This physical sign has not been previously reported in the literature (Fig. 7-86B).

Observe the shoulders from above. There is absence of the anterior contour of the shoulder on the dislocated side, and prominence posteriorly (Fig. 7-86).

On motion of the arm upward, the scapula moves simultaneously with the arm, as the humeral head is impaled over the posterior rim of the glenoid.

A chronic posterior dislocation can be easily missed, because the patient is able to elevate the arm in forward flexion due to scapular motion, and can easily reach the mouth, head, and the midline of the back, since the arm is fixed in internal rotation.

Another source of error is the "normal" appearance of the AP roentgenogram of a posterior dislocation (Fig. 7-87), whereas an anterior dislocation is evident on anterior-posterior views. Seventy-five percent of posterior dislocations in our series were missed by the patients' referring doctors[119] and 79 percent were missed in McLaughlin's series.[81] It should be noted that in the anterior-posterior view of a posterior dislocation the humeral head is *always* in internal rotation and the overlapping of the humeral head on the glenoid rim, or the "half-moon" appearance, is usually absent or diminished (Fig. 7-88A, B). An anterior-posterior view may also demonstrate the reverse Hill-Sachs or medial head defect (Fig. 7-88A, B).

An *axillary view will always give the answer* (Fig. 7-88C). There are a number of satisfactory views for the axillary technique (see Chap. 5). The Y-lateral view can be taken if the arm cannot be abducted. The transthoracic view, which is so frequently used, is unsatisfactory. A computed axial tomographic (CAT) scan will clearly demonstrate a posterior dislocation, as well as the head defect.

A good rule is to take an axillary view whenever a patient who has experienced an injury to the shoulder, or has a history of epilepsy, and complains of a stiff painful shoulder afterwards, does *not* respond to physical therapy, injections, or even manipulation, and when the anterior-posterior radiographs are interpreted as "negative." Although there are a number of techniques for obtaining an axillary view, we prefer the view taken with the patient in supination (see Chap. 5).

Classification

As with anterior dislocations, posterior dislocations are similarly classified:

1. Traumatic
   a. Acute
   b. Recurrent

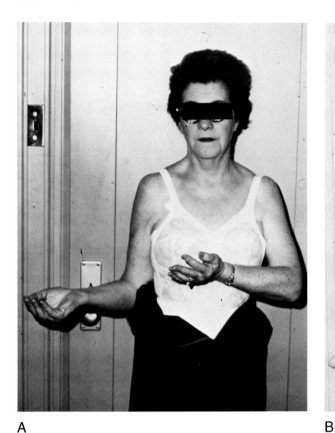

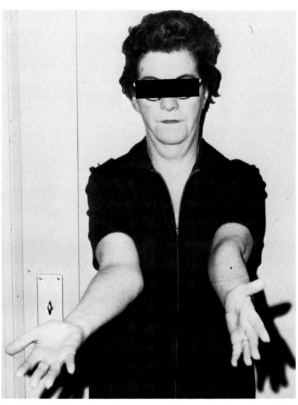

A   B

Fig. 7-85. The posterior dislocation of the patient's left shoulder had been unrecognized for 2 years, and treated for a "frozen" shoulder. **(A)** The fixed internal rotation of the left shoulder is evident when the patient flexes the elbows to 90°. **(B)** With extension of the arms, the patient is unable to turn her left palm up even though the arm is in complete supination (Rowe sign). (Rowe CR: Chronic unreduced dislocations of the shoulder. J Bone Joint Surg 64A:494, 1982.)

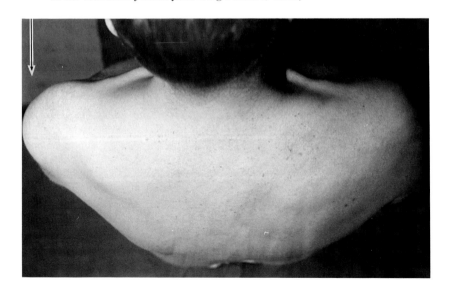

Fig. 7-86. Observation of the patient from above demonstrates posterior prominence and absence of anterior contour on the left. (Note arrow.)

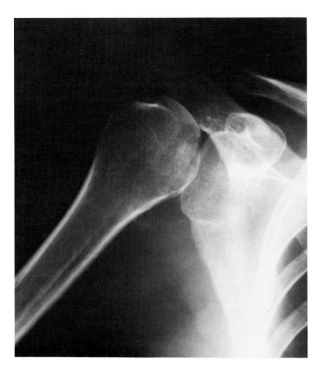

Fig. 7-87. These AP views were read as normal by a qualified roentgenologist. Note the absence of the "half moon" of the left shoulder.

Pathologic Findings

1. Detachment of the capsule and labrum from the posterior rim of the glenoid (a "reverse" Bankart lesion) is the most common lesion. It should be noted, however, that the posterior labrum and capsule are not as well developed as they are anteriorly. This influences the operative technique of restoring stability.
2. Excessive laxity or redundancy of the posterior capsule is usually present in recurrent dislocation.
3. An impacted head defect (the opposite of the Hill-Sachs lesion) on the anterior-medial aspect of the humeral head, may be present. Figure 7-88A and B shows examples of a medium and a sever head defect produced by posterior dislocation.
4. Fracture of the posterior rim of the glenoid is uncommon.
5. Congenital or developmental defects of the glenoid fossa (excessive retrotilt or version) may occur but are unusual. Damage to the neurovascular structures is rare.
6. In patients with generalized ligament laxity, particularly in gymnasts and ballet dancers, some degree of posterior and anterior multidirectional instability is physiological

Treatment

CLOSED REDUCTION

Indications

As noted, a posterior dislocation, as with an anterior dislocation, may be traumatic, atraumatic, voluntary, or involuntary. The humeral head in a recurrent posterior atraumatic dislocation may rest on the posterior surface of the scapula. If it is a chronic unreduced dislocation, the head will be impaled or "locked" over the posterior glenoid rim. A true axillary view will demonstrate which type is present. Transient, atraumatic, or voluntary subluxations are usually easy to reduce, or may reduce spontaneously. The complete recurrent dislocation, or the impaled unreduced dislocation, may require intravenous relaxant or light anesthesia for reduction. I have found that the reduction of a posterior dislocation is a bit more difficult than an anterior dislocation. One should visualize the mechanism of the production of a posterior dislocation

c. Chronic
    d. Transient
2. Atraumatic
    a. Acute
    b. Recurrent
    c. Involuntary and multidirectional
3. Voluntary
4. Congenital, paralytic, cerebral palsy

Mechanism of Injury

A posterior dislocation is usually produced by a fall on the outstretched arm in forward flexion and internal rotation, or in adduction. It may also be produced by a direct blow to the anterior aspect of the shoulder. A third mechanism is convulsive seizures such as electric shock, or an epileptic seizure. These may be bilateral.

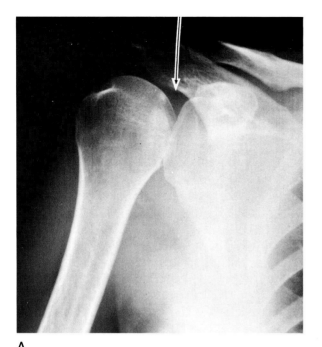

A

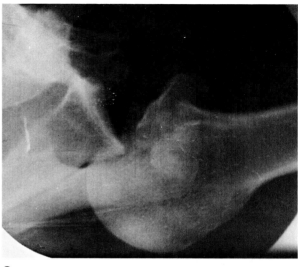

C

B

Fig. 7-88. Note the "reverse" Hill-Sachs lesion of the humeral head on the medial border of the head, typical of a posterior dislocation. (A) Moderate-size head defect (arrow). (B) Severe head defect. (C) Axillary view.

and reverse it; in other words, apply forward traction with the arm in forward flexion and internal rotation with some adduction and gently "work" the head loose from its posterior position by gradually elevating the arm. Pressure is then applied posteriorly to the head, with continued traction in elevation and internal rota-tion. This is usually successful, unless the head is too firmly locked over the posterior rim. If one or two trials do not unlock the impaled head, rather than applying more manipulative force, open reduction would be the safest method. Rockwood also stresses this point.[109]

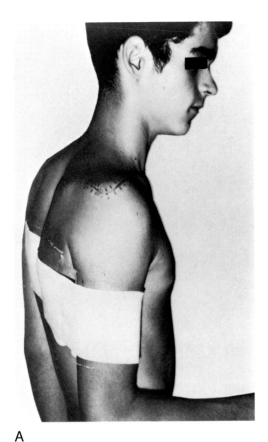

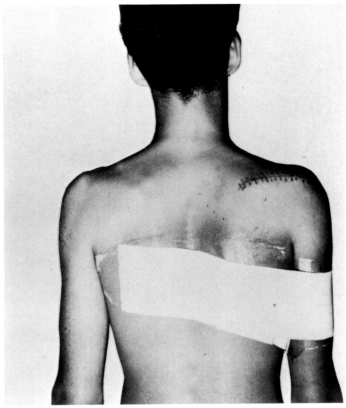

A   B

Fig. 7-89. This simple, comfortable method of support has maintained all of our posterior dislocations safely reduced following closed reduction or operative reductions. **(A)** As long as the arm does not cross the coronal plane anteriorly, the shoulder has not dislocated. The patient may flex the elbow, and move the shoulder in extension. **(B)** The elastoplast can be applied at surgery and extends across the back. This can be changed when needed. **(C)** We have found that cast immobilization or keeping the arm in internal rotation with a brace is *not* necessary. The patients are happy not to have a cast or a brace with which to contend. (See Fig. 7-75E for canvas strapping that can be worn during the day or night.) (Fig. A from Rowe CR: Chronic unreduced dislocations of the shoulder. J Bone Joint Surg 64A: 494, 1982.)

Postreduction Support

Once the dislocation is reduced, the simple, effective method of applying elastoplast around the arm and onto the back, so that the arm does not extend forward beyond the coronal plane, has proved successful (Fig. 7-89A, B). I have not found it necessary to hold the arm in external rotation, nor has it been necessary to use a plaster cast (Fig. 7-89C), splint, braces, or transfixing with pins or screws (Fig. 7-90B). With the elastoplast support, the patient is free to flex the elbow and move the arm in extension for early motion, which is so necessary for the health of the joint cartilage. We stress again that it is not necessary to immobilize the arm. As a rule, at 3 weeks the strapping can be removed and the arm allowed gradually to regain flexion, abduction, and rotation. A stock restrainer for sleeping may be used for 3 weeks. After an initial or recurrent dislocation or subluxation, the patient should be put on a program of specific resistive exercises with emphasis on external rotation to strengthen the infraspinatus, teres minor, and capsule. The patient should avoid forward flexion

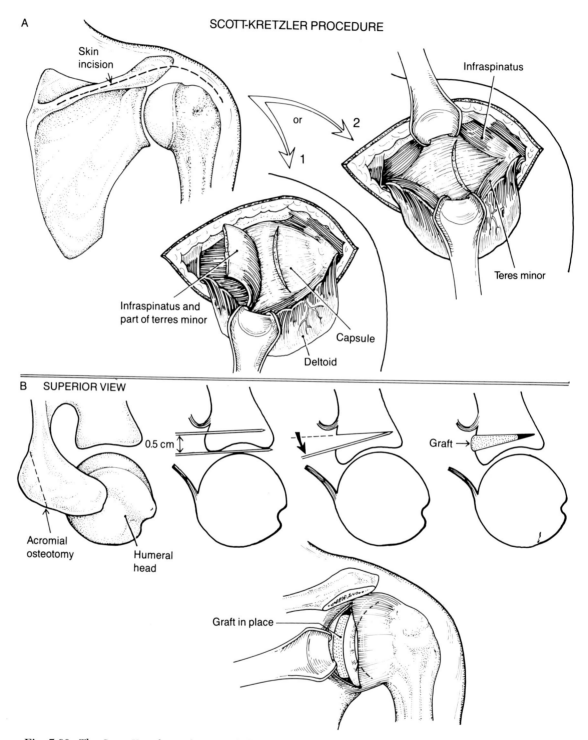

Fig. 7-90. The Scott-Kretzler technique of glenoid osteotomy. **(A)** The surgical approach. (1) Entering the joint by separating the infraspinatus from the capsule, or, (2) by splitting the interval between the infraspinatus and teres minor. **(B)** It is important to have a humeral head retractor in the joint. The osteotomy is made 0.5 cm from the rim of the glenoid. Avoid entering the joint.

and internal rotation of the arm or adduction across the body until the arm has regained stabilizing strength, and there is no apprehension on motion, which usually takes 6 weeks. Exercises are especially effective with the voluntary and multidirectional types of instabilities.

SURGICAL

Recurrent Posterior Dislocations

It is most important, before deciding upon surgery, to identify clearly the type of recurrent dislocation the patient has. If it is a true traumatic recurrent dislocation, or an atraumatic type, in which there is no evidence of voluntary dislocation, the prognosis for surgical treatment is favorable. If the voluntary type has caused stretching of the posterior capsule to a degree that the shoulder slips out involuntarily and the patient is cooperative, with no emotional or psychiatric problems, the prognosis should be good with surgery. However, one should *avoid* surgery on uncooperative patients with personality or emotional problems, since they are apt to destroy any type of reconstructive procedure carried out on their shoulder.[122]

There are a number of surgical approaches and techniques for recurrent posterior dislocations.

Posterior Deltoid Turned-Down Approach (**Fig. 7-90**). The skin incision extends along the spine of the scapula, curving down over the junction of the mid and posterior deltoid.

The deltoid with its osteoperiosteal attachment is separated by sharp dissection from the spine of the scapula. Care must be taken to avoid incising the infraspinatus muscle, which lies immediately below the deltoid insertion. The deltoid is split for a distance of 5 to 8 cm in line of its fibers over its posterior extent and over its lateral insertions, to allow the muscle to be turned down.

This gives excellent exposure to the infraspinatus and teres minor muscles.

Once the deltoid has been retracted, two approaches may be used to expose the capsule. The capsule may be reached by separating the interval between the infraspinatus and teres minor muscles. The suprascapular nerve must be kept in mind, as it enters the infraspinatus muscle parallel to the suprascapular notch superiorly. The second approach

is by removing the infraspinatus and teres minor muscles from the posterior capsule by sharp dissection, similarly to removing the subscapularis from the anterior capsule. A portion of the teres minor insertion should be left intact, to protect the axillary nerve that exits from the quadrilateral space. My preference is to remove the infraspinatus and a portion of the teres minor from the capsule rather than splitting the interval between the infraspinatus and teres minor. The former gives a better exposure of the capsule and the suprascapular nerve is protected by turning it back with the muscle. The infraspinatus can also be advanced as needed in closure. The capsule is opened vertically 0.5 cm lateral to the posterior glenoid rim. A humeral head retractor is inserted to expose the glenoid fossa.

Rockwood Posterior Shoulder Approach[109] (*see Chap. 3*). This approach has the advantage of relatively little blood loss, although it gives a smaller exposure. I have not used this approach, but it does have its appealing application. I would, however, advise the uninitiated surgeon first to try this on a fresh cadaver due to this approach's more limited space than the turn-down deltoid approach.

"Utility" Approach. The reader is referred to the section on chronic unreduced shoulder dislocations and Chapter 3. Greater exposure is needed for the chronic unreduced dislocation than for the fresh or recurrent posterior dislocations, due to scar tissue, displaced nerve and vascular supply, and for protection of the humeral head in freeing it from the glenoid rim.

McLaughlin recommended an anterior approach.[82] Rockwood uses his posterior approach.[115] In chronic dislocations, we prefer the "utility" approach, which gives excellent exposure of the humeral head and the joint[119] anteriorly, laterally, and posteriorly. This is necessary to avoid further injury to the humeral head.

Soft Tissue Procedures. Posterior Bankart or Putti-Platt procedures are not as stable or supportive as they are anteriorly. This is due to the fact that the posterior capsule and muscle are not as strong as the anterior capsule, with its reinforcing capsular ligaments and the subscapularis muscle. Tibone[139] reported 30 percent failures in 10 patients in whom posterior staple capsulorrhaphies were used. Neer

BOYD PROCEDURE

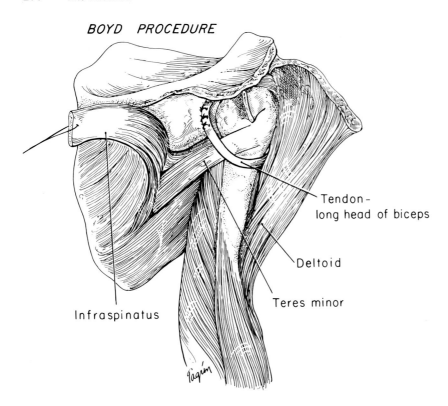

Tendon - long head of biceps

Deltoid

Teres minor

Infraspinatus

Fig. 7-91. The Boyd technique of transplanting the long head of biceps tendon posteriorly. (Boyd HB, Anderson LD: A method for reinsertion of the distal biceps brachii tendon. J Bone Joint Surg 43A:1041, 1961.)

in 1980 reported satisfactory results using his inferior capsular shift technique posteriorly, which is similar to his anterior capsular shift, principally for involuntary recurrent dislocations.[97]

Boyd[20] in 1972 reported an unusual technique of transplanting the tendon of the long head of biceps around the neck of the humerus to the posterior glenoid rim (Fig. 7-91), thus supporting the posterior structures. This procedure has worked very effectively; however, it is an extensive surgical procedure requiring an anterior and posterior exposure of the glenohumeral joint. Also, we do not favor removing the tendon of the long head of biceps when other techniques are available.

Scott[131] or Kretzler[70] Procedure (Fig. 7-90). This technique, although demanding, has proved to be the most effective and reliable for me. The deltoid is turned down from the spine of the scapula and the infraspinatus is separated from the posterior capsule, as recommended by Scott, and turned back, protecting the suprascapular nerve (Fig. 7-90). Kretzler exposes the capsule by retracting the infraspinatus upward. We use the curvature of the posterior acro-

mion as our bone graft. Rockwood[115] prefers to take the graft horizontally from the posterior acromion. If the capsule has been avulsed from the posterior glenoid rim, the osteotomy is made intrascapular. If the capsule is not separated from the rim, the osteotomy is made extracapsular if the capsule cannot be separated from the neck. Adequate exposure is necessary. Complications arise when exposure is poor. The use of the humeral head retractor is mandatory, so that there is complete exposure of the glenoid fossa.

The osteotome should enter the neck 0.5 cm from the articular surface, in the same plane as the joint surface to avoid entering the fossa. It is helpful to leave the upper edge of the osteotome exposed to aid in the direction and depth of the blade. The osteotome blade should be tapped carefully approximately four-fifths of the way across the neck, which is then gently pried open. If the blade is not far enough across the neck, the glenoid may fracture when pried. If the blade goes too far, the glenoid may be unstable, therefore an experienced touch is necessary. The graft is taken from the posterior angle of the acromion and should be prismatic in shape: thicker at the base than the leading edge. It should be carefully fashioned

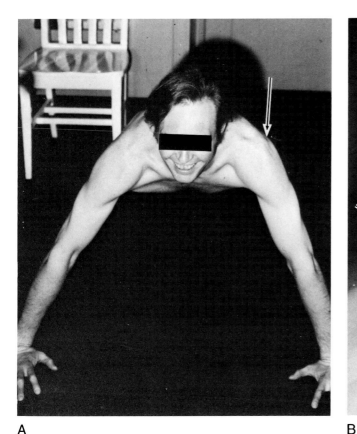

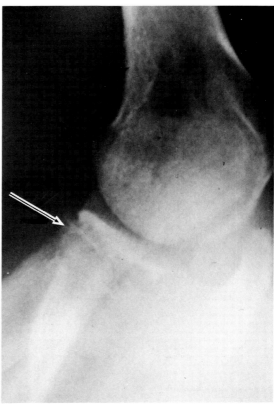

A   B

Fig. 7-92. Patient 1½ years after Scott osteotomy of glenoid neck for recurrent posterior dislocation of the left shoulder. The patient has no recurrences, does heavy work and push-ups, and is very happy with the results. **(A)** Push-ups. (Arrow indicates operated side.) **(B)** Viable bone graft (indicated by arrow).

and thinned down to fit snugly into the opening. It should not exceed 0.5 cm in width at its base. We have not found it necessary to secure the graft with screws or staples.

We have used the Scott-Kretzler technique in five patients, two with excellent and three with good results (Fig. 7-92). We have not had the complications from this procedure as reported by others, of 7 recurrences in 17 patients and complications of degenerative arthritis, muscle contracture, and osteonecrosis,[54] or of postoperative coracoid impingement. It is easy to understand how these complications could occur if the graft is too thick, or the osteotomy does not extend beyond the midline of the glenoid width, which would naturally displace the head anteriorly against the coracoid. We have had no recurrences, no degenerative joint changes, and no coracoid im-

pingement following surgery. English[43] reported good results using the Scott-Kretzler osteotomy in five patients, as did Hernandez and Drez.[57] Bestard reported 12 posterior glenoplasties in 1986[13] using the Scott-Kretzler technique with good results. They stress attention to technique. We emphasize again that the Scott-Kretzler technique requires precise attention to detail, the use of the humeral head retractor, and adequate exposure.

One should keep in mind the suprascapular nerve as it exits through the suprascapular notch into the infraspinatus muscle. The nerve is more apt to be compromised if the muscle is split. Also, the capsule should not be closed too tightly or internal rotation of the shoulder may be limited. The infraspinatus muscle is reattached to its original insertion. The deltoid is then reattached to its osteoperiosteal and muscular origins. If you are in doubt, a few drill holes may be made through the spine of the scapula for more secure fixation, although we have not found this necessary. Only when the deltoid is turned down from the lateral border of the acromion, where the central tendon inserts, does one have to osteotomize the rim of the acromion and leave the deltoid muscle attached.

The reverse Hybbinette-Eden onlay graft technique is an alternative to the Scott-Kretzler glenoplasty. This has not been as dependable for me as the Scott-Kretzler procedure, especially when a large Bankart lesion is not present. In this case, it is difficult to develop a solid bony bed for the onlay graft. With the glenoplasty, the graft is inserted securely into the neck of the glenoid. However, Mowery et al., in a recent publication,[93] reported favorably on five patients treated with an onlay iliac graft 2 × 3 cm placed 1.5 to 2.0 cm lateral to the glenoid rim. If a Bankart lesion is not present, they separate the capsule from the neck of the glenoid with a periosteal elevator, applying the graft to the neck of the glenoid and stabilizing it with one lag screw. The capsule is closed over the graft. A cast is applied for 6 weeks. One shoulder was complicated by an anterior dislocation; the other four patients returned to unrestricted activities and recreational sports. The authors do express a concern about late osteoarthritic changes of the joint.

See the previous sections for discussion of surgical treatment of chronic (unreduced) posterior dislocations.

TREATMENT OF FAILED SURGERY FOR RECURRENT ANTERIOR DISLOCATION

Much has been written about initial surgical procedures for recurrent anterior dislocations of the shoulder, but very little has been written about the causes of failure of primary repair. A number of questions have arisen: What were the specific cause of failure of the initial surgery? What additional procedures could be used to restore the shoulder's stability? What are the chances of success if a second procedure is performed?

Since 1962, we have treated 45 patients whose shoulder dislocation recurred after primary surgery; 39 were reported in 1984[126] and 6 since then. These were patients whose dislocations recurred but whose joints were not destroyed, which would require a joint replacement or arthrodesis. Studying this section very carefully will help us to analyze the causes of failure and determine what can be done to restore stability to the shoulder after previous failed surgery. We recommend also that the reader review the reports by Norris and Bigliani,[103] Zuckerman and Matsen,[149] and Rockwood.[114]

History

When a patient is seen for a failed surgical procedure, it is most important to document all events relative to the dislocation. First, carefully determine the specific type of initial dislocation. Was it traumatic, atraumatic, voluntary, or involuntary recurrent? By determining the specific type, the surgeon will get a lead as to whether the patient should have been treated initially by exercises or by surgery. We have found this most important, because a number of failed surgical procedures were performed on patient who would have responded to specific resistive exercises (atraumatic type) or in whom surgery was contraindicated (voluntary type).

If the initial dislocation was traumatic, with radiographic evidence of a Hill-Sachs lesion, one would expect definite traumatic lesions to be corrected. If the initial dislocation was the result of the functional use of the arm, or an atraumatic experience, or was produced by muscle action (voluntary dislocation), one would suspect the cause to be increased laxity of the supporting soft tissues with a redundant capsule, with or without unidirectional or multidirectional instabilities. If the recurrence was the result of a forceful hyperextension of the arm, or a direct blow, more extensive damage to the capsule, muscle, and bone can be expected. The type of previous treatment the patient received is also important. A copy of the previous operative report and radiograms is needed. Did reduction occur easily or with difficulty? If recurrences had occurred with little trauma, and reduction was spontaneous or self-reduced, the patient might respond to a schedule of specific resistive exercises instead of surgery.

Physical Examination

It is important to note the physical type of the patient, particularly whether the patient has generalized ligament laxity of the joints. The patient should also be checked carefully for motor or sensory nerve deficits, muscle atrophy, weakness, or bony abnormalities. The radial pulse is checked in different positions of elevation and extension of the arm. It is helpful to have the patient demonstrate the position of the extremity that he or she avoids for fear that the shoulder may "slip out." The "apprehension" test is an excellent maneuver to indicate whether there is recurrent weakness of the anterior capsule mechanism.

Diagnostic Aids

Careful radiologic examination is most important to identify bone or joint injury or the presence of metal implants. Anterior–posterior views in neutral, in 60° of internal rotation, and 60° of external rotation, plus a true axillary view, should be taken to outline the anterior glenoid rim or the position or displacement of metal implants. When indicated, other diagnostic procedures such as arthroscopy, arthrotomograms, apical oblique views, or CAT scans are used.

Pathologic Findings: Causes of Failure

The causes of failure of previous surgery are listed in Table 7-7. In our 1984 study[126] and our experience

Table 7-7. Pathologic Findings: Causes of Failure of 38 Previous Operations

	N	%
Unrepaired initial Bankart lesions	17 (45%)	
		74%
Recurred Bankart lesions	11 (29%)	
Excessive laxity of capsule	24	63
Primary cause of recurrence—5		
Hill-Sachs lesions	21	55
Primary cause of recurrence—2		
Excessive *scarring* of subscapularis muscle	7	18
Metal failure	5	13
3 duToit procedures		
2 Bristow procedures		

since then, in 38 failed shoulders there were 17 Bankart lesions not corrected at the time of initial surgery (45 percent) and 11 Bankart lesions that were repaired but recurred (29 percent) or a total of 74 percent. This was comparable to the incidence of Bankart lesions (85 percent) for primary surgery in a study reported in 1978.[121] Excessive laxity of the capsule was found in four shoulders and considered the primary cause of recurrence in two. Metal failures occurred in 13 percent of the failed procedures. Norris found unrepaired Bankart lesions in 35 percent of his reoperations.[103]

Treatment

CLOSED

Seven (16 percent) of the 45 patients responded to a program of specific resistive exercises in abduction, external rotation, and internal rotation. For best results, the exercises (as outlined previously) should be carried out with the arm at the side of the body to eliminate the action of the pectoral muscles. We found that routine shoulder exercises including the scapulothoracic and thoracohumeral muscles were not effective in increasing the stability of the shoulder joint per se. Whether or not the program of resistive exercises eliminates the shoulder instability, the shoulders will benefit from a trial of resistive exercises.

OPERATIVE

Thirty-eight shoulders were reoperated upon. Of these, 31 had experienced 1 previous failed procedure, five had undergone 2 previous unsuccessful procedures, and 2 had had 3 previous failed procedures. The same surgical principles apply to reoperation as primary procedures:

Layer-by-layer exploration
Identification of the causative pathologic lesions
Correction of the lesion

Previous surgery presented a number of problems one should be prepared to meet:

Prior skin incisions
Altered anatomy

Scarring of the subcapularis muscle and capsule

Restricted joint motion due to postoperative scar tissue and adhesions

Articular damage

Failed metal, such as staples, screws, or pins that may have loosened, broken, or become displaced

An apprehensive, and at times, depressed, patient

FINDINGS FROM PREVIOUS SURGICAL PROCEDURES

The condition of tissues found at secondary surgery varied according to the method of repair performed initially. Of the failed procedures, the procedures that we found disturbed the subscapularis muscle and capsule the least, were the Magnuson-Stack and Nicola procedures. Although the subscapularis muscle had been transplanted in the five failed Magnuson-Stack procedures, there was very little scarring of the muscle or capsule (see Fig. 7-101). The muscle could be easily turned back and the Bankart lesion repaired. In the three Nicola procedures the subcapularis muscle had not been disturbed. The pathologic lesions were easily corrected in each group.

Of the 13 failed Bankart procedures, the subscapularis muscle and capsule were unscarred in 2, only mild scarring was present in 8, and moderate scarring

in 3. It was significant that in all 13 the subscapularis muscle could be carefully separated from the underlying capsule (so important in reconstructive procedures). The primary cause of failure of the previous procedures was recurrence or unrepaired Bankart lesions in nine, severe laxity of the capsule in three, and a severe Hill-Sachs lesion of the humeral head in one.

In the nine Putti-Platt procedures, the subscapular muscle and capsule did not fare quite as well, since the muscle was scarred severely in three, moderately in four, and mildly in two. However, it was possible to separate the muscle from the capsule in all nine patients. The primary cause of failure was eight unrepaired Bankart lesions and one severe Hill-Sachs lesion.

Of the four failed duToit procedures, recurrence of Bankart lesions was present in two (one of these with a severe Hill-Sachs lesion) (Fig. 7-93), and loosening of the staples in three (Fig. 7-94). The staple was found in the joint in one shoulder and severe degenerative joint disease in two shoulders (Fig. 7-95). The subscapularis muscle was preserved and could be separated from the capsule in all four shoulders.

The four failed Bristow procedures, however, had severe scarring of the subscapularis muscle and cap-

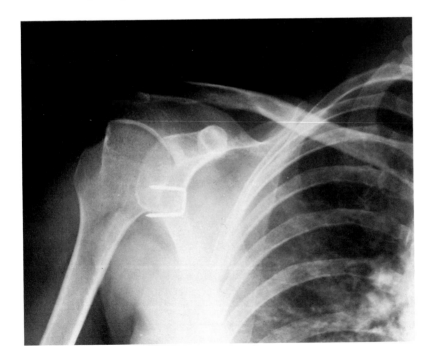

Fig. 7-93. A failed duToit procedure with a severe Hill-Sachs lesion and a loose staple.

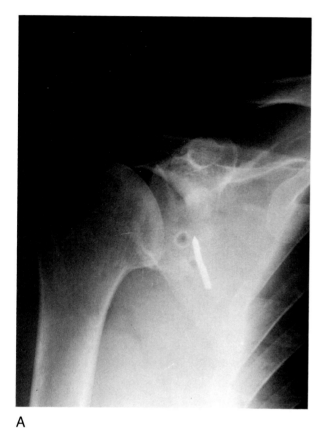

A

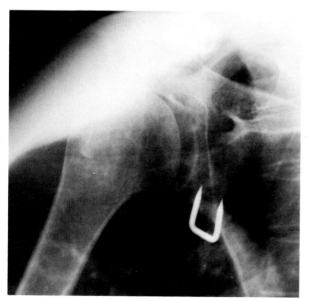

B

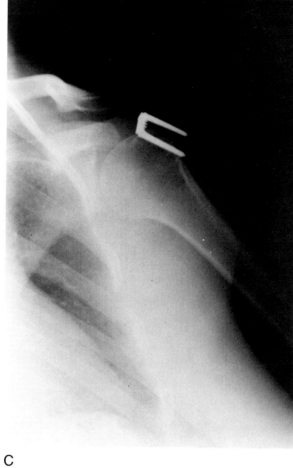

C

Fig. 7-94. (**A**) An example of an avulsed staple as the result of an automobile accident. (**B**) Another loose staple was the result of heavy lifting. At surgery, it was found adjacent to the axillary artery. (**C**) Once metal loosens about the shoulder, it tends to travel. (Figs. A and B from Rowe CR, Zarins B, Ciulli JV: Recurrent anterior dislocation of the shoulder after surgical repair. Apparent causes of failure and treatment. J Bone Joint Surg 66A:166, 1984.)

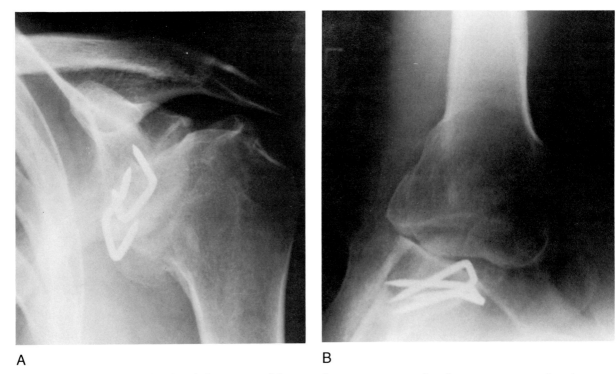

A   B

Fig. 7-95. An example of total destruction of the joint from impinging staples. It was necessary to insert a replacement prosthesis. **(A)** AP view. **(B)** Axillary view.

sule in all four shoulders, due to the transplanted coracoid tendon through the subscapularis muscle. The subscapularis muscle plane was destroyed in all four shoulders. This complicated efforts to separate the subscapularis muscle from the scarred capsule and to restore stability to the joint. The coracoid transplant was too high in three (above the "equator") (Fig. 7-96), not united in two (Fig. 7-97), with one loose screw and one broken screw (Fig. 7-98). It was interesting that unrepaired Bankart lesions were present in all four shoulders. Consequently, the causes of failure in the Bristow procedures were multiple: unrepaired Bankart lesions, failed metal, nonunion of the coracoid, and severe scarring of the subscapularis muscle and capsule. Norris[103] reports that 18 of 20 failed Bristow procedures in his series had symptomatic nonunion of the coracoid transplant, 8 had unrepaired Bankart lesions, and 6 had developed degenerative arthritis.

Zuckerman and Matson[149] report 37 patients with complications due to implants (screws and staples).

Forty-one percent had sustained significant injury to the articular surface of the glenoid or humerus. They noted that "the results in this group of patients indicated that screws and staples can produce complications that require re-operations." Twenty-one had had Bristow procedures, 10 had had duToit procedures, and 4 had had Magnuson procedures. In one Bristow procedure the loose screw had eroded the axillary artery, necessitating vascular reconstruction. Rockwood concluded from his study "for that reason I prefer to perform reconstructions without the use of metal—especially staples."[114] Although we see many complications, we must remember there are many surgeons with few complications.

SURGICAL TREATMENT USED AT REOPERATION

Although we have seen many complications of surgical procedures for recurrent dislocation of the shoulder, this report concerns only the failed procedures

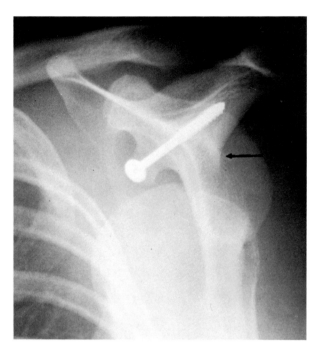

Fig. 7-96. The transplant in the patient was "above the equator" of the glenoid, and too high to prevent dislocation.

in which joints were not destroyed and had a chance to be helped by reoperation. Patients whose joints came to arthrodesis, joint replacement, or were septic were omitted. These complications are reviewed in another category.[114]

Of the surgical procedures used in reoperation on the 38 failed cases, the Bankart procedure was used when the subscapularis muscle could be separated from the capsule. This was possible in 30 shoulders (79 percent). Four Putti-Platt procedures were carried out when the subscapularis could not be separated from the capsule. Modified capsulorrhaphy was carried out in four shoulders with severe laxity of the capsule and in which a Bankart lesion was absent.

OPERATIVE TECHNIQUES

When it is possible to separate the subscapularis muscle from the joint capsule we would recommend the following:

1. A standard Bankart procedure when a Bankart lesion is present, as in the patient with a failed Magnuson procedure in Figure 7-99.
2. If no Bankart lesion is present, a modified capsulorrhaphy is recommended. Norris[103] and Rockwood[114] recommend the capsular shift procedure

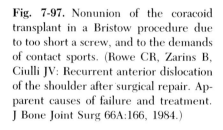

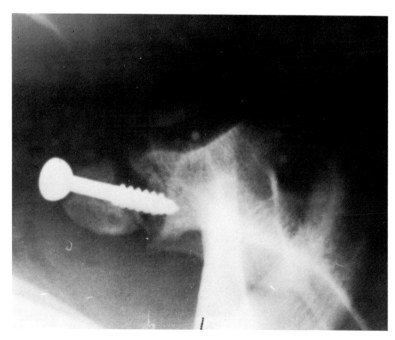

Fig. 7-97. Nonunion of the coracoid transplant in a Bristow procedure due to too short a screw, and to the demands of contact sports. (Rowe CR, Zarins B, Ciulli JV: Recurrent anterior dislocation of the shoulder after surgical repair. Apparent causes of failure and treatment. J Bone Joint Surg 66A:166, 1984.)

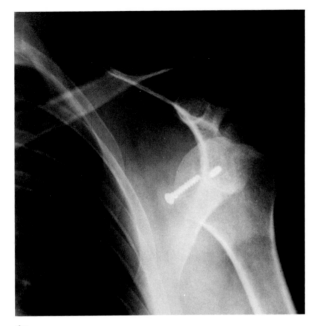

A.

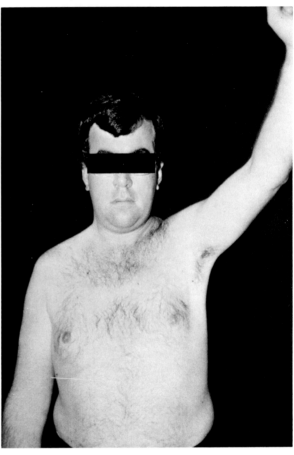

B

Fig. 7-98. (A) Radiograph of a 29-year-old man who had undergone the following procedures: 1977: A Putti-Platt procedure, left shoulder, was performed (recurred). 1982: Bristow procedure carried out. Recurred with broken screw and nonunion of coracoid. 1984: Exploration of shoulder, removal of screw. Large Bankart lesion, repaired with Bankart procedure. (B) Patient has a stable, strong shoulder, with no recurrence and no pain following reoperation.

but caution that, with the scar tissue from previous surgery, it may tighten the capsule too much.

If the subscapularis muscle and capsule are severely scarred and cannot be separated, a modified Putti-Platt procedure is recommended. The double layers should be breasted, as outlined previously. In some instances, some of the layers could be reattached to the glenoid rim.

In the failed Bristow procedures, we have not attempted to reattach the coracoid back to its original base because of scar tissue. Rather than attempt to screw the nonunion to the neck of the glenoid again, we leave the transplant in situ and repair the capsule to the rim of the glenoid throughout the extent of its avulsion. When possible, the transplanted tendons

were reattached to surrounding muscle and tendon tissue.

Unusual problems may be encountered. Two patients, each of whom had undergone two unsuccessful procedures, and had severe Hill-Sachs lesions, were reoperated upon. Both patients were so apprehensive when examined that they were too fearful to elevate their arm beyond the level of the shoulder. One of the patients strapped her shoulder to her side when she went to bed for fear of dislocating it during her sleep (Fig. 7-100). Each patient responded successfully to a combination of an anterior Bankart repair plus a Connolly procedure[30] (transplantation of the infraspinatus muscle into the Hill-Sachs lesion) through a second superior incision. This changed the Hill-Sachs lesion from an intraarticular to an extraar-

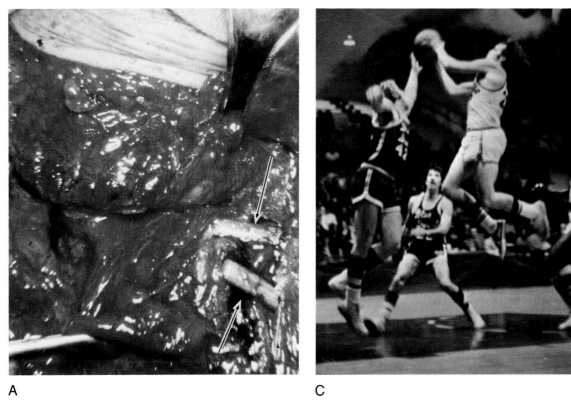

A

C

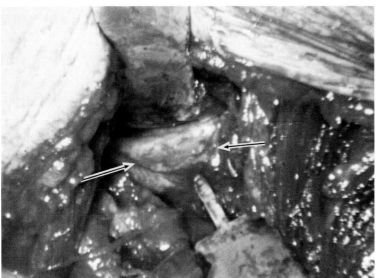

B

Fig. 7-99. A recurrent Magnuson procedure in a promising basketball player. (**A**) View of the transplanted subscapularis muscle to the humerus and loose staples. The staples were removed (see arrows) and the subscapularis turned up. (**B**) A large Bankart lesion was present (arrows). (**C**) Patient (the player with the ball) has returned to basketball at New England College. (Fig. C from Rowe CR, Patel D, Southmayd WW: The Bankart procedure. A long-term end-result study. J Bone Joint Surg 60A:13, 1978.)

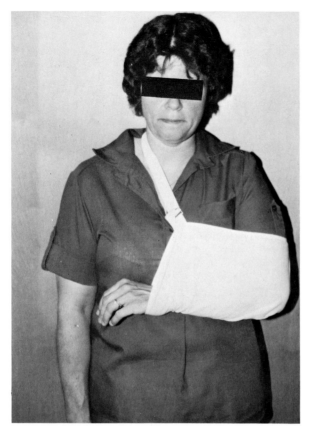

A

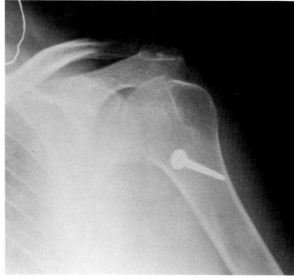

B

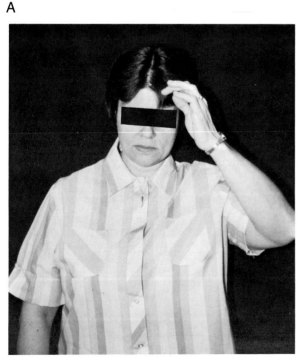

C

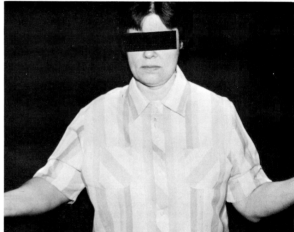

D

Fig. 7-100. A 37-year-old woman with a severe Hill-Sachs lesion underwent the following surgical procedures. 1980: Magnuson procedure on left shoulder (recurred). 1981: Removal of nail. 1982: Putti-Platt procedure. (recurred). **(A)** On examination, her shoulder was so unstable she did not wish to release her arm. She strapped her arm to her body at night. **(B)** Radiograph shows a severe Hill-Sachs lesion. Exploration of her shoulder in 1984: (1) Anterior exploration, with repair of large Bankart lesion and severe adhesions (2) plus a superior incision, with transplantation of infraspinatus to the Hill-Sachs lesion (Connolly procedure). **(C,D)** She now has a stable shoulder and useful arm although limited elevation. She is happy and back at work. Her pain and instability have been relieved.

Table 7-8. Results of 30 Reoperations

Findings	N	%
Excellent	10	(33)
Good	18	(60)
Fair	0	
Poor	2	(7)

Recurrence of instability following surgery

Subluxation	1
Dislocation	1

Seven treated by exercises

Excellent	1
Good	4
Fair	1
Poor	1

ticular lesion. We agree with Connolly that the Bankart lesion should be repaired when possible and the infraspinatus muscle transferred. This combination is highly recommended for the patient whose routine procedure has failed and in whom a severe Hill-Sachs lesion is present in the humeral head. An alternative procedure would be the Weber technique,[144] in which the humeral head is rotated, displacing the Hill-Sachs lesion away from the glenoid rim, by a proximal humeral osteotomy, or an anterior bone block procedure using the Hybbinette-Eden technique.

Results

Our results (Table 7-8) were evaluated on a 100-point scoring system, in which 50 points are assigned for stability, 30 points to function, and 20 to motion. The results of reoperation on 30 shoulders whose joints had not been destroyed by previous surgery have been *surprisingly good*. These patients were evaluated for an average of 4 years (from 2 to 10 years). Ten patients (33 percent) were graded excellent, 18 patients (60 percent) were rated good, and 2 (7 percent) poor. Recurrence following reoperation was 7 percent (one subluxation and one dislocation). Thus, 93 percent were excellent and good. This encouraging result was consistent with Norris's results in 1985 of 81 percent good and excellent results in 51 evaluated reoperations.[30] Of the seven patients treated by specific resistive exercises, one result was excellent, four were good, one was fair, and one was poor.

REFERENCES

1. Adams JC: Recurrent dislocation of the shoulder. J Bone Joint Surg 30B:26, 1948
2. Allman FL: Report of more than 300 Bristow procedures in athletes for recurrent dislocation/subluxation of the shoulder. J Bone Joint Surg 33A:261, 1978
3. Anderson D Zvirbulis R, Ciullo J: Scapular manipulation for reducation of anterior shoulder dislocations. Clin Orthop Rel Res 181, April 1962
4. Auger B: Traite' Incanographique des Maladies Chirurgicales, Bailliere, Paris, 1865
5. Aronen JG: Decreasing the incidence of recurrence of first time anterior shoulder dislocations with rehabilitation. Read at the American Shoulder and Elbow Surgeons, Fourth Annual Meeting, Las Vegas, Nevada, January 23, 1985
6. Artz T, Huffer JM: A major complication of the modified Bristow procedure for recurrent dislocation of the shoulder. J Bone Joint Surg 54A:1293, 1972
7. Badgley CE, O'Connor GA: A combined procedure for repair of recurrent anterior dislocations of the shoulder. J Bone Joint Surg 47A:1283, 1965
8. Bailey RW: Acute and recurrent dislocations of the shoulder. J Bone Joint Surg 49A:767, 1967
9. Bankart ASB: Recurrent or habitual dislocation of the shoulder. Br Med J 2:1132, 1923
10. Bankart ASB: The pathology and treatment of the recurrent dislocations of the shoulder joint. Br J Surg 23, 1938
11. Bateman JE: The Shoulder and Neck, 2nd Ed. W.B. Saunders, Philadelphia, 1978
12. Bennett GE: Old dislocations of the shoulder. J Bone Joint Surg 18:594, 1936
13. Bestard EA, Schoene HR, Bestard EH: Glenoplasty in management of recurrent shoulder dislocations. Contemp Orthop 12:47, 1986
14. Blazina ME, Satzman JS: Recurrent anterior subluxation of the shoulder in athletes—a distinct entity. Proceedings of the American Academy of Orthopaedic Surgeons. J Bone Joint Surg 51A:1037, 1969
15. Blom S, Dahback LD: Nerve injuries in dislocations of the shoulder joint. Acta Chir Scand 136:461, 1970
16. Bonnin JG: Transplantation of the coracoid tip: a definitive operation for recurrent anterior dislocation of the shoulder. Proc R Soc Med 66:755, 1973
17. Bosley RC, Miles JS: Scapular manipulation for reduction of anterior inferior shoulder dislocations. Read at Annual Meeting of American Academy of Orthopaedic Surgeons, San Francisco, CA, February 24, 1979
18. Bost FE, Inman VT: The pathological changes in recurrent dislocation of the shoulder. J Bone Joint Surg 24:595, 1942

19. Boyd HB, Hunt HO: Recurrent dislocations of the shoulder. The staple capsulorrhaphy. J Bone Joint Surg 47A:1514, 1965

20. Boyd HB, Sisk TD: Recurrent posterior dislocation of the shoulder: J Bone Joint Surg 54A:779, 1972

21. Bracker MD: New treatment for dislocated shoulders. Phys Sports Med 12:155, 1984

22. Braly WG, Tullos HS: A modification of the Bristow procedure for recurrent anterior shoulder dislocations and subluxations. AM J Sports Med 13:81, 1985

23. Broca A, Hartman H: Contribution a l'étude des luxations de l'épaule. Bull Soc Anat 4:416, 1890

24. Brockbank W, Griffith D: Orthopaedic surgery in the sixteenth and seventeenth centuries, luxations of the shoulder. J Bone Joint Surg 30B:365, 1948

25. Caird FM: The shoulder joint in relation to certain dislocations and fractures. Edinburgh Med J 32:708, 1887

26. Caspari R: Fascial repair of recurrent anterior dislocation of the shoulder. Read at the Annual Meeting of the Arthroscopy Association of North America, Boston, April 13, 1985

27. Codman EA: The Shoulder. T. Todd, Boston, 1934 Reprinted, Robert E. Kreiger Publishing, Malabar, Florida, 1984

28. Codman EA: Anatomy of the subdeltoid bursa and its clinical importance. Boston Med Surg J 613:22, 1906

28a. Cofield RH, Kavanagh BF, Frassica FJ: Anterior shoulder instability. Instructional Course Lectures 210–227. CV Mosby, St. Louis, 1985

29. Conforti B: Boytchev's procedure for recurrent dislocation of the shoulder. J Bone Joint Surg 56:386, 1974 Conforti B: The results of Boytchev procedure for treatment of recurrent dislocation of the shoulder. Int Orthop 4:127, 1980

30. Connolly JF: Humeral head defects associated with shoulder dislocations. Their diagnostic and surgical significance. p. 42. In Instructional Course Lectures. The American Academy of Orthopaedic Surgeons. C.V. Mosby, St. Louis, 1972

31. Cooper A: A Treatise on Dislocations and Fractures of Joints. Carey & Lea, Philadelphia, 1825

32. Cubbins WR, Callahan JJ, Scuderi CS: The reduction of old or irreducible dislocations of the shoulder joint. Surg Gynecol Obstet 58:129, 1934

33. D'Angelo D: Lussazione voluntaria della spalla. Arch Putti 17:142, 1962

34. Danzl DF, Vicario SJ, Gleis GL: Reduction of anterior subcoracoid shoulder dislocation. Clin Orthop 1985

35. DeAnquin CE: Recurrent dislocation of the shoulder: roentgenographic study. Proceedings of the American Academy of Orthopaedic Surgeons. J Bone Joint Surg 47A:1085, 1965

36. DeAnquin CE: Comparative study of bone lesions in traumatic recurrent dislocation of the shoulder. p. 303. In: Surgery of the Shoulder. BC Decker, Toronto, 1984

37. Debevoise NT, Hyatt GW: Humeral torsion in recurrent shoulder dislocation. Clin Orthop 76:87, 1971

38. DePalma AF: Factors influencing the choice of a modified Magnuson procedure for recurrent anterior dislocation of the shoulder. Surg Clin North Am 43:1647, 1963

39. DePalma AF: Surgery of the Shoulder, 2nd Ed. J.B. Lippincott, Philadelphia, 1978

40. duToit GT, Roux D: Recurrent dislocation of the shoulder. Johannesburg stapling operation. J Bone Joint Surg 37A:633, 1965

41. Eden R: Zur operation behandlung der habituellen schulterluxation. Zentralbl Chir 47:1002. 1920

42. Ellison AE: Inside-out Bankart procedure. Read at the Meeting of the American Orthopaedic Association, Hot Springs, Virginia, June 1986

43. English E, MacNab I: Recurrent posterior dislocations of the shoulder. Can J Surg 17:147, 1974

44. Eyre-Brook AL: Recurrent dislocation of the shoulder. Lesions discovered in seventeen cases, surgery employed, and immediate report of results. J Bone Joint Surg 30B:39, 1948

45. Fahey JJ, DeCosola M: Pathology of the Shoulder After Experimental Dislocation at Autopsy. AAOS Scientific Exhibit, Chicago 1947. Cited in ref. 92.

46. Flower WH: On the pathological changes produced in the shoulder joint by traumatic dislocation. Trans Pathol Soc London 12:179, 1961

47. Foster WS, Ford TB, Drez D: Isolated posterior shoulder dislocations in a child. Am J Sports Med 13:198, 1985

48. Franklin TH: Injury to the musculocutaneous nerve as a complication of operations for recurrent dislocations of the shoulder. J Bone Joint Surg 66B:449, 1984

49. Fried A: Habitual posterior dislocation of the shoulder joint. A report on five operated cases. Acta Orthop Scand 18:329, 1949

50. Gallie WE, LeMesurier AB: Recurring dislocation of the shoulder. J Bone Joint Surg 30B:9, 1948

51. Genovesi A: Contributo alla conoscenza della Lussazione Volontaria della spalla. Arch Putti 17:268, 1962

52. Gerber C, Ganz R: Clinical assessment of instability of the shoulder. J Bone Joint Surg 66B:551, 1984

53. Gitlin G, Schwartz A, Welner A: Voluntary bilateral posterior dislocation of the shoulder joint. Am J Surg 97:777, 1959

54. Hawkins RJ, Neer CS: Missed posterior dislocations of the shoulder. p. 848. In Bateman, Welsh (eds); Surgery of the Shoulder. J.B. Lippincott, Philadelphia, 1975

55. Helfet AJ: Caracoid transplantation for recurring dislocation of the shoulder. The Rowley Bristow operation. J Bone Joint Surg 40B:198, 1958

56. Henry JH, Genung JA: Natural history of glenohumeral dislocation, revisited. Am J Sports Med 10:135, 1982

57. Hernandez A, Drez D: Operative treatment of posterior shoulder dislocations by posterior glenoplasty. Read at meeting of the Am Orthopaedic Society for Sports Medicine, February 1986, New Orleans

58. Hill SA, Sachs MD: The grooved defect of the humeral head. A frequently unrecognized complication of dislocation of the shoulder joint. Radiology 35:690, 1940

59. Hill JA, Lombardo SJ, Kerlan RK et al: The modified Bristow-Helfet procedure for recurrent anterior subluxation and dislocation. Am J Sports Med 9:283, 1981

60. Hindmarsh J, Lindberg A: Eden-Hybbinette's operation for recurrent dislocation of the humero-scapular joint. Acta Orthop Scand 38:459, 1967

61. Hippocrates: The Genuine Works of Hippocrates. Translated by Adams F. Williams & Wilkins, Baltimore, 1946

62. Hovelius L: Anterior dislocation of the shoulder. A clinical study on incidence, prognosis and operative treatment of the Bristow-Laterjet procedure. Linkoping University Medical Dissertation, 1982

63. Howarth MB: General subluxation of the ligaments with special reference to the knee and shoulder. Clin Orthop 30:133, 1963

64. Hussein MK: Kocher's method is 3,000 years old. J Bone Joint Surg 50B:669, 1968

65. Hybbinette S: Transplantation d'un fragment osseux pour remedier aux luxations recidivante de l'épaule. Acta Scand 17:411, 1932

66. Jones L: The shoulder joint—observations on the anatomy and physiology. With an analysis of a reconstructive operation following extensive injury. Surg Gynecol Obstet 75:433, 1942

67. Keiser RP, Wilson CL: Bilateral recurrent dislocation of the shoulder (atraumatic) in a thirteen year old girl. J Bone Joint Surg 43A:553, 1961

68. Kocher T: Eine neue Reductionsmethode fur Schulterverenkurg. Berlin Klin Wochenschr, 7:101, 1870

69. Krazar B, Relovszky E: Prognosis of primary dislocations of the shoulder. Acta Orthop Scand 40:216, 1969

70. Kretzler HH, Blue AR: Recurrent posterior dislocations of the shoulder in cerebral palsy. J Bone Joint Surg 48A:1221, 1966

71. Lange M: Orthopadische-Chirurgische. J.F. Bergmann, Munich, 1951

72. Latarjet J: A propos du traitement des luxations recidivantes de l'epaule. Lyon Chir 49:994, 1954

73. LeClerc J: Chronic subluxation of the shoulder. Proceedings of Dewar Orthopaedic Club. J Bone Joint Surg 51B:778, 1969

74. Leffert RD, Rowe CR, Kozlowski B, Meister M: Treatment of voluntary dislocation of the shoulder by therapeutic exercises based on video-electromyographic analysis. J Bone Joint Surg 7:141, 1983

75. Leidelmeyer R: Reduced: shoulder, subtly and painlessly. Emergency Med 9:233, 1977

76. Lombardo SJ, Kerlan RK, Jobe FW et al: The modified Bristow procedure for recurrent dislocation of the shoulder. J Bone Joint Surg, 58A:256, 1976

77. Luckey CA: Recurrent dislocation of the shoulder. Modification of the Bankart capsulorrhaphy. Am J Surg 77:220, 1949

78. MacKenzie DB: The Bristow-Helfet operation for recurrent anterior dislocation of the shoulder. J Bone Joint Surg 62B:273, 1980

79. Magnuson PB, Stack JK: Recurrent dislocation of the shoulder. JAMA 123:889, 1943

79a. Matsen FA: Instructional Course on the Shoulder. American Academy of Orthopaedic Surgery, January, 1987, San Francisco

80. May VR: A modified Bristow operation for anterior recurrent dislocation of the shoulder. J Bone Joint Surg 52A:1010, 1970

81. McLaughlin HL: Posterior dislocation of the shoulder. J Bone Joint Surg 34A:584, 1952

82. McLaughlin HL, Cavallaro WW: Primary anterior dislocation of the shoulder. Am J Surg 80:615, 1950

83. McLaughlin HL, MacLellan D: Recurrent anterior dislocation of shoulder II, A comparative study. J Trauma 7:191, 1967

84. McMurray TB: Recurrent dislocation of the shoulder. J Bone Joint Surg 43B:402, 1961

85. Mead NC, Sweeney HJ: Bristow procedure. Spectator July 9, 1964

86. Milch H: Pulsion–traction in reduction of dislocation in fracture–dislocation of the humerus. Bull Hosp Joint Dis 24:147, 1963

87. Milton GW: The mechanism of circumflex and other nerve injuries in dislocation of the shoulder and the possible mechanism of nerve injuries during reduction of dislocation. Aust NZ J Surg 23:24, 1955

88. Mirick MJ, Clinton JE, Ruiz E: External rotation method of shoulder dislocation. J Am Col Emergency Phys 8:528, 1979

89. Mollerud A: A case of bilateral habitual luxation in the posterior part of the dislocation joint. Acta Chir Scand 94:181, 1946

90. Morton KS: The unstable shoulder: recurrent subluxation. Proceedings of the Canadian Orthopaedic Association. J Bone Joint Surg 59B:508, 1977

91. Moseley HF, Overgaard B: The anterior capsular

mechanism in recurrent anterior dislocations of the shoulder. J Bone Joint Surg, 44B:913, 1962

92. Moseley HF: Shoulder Lesions, 3rd ed. E & S Livingstone, Edinburgh, 1969

93. Mowery CA, Garfin SR, Booth RE, Rathman RH: Recurrent posterior dislocation of the shoulder: Treatment with bone graft. J Bone Joint Surg 67A:777, 1985

94. Myer-Burgdorff H: Die Behandlung der habituellen shulterluxation. Zentralbl Chir 60:827, 1939

95. Neer CS II: Articular replacement for the humeral head. J Bone Joint Surg 37A:215, 1955

96. Neer CS: Replacement arthroplasty for glenohumeral osteoarthritis. J Bone Joint Surg 56A:1, 1974

97. Neer CS, Foster CR: Inferior capsular shift for involuntary inferior and multidirectional instability of the shoulder. A preliminary report. J Bone Joint Surg 62A:897, 1980

98. Neviaser JS: Treatment of old unreduced dislocations of the shoulder. Surg Clin North Am 43:1671, 1963

99. Nicola T: Recurrent dislocation of the shoulder. J Bone Joint Surg 16:663, 1934

100. Nicola T: Anterior dislocation of the shoulder. The role of the articular capsule. J Bone Joint Surg 25:614, 1942

101. Nielsen AB, Nielsen K: The modified Bristow procedure for recurrent anterior dislocation of the shoulder. Acta Orthop Scand 53:229, 1982

102. Norris TR, Bigliani LU: Analysis of failed repair for shoulder instability—a preliminary report. p. 111. In Bateman, Welsh (eds): Surgery of the Shoulder. Philadelphia, C.V. Mosby, 1984

103. Norris TR, Bigliani LU, Niebauer JJ: Treatment for shoulder instability following failed surgery. Read at 98th Annual Meeting of the American Orthopaedic Association, San Diego, California, June 12, 1985

104. Osmond-Clarke H: Habitual dislocation of the shoulder. The Putti-Platt operation. J Bone Joint Surg 30B:19, 1948

105. Oster A: Recurrent anterior dislocation of the shoulder treated by the Eden-Hybbinette operation. Follow-up of 78 cases. Acta Orthop Scand 40:43, 1969

106. Palmer I, Widen A: The bone block method for recurrent dislocation of the shoulder joint. J Bone Joint Surg 30B:53, 1948

107. Pasila M, Kiviluoto O, Jaroma H, Sundholm A: Recover from primary shoulder dislocations and its complications. Acta Orthop Scand 51:25, 1980

108. Perthes G: Uber operationen der habituellen Schulterluxation. D.T.Z., Chir. 85:199, 1906

109. Post M: Recurrent Posterior Dislocations in the Shoulder. Surgical and Non Surgical Management. Lea & Febiger, Philadelphia, 1978

110. Protzman RR: Anterior instability of the shoulder. J Bone Joint Surg 62A:909, 1980

111. Reischauer F: Ueber wilkurliche Schulteruerrkungen (rein wilkurliche, habituell wilkurliche und Pendel-Luxationen) und "schnapende Schulter." Arch Orthop Unfall Chir 22:45, 1923

112. Ricard: Traitement des luxations recidivantes de l'epaule par la suture de la capsule articulare on arthrorrophie AZ des Hop, 49, 1894. p. 179. In Bick EM (ed): History and Source Book of Orthopaedic Surgery. Hospital for Joint Disease, New York, 1933

113. Rockwood CA: Subluxation of the shoulder—the classification, diagnosis and treatment. Orthop Trans 4:306, 1979

114. Rockwood CA: Analysis of failed surgical procedures for anterior shoulder instability. Read at the 4th Annual Meeting of the American Shoulder and Elbow Surgeons, Las Vegas, Nevada, January 27, 1985

115. Rockwood CA, Green DP: Fracture–Dislocations of Shoulder Fractures. J.B. Lippincott, Philadelphia, 1975

116. Rockwood CA, Green DP: Fractures in Adults. J.B. Lippincott, Philadelphia, 1984

117. Rowe CR: Prognosis of dislocations of the shoulder. J Bone Joint Surg 38A:957, 1956

118. Rowe CR: Complicated dislocations of the shoulder—guidelines in treatment. Am J Surg 117:549, 1969

119. Rowe CR: Chronic unreduced dislocations of the shoulder. J Bone Joint Surg 64A:494, 1982

120. Rowe CR, Marble AC: Shoulder girdle injuries. p. 254. In Cave EF (ed): Fractures and Other Injuries. Year Book Publishers, Chicago, 1958

121. Rowe CR, Patel D, Southmayd WW: The Bankart procedure. A long term end-result study. J Bone Joint Surg 60A:1, 1978

122. Rowe CR, Pierce DS, Clark DG: Voluntary dislocation of the shoulder. J Bone Joint Surg 55A(3):445, 1973

123. Rowe CR, Sakellarides HT: Factors related to recurrences of anterior dislocation of the shoulder. Clin Orthop 20:40, 1961

124. Rowe CR, Zarins B: Recurrent transient subluxation of the shoulder. J Bone Joint Surg 63A:863, 1981

125. Rowe CR, Zarins B: Chronic unreduced dislocations of the shoulder. J Bone Joint Surg 64A:494, 1982

126. Rowe CR, Zarins B, Ciullo J: Recurrent anterior dislocation of the shoulder after surgical repair. Apparent cause of failure and treatment. J Bone Joint Surg 66A:159, 1984

127. Saha AK: Recurrent Anterior Dislocation of the Shoulder: A New Concept. Academic Publishers, Calcutta, India, 1969

128. Samilson RL: Severe degenerative arthritis of the shoulder following repair of recurrent anterior dislocations. J Bone Joint Surg 64A:634, 1982

129. Samilson RL: Dislocation arthropathy of the shoulder. J Bone Joint Surg 65A:456, 1983

130. Schulz TJ, et al: Unrecognized dislocations of the shoulder. J Trauma 9:1009, 1969

131. Scott DJ: Treatment of recurrent posterior dislocation of the shoulder by glenoplasty. J Bone Joint Surg 49A:471, 1967

132. Simonet WT, Melton LJ, Cofield RH, Iltrup DM: Incidence of anterior shoulder dislocation in Olmsted County, Minn. Clin Orthop Rel Res 186:186, 1984

133. Souchon E: Operative treatment of irreducible dislocations of the shoulder joint, recent or old, simple or complicated. Trans Am Surg Assoc 15:311, 1891

134. Stimson LA: A Practical Treatise on Fractures and Dislocations. Lea Brothers, New York, 1907

135. Sverdlov IM, Arenberg AA, Ahitnitsky RE: Voluntary subluxation of the shoulder. Central Institute Traumatology and Orthopaedics, 1962

136. Sweeney JH, Mead NC, Dawson WJ: Fourteen years experience with the modified Bristow procedure. Presented at the Annual Meeting of American Academy of Orthopaedic Surgeons, March 1975

137. Symeonides PP: The significance of the subscapularis muscle in the pathogenesis of recurrent anterior dislocation of the shoulder. J Bone Joint Surg 54B:476, 1972

138. Thompson FR, Moga JJ: The combined operative repair of anterior and posterior shoulder subluxation. Audiovisual program. Am Academy of Orthopaedic Surgeons, January 10, 1965

139. Tibone J, Prietto, Jobe F et al: Staple capsulorrhaphy for recurrent posterior shoulder dislocation. Am J Sports Med 9:135, 1981

140. Townley CO: The capsular mechanism in recurrent dislocation of the shoulder. J Bone Joint Surg 32A:370, 1950

141. Turkel SJ, Panio MW, Marshall JL et al: Stabilizing mechanisms preventing anterior dislocation of the glenohumeral joint. J Bone Joint Surg 63A:1208, 1981

142. Viek P, Bill BT: The Bankart shoulder reconstruction—the use of pullout wires and other practical details. J Bone Joint Surg 41A:236, 1959

143. Watson-Jones JR: Recurrent dislocations of the shoulder (editorial). J Bone Joint Surg 30B:6, 1948

144. Weber BG, Simpson A, Hardegger F: Rotational osteotomy for recurrent anterior dislocation of the shoulder, associated with large Hill-Sachs lesions. J Bone Joint Surg 66A:1443, 1984

145. White M: Late results of shoulder dislocations. Trans R Med Chir Soc 22:243, 1929

146. Willis JB, Meyn MA, Miller EH: Infraspinatus transfer for recurrent anterior dislocation of the shoulder. Read at the Annual Meeting of the American Academy of Orthopaedic Surgeons, Las Vegas, Nevada, February 27, 1981

147. Wilson JC, McKeever FM: Traumatic posterior (retroglenoid) dislocation of the humerus. J Bone Joint Surg 31A:160, 1949

148. Yoneda B, Walsh RP, MacIntosh DL: Conservative treatment of shoulder dislocation in young males. J Bone Joint Surg.

149. Zuckerman JD, Matsen FA: Complications about the glenohumeral joint related to the use of screws and staples. J Bone Joint Surg 66A:175, 1984

Acromioclavicular and Sternoclavicular Joints

8

Carter R. Rowe

ACROMIOCLAVICULAR JOINT

There has been more controversy concerning the acromioclavicular joint regarding treatment for injuries and complications than that for any other joint of its size in the body. Located on the outer angle of the shoulder, it is exposed to repeated trauma, in contrast to the more protected sternoclavicular joint.

Injuries

Injuries to the acromioclavicular joint may occur from direct blows to the point of the shoulder or to its anterior or posterior surfaces. Occasionally, the joint may be displaced by an indirect force transmitted from a fall on the elbow or outstretched arm. Nielson[52] reviewed 101 injuries to the acromioclavicular joint and found that 70 percent were caused by a direct blow to the shoulder.

Depending on the mechanism of injury, the clavicle may be dislocated superiorly (the usual direction), or posteriorly[3] and at times inferiorly.[57] Beckman[8] reported a patient in whom both ends of the clavicle dislocated simultaneously. Observations vary as to the incidence and degree of rupture of the coracoclavicular ligaments. I have observed, at surgery, some complete superior dislocations of the clavicle in which the coracoclavicular ligaments were not ruptured; in others, however—usually those that "tent" the skin—the coracoclavicular ligaments were ruptured. Gurd also made this observation.[33] Rosenorm,[62] based on his study of postmortem dissections, demonstrated that the clavicle could dislocate superiorly without rupture of the coracoclavicular ligament. Division of the coracoclavicular ligaments merely increased the extent of upward dislocation. This has been our experience. In a recent in-depth biomechanical study by Fukuda et al.,[28] many of Urist's findings in 1946[72] were confirmed, specifically, that the acromioclavicular ligament contributed approximately two-thirds of the constraining force to superior and posterior displacement. With large displacements and increased load, the coracoclavicular ligament contributed the major share of constraint. This article is an excellent study.

Classification

Classification of acromioclavicular injuries is somewhat arbitrary, due to variations in ligament injury. A classification that has worked successfully for us is as follows (Fig. 8-1):

293

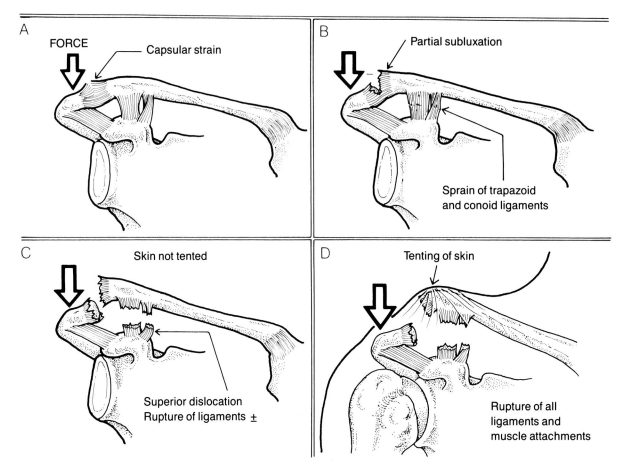

Fig. 8-1. Classification of acromioclavicular injuries. (**A**) Capsular sprain. (**B**) Partial subluxation. (**C**) Superior dislocation (*without* tenting of the skin). Rupture of coracoclavicular ligaments in majority of patients. (**D**) Severe superior dislocation (*with* tenting of the skin). Rupture of all ligaments and muscle attachments (see Fig. 8-2 also). (*Figure continues.*)

1. *Sprain* (Fig. 8-1A): no displacement of the joint occurs, merely sprain of the acromioclavicular capsule and ligaments.
2. *Partial subluxation* (Fig. 8-1B): Usually the superior acromioclavicular ligament is ruptured, with partial rupture of capsule and sprain of coracoclavicular ligaments.
3. *Complete superior dislocations* (*without* tenting of the skin) (Figs. 8-1C, 8-2): the acromioclavicular joint is disrupted and the coracoclavicular ligaments are usually ruptured, although they may not be, depending on the severity of the dislocation.
4. *Severe superior dislocations* (*with* "tenting" of the skin) (Fig. 8-1D; see Fig. 8-14): disruption of the acromioclavicular joint occurs with complete rupture of the coracoclavicular ligaments and muscle attachments.
5. *Posterior dislocations* (Fig. 8-1E): In the posterior dislocation, the coracoclavicular ligament is usually not ruptured. There is no increase in the space between the clavicle and the coracoid; in fact, the space may be less than on the opposite side. Fracture of the end of the clavicle may occur.
6. *Inferior dislocation:* the coracoclavicular ligament remains intact.[57] The clavicle, in rare instances, may displace inferior to the coracoid process (Figs. 8-1F, and 8-3).

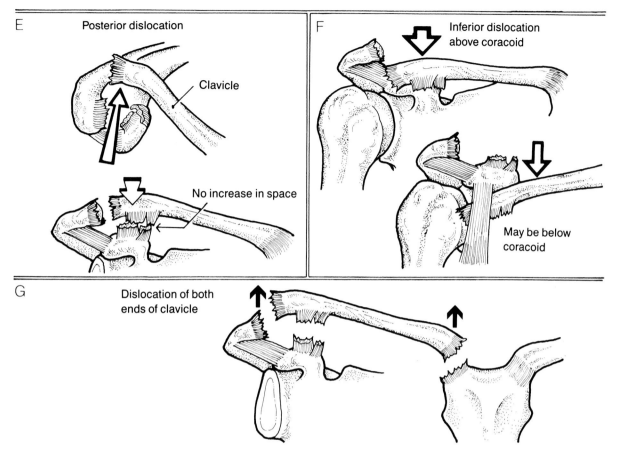

Fig. 8-1 (*Continued*). (**E**) Posterior dislocation. The space between the clavicle and coracoid is narrower than normal. (**F**) Inferior dislocation. May be above or below the coracoid process (Fig. 8-3). (**G**) Simultaneous dislocation of both ends of the clavicle.

7. *Complete and simultaneous dislocation of both ends of the clavicle*[8] (Fig. 8-1G).

Diagnosis

Superior dislocations of the acromioclavicular joint are clearly identified clinically by the prominence of the end of the clavicle, and by radiograms that outline the upward dislocation of the clavicle, as well as the increased distance between the undersurface of the clavicle and the coracoid process. Inferior dislocation is diagnosed by depression of the distal end of the clavicle by AP radiographs. Posterior dislocation, however, is more difficult to identify due to the absence of deformity superiorly. On close examination, there is palpable prominence of the end of the clavicle

posteriorly. Also, the AP radiographs will show narrowing of the space between the undersurface of the clavicle and the coracoid, rather than an increase in the space, compared to the opposite shoulder. Posterior dislocations can also be identified on true axillary views or by computed axial tomographic (CAT) scans. The distal end of the clavicle may be widened due to fracture.

Treatment

TYPES I AND II

There has been little change in the treatment of types I and II injuries over the years. Both are treated conservatively with ice packs to the shoulder initially

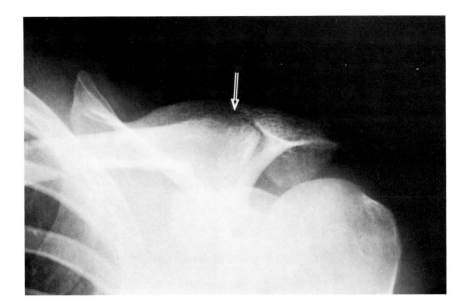

Fig. 8-2. Radiograph showing an inferior dislocation of the left clavicle.

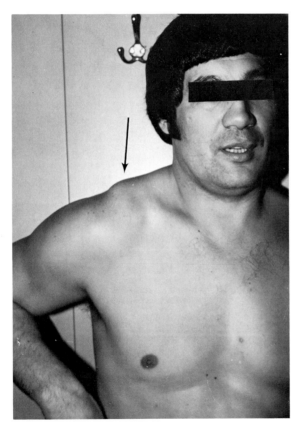

Fig. 8-3. J.B. played for 22 years in the National Hockey League with complete superior dislocation of right clavicle (type III) with no treatment and no complaints.

as needed and temporary support to the arm. Limiting pain may persist for 3 weeks or more. A soccer player with protective shoulder pads may return to playing sooner than the tennis player, swimmer, or javelin thrower whose dominant arm is injured. Although the prognosis is usually good, some type II injuries may develop late traumatic changes in the joint due to uneven contact of the joint surfaces. These will necessitate resection of the distal end of the clavicle for relief.

TYPE III

In general, there are three different schools of thought in the treatment of complete superior dislocations (without tenting of the skin) in this category (Figs. 8-2, 8-4) each with their loyal supporters. If the skin is tented, internal fixation is indicated.

The Do-Nothing School

No attempt is made to reduce the dislocation or stabilize its position. A sling is advised for a few days for comfort, but not for reduction. Ice is applied to the shoulder as needed. Discomfort may be present for 10 days to 2 weeks. From 3 to 6 weeks, activities are allowed as tolerated. This approach has become more popular during the past 10 years, as the patient loses little time from work or athletics, and does not have to be hospitalized. If surgery is necessary later, it can be scheduled at a time that is more convenient

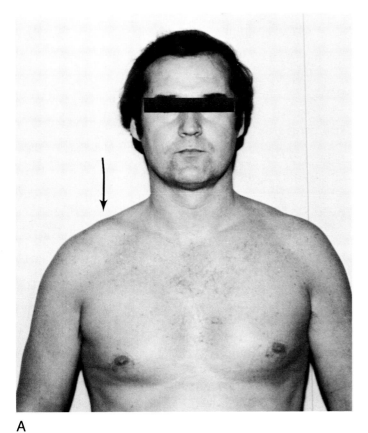

A

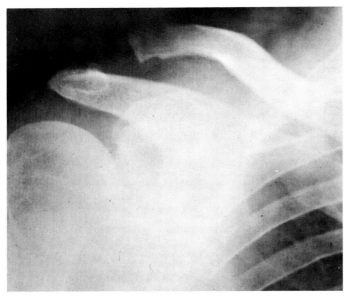

B

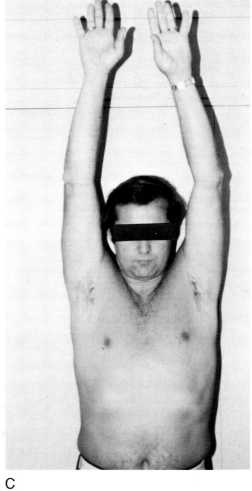

C

Fig. 8-4. J.T. had complete superior dislocation of his right acromioclavicular joint (type III). He received no sling, no support, no surgery. **(A)** The injury occurred in February of 1977. **(B)** Radiograph at initial examination. **(C)** Three months following injury, has been playing golf, has "no pain," and no loss of time from work.

for the patient. Cox[21] reports improved results with no support to the arm in 62 percent of his patients, whereas with immobilization and sling, only 25 percent improved at 3 to 6 weeks. He operated on only 11 percent. We agree and would favor active use of the arm and shoulder as soon as tolerated.

Walsh et al.[61] report on nine patients with superior dislocation treated nonsurgically and nine treated surgically. They concluded that "grade III injuries treated nonoperatively showed no significant strength deficits. Surgically treated, grade III injuries had a significant deficit." However, grade III injuries treated conservatively had more discomfort. Comparative studies have been carried out by Hawkins[34] and Imatani et al.[36] of operative versus nonoperative treatment. They also concluded that nonoperative treatment yielded as good, if not better, results than surgical treatment. Weaver and Dunn in 1972[75] supported conservative treatment for complete dislocation, except for grade III injuries or those that tent the skin. With this we would also agree.

Glick et al.[32] describes weakness of forward flexion and abduction in 8 of 34 complete dislocations treated nonoperatively, but favored no treatment, especially in athletes, since it allowed them to return to their sport more rapidly and safely. They concluded that complete reduction is not necessary since none of the athletes they treated were disabled at follow-up examination.

Larsen et al.[41] report an interesting prospective study comparing 41 patients operated upon and 43 patients treated conservatively. The rehabilitation period was shorter with nonoperative treatment. "About half of the patients who were operated on had problems with the metallic devices. . . . In our opinion, however, most other patients (other than those who tent the skin, or heavy weight lifters) should be treated conservatively with a sling until they are pain free."

Our conservative treatment for type III dislocation (superior dislocation without tenting of the skin), has been encouraging. Sixty percent of patients were satisfied with their shoulder as far as function was concerned. They accepted the deformity which, incidentally, tends to become less in time. Many forgot about their shoulder. Figure 8-3 illustrates a complete dislocation of the right acromioclavicular joint in a National League Hockey player who had played with complete superior dislocation of his acromioclavicular joint for

20 years and had absolutely no problem with his shoulder. Only when someone remarked about the "bump" was he aware of his shoulder.

Figure 8-4A shows a 32-year-old radiology technician (J.T) who came to us a few days after he had experienced complete dislocation of his right acromioclavicular joint (Fig. 8-4B). Immediate surgery had been advised. He stated that he had observed, on a number of routine chest films taken in his hospital, complete dislocations of the acromioclavicular joint that the patient either was not aware of or had no complaints about. We advised him that he could return to work the next day and we would see him at intervals. At 6 weeks, he was much improved and had started playing golf. At 3 months (Fig. 8-4C) he had full activity and stated that his golf was much better than it had been before injury!

Twenty percent of the group were somewhat disturbed by their shoulder, but not to the extent that they wished to have surgery. They accepted the bump, with some discomfort at times, but were taking part in athletics and work. *Twenty percent* were unhappy with the cosmetic appearance, or were experiencing disturbing degrees of discomfort, and wished to have surgical help. In those who needed surgery, the technique we have used consists of resection of the distal 1 cm of the clavicle with reinforcing closure (see below for section on technique). Our experience with this technique for superior dislocation that does not "tent" the skin (groups I, II, III) has been most successful. When the clavicle sticks up under the skin, internal fixation is advised.

Closed Reduction and External Support

If closed reduction and external support are used, the clavicle should be reduced *as soon as possible*, and maintained reduced with some type of shoulder support. The most popular type of support now is the Kenny-Howard halter, which is very effective (Fig. 8-5A). If it is used, however, the support straps should be tightened or adjusted daily to maintain reduction as recommended by Allman.[3] Unfortunately, patients may lose some of the reduction when they lie down; therefore, two or three pillows are recommended for sleep at night. Also, the halter must not be removed when the patient takes a shower, for at least 3 to 4 weeks. Even under ideal circumstances, the clavicle may become partially subluxated, or lose

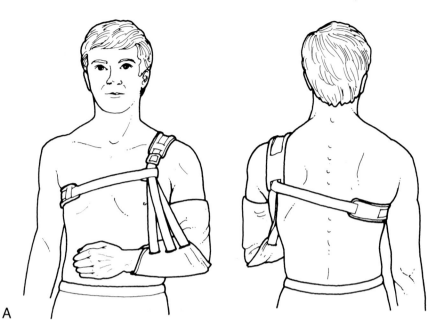

Fig. 8-5. (**A**) The Kenny-Howard shoulder halter for acromioclavicular separations is the choice today. (**B**) Old method used in 1952, which was much less effective.

A

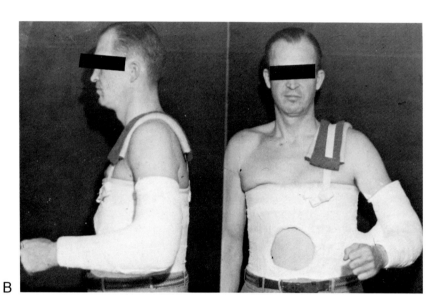

B

its reduction completely, if every detail of treatment is not carried out. Sage et al. reported a 57.9 percent recurrence of subluxation in shoulders with external immobilization for 3.4 weeks.[62] In the 1950s, before the advent of improved shoulder halters such as the Kenny-Howard type, orthopaedic surgeons tried many ingenious methods to maintain reduction. Figure 8-5B shows an example of determined efforts to maintain reduction of a dislocated acromioclavicular joint in the past (1950). Happily, more comfortable and acceptable methods of maintaining reduction of the clavicle have been devised.

Open Reduction and Internal Fixation

A multitude of fixation devices and techniques have been devised to stabilize this challenging and recalcitrant joint.

1. Transfixation of the acromioclavicular joint with various types of pins and screws[1,6,11,53,54,66,77]
2. Stabilization of the clavicle to the coracoid process
   With screws[9,60]
   With wire loops[7,58]
   With Dacron vascular graft loops and other types of artificial ligaments[23,27,37,52]
   With transplant of the coracoacromial ligament to the clavicle[13,19,49,54,75]
   By transplanting the coracoid process with its muscular attachments to the clavicle[4,16,24,39]
   With short head of biceps[73]
   With arthrodesis of the acromioclavicular joint[15,17]
3. Resection of the distal end of the clavicle.[33,49,60]
   Of the above surgical procedures, the more commonly used are the following:

Transfixation of the Acromioclavicular Joint.
Some surgeons prefer one or two 3/32-inch Kirshner pins (Fig. 8-6). Threaded pins have the advantage of not working out; however, if they become bent or broken, removal may be very difficult. Smooth pins are easily removed but may extrude before they

should. A very effective and strong pin is the Simmons-Martin[64] pin, designed as a single pin fixation with minimum injury to the joint surfaces (Fig. 8-7). The uninitiated surgeon should be reminded that *the proximal end of the transfixing pin should not perforate the medial cortex of the clavicle,* as pins may migrate medially into the chest or lungs (see section on complications below). Bending the distal end of the pin has been used as a safeguard. A check-up radiograph at the time of surgery, to be certain that the pin has been properly placed, may prevent much embarrassment to the surgeon. In addition to transfixing pins, Neviaser reinforces the joint by freeing the coracoacromial ligament from the coracoid and turning it up and over the joint to reinforce the damaged superior ligament[52] (Fig. 8-8C). If the dislocation is an old one, the distal end of the clavicle can also be removed and the clavicle stabilized by pinning or by screw fixation of the clavicle to the coracoid. The surgeon should remember that the clavicle assumes a gradual S-curve. The pins must be introduced to take advantage of the S-curve of the outer third of the clavicle. The pins are usually left in for 6 weeks. The patient should be cautioned not

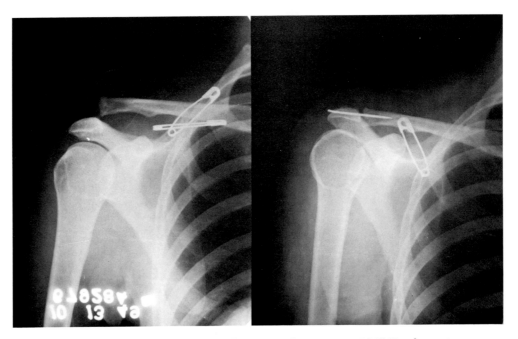

Fig. 8-6. Fixation of acromioclavicular joint with one or two 3/32″ Kirschner pins.

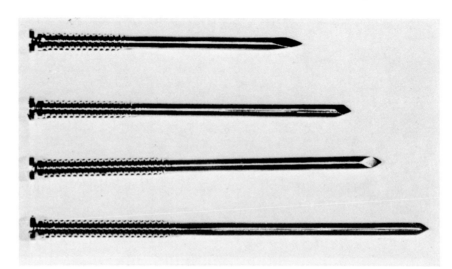

Fig. 8-7. The Simmons-Martin pins for single pin fixation.

to carry the arm through full ranges of motion or to push or lift heavy objects until the pins have been removed, to avoid bending or extruding the pins.

Screw Fixation of the Clavicle to the Coracoid Process. Bosworth (1941) popularized the screw fixation of the clavicle to the coracoid process.[9] More recently, Rockwood[60] has devised a clavicular–coracoid lag screw that is inserted 1 inch medial to the acromioclavicular joint so that it enters the base of the coracoid process (Fig. 8-8D). In chronic cases, he recommends resection of the distal end of the clavicle, release of the coracoacromial ligament from the acromion, and its transplantation into the open end of the clavicle according to the Weaver-Dunn technique. For extra strength, the coracoacromial ligament may be turned up directly to the undersurface of the clavicle,[13] or Dacron vascular or fascial grafts may be passed around the clavicle and the coracoid. We do not recommend silk or wire, or even Dacron graft, as either might cause pressure necrosis and cut through the cortical bone of the clavicle. Dahl[23] reports a case in which the Dacron graft around the clavicle eroded through the entire clavicle.

"Dynamic" Transfers of Coracoid to Clavicle. Dewar and Barrington have recommended transplanting the osteotomized coracoid with its muscular attachments of short head of biceps and coracobrachialis to the undersurface of the clavicle by screw fixation[24] (Fig. 8-9). They report five patients with no complications. However, Caspi and associates warn of injury to the musculocutaneous nerve with use of this technique.[16]

Resection of Distal End of the Clavicle. McLaughlin[47] credits Fracassini with first describing resection of the outer end of the clavicle in 1902. This procedure was later popularized by Gurd[33] and Mumford[50] in 1941. Gurd emphasized its indications in complete dislocations of the clavicle and Mumford for the incomplete dislocations with traumatic changes of the acromioclavicular joint. The tendency with both authors, however, was to remove too much of the clavicle and perhaps not give more attention to smoothing the end of the bone and securing the distal end by double breasting the capsule, the osteoperiosteal flaps, and muscles.

Weaver and Dunn Technique. The Weaver and Dunn technique combines an oblique resection of the distal end of the clavicle with intramedullary transfer of the coracoacromial ligament to the clavicle (Fig. 8-10). The ligament is freed from the acromion. The authors remove 2 cm of distal clavicle (instead of 1 cm): this places the open end of the clavicle directly over the coracoid process, facilitating the introduction of the ligament into the medullary portion of the clavicle. When performed as the authors advise, this is a very dependable technique.[75]

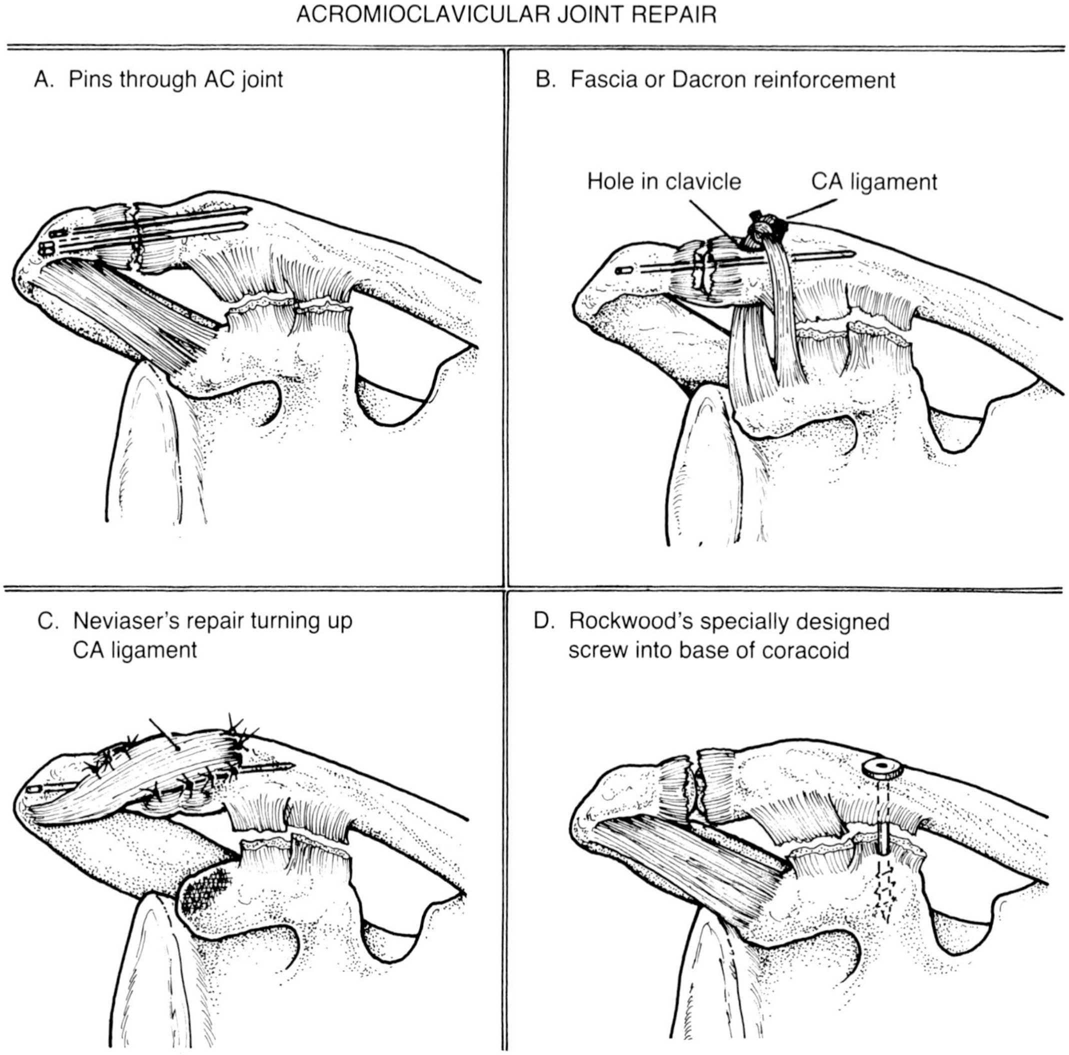

ACROMIOCLAVICULAR JOINT REPAIR

Fig. 8-8. Methods of repairing the acromioclavicular joint. (**A**) Transarticular pin fixation. (**B**) Pin fixation plus reinforcement by turning up the coracoacromial ligament over the clavicle, or through the end of the clavicle Weaver-Dunn technique (see Fig. 8-11). (**C**) Pin fixation plus Neviaser technique of turning up the coracoacromial ligament to reinforce the superior capsular ligament. (**D**) Rockwood's technique of using a specially designed lag screw introduced into the base of the coracoid.

Author's Technique

We have revised the technique of removal of the distal end of the clavicle and have used it successfully in acute as well as chronic dislocations of the acromioclavicular joint when indicated (Fig. 8-11). However, for this to be successful it must be performed correctly. It is not recommended in severe dislocations that tent the skin; we would use the Weaver-

Dunn technique or transfixing pins in such a case. We no longer find it necessary to explore the trapezoid and coronoid ligaments to see whether the ligaments have ruptured or not. Several points in technique are most important:

1. A short saber incision will give the best skin closure and less spread of the incision.

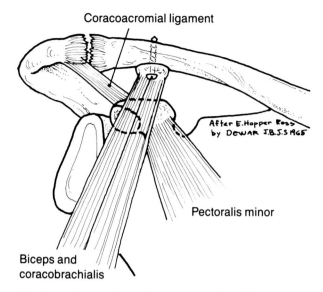

Fig. 8-9. The Dewar technique: transfer of the coracoid process with attached muscles by screw fixation to the undersurface of the clavicle—the "dynamic" transfer.

2. Once through the skin, the incision is made in line with the clavicle along the superior surface, *directly* down to bone, turning back *in one layer* the trapezius and deltoid attachments, the osteoperiosteal covering of the bone, and the capsule (Fig. 8-11B). When the layers are overlapped in closure, this ensures a strong and secure closure.

3. Only 1 cm of clavicle should be removed (Fig. 8-11C). This is also most important in preserving stability. The more clavicle removed, the more unstable the end of the bone may become. A mini pneumatic oscillating saw is used to remove the distal 1 cm of clavicle. Care is taken to rongeur off smoothly the superior cortex of the clavicle and the bone or periosteal tissue inferiorly. The clavicle is also narrowed slightly on either side.

4. Next, the arm is carried through a full range of motion in abduction, adduction, and elevation. There should be *no* impingement or contact of clavicle against the acromion. If there is, and more room is needed, a small portion of the inner acromion is removed rather than more clavicle.

5. Repair is carried out by overlapping, *in one layer*, the trapezius and deltoid muscles, the osteoperiosteal sleeves, and acromioclavicular capsule (Fig. 8-11D). This depresses the end of the clavicle and gives the clavicle remarkable stability. Witness to

this are the athletes who have returned to full involvement and have continued playing. The investigations of Urist[71] and Fukuda[28] also emphasize the strength of the capsule. When properly performed, this procedure leaves the shoulder strong.

6. The arm is not immobilized postoperatively. Instead, early gentle motion of the extremity is encouraged. A sling may be used for a few days for comfort, but discarded soon afterwards. Heavy lifting or strenuous activities, however, are avoided for 3 to 4 weeks. Some athletes have returned to activities at the end of 3 weeks. Others have waited 6 weeks, by which time heavy labor and contact sports are possible.

RESULTS

The rewarding aspects of this procedure are the elimination of urgency for surgery, the lack of complications, and its good results. The deformity is removed and should not return. There is no metal to break, bend, or migrate. No second operations are necessary to remove screws, pins, or wires. No immobilization is needed. The patient returns to active participation in sports as tolerated. Some orthopaedic surgeons have stated that following this technique the patient should not return to football or contact sports, and that the clavicle will be unstable. This is possible if the end of the clavicle is incorrectly removed and poorly repaired, or if too much removed. Our experience has been entirely different, with 90 percent good to excellent results. The result will depend on the technique employed. We have had college and professional football players and National Hockey League players continue at top performance following this technique. Again, it must be carried out correctly: preserve the osteoperiosteal sleeve, muscle attachment, and the joint capsule, and remove no more than 1 cm of clavicle. Exceptions to the above are instances when the end of the clavicle tents the skin, in which cases internal fixation is indicated.

Patient J. McK.

A professional National Hockey League player suffered a complete superior dislocation of the left acromioclavicular joint (Fig. 8-12). Resection of the distal clavicle was carried out initially by our technique. In 3 weeks he was skating, and 5 weeks after the operation he was back on his line, playing in the

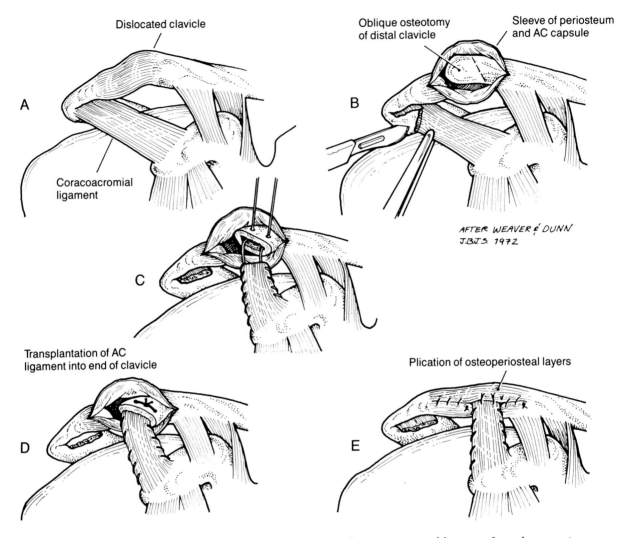

Dislocated clavicle

Coracoacromial ligament

A

Oblique osteotomy of distal clavicle

Sleeve of periosteum and AC capsule

B

AFTER WEAVER & DUNN
J.B.J.S. 1972

C

Transplantation of AC ligament into end of clavicle

D

Plication of osteoperiosteal layers

E

Fig. 8-10. (A–E) The Weaver-Dunn technique of releasing the coracoacromial ligament from the acromion, obliquely osteotomizing the distal clavicle, and transplanting the coracoacromial ligament into the end of the clavicle. Plication of the osteoperiosteal flaps gives extra support.

Stanley Cup playoffs. The player continued with a successful career for 10 more years.

Patient D.E.

Another National Hockey League player suffered a complete dislocation of his left acromioclavicular joint in 1971. The distal end of his clavicle was removed. He was skating in 2 weeks and back on his line in 3½ weeks. This was earlier than we had advised. However, he demonstrated that this was possi-

ble. He continues to the present time as an active player for one of the Eastern Division National Hockey League teams.

Patient W.A. (Fig. 8-13)

He underwent removal of the distal 1 cm centimeter of the clavicle for complete superior dislocation. He performed in college as a quarterback with minimal complaints and was happy with the outcome of surgery.

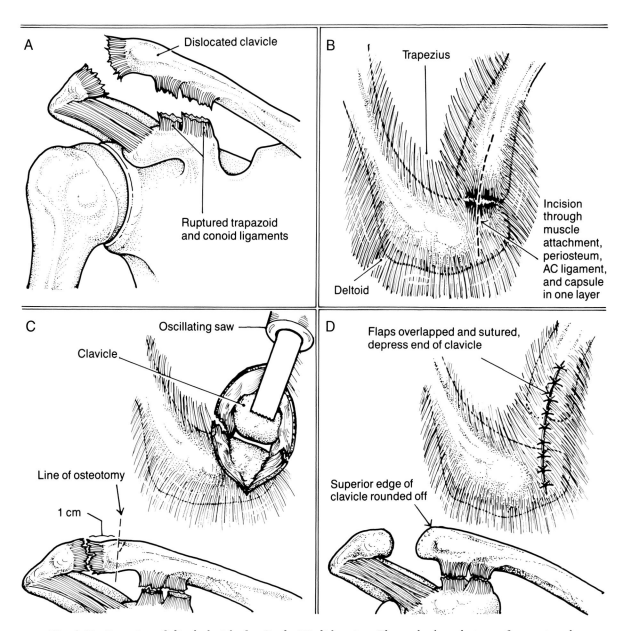

Fig. 8-11. Resection of distal clavicle for Grade III dislocation. The author's technique of removing the distal 1 cm of clavicle and double-breasting the osteoperiosteal, capsular, and muscle flaps over for stability. **(A)** The dislocation. **(B)** Incision in one layer of the osteoperiosteal layer, muscle attachments, and capsule. **(C)** Removal of 1 cm of the distal clavicle, no more. If more space is needed, remove a portion of the opposing acromion. **(D)** The superior cortex of clavicle is rounded off and the flaps of osteoperiosteal, capsule, and muscle attachments double breasted in one layer. This depresses the end of the clavicle. This technique can be used for recent or chronic painful dislocations.

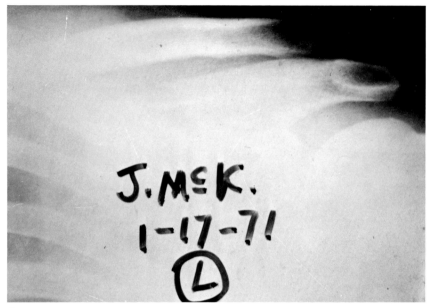

A

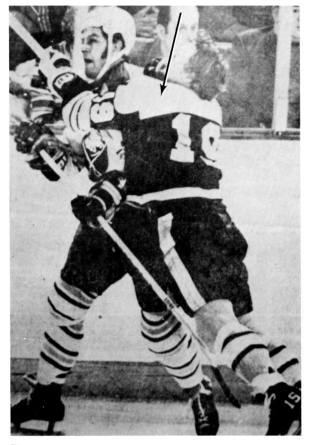

B

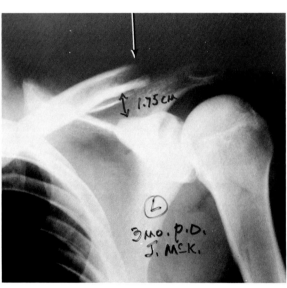

C

Fig. 8-12. (**A**) Acute superior dislocation of the left acromioclavicular joint in a National Hockey League player thrown against the boards. (**B**) Back on his line for the Stanley Cup play-off 5 weeks after removal of 1 cm of clavicle (see arrow). (**C**) Three months postoperative: note the good relation with acromion.

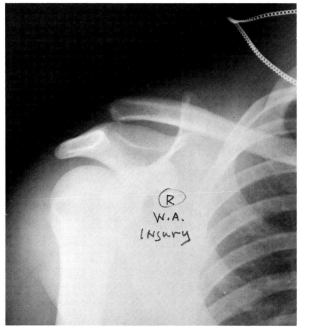
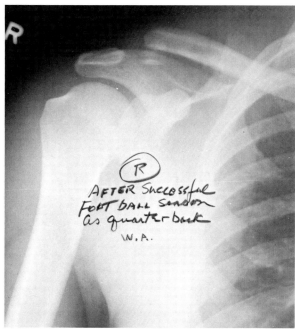

A   B

Fig. 8-13. (A) Complete superior acromioclavicular dislocation of the right clavicle in a football player. (B) Resection of the distal 1 cm eliminated "the bump." He then successfully completed his football season as quarterback on his college team.

Type IIIB (with Tenting under the Skin (Fig. 8-14)

This is best treated with open reduction and with some type of internal fixation of the joint, or with the Weaver-Dunn procedure. If the surgeon has the correct instruments and follows Rockwood's technique closely, he or she should have a very good result with screw fixation to the coracoid. We have had good results with transfixing the joint with one or two 3/32 inch Kirschner pins, which should be removed in 6 weeks.

Posterior Dislocations of the Clavicle

These may go unrecognized for long periods of time, since there is absence of the deformity clinically on radiographs. The only physical finding is a palpable prominence posteriorly, and narrowing of the coracoclavicular space on the radiograph. This can be missed very easily on physical examination. Resection of the bony prominence of the distal 1 cm of the clavicle, and of a small amount of opposing acromion if neces-

sary, reshaping the end of the clavicle to eliminate the posterior prominence, has been consistently successful in all those we have operated upon. Not infrequently, the end of the clavicle is fractured and widened in posterior dislocations. It is necessary to narrow the clavicle when widened by fracture. This should be appreciated and looked for. When this is not recognized, reduction is not successful with either closed or open treatment.

DISCUSSION

For the acute complete dislocation, the surgeon has a variety of methods of treatment from which to choose. As pointed out, most orthopaedic surgeons stick to one technique for all types of dislocations. Unfortunately, this does not permit selectivity in treatment, and may expose many patients to unnecessary surgery. If the dislocation is superior, but not "tenting" the skin, we would suggest two options:

(1) The no-treatment regimen is preferred, especially if the patient is an athlete. With this treatment,

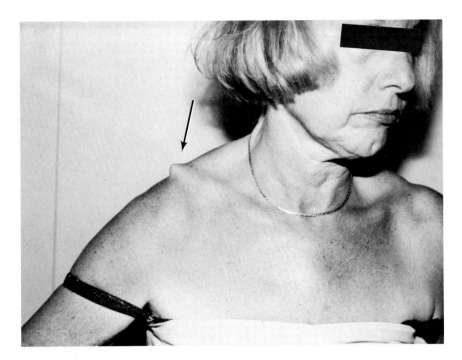

Fig. 8-14. An example of type IIIB "tenting" under the skin. Surgical fixation is indicated in this type.

the shoulder is not immobilized except for a short period of time, for comfort, in a sling. Patients are not taken out of circulation or hospitalized. They are allowed to keep physically active by running, skating, biking, or using the arm as tolerated, for 4 to 6 weeks, after which they may return to full contact sports. Patients are told that they have a 60 percent chance of being satisfied with their shoulder. If they have problems with their shoulder later, the shoulder can be operated on electively for resection of the end of the clavicle.

(2) The patient may elect to be rid of the clavicular prominence initially and not face a possible later operation. Again, with the dislocation that is prominent but does not tent the skin, we would advise removal of the distal end of the clavicle by the technique previously described. We stress again that results will depend on technique and attention to detail.

If the superior dislocation is extreme and "tents" the skin, we would recommend:

1. Early reduction with transfixing pins across the acromioclavicular joint.
2. The Weaver-Dunn transplant of the coracoacromial ligament, with removal of the distal 1 cm of clavicle (Fig. 8-10).

3. The Rockwood clavicular screw to the coracoid (if the surgeon is familiar with this technique and has the necessary equipment) (see Fig. 8-D).

Complications

CALCIFICATION

A common complication, and fortunately not a bothersome one, is calcification, or even ossification, as reported by Soule, of the coracoclavicular ligament.[64] Interestingly, this does not restrict motion of the shoulder and is usually symptom-less. It occurs more commonly following operative treatment, but can occur on occasions with closed treatment, as well as with no treatment. This is a complication seen by all of us. Fortunately, it is benign.

IATROGENIC

An *iatrogenic* complication of surgery of the acromioclavicular joint is *excessive* removal of the distal end of the clavicle (Fig. 8-15). In our opinion, removal of over 1 cm is not necessary. Only the amount of clavicle that impinges on the acromion should be removed. Beyond 1.0 cm there may be a gap between

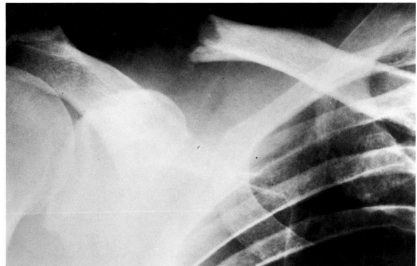

A

Fig. 8-15. (**A**) A radiograph showing removal of *too much* clavicle for an acromioclavicular dislocation. Not only has too much clavicle been removed, but also a spur remains on the inferior cortex. The patient has pain and a disturbing defect. (**B**) With secondary ossification of the coracoclavicular ligament. (**C**) Another example of excessive removal of the end of the clavicle. This was painful and disfiguring.

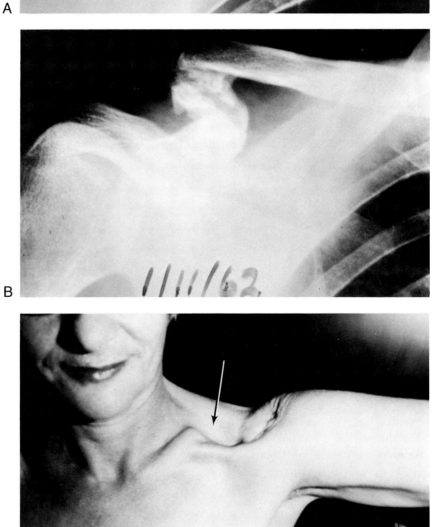

B

C

the clavicle and acromion. This very likely has accounted for reluctance to use this technique in the past. Unfortunately, this is seen too commonly. If the surgeon believes that removal of more than 1 cm of clavicle is indicated, as pointed out, removal of a small portion of opposing acromion would be safer and more effective.

MISPLACEMENT OF PINS ACROSS THE ACROMIOCLAVICULAR JOINT

As shown in Figure 8-16A, the surgeon pinned the clavicle but missed the acromion. As shown in Figure 8-16B, the surgeon missed the clavicle but pinned the acromion. After the pins were removed, both patients had good results, we might add, in spite of surgery.

MIGRATION OF PINS

Again, avoid perforating the proximal cortex of the clavicle with transfixing pins, since motion of the shoulder may cause the pins to migrate medially into the brachial plexus or mediastinum. If the medial cortex of the bone is not perforated, the pin will not migrate inward. Lindsey and Gutowski have recently reported a patient in whom the pin broke and the proximal section migrated into the neck.[42] Other surgeons report migration of a threaded Steinmann pin into the spinal canal[41] and another of migration of pins to the lung.[70] Restricting the activities of your patient, examining check-up radiographs, and being certain the medial end of the pin does not perforate the medial cortex of the bone are necessary precautions.

MULTIPLE UNSUCCESSFUL PROCEDURES

When surgeons are too aggressive multiple unsuccessful procedures may be performed. The patient in Figure 8-17 had experienced four unsuccessful procedures for a dislocation of the left acromioclavicular joint, and was totally disabled with chronic pain and loss of shoulder motion and function, as a result of repeated failed surgery. How much better off this patient may have been, if he had received no treatment.

SCREW FIXATION OF THE CLAVICLE TO THE CORACOID PROCESS

Pulling out of the screw from the coracoid, erosion of the screw in the clavicle, or fracture of the screw as a result of excessive shoulder motion may occur.

STRETCHED INJURY

Caspi et al.[16] report three patients who experienced stretched injury to the musculocutaneous nerve following dynamic fixation of the coracoid to the clavicle for acromioclavicular separation. Fortunately, with rest, all three eventually recovered.

PRESSURE NECROSIS

This may occur secondary to lashing the clavicle to the coracoid. The use of wires, silk, or, at times, Dacron around the clavicle may cause pressure necrosis of the clavicle. To avoid this, the Dacron may be pulled through the clavicle via drill holes rather than around it.

CLAVICLECTOMY

This has been reported after multiple unsuccessful attempts to stabilize nonunions of the clavicle or with repeated removal of excess clavicle. In patients who are badly disabled or deformed, claviclectomy may be considered (see section on sternoclavicular joint, below).

OSTEOLYSIS OF DISTAL END OF CLAVICLE

As pointed out by Rockwood,[60] a series of 100 cases have been reported in the literature. None have been reported in women and the majority have been weight-lifters. Madsen[45] in 1963 reported seven patients and cited an acute injury or repeated stress in the shoulder as causative factors. Cahill[14] in 1982 reported 46 cases in athletes, none of whom had an acute injury. Forty-five of the 46 were weight-lifters. None of the patients we have seen had an acute injury; all were associated with weight-lifting (Fig. 8-18). The patients complain of a dull ache, usually in the early period of the syndrome, and weakness. Usually, local discomfort lessens as the clavicle reforms. If symptoms continue, or the osteoporosis increases, one should rule out possible multiple myeloma, hyper-

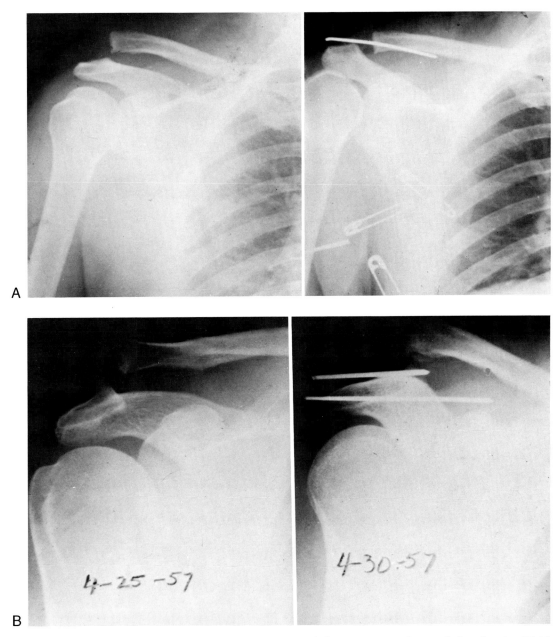

Fig. 8-16. Misplacement of pins. (**A**) The surgeon missed the acromion and pinned the clavicle. (**B**) The surgeon pinned the acromion, but missed the clavicle. Interestingly, both patients were happy after their pins were removed.

parathyroid disease, scleroderma, infection, or "disappearing bone disease." Microscopic studies have been reported by Lamont and also by Murphy et al.[51] Murphy reported patients (one female) all of whom had the distal end of the clavicle removed. Microscopic findings revealed destruction of the distal end of the clavicle including cartilage and bone. The cartilage of the acromion was not involved. Sections

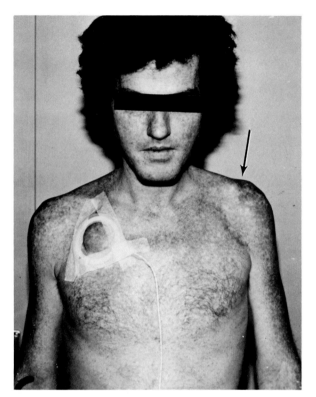

A

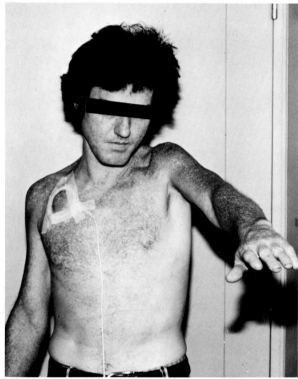

B

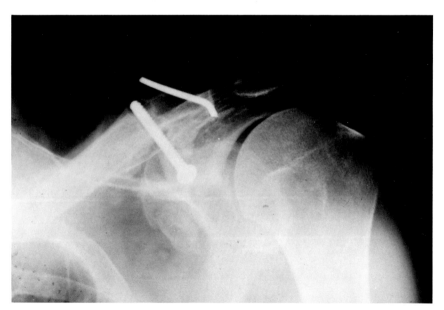

C

Fig. 8-17. A surgical disaster as the result of four unsuccessful operations for a dislocated left acromioclavicular joint. **(A,B)** The patient is totally disabled with chronic pain and loss of function of his left shoulder. **(C)** Radiographs of the left shoulder.

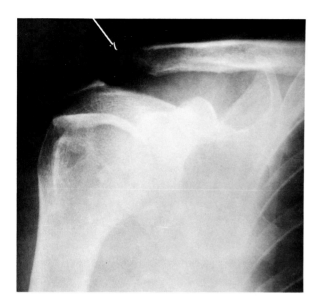

Fig. 8-18. A 25-year-old man with osteolysis of distal end of clavicle from weight-lifting.

of the clavicle showed only "sclerotic bone," "aseptic necrosis," and "fibrous reaction." They conclude "the mechanism of this bone and cartilage resorption is unknown—possibly this represents a disorder of one or more 'bone remodeling' units activated by trauma." Their patients' conditions were relieved by surgical removal of the distal end of the clavicle. None of the patients we have seen required resection of the end of the clavicle. Some clavicles have recalcified, others have continued unchanged with few or no symptoms for years.

STERNOCLAVICULAR JOINT

Dislocations and subluxations of the sternoclavicular joint are uncommon. In a review of 1,603 shoulder injuries by the author in 1958, there were only 13 sternoclavicular injuries[63]; since then, we have seen a total of 34 sternoclavicular dislocations (Table 8-1). In 1825, Sir Astley Cooper[18] recognized and treated dislocations of the sternoclavicular joint. In 1843, Rodrigues[61] reported his experience with a posterior dislocation of the clavicle. The first reports in the

Table 8-1. Sternoclavicular Dislocations: 40 Years' Experience

34 Dislocations
30 Superior
4 Posterior
11 Acute
12 Chronic (1 "floating" clavicle)
11 Recurrent (4 voluntary dislocations)

American literature were by Cotton,[20] followed by Duggan,[25] Lowman,[43] later by Howard and Shafer,[35] and more recently by Rockwood.[60]

Anatomy

The sternoclavicular joint is a diarthrodial joint with the distinction of being the sole articulation between the upper extremity and the axial skeleton. It is an odd joint for such an important fulcrum, as much of the medial clavicle rides above its sternal junction and, except for its strong ligaments, it would be a very unstable joint. The sternoclavicular capsular ligament borders the anterior and posterior aspects of the joint. The interclavicular ligament supports the superior surface. The costoclavicular ligament supports the inferior joint (between the clavicle and the first rib). The intraarticular disc, which arises from the first rib and inserts on the superior surface of the clavicle, divides the joint into two compartments, and acts as a check-rein superiorly and medially. The joint has a very functional range of motion, with 35° of elevation, 35° of forward and backward horizontal motion, and 45° to 50° of rotation.

Among the concerns with injuries to the sternoclavicular joint are the vital structures that lie directly posterior to the medial end of the clavicle: the subclavian veins, innominate arteries, trachea, esophagus, and mediastinum (Fig. 8-19).

Mechanism of Injury

Injury to the sternoclavicular joint may result from a transmitted blow to the point of the shoulder or a direct blow to the clavicle or chest. A transmitted blow to the point of the shoulder in extension would

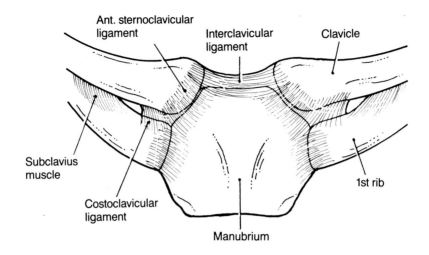

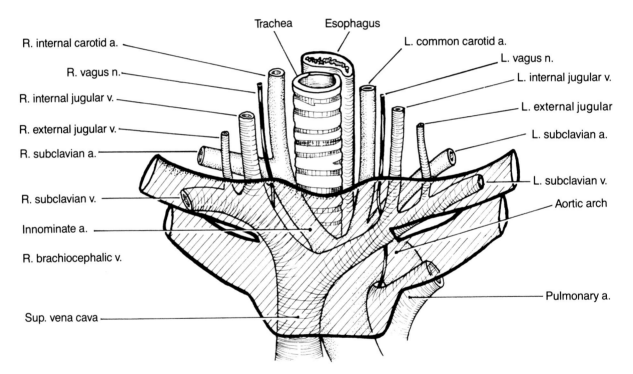

Fig. 8-19. Anatomy of the sternoclavicular joint. The vulnerable posterior structures should be constantly kept in mind.

predispose to an anterior or superior dislocation, whereas a blow to the anterior chest or clavicle would predispose to a posterior or retrosternal dislocation. Omer[56] reported on 82 cases from 14 military hospitals. Vehicular accidents accounted for 47 percent and athletics for 31 percent.

Classification

TRAUMATIC

1. Sprain: partial tear of the capsular ligament but no displacement.

2. Partial subluxation: rupture of the sternoclavicular capsular ligament, without rupture of the costoclavicular ligament or intraarticular disc.
3. Complete dislocation: rupture of the sternoclavicular and costoclavicular ligaments and, most likely, the intraarticular disc.
    a. Anterior–superior
    b. Posterior (substernal)
4. Complete dislocation with fracture of the medial end of the clavicle
5. Complete dislocation of both ends of the clavicle: panclavicular dislocation.

VOLUNTARY

Voluntary subluxation or dislocation of the sternoclavicular joint anteriorly and superiorly may occur as with the glenohumeral joint and the scapula, and accounts for a small number of dislocations. The ligaments of the joint remain intact, but are abnormally lax (see Fig. 8-30). See section on Voluntary Recurrent Dislocations for cautions in treatment.

Diagnosis

Patients who have injured their sternoclavicular joint give a history of a blow to the point of the shoulder or a direct blow to the chest or clavicle, with resultant discomfort of the joint or sternum. Soft tissue swelling may initially conceal an anterior or superior dislocation, but once the swelling has subsided the deformity is evident. Much more difficult to recognize clinically is the retrosternal or posterior dislocation, which may show little surface abnormality except possibly a slight depression of the inner clavicle. The patient, however, will complain of local sternoclavicular discomfort and of difficulty in breathing or swallowing. Jockeys describe this as "a brush with death."

Radiographic Examination

Anteroposterior radiographs may be difficult to interpret. Oblique views and tomograms are helpful. More recently, CAT scans have proven most successful and should be taken especially when there is a question of a posterior dislocation. Rockwood has found his "serendipity" view a very helpful one, in which the x-ray tube is tilted 40° from the vertical and is aimed directly at the manubrium. It is recommended that the cassette be large enough to cover the shoulder[60] (Fig. 8-20).

Treatment (Table 8-2)

SPRAINS AND PARTIAL SUBLUXATIONS

These respond to conservative measures consisting of ice locally for the first 48 hours, a sling if needed, and rest of the extremity. As a rule, by the second or third week much of the discomfort will have subsided and increasing use of the arm and shoulder is allowed as tolerated.

COMPLETE ANTERIOR–SUPERIOR DISLOCATION

Anterior dislocations, if seen early, have a good chance of being reduced by manipulation. Success depends on the condition of the intraarticular disc.

Manipulation

This is carried out under intravenous medication or light relaxant anesthesia. A roll is placed between the shoulder blades so that the shoulders can be elevated and hyperextended (Fig. 8-21). The clavicle is then reduced by manual assistance. Reduction is accompanied usually by a "thud" and, in most instances, is stable. A comfortable postoperative support is indicated for a period of a week to 10 days. The support we prefer is shown in Fig. 7-76. A figure-of-eight may also be used. In either case, complete elevation in extension of the arm should be avoided for 3 weeks. If, however, the reduction is incomplete, we have found that the majority of anterior dislocations will, in time, do very well conservatively without further attempts at reduction or operation unless they become recurrent. Rockwood calls attention to physis injuries in adolescents of the medial end of the clavicle, which can easily be misdiagnosed as an anterior dislocation of the joint because the epiphysis is the last to close, usually in the 23rd to 25th year (Fig. 8-22). He rightly advises a careful investigation and conservative treatment program. His historical review of this injury and his personal experience are well worth reading.

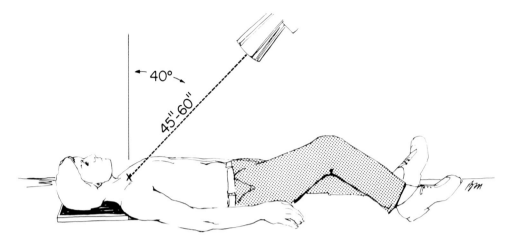

Fig. 8-20. The Rockwood view of the sternoclavicular joint. The cassette should be large enough to receive the projected images of medial halves of both clavicles. In children, the tube distance should be approximately 45°, with thicker-chested adults, the distance should be 60°. (Rockwood CA, Jr., Green DP: Fractures in Adults, 2nd. ed. JB Lippincott, Philadelphia, 1984.)

Open Reduction of Superior Dislocation

For recurrent anterior dislocation or for symptomatic unreduced dislocations, open reduction may be indicated. The surgeon should remember to inform the patient that the trade-offs for an open reduction of the sternoclavicular joint are operative risks and a rather unsightly scar in a very exposed area. A more acceptable incision results if it is kept straight in line with the clavicle and sternoclavicular joint; however, the exposure is better with a curved incision.

Capsular Repair.   If, on exposure of the joint, the intraarticular disc remains attached deep to the first rib, it may be used to repair the superior capsular ligament and the interclavicular ligament, or it may

be split: bring its arms up around the clavicle and repair superiorly for added support (Fig. 8-23).

We do not use temporary pin fixation; however, if this is done, the pin should *not* perforate the medial cortex of the manubrium. Also, it should be left so that its end can be palpated subcutaneously. It should be checked each day by the patient and by radiographs when indicated. It is removed in 3 weeks. It is important to instruct patients not to elevate their arms above 90° until the pin has been removed. Rockwood[60] does not recommend open reduction of the sternoclavicular joint, and strongly advises against the use of transfixing pins.

Fascial Repairs.   My choice of the three is the Speed technique, with a strip of fascia around the

Table 8-2. Results of Treatment

	Number	Excellent	Good	Fair	Poor
No treatment	13	5	6	2[a]	
Manipulative reduction	3	2	1		
Open reduction					
Capsular repair	2	0	0	1	1[a]
Fascial repair	7	3	2	0	2[b]
Resection, medial					
End of clavicle	4	0	2	0	2[a]
Claviclectomy	5	4	1	0	0

[a] One voluntary dislocator in each category.
[b] One was a compensation case.

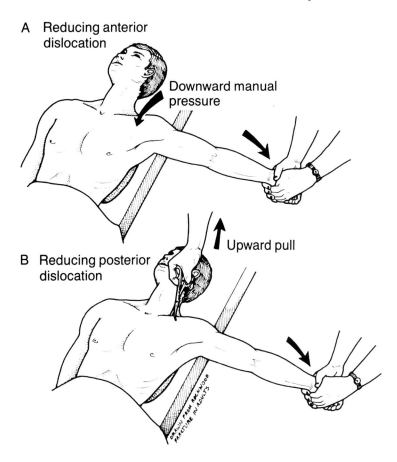

A Reducing anterior dislocation

Downward manual pressure

B Reducing posterior dislocation

Upward pull

Fig. 8-21. Manipulative reduction of the sternoclavicular joint in abduction. (**A**) For an anterior dislocation. (**B**) For a posterior dislocation. (Redrawn from Rockwood CA, Jr., Green DP: Fractures in Adults, 2nd ed. JB Lippincott, Philadelphia, 1975.)

second rib instead of the first.[5,43,62,68] It is safer and stronger. Patient R.S., a jockey 3 months following the Speed technique for recurrent superior dislocation of his left sternoclavicular joint is shown in Figure 8-23C.

Omer Technique. This consists of a step osteotomy at the attachment of the sternocleidomastoid

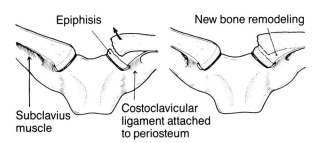

Epiphisis

New bone remodeling

Subclavius muscle

Costoclavicular ligament attached to periosteum

Fig. 8-22. Separation of the medial epiphysis, which may be misdiagnosed as an anterior sternoclavicular dislocation.

muscle. After the clavicle is shortened; the deformity is eliminated and healing is facilitated.[56]

Resection of the Inner 1.5 to 2 cm of Clavicle. It is most important that the periosteum be removed proximally, otherwise a mass of bone and cartilage may reform later and be as prominent and bothersome as the original end of the clavicle. This word of caution is also voiced by Moseley.[48]

POSTERIOR (RETROSTERNAL) DISLOCATIONS

Thorough clinical and radiographic studies must be carried out before treatment is begun. The dangers and complications of treatment should be reviewed with the patient.

Closed Manipulation

The usual method of closed reduction recommended in textbooks is to place a sandbag or bolster between the scapulae and apply traction to the ab-

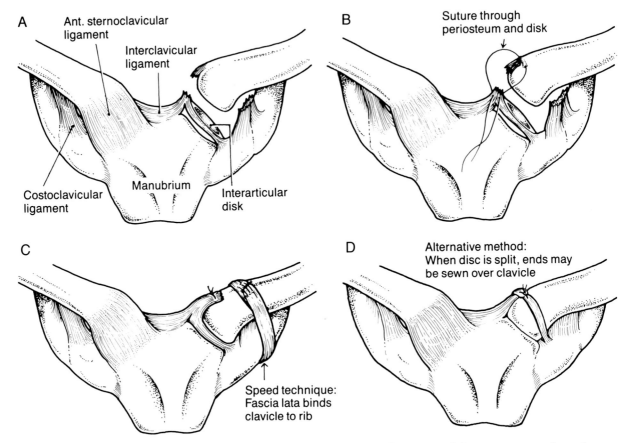

Fig. 8-23. Repair of sternoclavicular dislocation. (**A**) Dislocation with rupture of the superior capsular and the costoclavicular ligaments. (**B**) Repair of the superior interclavicular and the costoclavicular ligaments. (**C**) The Speed technique, using a strip of fascia lata. (**D**) An option for securing the joint.

ducted arm in extension. Percutaneous traction is used if needed.[25,26,44,46,56] This technique is reported in general to be successful in the majority of reports (Fig. 8-21B).

Buckerfield and Castle,[10] however, in 1984, reviewed the literature and found that of a total of 40 retrosternal dislocations for which reduction had been attempted by applying traction to the abducted arm, only 26 (68 percent) had a successful result. They reported more successful results by applying traction with the arm in adduction, and suggested the following technique (Fig. 8-24).

A substantial bolster is placed between the shoulders, which improves the retraction of the shoulders. Because the shoulders are fully retracted, the clavicle is brought out from behind the manubrium more easily, which is necessary to reduce the clavicle.

By adducting the arm, the retraction force is only 20° above the horizontal, the pectoralis major is relaxed, and the medial end of the clavicle can be effectively levered over the first rib and reduced. If the arm is retracted in abduction, the angle of the clavicle is greater, which eliminates much of the direct pull on the clavicle, therefore increasing the difficulty of reduction. Less force is needed in adduction than in abduction. Six of their seven posterior dislocations were successful. One of the successful shoulders was not manipulated until 96 hours after the injury.

This article deserves careful study. Its principles are sound. The technique should be considered whenever a posterior dislocation of the clavicle is treated. The authors summarize: "our method utilizes a levering principle instead. Caudal traction applied to the adducted arm depresses the lateral end of the

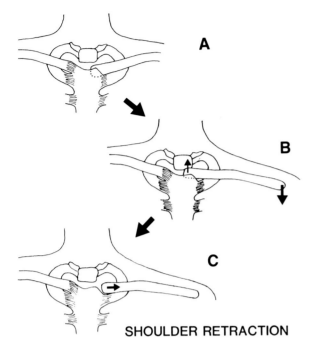

SHOULDER RETRACTION

Fig. 8-24. Manipulative reduction of a posterior dislocation in adduction (Buckerfield technique). **(A)** The retrosternal dislocation. **(B)** Caudal traction on the arm levers the medial end of the clavicle superiorly. **(C)** With shoulder retraction, the medial end of the clavicle is drawn anteriorly and laterally into a reduced position. (Buckerfield CT, Castle ME: Acute traumatic retrosternal dislocation of the clavicle. J Bone Joint Surg 66A:379, 1984.)

clavicle to the horizontal position while the medial end of the clavicle tends to be levered superiorly with the first rib acting as the fulcrum."

Open Reduction for Posterior (Substernal) Dislocation

The surgeon and patient must be aware of the risks and complications of open reduction. If the patient is not having difficulty, open reduction may not be necessary. If open reduction is indicated, adequate blood replacement should be available, as well as a thoracic surgeon. The entire arm should be surgically prepped and draped. A curved incision is made over the medial end of the clavicle. The safest exposure for a posterior dislocation of the clavicle is to remain subperiosteal. If there is irregularity or fracture of the medial end of the clavicle, this can be gently

released subperiosteally. One is relatively safe if all dissection is subperiosteal. The joint space is inspected and the disc removed if damaged.

Traction is applied to the arm in abduction or adduction and extension. A towel clip may be helpful in grasping the clavicle. If the joint portion of the clavicle is traumatized and the tissues are fibrotic, then the medial 1 cm of clavicle can be resected to allow reduction. It is safer to do this after reduction (Fig. 25A, B). The fractured medial end of the left clavicle that was removed because of an unreduced substernal dislocation is shown in Figure 8-25B. Various methods of stabilizing the clavicle are used. My preference is the Speed technique (Fig. 8-23C), as with an anterior dislocation. If pin fixation is necessary, we would caution the surgeon to use threaded pins of adequate strength (3/32 inches) and not to perforate the inner cortex of the manubrium. Interval radiographs should be taken to be certain that there is no migration of the pins. The patient should be cautioned to not carry his or her extremity above shoulder level. Support should be a figure-of-eight or a modified plaster spica cast.

CLAVICLECTOMY: RECURRENT POSTERIOR DISLOCATION OF THE CLAVICLE FOLLOWING CLOSED OR OPEN REDUCTION

On several occasions, patients who have had persistent nonunion of the clavicle after surgical failure or recurrence of a retrosternal dislocation of their clavicle following closed or open reduction have experienced pressure on the trachea. They agree that they did not want "another brush with death" and have requested surgical removal of the clavicle. Their requests were carried out on five occasions with surprisingly excellent results. The *old warning* that the shoulder will drop, or foreshorten, or be weak if the clavicle is removed has not been our experience. Attention to technique is, however, most important. The incision is made just above the clavicle, directly down to bone. The clavicle is removed subperiosteally; preserving the intact osteoperiosteal sheath and muscle attachments. A strip of fibrin foam is placed in the periosteal sac and the sheath with its muscle attachments are carefully resutured. A sling is worn for 3 weeks, followed by gradual use of the arm as tolerated. In each instance of total removal

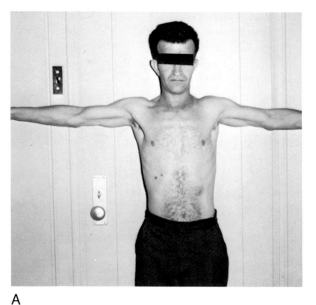

A

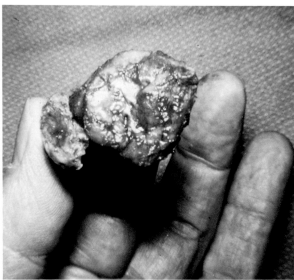

B

Fig. 8-25. (A) Four months after resection of the medial end of the clavicle for chronic fracture and posterior dislocation. **(B)** End of the clavicle showing traumatized fractured joint.

of the clavicle, within 6 weeks pressure applied over the course of the periosteal tube was firm. There is no depression. The muscles were well attached and strong. One jockey was back riding within 10 weeks with good functional strength, no discomfort, no drooping of the shoulder or depression, and without fear of a repeat injury.

Mrs. S., a right-handed woman, was seen because of repeated unsuccessful resection of the medial portion of her right clavicle. She was unable to play golf, fly cast or shoot a gun. Her right clavicle was removed. In Figure 8-26, she is shown 1 year after surgery and has returned to all of her activities; she shoots a 12-gauge shot gun with her *right* shoulder. She has ⅜ of an inch shortening and no droop to her right shoulder. Cosmetic result is excellent.

Mrs. G.L. (Fig. 8-27) is shown 1 year following a right claviclectomy for a chronic unreduced posterior dislocation and fracture of the medial end of the clavicle. She is free of difficult breathing and swallowing, and is most grateful that she has a "perfectly normal shoulder." Mr. F's left clavicle was removed because of chronic pain and brachial plexus pressure following fracture of his left clavicle. He has returned to work. His symptoms are minor. Notice his level shoulders

and only 0.5 cm shortening of his shoulder breadth (Fig. 8-28).

The patients have shown that removal of the clavicle, if performed correctly, carries little disfigurement or disfunction.

VOLUNTARY RECURRENT DISLOCATION

The surgeon should be aware that voluntary recurrent dislocations of the sternoclavicular joint can occur. We have seen several incidences of this in patients who have had one or two *unsuccessful* surgical attempts to stabilize the joint. In each instance, the patient has been able to dislocate the clavicle freely after surgery. This has also been reported by Rockwood and Moseley. This voluntary dislocator demonstrates her ability to dislocate her right sternoclavicular joint superiorly following three unsuccessful repairs (one fascial and two resection of medial end of clavicle) (Fig. 8-29). As with voluntary dislocations of the glenohumeral joint, these patients prove a great embarrassment to the surgeon. It is most important to identify this syndrome and avoid surgery. It is interesting that voluntary recurrent subluxation or dislocations is not painful (unless operated upon), and are produced only by the wish of the patient.

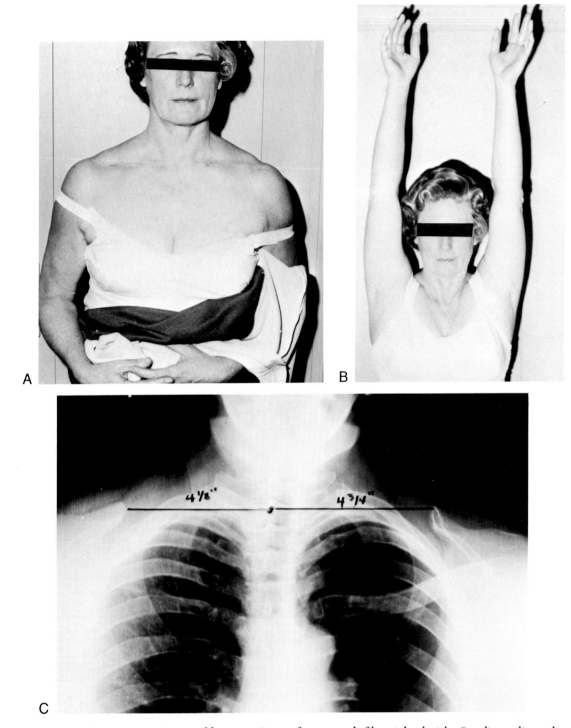

Fig. 8-26. (**A**) Patient S., a 50-year-old woman, 1 year after removal of her right clavicle. Standing radiograph shows only 3/8 inch shortening of shoulder breadth, and no droop of the shoulder. (**B**) She has returned to fly casting, golf, and shoots a 12-gauge shot gun on her right shoulder. (**C**) Measurements and level of her shoulders.

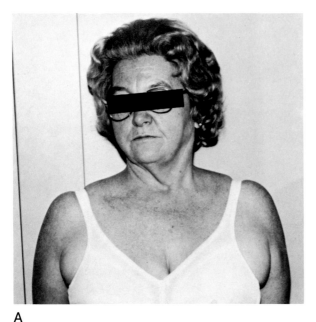

A

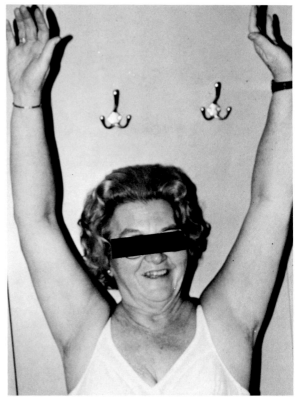

B

Fig. 8-27. (**A**) Patient G.L., 1 year following resection of her right clavicle for a chronic unreduced posterior dislocation. (**B**) She is free of difficulty in breathing and swallowing, and considers her shoulder "perfectly normal," and is very happy with cosmetic appearance.

CHRONIC UNREDUCED DISLOCATION

We have seen a number of unreduced anterior or superior dislocations of the sternoclavicular joint remain without pain, with full range of motion and strength. This has been the experience of others as well.[44,48,56,59,60,69] An occasional patient with unreduced posterior dislocation may elect conservative treatment. Stankler[68] reports two unreduced posterior dislocations. One patient was diagnosed 2½ years after injury. He had been "symptom free" apart from cramps and cyanosis of the hand and venous distention of the forearm following excessive use of the arm. The second patient, a 19-year-old medical student, experienced a rugby injury 4½ years before examination. Initially, he experienced pain in his left shoulder radiating up the left side of his neck. He too experienced partial venous engorgement of his hand when it was dependent. One month after injury a venogram showed complete obstruction of the left subclavian vein. This responded sufficiently to anticoagulants; gradually the patient improved and was symptom free for 4½ years. During the past year, I saw a 26-year-old physical therapist because of a chronic unrecognized posterior dislocation of her left clavicle. She was experiencing only mild discomfort, usually when lifting a patient. She had no complaints of dyspnea or dysphagia. There was no congestion nor any sensory changes of her extremity. She is being observed.

TRAUMATIC "FLOATING" CLAVICLE: PANCLAVICULAR DISLOCATION

Beckman[8] in 1923 is reported to have seen the sixteenth case of complete dislocation of the clavicle. Gearen[29] in 1982 and Jains[38] in 1984 added reports on single cases. Both patients did well on closed treatment. Jains' case was not manipulated and was treated only with a sling. In 6 months the patient had complete, painless motion of the shoulder. Gearen's pa-

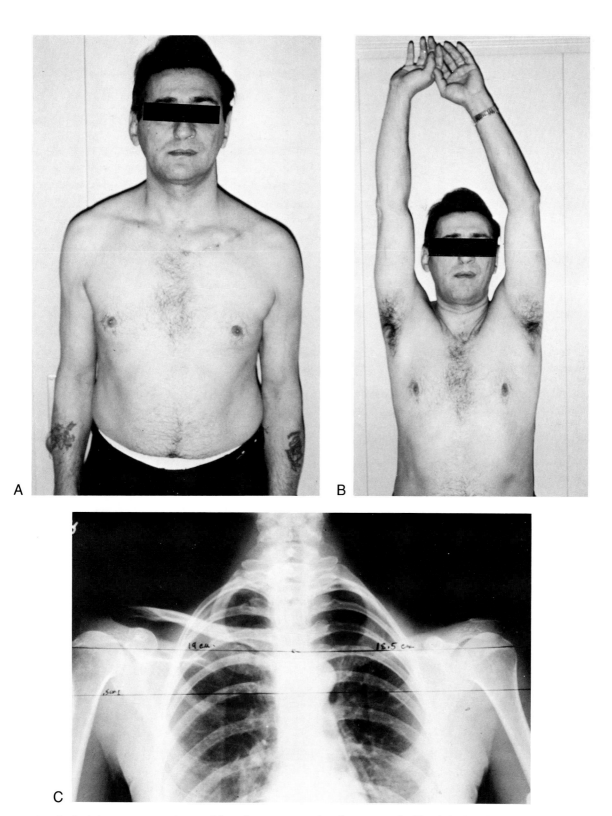

Fig. 8-28. (**A**) Patient F., 45-year-old workman, 6 months after removal of his left clavicle because of an old fracture of clavicle with brachial plexus pressure. Only minimal symptoms are evident. He has returned to heavy work. (**B**) Complete range of motion. (**C**) Radiograph taken with patient standing. Only 0.5 cm shortening of his shoulder breadth. Slight droop to shoulder.

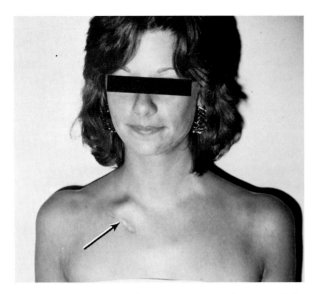

tient was manipulated with reduction of the acromio-clavicular joint but not of the sternoclavicular joint; however, the result was good at both ends of the clavicle. In general, closed treatment is preferred to open reduction. Because of other multiple injuries, this patient's right "floating clavicle" was treated conservatively with a very satisfactory result (Fig. 8-30). Of interest is that the majority of complete dislocations of the clavicle were caused by a direct blow to the spine of the scapula. Rockwood[60] treated four patients with complete dislocation of the clavicle using "skillful neglect" and reports good functional result.

Summary

Fig. 8-29. Recurrent voluntary anterior dislocation of the right shoulder following three unsuccessful surgical repairs.

We have been impressed with the acceptable result of leaving untreated the anterior-superior dislocation, unless it is recurrent and is also not voluntary. If

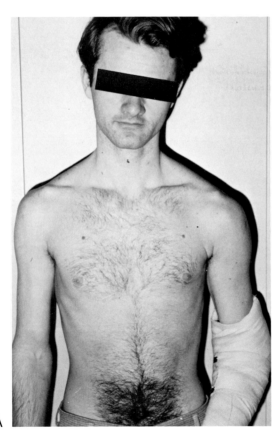

A

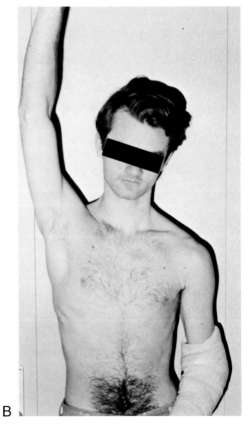

B

Fig. 8-30. **(A)** A right "floating clavicle," untreated. **(B)** Clavicle with complete range of motion and minimal complaints.

acute, a manipulation may be attempted; if unsuccessful, open reduction is an option. If the clavicle has undergone repeated unsuccessful surgical procedures, removal of the medial end is an option. A last option for nonunion pressure on the brachial plexus or recurrent posterior dislocation in clavicletomy. Strong, useful shoulders have resulted, with no disturbing droop or shortening of contour in our series of claviclectomies.

We should not end the chapter on the sternoclavicular joint without a reference to Jackson Burrows[12] of London, England, a master of orthopaedic surgery, who recommended stabilizing the clavicle with tenodesis of the subclavius tendon. Although we have not used this technique, we appreciate Jackson Burrows innovation, and especially his comment, "here it seems simpler, safer, and easier to pick up a mooring, than to drop anchor."

REFERENCES

1. Ahstrom JP: Surgical repair of complete acromioclavicular separation. JAMA 217:785, 1971
2. Alldredge RH: Surgical treatment of acromioclavicular dislocation. J Bone Joint Surg 47A:1278, 1965
3. Allman FL: Fractures and ligamentous injuries of the clavicle and its articulations. J Bone Joint Surg 49A:774, 1967
4. Bailey RW, et al: A dynamic repair for acute and chronic injuries of the acromioclavicular area. J Bone Joint Surg 54A:1802, 1972
5. Bankart AS: An operation for recurrent dislocation of the sternoclavicular joint. Br J Surg 26:320, 1938
6. Bateman JE: Athletic injuries about the shoulder in throwing and body contact sports. Clin Orthop 27:75, 1962
7. Bearden JM, Hughston JC, Whatley GS: Acromioclavicular dislocation, a method of treatment. J Sports Med 1:5, 1973
8. Beckman T: A case of simultaneous luxation in both ends of the clavicle. Acta Chir Scand 56:156, 1923
9. Bosworth BM: Acromioclavicular separation: new method of repair. Surg Gynecol Obstet 73:866, 1941
10. Buckerfield CT, Castle ME: Acute traumatic retrosternal dislocation of the clavicle. J Bone Joint Surg 66A:379, 1984
11. Bundens WD, Cook JI: Repair of acromioclavicular separations by deltoid-trapezius imbrication. Clin Orthop 20:109, 1961
12. Burrows J: Tenodesis of subclavius in the treatment of recurrent dislocation of the sternoclavicular joint. J Bone Joint Surg 33B:240, 1951
13. Burton ME: Operative treatment of acromioclavicular dislocations. Bull Hosp Joint Dis 36:109, 1975
14. Cahill BR: Osteolysis in the distal part of the clavicle in male athletes. J Bone Joint Surg 64A:1053, 1962
15. Caldwell GD: Treatment of complete permanent acromioclavicular dislocation by surgical arthrodesis. J Bone Joint Surg 25:368, 1943
16. Caspi I, Ezra E, Neurbay J, Horoszovski H: Musculocutaneous nerve injury following dynamic fixature of distal clavicle. Clin Orthop Rel Research 1985
17. Campos OP: Acromioclavicular dislocation. Am J Surg 43:287, 1939
18. Cooper A: A Treatise on Fractures and Dislocations of the Joints, 2nd American ed, from the 6th London ed. Lilly and Wait, Carter and Herdee, Boston, 1932
19. Copeland S, Kessel L: Disruption of the acromioclavicular joint: surgical anatomy and biological reconstruction. Injury 11:208, 1980
20. Cotton FJ: Dislocations and Joint Fractures. WB Saunders, Philadelphia, 1910
21. Cox JS: The fate of the acromioclavicular joint in athletic injuries. Am J Sports Med 9:50, 1981
22. Currie DI: An apparatus for dislocation of the acromial end of the clavicle. Br Med J 1:570, 1924
23. Dahl E: Velour prosthesis in fractures and dislocations in the clavicular region. Chirurgerie 53:120, 1982
24. Dewar FP, Barrington TW: The treatment of chronic acromioclavicular dislocation. J Bone Joint Surg 47B:32, 1965
25. Duggan N: Recurrent dislocation of the sternoclavicular cartilage. J Bone Joint Surg 13:365, 1931
26. Ferry AM, Rook FW, Masterson JH: Retrosternal dislocation of the clavicle. J Bone Joint Surg 905, 1957
27. Fleming RE, Tomberg DN, Kiernan HA: An operative repair of acromioclavicular separation. J Trauma 18:709, 1978
28. Fukuda K, Craig EV, An KA et al: Biomechanical study of the ligamentous system of the acromioclavicular joint. J Bone Joint Surg 68A:434, 1986
29. Gearen PF, Petty W: Panclavicular dislocation. J Bone Joint Surg 64A:454, 1982
30. Giannestras NJ: A method of immobilization of acute acromioclavicular separation. J Bone Joint Surg 26:597, 1944
31. Gibbons ME: An appliance for conservative treatment of acromioclavicular dislocation. J Bone Joint Surg 28:164, 1944
32. Glick JM, Melburn CJ, Haggerty JF et al: Dislocation

of the acromioclavicular joint. Am J Sports Med 6:263, 1977

33. Gurd FB: The treatment of complete dislocation of the outer end of the clavicle. Ann Surg 113:1094, 1941

34. Hawkins RJ: The acromioclavicular joint. Paper presented at the AAOS Summer Institute, Chicago, July 10, 1980

35. Howard FM, Shafer SJ: Injuries to the clavicle with neurovascular complications. J Bone Joint Surg 47A:1335, 1965

36. Imatani RJ, Hanlon JJ, Cady GW: Acute complete acromioclavicular. J Bone Joint Surg 57A:328, 1975

37. Jacobs B, Wade PA: Acromioclavicular joint injury. J Bone Joint Surg 48A:475, 1968

38. Jains AS: Traumatic floating clavicle. J Bone Joint Surg 66B:560, 1984

39. Laing PG: Transplantation of long head of biceps in complete acromioclavicular separations. J Bone Joint Surg 41A:1667, 1969

40. Lamont MK: Osteolysis of the outer end of the clavicle. NZ Med J 95:241, 1982

41. Larsen E, Bjerg-Nielsen A et al: Conservative or surgical treatment of acromioclavicular dislocation. J Bone Joint Surg 68A:552, 1986

42. Lindsey RW, Gutowski WT: The migration of a broken pin following fixation of the acromioclavicular joint. Orthopaedics 9:413, 1986

43. Lowman CL: Operative correction of old sternoclavicular dislocation. J Bone Joint Surg 10:740, 1928

44. Lunseth PA, Chapman KW, Frankel VH: Surgical treatment of clavicular joint. J Bone Joint Surg 57B:193, 1975

45. Madsen B: Osteolysis of the acromial end of the clavicle following trauma. Br J Radiol 36:822, 1963

46. McKenzie JMM: Retrosternal dislocation of the clavicle. J Bone Joint Surg 45B:138, 1963

47. McLaughlin HL: Trauma. WB Saunders, Philadelphia, 1959

48. Moseley HF: Shoulder Lesions. E & S Livingstone, Edinburgh, 1969

49. Moshein J, Elconin KB: Repair of acute acromioclavicular dislocations utilizing the coraco-acromial ligament. J Bone Joint Surg 51A:812, 1969

50. Mumford EB: Acromioclavicular dislocation. J Bone Joint Surg 23:799, 1941

51. Murphy GB et al: Post-traumatic osteolysis of distal clavicle. Clin Orthop 109:114, 1975

52. Nielson CL: Repair of acromioclavicular separation with knotted dacron graft. Clin Orthop 143:289, 1979

53. Nielson WB: Injury to the acromioclavicular joint. J Bone Joint Surg 45B:207, 1963

54. Neviaser JS: Acromioclavicular dislocation treated by transference of the coraco-acromial ligament. Clin Orthop 58:57, 1968

55. Norrell H, Llewellyn RC: Migration of threaded Steinmann from AC joint into the spinal canal. J Bone Joint Surg 47A:1024, 1965

56. Omer GE: Osteotomy of the clavicle in surgical reduction of anterior sternoclavicular dislocation. J Trauma 7:584, 1967

57. Patterson WR: Inferior dislocations of the distal end of the clavicle. J Bone Joint Surg 49A:1184, 1967

58. Phemister DB: The treatment of dislocation of the acromioclavicular joint by open reduction and threaded wire fixation. J Bone Joint Surg 24:166, 1942

59. Post M: The Shoulder—Surgical and Nonsurgical Management. Lea & Febiger, Philadelphia, 1978

60. Rockwood CA, Green DP: Fractures in Adults. JB Lippincott, Philadelphia, 1984

61. Rodrigues H: Case of dislocation inwards of the internal extremity of the clavicle. Lancet: 1:309, 1843

62. Rosenorm M, Pedersen EB: Comparison between conservative and operative treatment of acute acromioclavicular dislocation. Acta Orthop Scand 45:50, 1974

63. Rowe CR: Shoulder girdle injuries. p. 254. In Cave EF (ed): Fractures and Other Injuries. Year Book Publishers, Chicago, 1958

64. Rowe CR: Trends in treatment of complete acromioclavicular dislocations. In Surgery of Shoulder, Toronto, 1973–78, 1984

65. Sage FP, Salvatore JE: Injuries of the acromioclavicular joint. South Med J 56:486, 1963

66. Simmons EH, Martin RF: Acute dislocation of the acromioclavicular joint. Can J Surg 473: 1968

67. Soule AB: Ossification of the coracoclavicular joint following dislocation of the acromioclavicular articulation. Am J Roentgenol 56:607, 1946

68. Speed JK: Recurrent anterior dislocation of the shoulder. Operative care by bone grafts. Surg Gynecol Obstet 44:468, 1927

69. Stankler L: Posterior dislocation of the clavicle: a report of two (unreduced) cases. Br J Surg 50:164, 1962

70. Tristan TA, Daughridge TG: Migration of a metallic pin from the humerus into the lung. N Engl J Med 270:987, 1964

71. Tyler GT: Acromioclavicular dislocation fixed by vitallium screw through the joint. Am J Surg 57:245, 1942

72. Urist MR: Complete dislocations of the acromioclavicular joint. J Bone Joint Surg 28:813, 1946

73. Vargus L: Repair of complete acromioclavicular dislocation utilizing the short head of biceps. J Bone Joint Surg 24:772, 1942

74. Walsh WM, Petersen DA, Shelton G, Neumann RD: Shoulder strength following acromioclavicular injury. Am J Sports Med 13:153, 1985

75. Weaver JK, Dunn HK: Treatment of acromioclavicular injuries. J Bone Joint Surg 54A:1187, 1972

76. Weitzman G: Treatment of acute acromioclavicular joint dislocation by a modified Bosworth method. J Bone Joint Surg 49A:1167, 1967

77. Wolen I: Acute acromioclavicular dislocation. J Bone Joint Surg 26:589, 1944

9

FRACTURES
OF THE ADULT SHOULDER

The Glenohumeral Joint

Carter R. Rowe
Mark Colville

Fractures of the proximal humerus are relatively common in adults, forming 4 to 5 percent of all fractures whereas in children they are relatively uncommon. Approximately 80 percent of adult proximal humeral fractures, despite frequent comminution, are minimally displaced and satisfactory results may be obtained with nonoperative treatment and early motion. Displaced fractures of a high-energy injury pose the greatest challenges to successful treatment and functional recovery.

SURGICAL ANATOMY

Mobility and stability of the glenohumeral joint are provided by the dynamic actions of the muscles of the rotator cuff. The intrinsic pull of these muscles at their sites of bony attachment to the proximal humerus dictates the pattern and direction of displacement seen in fractures in this area.

It is important to picture the anatomy of the shoulder when manipulating proximal humeral fractures and the pull of the attached muscles when the arm is in different positions (Fig. 9-1). With the arm in neutral position at the side of the body, the muscles attached to the head and upper shaft are relaxed. With the arm at 90° of abduction (the airplane splint position), the pull of the pectoralis major may displace the humeral shaft medially. When the entire rotator cuff is intact, as in fractures of the surgical neck, the forces on the humeral head are relatively well balanced. Rotation is minimal and the head may be flexed slightly forward. The greatest rotational deformity occurs when one of the tuberosities is displaced, leaving the pull of the remaining rotator cuff unopposed. These are the most difficult fractures to reduce by closed means, and the most likely to redisplace. Manual manipulations may be successful, in full elevation, as the muscle actions of the rotator cuff are neutralized and the attached cuff tends to cone the fragments into anatomical alignment, around the tendon of the long head of biceps (Fig. 9-1B).

Anatomical studies by Laing[8] have shown that the blood supply to the humeral head is primarily derived from the ascending branch of the anterior humeral circumflex artery. It enters the bone either at the upper end of the bicipital groove or by branches to the greater and lesser tuberosities. To a lesser extent, the posterior humeral circumflex artery also was dem-

331

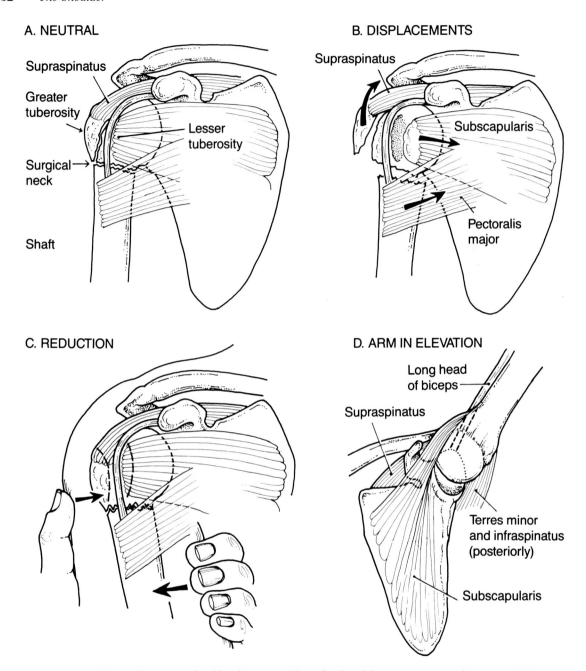

Fig. 9-1. Muscle attachments in shoulder fractures. (**A**) Undisplaced fractures in neutral position. (**B**) Direction of displaced fractures. (**C**) Manual reduction; arm at side of body. (**D**) In elevation, the muscles "cone" the displaced fractures with the aid of the long head of biceps in alignment.

onstrated to contribute through posteromedial branches. Displaced fractures of both tuberosities and the surgical neck without rotator cuff attachment therefore may result in osteonecrosis of the humeral head fragment. When attempting open reduction of proximal humeral fractures, it is critical to avoid damaging remaining soft tissues attached to the humeral head.

Injury to the neurovascular bundle, which lies anteromedially, may occur in higher-energy fractures and fracture dislocations.

CLASSIFICATION

Although fractures of the humeral head and neck are mentioned briefly by Hippocrates,[6] by Cooper[4] in 1825, and by Cotton[5] in 1910, it was not until Codman[3] in 1934 that fractures of the shoulder were classified into four parts: the greater tuberosity, the lesser tuberosity, the head, and the shaft (Fig. 9-2). This introduced the modern approach to the treatment of the fractured shoulder. The principles of this classification continue to be used, and are the basis of Neer's[11] classification introduced in 1970 (Fig. 9-3). Codman pointed out that in the majority of instances the rotator cuff remained attached to the tuberosities and aided in molding the fragments together when manipulated. This was a very important observation. He also illustrated the important part played by the long head of the biceps in realigning the fragments when the shoulder was manipulated in full elevation, or in the "pivotal position." Neer's classification is based not on the level of the fracture or the mechanism of injury but on the presence or absence of displacement of one or more of the four major segments: the humeral head, shaft, and greater and lesser tuberosities. Displacement is defined as significant if it is greater than 1 cm or angulated more than 45°.

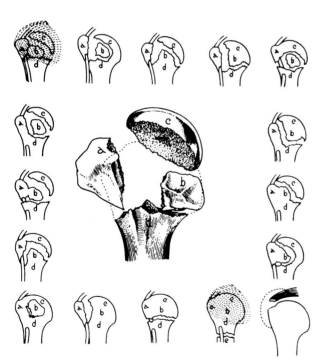

Fig. 9-2. Codman's (1934) classification of four part humeral head and neck fractures. (Codman EA: The Shoulder. Thomas Todd, Boston, 1934. © 1984 Robert E. Kreiger, Malabor, Florida)

DIAGNOSIS

An attempt should be made to determine the mechanism of injury. The history of previous injuries or surgical procedures to the involved shoulder and possible complicating medical problems are noted. A detailed history may alert the examining physician to the possibility of an otherwise frequently missed injury, such as posterior dislocation or fracture dislocation. A careful check of the surface anatomy is made and the involved upper extremity examined for any motor or sensory nerve or circulatory deficits. Injuries adjacent to the shoulder such as fractured ribs, pneumothorax, or subcutaneous emphysema are identified (see Fig. 9-40A).

TREATMENT

Decisions about treatment of a fractured shoulder should depend on a number of factors:

1. The age of the patient
2. The stability of the fracture
3. The number and displacement of fractured fragments

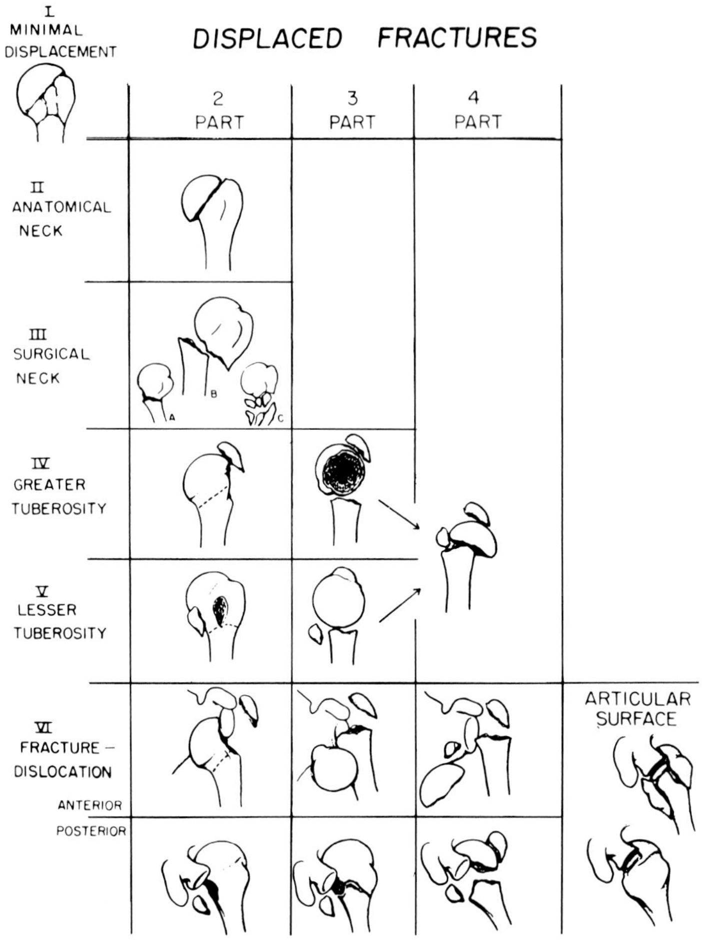

Fig. 9-3. Neer's (1970) classification of four part humeral head and neck fractures. (Neer CS: Displaced proximal humal fractures. Part I, Classification and evaluation. J Bone Joint Surg 52A:1077, 1970.)

4. The occupation of the patient and the projected functional demands on the shoulder

In arriving at a decision, one should remember that the shoulder will accept less than a perfect anatomical reduction for good function, as it is not a weight-bearing joint. Also, the rotator cuff covers the tuberosity fragments, thus presenting a smoother picture than one actually sees on the radiographs. If surgery is decided upon, the fragments should be of a size and consistency to accept internal fixation. Fortunately, the majority of shoulder fractures, despite degrees of comminution, are minimally displaced and satisfactory results, including early motion, may be obtained with nonoperative treatment.

Undisplaced Fractures

With an undisplaced or slightly displaced impacted fracture of the neck or tuberosity, a sling support to the arm and early pendulum motion are indicated, as Bigelow [1] advised in 1869:

3 essentials:

Pad in axilla
Elbow at side
Arm in sling

An ice cap to the shoulder every 2 hours reduces swelling and discomfort. The patient is encouraged to begin early gentle pendulum exercises in forward flexion. This puts little strain on the shoulder, lessens adhesion formation, and stimulates healing. Motion and function of the extremity are increased as tolerated. Physical therapy is usually not necessary, unless the patient has difficulty in initiating motion and use of the extremity. If progress is delayed, there may be a specific reason. In this case, an axillary view should be taken to be certain the patient does not have an unrecognized posterior dislocation or displacement of the shaft. This, unfortunately, has happened. Also, one should check closely to be certain that a tuberosity fracture is not displaced up under the acromion.

Displaced Fractures

ACCEPTABLE DISPLACEMENT: SUPPORT TO THE SHOULDER ONLY

Some displaced tuberosity and neck fractures may be acceptable without manipulation or open reduction. The decision for support only will depend on the occupation and age of the patient, and the risk of surgical interference. The tennis player or pitcher will require a more accurate reduction of a displaced

tuberosity fracture than a gardener or banker. As pointed out, although the radiographic appearance may be jagged and displaced, the fragments are, as a rule, covered with cuff attachments. Healing will occur if *not* disturbed by too early aggressive attempts to return motion or "strengthening exercises." In Figure 9-4, the position of this displaced fracture was acceptable after reduction of the shoulder. It was treated by support only. Complete healing and function of the arm were obtained. Although open reduction seemed indicated in Figure 9-5, the patient was treated with sling support only because of a chronic blood condition, and, surprisingly, won out with firm healing and a useful arm. Fortunately, the fragments were posterior and did not impinge under the acromion. The patient in Figure 9-6 demonstrates nature's determination to heal displaced fractures of the shoulder. The patient did not seek treatment initially, and came in sometime after his injury because of limited motion of his shoulder. Surgical reduction was discussed but the patient did not wish to undergo surgery, since his strength was good, he had little discomfort, and his shoulder answered his needs. He was satisfied to know why his shoulder motion was limited, and accepted it as such.

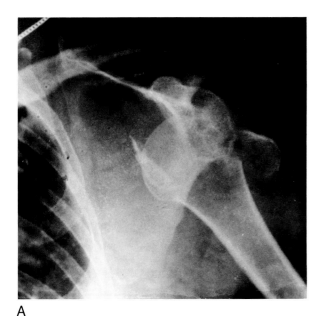

A

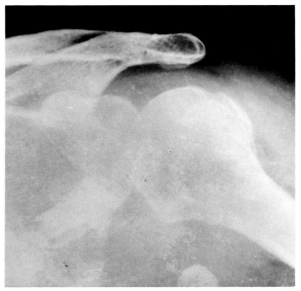

B

Fig. 9-4. (**A**) A displaced greater tuberosity fracture. (**B**) Fracture in acceptable position after reduction.

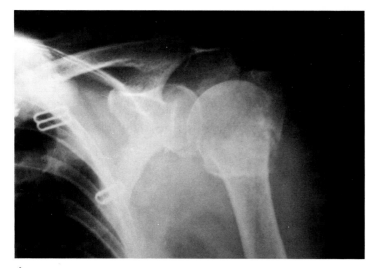

A

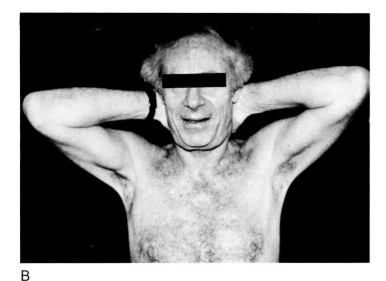

B

C

Fig. 9-5. (**A**) Although open reduction seemed indicated, because of a chronic blood condition the patient was given a chance to heal with closed treatment. (**B,C**) He recovered with a surprisingly excellent result.

MANIPULATION

When displacement is not acceptable, a trial with manipulation is a reasonable approach before deciding upon open reduction. Although manipulation may not result in perfect reduction, it may be acceptable. It is important to stress again that success with manipulative treatment *depends directly on the interest and care given by the treating surgeon.* Personal instruction is necessary. The patient's care and progress should not be delegated to someone else, particularly during the fragile early stage. Once the gluing stage

of callus formation has occurred, displacement of the fracture is less likely to occur and gentle pendulum motion may be begun. In some instances, plaster slab fixation of the shoulder girdle is indicated for comfort and stability (Fig. 9-7). However, the majority of patients may need only a sling support and careful instruction.

The alignment of the fracture in Figure 9-8 was improved by manipulation and progressed to mature healing, as did that in the patient in Figure 9-9. The 65-year-old patient in Figure 9-10 suffered a severely

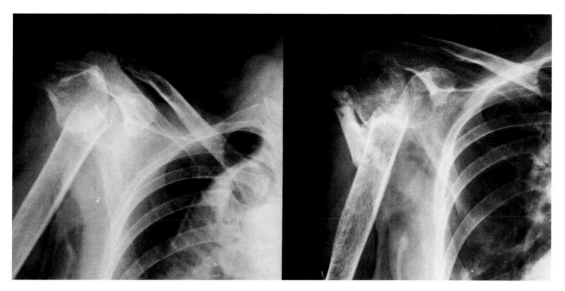

Fig. 9-6. Another example of nature's propensity to heal, if the arm is supported at the side of the body. Although manipulation or open reduction was indicated, the patient was satisfied leaving his arm as it was.

comminuted fracture of the right shoulder. We accepted the result of a closed manipulation. Her fracture healed and, although she had some restriction of motion, she was comfortable and pleased with her result. With the multiple small fragments, I doubt if we could have improved on her end result with open reduction.

Many multiple fractures of the shoulder girdle, as illustrated in Figure 9-10, will do well with manipulation and closed treatment. Success with this type of fracture depends on the surgeon taking care of the patient and *not* delegating their care to someone else. Also, therapy to regain motion and strength should be delayed until the fractured fragments have healed sufficiently. Early motion with little stress to the fractured fragments can be initiated by having the patient bend forward and gently carry out pendulum motion. Keep in mind, however, that manipulation of displaced comminuted fractures is frequently unsuccessful. Stableforth[16] failed to achieve satisfactory reduction in any of the 13 comminuted fractures manipulated in his series. Similarly, of five comminuted fractures manipulated by Young,[21] all subsequently redisplaced. Neer[12] also had a low success rate in his series. Although closed treatment of displaced comminuted fracture of the proximal humerus is advocated by some authors,[21] there seems to be a

growing body of literature reporting poor results from closed treatment. Clifford[2] reported that 46 percent of patients with three-part fractures treated by closed technique had a poor or unsatisfactory outcome. Svend-Hansen,[18] in a review of 49 patients with displaced proximal humeral fractures, reported a 61 percent incidence of unsatisfactory results or failures. It is important, therefore, to recognize when manipulation has failed to achieve satisfactory reduction so that open treatment may be undertaken, especially in the younger patient. It is also important to identify why manipulation was not successful. Was motion begun too early and too agressively?

OPEN REDUCTION

Isolated Two-Part Displaced Tuberosity Fractures

When displacement of the tuberosity impinges under the acromion, limiting abduction, open reduction is indicated. Anatomical reduction is specifically needed for those involved in sports such as tennis, basketball, throwing, or in occupations such as painters, carpenters, and plasterers as illustrated in Figure 9-11A,B,C; two screws can also be used (Fig. 9-11D,E).

The majority of tuberosity fractures can be ade-

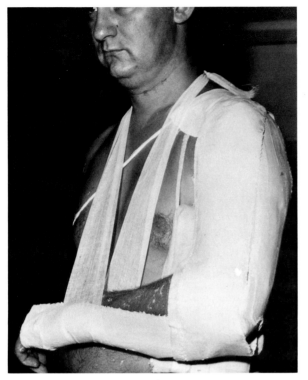

A

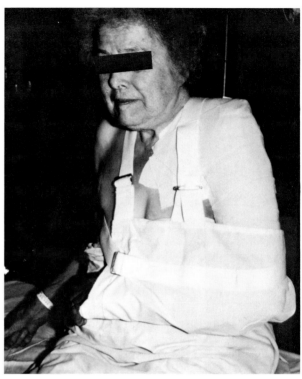

B

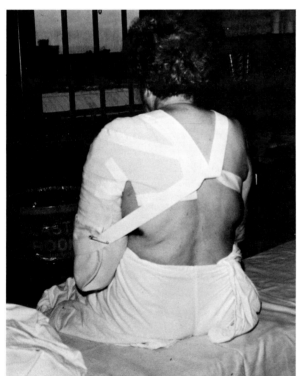

C

Fig. 9-7. Often the combination of plaster slabs (**A**) or slabs with a sling support (**B,C**) gives comfort and stability to the shoulder.

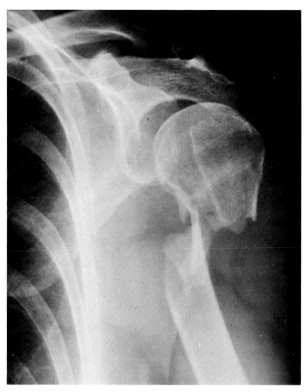

A

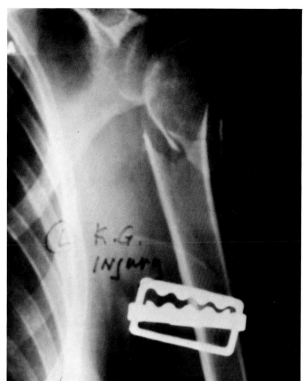

B

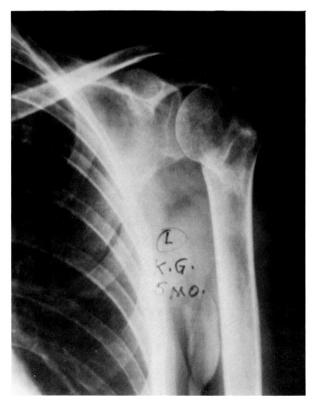

C

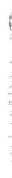

Fig. 9-8. (**A**) The alignment of this displaced fracture was improved by manipulation and treated with a simple sling support. (**B,C**) Although not perfectly reduced, the fracture progressed to mature healing and complete range of motion.

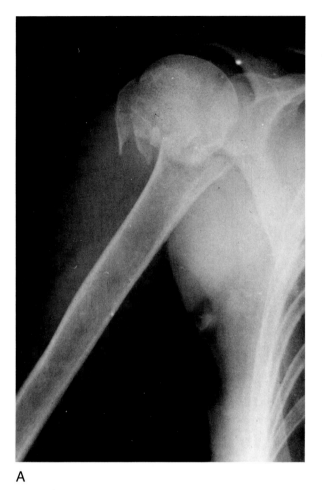

A

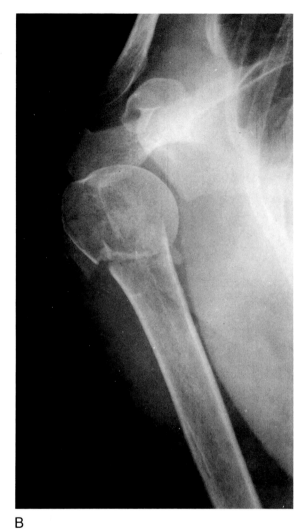

B

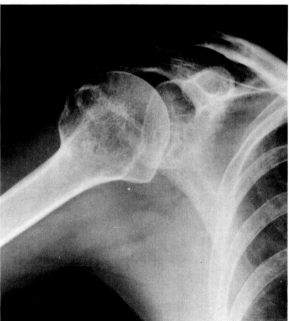

C

Fig. 9-9. (A–C) Another example of a displaced humeral neck fracture, improved by manipulation, which progressed to mature healing. We stress again that patients' shoulders should be allowed to heal before subjecting them to "therapy."

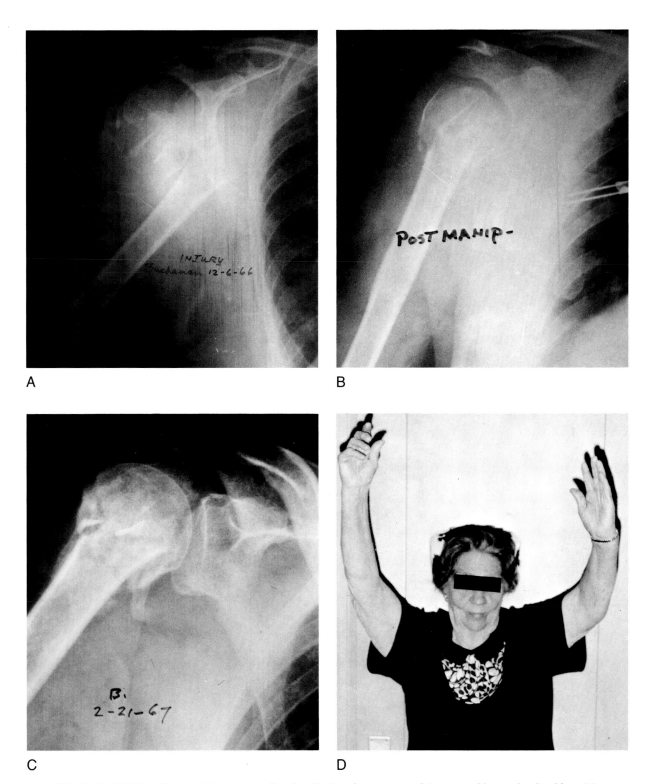

Fig. 9-10. (A) This 65-year-old patient suffered a displaced comminuted fracture of her right shoulder. (B) The fractured fragments were reduced by gently taking her arm in complete elevation, then down to her side. (C) Appearance 10 weeks after injury. (D) She was happy with her shoulder: she had a useful arm and minimal discomfort.

341

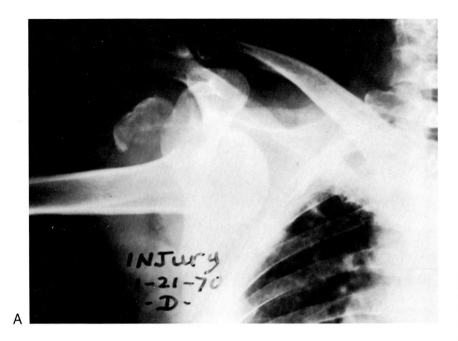

A

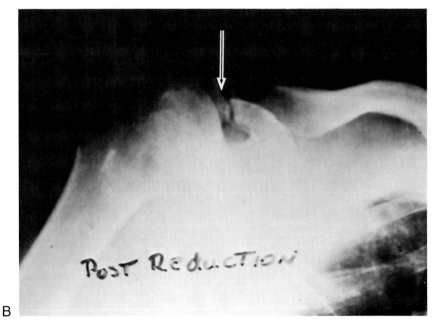

B

Fig. 9-11. (**A**) An anterior dislocation of the shoulder with a displaced fracture of the greater tuberosity in a laborer. (**B**) Following manipulation, the greater tuberosity (arrow) was displaced under the acromion. Such displacement can be easily missed initially. (*Figure continues.*)

quately exposed by an anterior deltoid muscle splitting incision without removing the deltoid from the clavicle or acromion (see Chap. 3). If additional exposure would be needed for nail and plate, the deltopec-toral approach should be used so that the incision can be extended down the arm. If the major position of the fracture is posterior, the Rockwood posterior approach is recommended (see Chap. 3).[14]

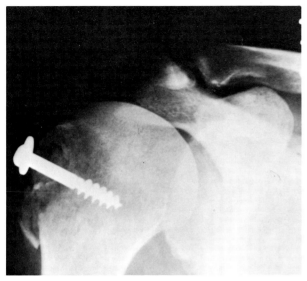

C

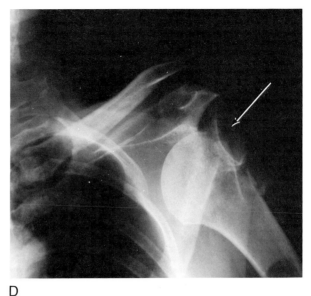

D

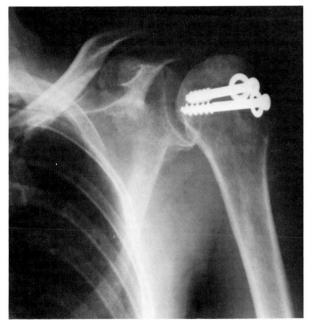

E

Fig. 9-11 *(Continued)*. (**C**) Open reduction with screw fixation was carried out. (**D**) Arrow points to displaced greater tuberosity in another fracture–dislocation. (**E**) Two-screw fixation was used to secure fixation.

Displaced Two-Part Fractures through the Surgical Neck (with Tuberosities and Head Intact)

This type of fracture may occur with dislocation of the humeral shaft and no displacement of the humeral head, or with displacement of the humeral head and no appreciable displacement of the humeral shaft (Fig. 9-12). Varying degrees of each can occur. An axillary view is necessary to give the degree and direction of displacement of the head or shaft. If an axillary view can not be taken, then the Y-lateral view would be helpful information. Again, we discourage the use of the transthoracic view, due to its poor detail and

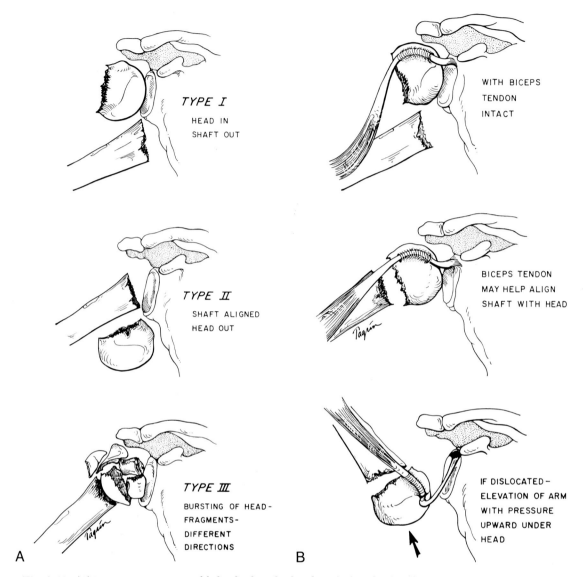

TYPE I
HEAD IN
SHAFT OUT

WITH BICEPS
TENDON
INTACT

TYPE II
SHAFT ALIGNED
HEAD OUT

BICEPS TENDON
MAY HELP ALIGN
SHAFT WITH HEAD

TYPE III
BURSTING OF HEAD-
FRAGMENTS-
DIFFERENT
DIRECTIONS

IF DISLOCATED-
ELEVATION OF ARM
WITH PRESSURE
UPWARD UNDER
HEAD

A   B

Fig. 9-12. (**A**) It is important to establish whether the head or shaft is displaced, as well as with comminuted fractures. (**B**) Visualizing that the long head of biceps tendon can be helpful in reducing displaced neck fractures.

unnecessary x-ray exposure. The long head of biceps may be very helpful in realigning the head and shaft. (Fig. 9-12B)

Surgical Technique. We have used with success the deltoid splitting approach for limited exposure of the head and neck, and for the insertion of a Rush rod, with minimal soft tissue exposure. In Figure 9-13, a deltoid splitting approach was used. The hu-

meral shaft had a long sharp end that was "shish-kebabed" into the head. This was stable and required no internal fixation. Rush rods can be inserted correctly and effectively through the deltoid splitting incision into the greater tuberosity and buried in the rotator cuff tendon for stability (Fig. 9-14). It is important that the rotator cuff is repaired over the rod. In Figure 9-15, the rods are incorrectly introduced

Fig. 9-13. (**A**) At surgery, the long, sharp distal fragment was shish-ke-babed into the head fragment. No metal fixation was necessary. (**B**) Natural healing and a strong arm resulted.

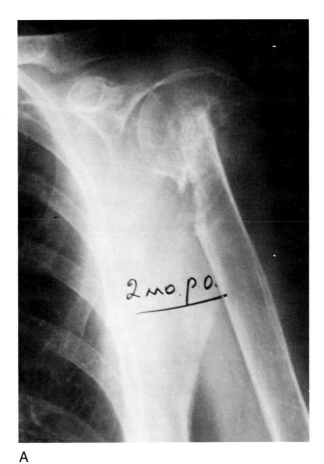

A

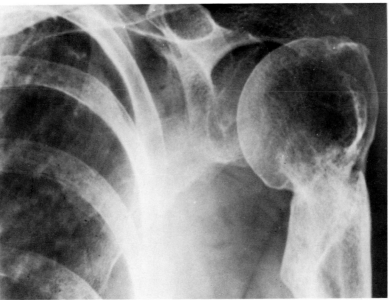

B

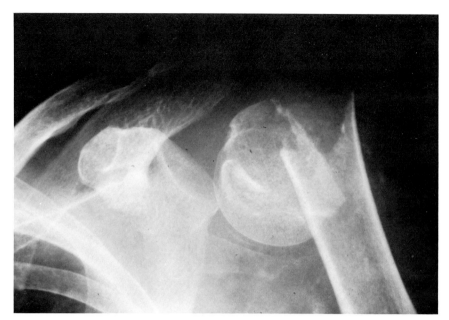

A

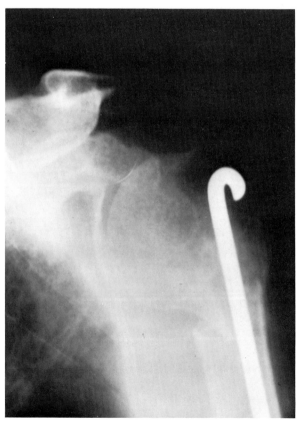

B

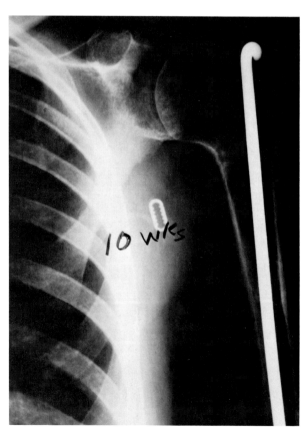

C

Fig. 9-14. Correct technique for insertion of Rush rod. **(A)** A displaced surgical neck fracture (left). **(B)** Correct application of a Rush rod through the grater tuberosity and *under* the rotator cuff. The rotator cuff should be sutured *over* the end of the rod for security. **(C)** Appearance 10 weeks later. (*Figure continues.*)

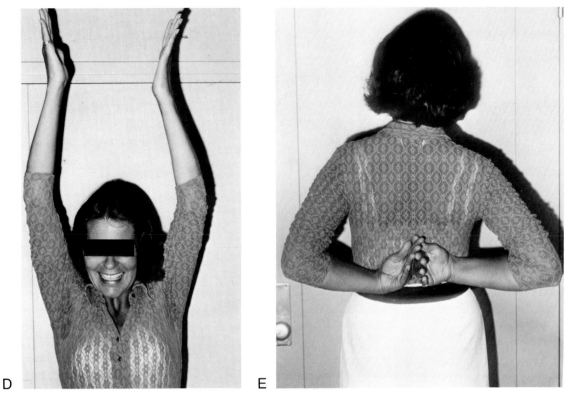

Fig. 9-14 (*Continued*). (**D,E**) End result (after removal of rod): complete healing, range of motion, and strength.

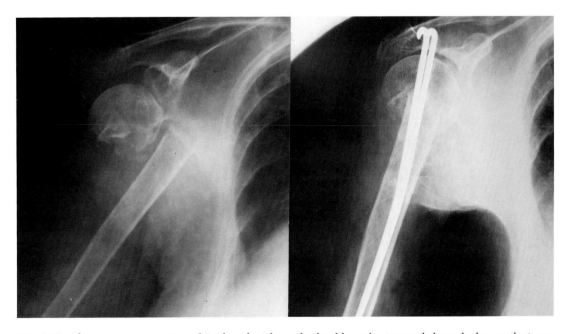

Fig. 9-15. The *incorrect* insertion of Rush rods. The rods should not be inserted through the cartilaginous dome of the humeral head.

through the cartilage of the humeral head rather than through the rotator cuff and tuberosity. Figure 9-16 A and B illustrate the Neer technique of using wire to secure the rod into the shaft. This is especially effective for nonunions. Two Rush rods with tension bands were used in this 72-year-old patient with non-union of 2 years' duration (Fig. 9-16C,D). On occasion, the Nicola procedure has been used to secure the humeral head.

Single Screw Fixation. A single compression screw can be used to great advantage in selected cases (Fig. 9-17). In introducing the screw, the drill hole must be made almost parallel to the axis of the shaft. Figure 9-18 illustrates the use of a long standard screw. The shoulder must be impacted to eliminate rotation. Be careful with screw fixation, because the fracture, although reduced, may be unstable for several weeks. Both of these patients healed and had good results.

Multiple Screws. Multiple screws (Fig. 9-19) can be used to stabilize principal fragments but should be used with caution, as the fixation is not strong. Nonabsorbable sutures through the major fragments may add support to the screws. Percutaneous fixation can be resorted to when indicated (Fig. 9-20) but, as demonstrated in Figure 9-21, may leave displaced fractures of the tuberosity unreduced.

Three-Part Fractures

DEFINITION AND TREATMENT

Three-part fractures are defined as those displaced fractures through the surgical neck accompanied by displacement of one of the tuberosities. The pull of the remaining attached rotator cuff causes severe rotational deformity of the proximal fragment, making closed reduction difficult to achieve and maintain.

Rosen[15] has recommended multiple Kirschner wire fixation and tension band wiring to obtain somewhat more rigid fixation while keeping soft tissue dissection to a minimum.

Use of the A-O T-plate or screw[10] (Figs. 9-22, 9-23), requires extensive soft tissue dissection and often fixation is difficult due to osteoporosis in the humeral head fragment. In a study of 27 multifragmented fractures of the proximal humerus, Sturzenegger et al.[17]

found gentle exploration and minimal osteosynthesis with a tension band wire or simple lag screw superior to plate fixation, with fewer complications and superior functional results. Prosthetic replacement is rarely indicated in three-part fractures, but may be considered in the elderly patient in whom stable fixation cannot be achieved at operation.[19]

POSTOPERATIVE TREATMENT

Passive assistive motions in the form of pendulum exercises should be started as soon as pain permits in fractures in which good fixation has been achieved. If fixation is tenuous, the arm should be immobilized in a sling and swathe for 2 to 3 weeks to allow the fracture to consolidate. Passive motion can then be started followed by graduated active exercises, usually at 6 weeks. Neer[12] has stressed the importance of the early recovery of external rotation in maximizing long-term functional results. Rehabilitation and recovery continue for several months. Continued gradual improvement in motion and strength for up to 2 years after surgery may be expected.

Four-Part Fractures

Displaced fractures of both tuberosities and the surgical neck are complicated by a high incidence of avascular necrosis of the humeral head. When the humeral head is a mere empty shell, with no tuberosity attachments to provide circulation, the chances of osteonecrosis occurring must be taken into consideration. The patient in Figure 9-24 presented with only a shell of humeral head at surgery. Consequently, a Neer[11,12] replacement prosthesis was carried out with attachment of the rotator cuff. When the upper shaft has been destroyed, bone grafting can be added to supplement the prosthesis (Fig. 9-24C). In Neer's series of 13 four-part fractures and fracture dislocations, the head was excised primarily five times and six of the remaining eight cases went on to late collapse. He found that the results of prosthetic replacement were superior to those of either closed or open reduction, with patients in the latter two groups showing uniformly poor results.

Sturzenegger et al.[17] reported a lower incidence of avascular necrosis, with 5 of 19 four-part fractures showing late collapse after open reduction, and only

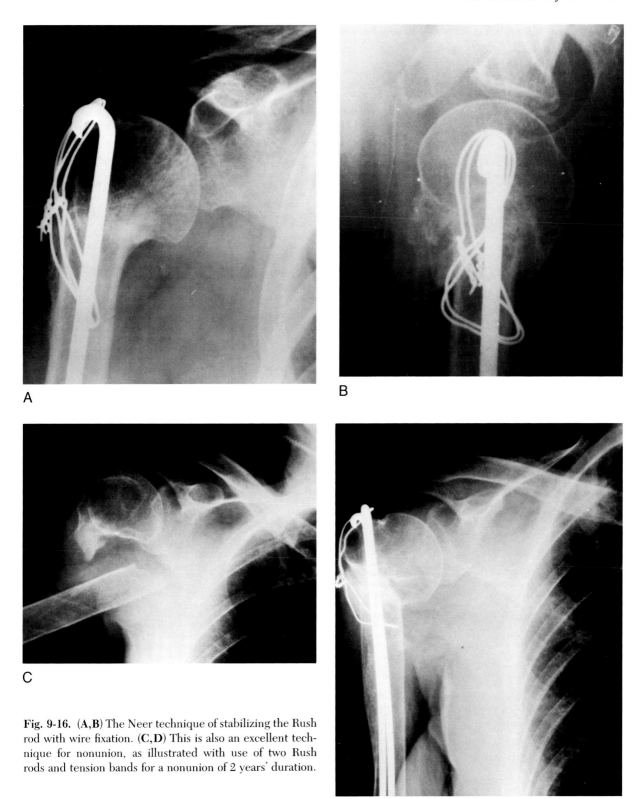

A

B

C

Fig. 9-16. (**A,B**) The Neer technique of stabilizing the Rush rod with wire fixation. (**C,D**) This is also an excellent technique for nonunion, as illustrated with use of two Rush rods and tension bands for a nonunion of 2 years' duration.

D

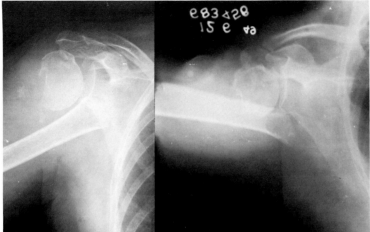

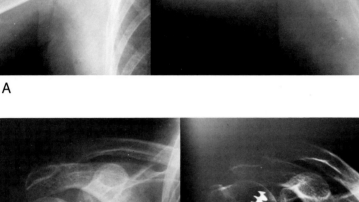

A

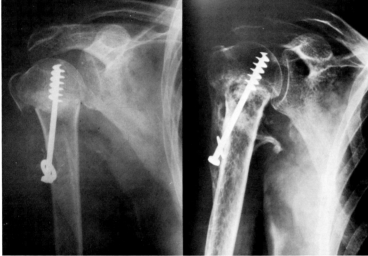

B

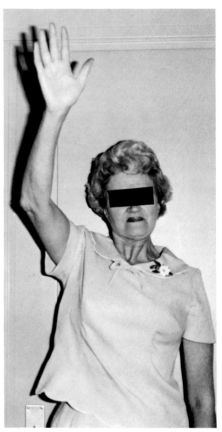

C

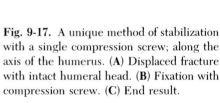

Fig. 9-17. A unique method of stabilization with a single compression screw; along the axis of the humerus. (**A**) Displaced fracture with intact humeral head. (**B**) Fixation with compression screw. (**C**) End result.

1 of these with late collapse after minimal osteosynthesis. Sixteen of 27 patients in their series achieved good or excellent results, leading the authors to recommend internal fixation for these injuries. Lee and Hansen [9] found no incidence of late collapse in 19 patients with displaced four-part fracture or fracture dislocation. We believe that although a majority of humeral heads in this injury develop avascular necrosis, some of the humeral heads will revascularize by creeping substitution. Collapse is less likely to occur because of the non-weight-bearing nature of the joint, and the rapid revascularization that takes place.

Another alternative to replacement prosthesis, especially if the patient has had previous surgery with wound complications, is the Laurence Jones [7] procedure. The patient in Figure 9-25 is an excellent example of the Laurence Jones procedure. It was performed in 1950, on her right shoulder, before the advent of shoulder replacement prostheses. She has a strong arm and excellent range of motion.

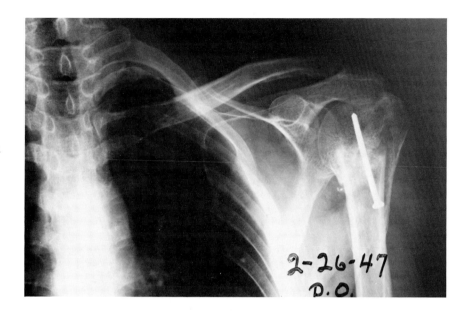

Fig. 9-18. Stabilization with a long standard screw.

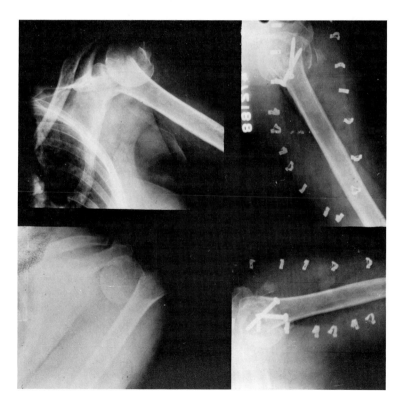

Fig. 9-19. Fixation with multiple screws.

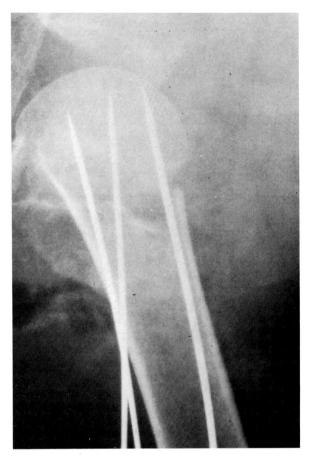

Fig. 9-20. Percutaneous fixation with 3/32 inch Steinmann pins.

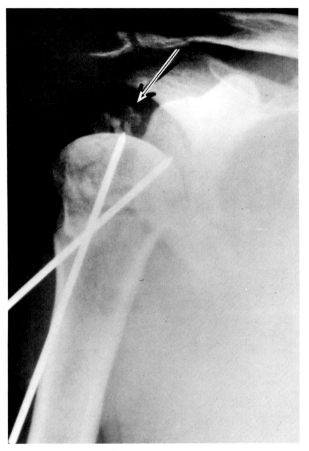

Fig. 9-21. The disadvantage of percutaneous pin is its inability to secure displaced fragments (arrow).

COMPLICATIONS

Decreased Motion

The most common complication of shoulder fracture is loss of function through restriction of motion from posttraumatic and/or postoperative adhesions. The key to functional recovery, as advocated by Codman[3] and Roberts,[13] is early motion, as soon as fracture stability permits, and the dedication of the patient and physician to a rehabilitation program that may continue over a period of several months. Forced manipulation is rarely indicated in these patients because of the risk of refracture through osteoporotic bone. Reflex sympathetic dystrophy may occur following shoulder fracture; this is characterized by dysesthesia, edema, and loss of motion in the entire upper extremity. This distressing complication occurs with overprotection of the extremity and can best be prevented by early use and function of the hand and elbow, even though motion of the shoulder is restricted.

Malunion

Malunions of displaced greater tuberosity fractures may cause pain and restriction of elevation in forward flexion and abduction. Surgical mobilization and distal advancement of the greater tuberosity may require extensive soft tissue dissection of the retracted rotators. Unfortunately, resection of the offending prominent bone fragments or tuberosities is not always asso-

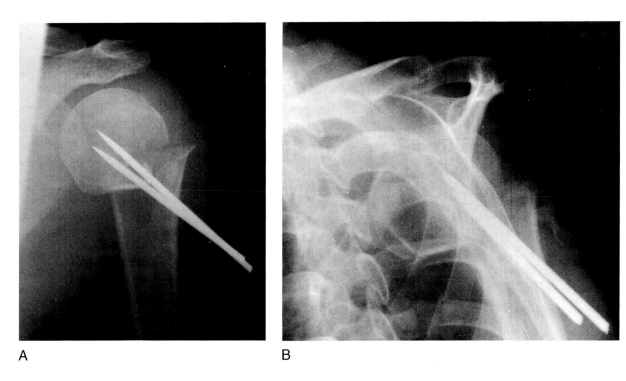

A

B

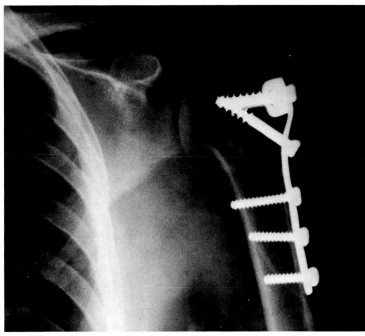

C

Fig. 9-22. (**A**) Displaced fracture with unstable pin fixation. (**B**) Progressive displacement. (**C**) Fixation with plate and screw.

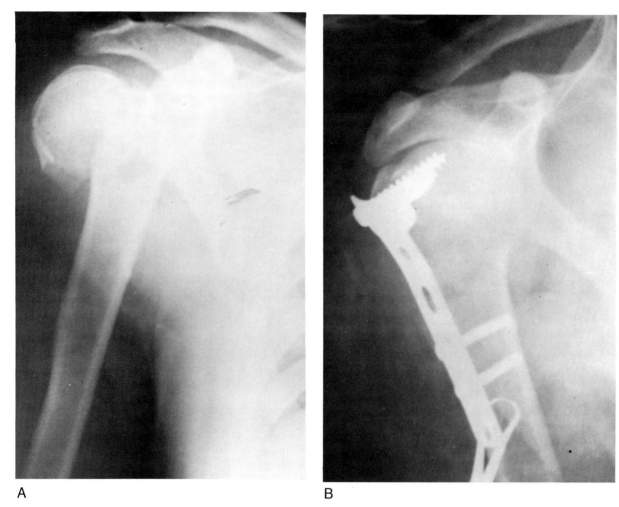

A   B

Fig. 9-23. (A) Displaced neck and tuberosity fracture. **(B)** Fracture stabilized with plate and screws. Although the screw was high, the end result was satisfactory.

ciated with rapid complete relief of pain due to chronic adhesions and secondary scar tissue.

In some instances, prosthetic replacement may be necessary; however, if chronic adhesions are present, discomfort and loss of motion may continue.

Shoulder arthrodesis for painful malunions and posttraumatic arthritis may be indicated in some individuals in whom the problem is associated with heavy lifting.

As noted the Laurence Jones procedure (Fig. 9-25) may be considered when a prosthesis cannot be used and arthrodesis is not possible. The presence of chronic adhesions, however, may be a cause of postoperative limited shoulder motion and pain, which occur with shoulder prosthesis.

Nonunions

Nonunions of surgical neck fractures are not rare and may be due to too early motion and too much traction, interposition of soft tissue (usually the biceps tendon), failure of fixation, or infection. Because the bone is usually osteoporotic, plate fixation is difficult. Tension band wiring with rush rod (Fig. 9-16A,B) as recommended by Neer, or Kirschner wire fixation

Fig. 9-24. With only a shell of humeral head and multiple fragments, the procedure of choice is a Neer replacement prosthesis. (**A**) The severely comminuted fracture. (**B**) The Neer replacement prosthesis, with attachment of the rotator cuff to the shaft. (**C**) Bone graft may be used to replace loss of bone stock of the proximal humerus, as recommended by Neer.

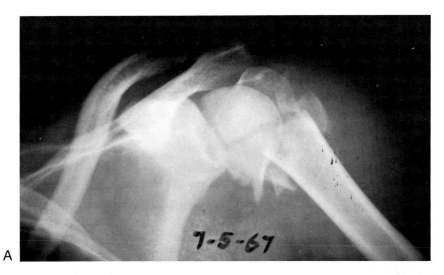

A

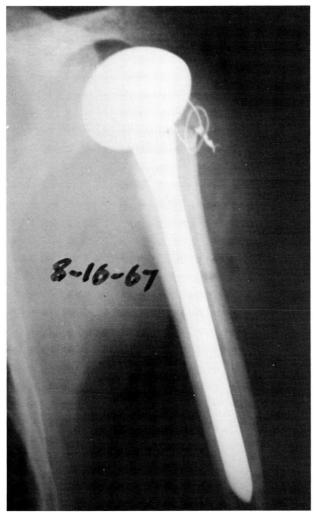

B

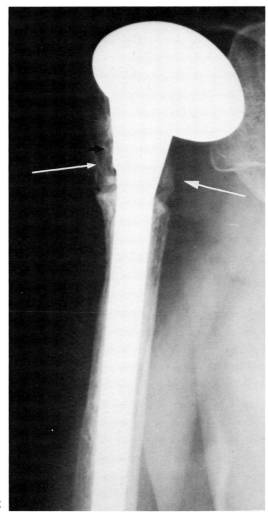

C

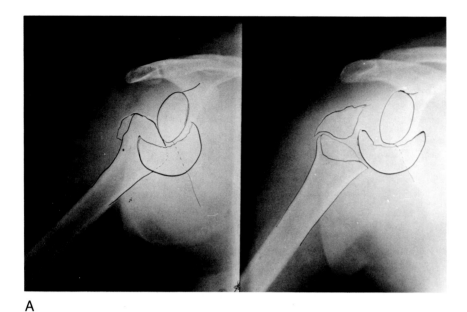

A

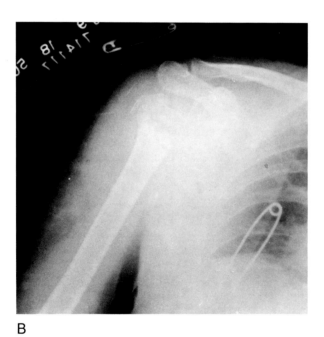

B

Fig. 9-25. A good back-up is the Jones procedure in cases with previous sepsis or lack of bony stock. **(A)** Comminuted fracture of the right shoulder with only a shell of head cartilage. This was in 1950, before the Neer prosthesis was available. **(B)** Postoperative Jones procedure resecting the cartilaginous head cap and reattaching the rotator cuff to the humeral shaft. (*Figure continues.*)

in combination with bone grafting, has been used with success. In Figure 9-16C, two Rush rods are used with tension band wiring in a 72-year-old woman with a 2 year history of nonunion. Complete healing was achieved.

Osteonecrosis

Osteonecrosis is a frequent complication of four part-fracture and fracture dislocations and may lead to late collapse of the humeral head.[9] Hemiarthro-

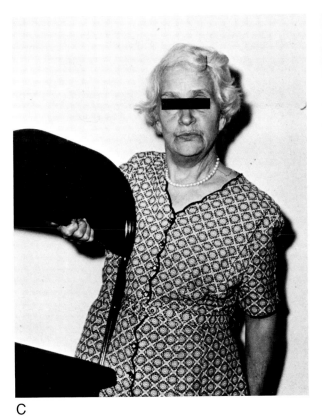

C

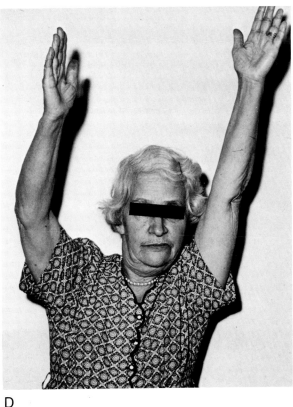

D

Fig. 9-25 (*Continued*). (**C,D**) A very good functional result, with ability to lift a heavy chair and good elevation. This patient has been happy with her result.

plasty, or total shoulder replacement, is indicated in patients with painful degenerative arthritis secondary to the resulting joint incongruity.

Brachial Plexus Injury

Although this is an uncommon incision it should be identified. Stableforth [16] reported an incidence of 6.1% in 81 patients with four-part fractures, also, a 4.9% incidence of vascular injury.

Infection

See Chapter 18 for a discussion of shoulder infections.

REFERENCES

1. Bigelow HJ: A Memoir of Henry Jacob Bigelow. Little Brown, Boston, 1900
2. Clifford PC: Fractures of the neck of the humerus; a review of the late results. Injury 12:91, 1980
3. Codman EA: The Shoulder. Thomas Todd, Boston, 1934
4. Cooper A: A Treatise in Dislocations and Fractures of the Joints. HC Carey & L Lea, Philadelphia, 1825
5. Cotton FJ: Dislocations and Joint Fractures. W B Saunders, Philadelphia, 1910
6. Hippocrates: The Genuine Works of Hippocrates. Williams & Wilkins, Baltimore, 1939
7. Jones L: The shoulder joint. Observations on the anatomy and physiology with analysis of reconstructive operation following extensive injury. Surg Gynecol Obstet 75:433, 1942

8. Laing PG: The arterial supply of the adult humerus. J Bone Joint Surg 38A:1105, 1956

9. Lee CK, Hansen HR: Post traumatic avascular necrosis of the humeral head in displaced proximal humeral fractures. J Trauma 21:788, 1981

10. Miller ME, Allogower M, Willenger, H: Manual of Internal Fixation. Springer-Verlag, New York, 1970

11. Neer CS: Displaced proximal humeral fractures. Part I. Classification and evaluation. J Bone Joint Surg 52A:1077, 1970

12. Neer CS: Displaced proximal humeral fractures, Part II. Treatment of four part and three part displacement. J Bone Joint Surg 52A:1090, 1970

13. Roberts SM: Fractures of the upper end of the humerus. An end result study which shows the advantage of early active motion. JAMA 98:367, 1932

14. Rockwood CA, Green DP (ed) Fractures, 2nd ed. JB Lippincott Philadelphia, 1984

15. Rosen H: Tension band wiring for fracture dislocation of the shoulder. Proceedings of the 12th Congress of the International Society of Orthopaedic Surgery and Traumatology, Tel Aviv, October 9–12, 1972, pp. 939–941. Exerpta Medica, Amsterdam.

16. Stableforth PG: Four part fractures of the neck of the humerus. J Bone Joint Surg 66B:104, 1984

17. Sturzenugger M, Ferraro E, Jakob RP: Results of surgical treatment of multifragmented fractures of the humeral head. Arch Orthop Trauma Surg 100:249, 1982

18. Svend-Hansen H: Displaced proximal humeral fractures: a review of 49 patients. Acta Orthop Scand 45:359, 1974

19. Tanner MW, Cofield RH: Prosthetic arthroplasty for fracture and fracture dislocation of the proximal humerus. Clin Orthop Rel Res 179:116, 1983

20. Whitson TB: Fractures of the surgical neck of the humerus. A study in reduction. J Bone Joint Surg 36B:423, 1954

21. Young TB, Wallace WA: Conservative treatment of fractures and fracture dislocation of the upper end of the humerus. J Bone Joint Surg 67B:373, 1985

The Clavicle

Carter R. Rowe

ANATOMY

Several anatomic characteristics of the clavicle should be noted:

1. The clavicle is unusual in being the only long bone to ossify by intramembranous process. It is the first bone in the body to ossify (fifth week of fetal life).
2. It has only one epiphysis, which is situated on the medial end of the clavicle.
3. The clavicle in the adult is dense, honeycombed, and lacks a true, well-defined medullary cavity. Gardner [1] describes the bone of the clavicle as "thick compacta." It is much more difficult to pass an intermedullary pin through the clavicle than one would expect.
4. The clavicle assumes the shape of an S-curve (Fig. 9-26) that is more curved in male than in female patients due to the increased strength of its muscle attachments. The straight middle third connects the outer and medial curves of the clavicle. This must be carefully evaluated when intramedullary fixation is used.
5. The clavicle is well supplied with blood and muscle attachments, which account for its marked ability to heal and its low incidence of nonunion.
6. The subclavian and axillary vessels and the nerves of the brachial plexus lie directly beneath the middle third of the clavicle. Although it provides a protection for the major vessels and nerves, injuries of the clavicle may also involve these structures.

INJURIES

The most common site of fracture of the clavicle is the middle third (82 percent). Forty-four percent of these occurred at the junction of the middle and outer thirds [7] (see Fig. 9-38). This is consistent with the functional anatomy of the clavicle, as the distal and proximal ends of the clavicle are secured firmly by strong ligaments and muscle attachments whereas the central section is relatively free of protective attachments. Twelve percent involved the outer end of the clavicle.

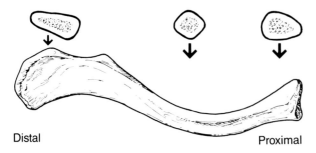

Distal   Proximal

Fig. 9-26. The bone of the clavicle is dense "thick compacta" without a well-defined medullary canal. It assumes an S-curve, more curved in male than in female patients.

the clavicle is also necessary to show the degree of inferior displacement of the fragments (Fig. 9-27).

CLINICAL EXAMINATION

The lungs should be checked by auscultation of the anterior and posterior chest. A careful examination of the extremities for nerve or vascular injury should also be carried out.

ROENTGENOGRAPHIC EXAMINATION

Because a fracture of the clavicle is caused by an appreciable direct or indirect blow to the shoulder, the fractured clavicle may be only one of the patient's shoulder injuries. One should *never* accept a small "postage stamp" film of a fractured clavicle, as other injuries may be missed. The radiograph requisition should read: "anterior posterior view of the clavicle on a large film to include the upper third of the humerus, the shoulder girdle, and the lung field." The fractured scapula and the subcutaneous emphysema of the lateral chest wall have been missed on a small film (see section on the scapula). A oblique view of

CLASSIFICATION

1. Undisplaced: The periosteal sleeve is intact and the fracture relatively stable
2. Displaced
   a. Mid-third (upward displacement) (see Fig. 9-34A)
   b. Distal (lateral) third (see Fig. 9-32)
   c. Inner third (rare)
3. Comminuted (Fig. 9-28A)
4. Involving the acromioclavicular joint (see Fig. 9-32)

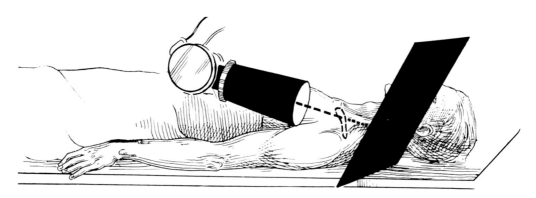

Fig. 9-27. An oblique view is often indicated to note the degree of inferior displacement of fragments. (Cave EF: Fractures and Other Injuries. Year Book Medical Publishers, Chicago, 1958.)

TREATMENT

Closed Reduction

The majority of middle third clavicular fractures should respond to closed treatment. This is supported by clinical experience.[4,8] The incidence of nonunion following closed treatment in our series was 0.8 percent and 3.7 percent after open treatment.[8] Neer reported 0.1 percent nonunion following closed treatment in 2,235 middle third fractures of the clavicle and 4.6 percent after open treatment.[4]

Support

The usual types of support for fractures of the middle third of the clavicle are illustrated in Figure 9-29A and B. In children, the clavicle heals rapidly and remodels so completely that very little treatment is needed, other than instructions to the parents to lift the child by the waist rather than by the arms or shoulders. Although the period of discomfort in children is very short, some children seem to feel better with a support of a hank of soft wool twisted in the form of a figure-of-eight dressing. In an adult with a stable, or not too badly displaced fracture of the midclavicle, perhaps the less binding and strapping used, the more comfortable the patient may be. A sling and the simple advice to "hold your shoulders back" may be sufficient. An ice cap applied just above or below the clavicle may eliminate much of the early "throbbing" discomfort. The use of at least three large pillows when in bed, semisitting, or lying completely flat, is recommended.

However, effective support to the shoulder is necessary in the adult with an unstable, displaced, or comminuted fracture. The typical displacement of a middle third fracture is upward displacement of the proximal fragment, due to the pull of the sternocleidomastoid muscle, and downward displacement of the distal fragment, due to the weight of the extremity (Fig. 9-28B). To reduce the fracture or correct its deformity, the arm and shoulder must be elevated and extended. This can be effectively obtained with the patients standing or sitting and asked to "hold the shoulder back and up."

The clavicular figure-of-eight is commonly used. However, care must be taken in its application. The figure-of-eight apparatus *can increase the deformity* if it is not properly applied. For instance, if the shoulder strap is allowed to slip laterally, it will further depress the lateral fragment thereby increasing the deformity, as illustrated in Figure 9-28. On admission to the emergency ward, this patient's fracture showed only slight displacement (Fig. 9-28A); after application of the figure-of-eight, the fracture was badly displaced downward due to the depression on the lateral fragment by the figure-of-eight (Fig. 9-28B). This was corrected by a cross-strap anteriorly to secure the figure-of-eight medially, thus eliminating its lateral displacement (Fig. 9-28C–E). In Figure 9-30A and B, the figure-of-eight has been correctly applied. An anterior cross-strap would be a safe precaution. It is most important that the figure-of-eight be checked several times a week for maintenance of reduction and for the presence of axillary irritation. Any numbness or tingling of the extremity should be reported immediately. The patient should be instructed to sleep semisitting for at least a week or so, preferably with a pillow between the shoulder blades. This is not always a comfortable arrangement for many adults, especially if they are restless sleepers.

A very effective and comfortable method of treatment of a displaced fracture is the modified half-shoulder spica, which has proved most helpful and satisfactory in our hospital (Fig. 9-31). This is applied with the patient sitting or lying supine on a metal strut, with the shoulders extended *backwards and upwards*. The plaster is carefully molded between the scapulae posteriorly and upward along the pectoralis major muscle anteriorly, thus supporting the shoulder upward and backward. One should carefully mold this and maintain gentle pressure with the hands until the plaster has set. The cast is cut at the level of the deltoid muscle insertion, allowing flexion and extension of the elbow. The young lady in Figure 9-31B wore this modified cast for a month in comfort, attended school, and kept up with her school work and activities. She entered the office to have the spica removed. The clavicle was stable enough to allow us to remove the spica at this time with excellent reduction. Clothing can be worn over the spica, allowing the patients to return safely to many of their usual activities. A special benefit of the shoulder spica is

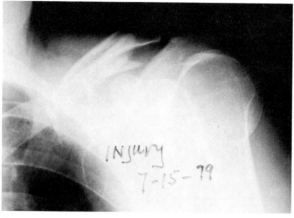

A

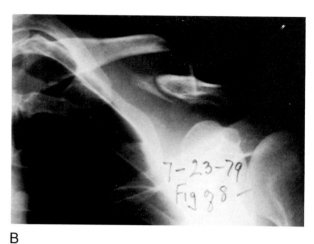

B

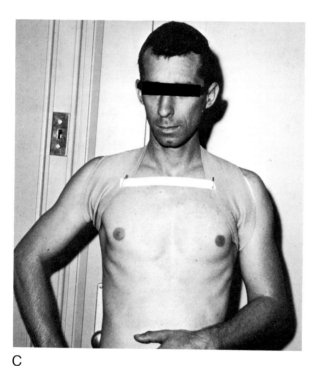

C

Fig. 9-28. **(A)** Appearance on admission to the emergency ward before application of figure-of-eight support. **(B)** After improper application of figure-of-eight support with depression of the distal fragment. **(C)** Improved position of fragments with correction of the figure-of-eight support. (*Figure continues.*)

that the patient is much more comfortable at night than with a clavicular cross or a figure-of-eight; also, it does not have to be adjusted or changed prior to removal. Rockwood also recommends a shoulder spica but includes both shoulders.[6] With careful molding of the half spica, we have not found it necessary to include both shoulders.

Fractures of the Outer Third of the Clavicle

Clavicular fractures of the distal clavicle, although less common, heal more slowly. Neer has called attention to this fracture and the importance of its two classifications.[5] In type I, the fracture is stable, the

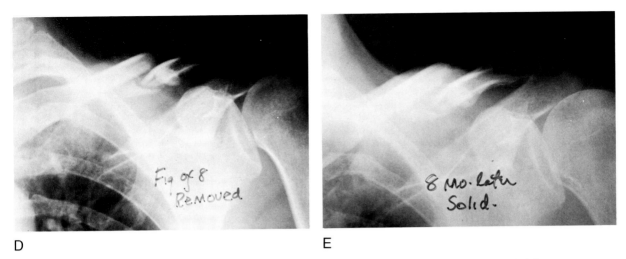

Fig. 9-28 (*Continued*). (**D**) Advancement of support medially with cross webbing. (**E**) Healed fracture.

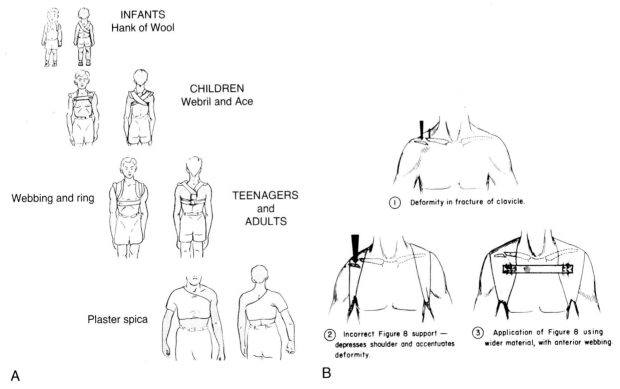

Fig. 9-29. (**A**) The usual types of supports for the clavicle. (**B**) With figure-of-eight supports, use anterior webbing to keep the support from slipping laterally and displacing the fracture.

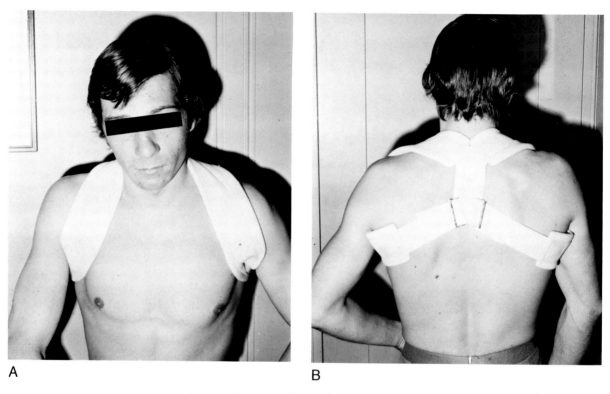

A   B

Fig. 9-30. **(A,B)** Example of a properly applied figure-of-eight support with the straps mesially placed.

coracoclavicular ligaments to the clavicle remain intact, and the fracture heals promptly. In type II, the coracoclavicular ligaments remain attached to the distal fragment and are detached from the medial segment, allowing upward displacement of the proximal fragment. In type II, it is very difficult to eliminate motion at the fracture site with conservative treatment, and the rate of nonunion of this type is higher. In fact, Neer states that this fracture accounted for one-half of the ununited clavicle fractures treated by closed methods in his series. In Figure 9-32, the inferior cortex remained intact with the coracoclavicular ligament, although the fracture involved the acromioclavicular joint. The fracture was openly reduced with circular sutures that restored the acromioclavicular joint and allowed good reduction of the fracture.

COMPLICATIONS OF CLOSED TREATMENT

Malunion

Failure to obtain accurate anatomical reduction with closed treatment is common. Healing may take place with more prominence under the skin than one would wish. However, in time, the prominence of the callus tends to become less. If the prominence remains disturbing, it can be removed by a fairly simple operation later, rather than carrying out a complete open reduction initially. Two patients seen by us with middle third fractures of the clavicle had excess callus formation at the fracture site with later

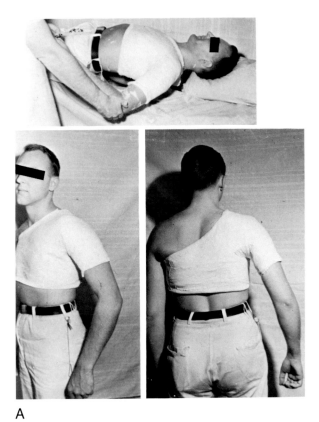

Fig. 9-31. **(A)** The half shoulder spica for comminuted fracture of the clavicle in the adult. The plaster is carefully molded anteriorly and posteriorly to keep the shoulder up and back. **(B)** This young lady has worn the shoulder support for a month, and has attended school with comfort and security. Note that her right shoulder has been maintained elevated and extended.

A

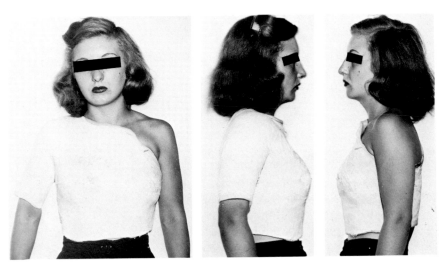

B

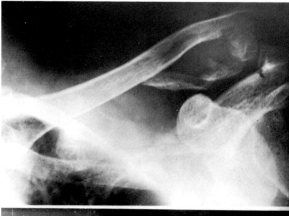

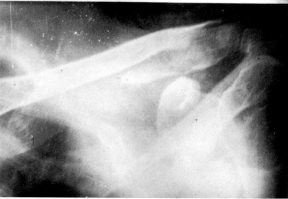

Fig. 9-32. Note that the inferior cortex remained attached to the coracoclavicular ligaments, and that the acromioclavicular joint is involved. Open reduction restored the acromioclavicular joint, with good reduction of the fracture.

neurovascular complications. Both of these were relieved by excision of the offending callus. No major vascular complications occurred in our series of closed or operative treatment.

Delayed Union

This may occur particularly with fractures of the outer third of the clavicle and, at times, with displaced middle third fractures. An interesting case in point is illustrated in Figure 9-33. Had this boy's admission to the hospital for bone grafting in February not been delayed by bronchial pneumonia, he would have been operated on for nonunion. In May we admitted him for bone grafting, and found to our surprise, on preoperative films, that his "nonunion" had completely

healed. Nature had performed an excellent bone grafting!

Nonunion

As pointed out, the incidence of nonunion is very low: 0.1 percent in Neer's series and 0.8 percent in our series. Nonunion following open reduction occurred in 4.6 percent in Neer's series and 3.7 percent in our series. These figures, however, came from the 1960s or 1970s. With improved techniques for internal fixation, the incidence of nonunion following open reduction should be lower. We have not found electrical stimulation for nonunion of the clavicle effective. Perhaps if we give nature more time, some of the "nonunions," at least in younger patients, would heal without surgery. Jupiter and Leffert's recent study of 23 nonunions treated at the Massachusetts General Hospital,[2] revealed that 87 percent were located in the middle third of the clavicle and 13 percent in the outer third. Sixteen of the 19 nonunions were treated with dynamic compression contoured plate fixation, to the superior surface of the clavicle in 13 and the inferior surface in 3. Iliac bone grafts were used in 13 cases. Surgery was successful in 89.4 percent. Failures were due to inadequate skeletal fixation.

Open Reduction

INDICATIONS

1. *Marked displacement* and angulation of the bone ends that cannot be reduced by closed methods, and may perforate the skin or damage the subclavian structures, are indications for open reduction.

2. Establish which cases are symptomatic nonunions. Although there is no definite definition of "nonunion" or "delayed union," there comes a time when open reduction may be considered for the fractured clavicle that has not healed.

TECHNIQUES

The two most commonly used methods of open reduction are onlay tubular plate and screws, and intramedullary pin fixation.

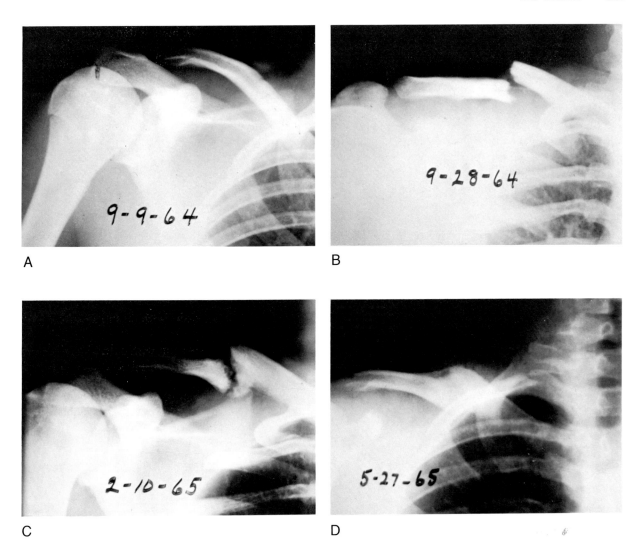

Fig. 9-33. (A) An undisplaced midclavicular fracture in a 17-year-old boy (**B**) who fell and completed the fracture 19 days later. (**C**) When seen again he had what appeared clinically as a painful nonunion. There was free painful motion. We arranged admission for a nonunion, but because of pneumonia, surgery was cancelled in February. (**D**) When he was seen in May, nature had done a better job than we might have performed.

Onlay Tubular Plate Fixation

With improvement in plate design and technique during the past 10 years, this would be the method of choice for open reduction of the clavicle, using the thin tubular plate and smaller than standard screws.

Position of the Patient. The patient is placed in a slightly semisitting position with a folded blanket or air bag beneath the shoulder. The entire extremity is prepped and draped surgically.

Exposure of the Fracture. An 8 cm incision is made just above or just below the clavicle, but not directly on the clavicle. Extreme care must be taken in exposing displaced fragments. Dissection should be subperiosteal to avoid injury to the vessels and nerves. Selected tubular plates and screws should be available that contour to the round surface of the clavicle. In the case of nonunion, bone may be added superiorly or posteriorly, but not inferiorly, to avoid contact with the vessels or nerves of the brachial area. The plate should be left in situ until union is established radiographically. This may take 10 to 12 weeks. During this time, the patient should be cautioned to avoid any type of excessive use of the arm or abuse of the shoulder. A protective sling or modified shoulder spica would be indicated for the first 3 weeks. The plate and screws can be removed through the same incision at a later date. Figure 9-34 illustrates the use of a tubular plate with precise reduction and fixation in a concert violinist. She has had an excellent result, with full use of her dominant right arm.

Intramedullary Fixation

This technique was more popular in the 1960s than it is now. It is now used more specifically for outer third fractures of the clavicle. There are, however, some considerations the uninitiated surgeon should be aware of:

1. It is difficult to introduce an intramedullary pin through the clavicle due to the absence of a true medullary space. The bone is dense and very difficult to perforate.
2. The surgeon should be aware of the curvature of the clavicle. The pin should be introduced to take advantage of the straight middle third of the clavicle; take care *not to perforate the medial cortex.* If the medial cortex is not perforated, the pin will *not* migrate into the body.

The surgeon must make a choice of the type of pin to use. The pin should be large enough to avoid bending or breakage. A smooth pin is stronger than a threaded pin, and is also easier to remove if it becomes bent or broken. Surgeons differ as in their technique; some prefer Knowles or Simmons pins. The author's preference for intramedullary pinning is as follows (Fig. 9-35):

1. Skin incision is made with a subperiosteal approach.
2. A 3/32 inch Kirschner pin with a drill tip is passed retrograde through the distal fragment and out through the skin.
3. Since the bone of the distal clavicle is dense, the drill tip is helpful. The acromioclavicular joint should be avoided.

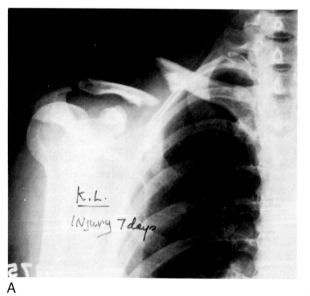

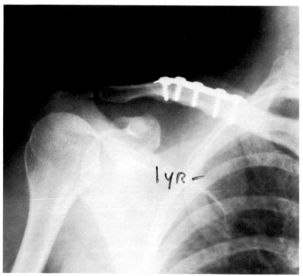

A   B

Fig. 9-34. (A) A badly displaced midclavicular fracture piercing the skin in a concert violinist. **(B)** Anatomic reduction and union were obtained with a tubular plate. The screws and plate were removed at 1 year. She has complete function of her dominant right shoulder.

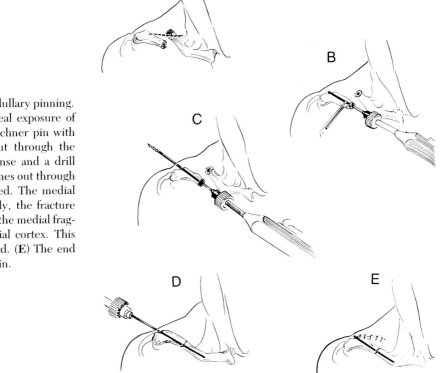

Fig. 9-35. Technique of intramedullary pinning. (**A**) Skin incision and subperiosteal exposure of the fracture (**B**) A 3/32 inch Kirschner pin with drill tip is passed retrograde out through the distal fragment. The bone is dense and a drill tip is needed. (**C**) The drill tip comes out through the skin. (**D**) The drill is removed. The medial end of the pin is cut off obliquely, the fracture reduced, and the pin passed into the medial fragment, but *not* through the medial cortex. This prevents it from migrating inward. (**E**) The end of the pin is cut off below the skin.

4. The drill is then removed. The medial end of the pin should be cut off obliquely, to facilitate its passage into the proximal clavicle. The fracture is reduced anatomically and the drill is attached to the distal end of the pin.

5. The pin is then drilled into the proximal fragment, as far as it will go, *but not through the cortex.* The cortex will limit the inner passage of the pin, making medial migration of the pin impossible. Its only migration would be outward. It is emphasized again that intramedullary drilling of the clavicle is difficult. The drilled tip of the pin assists in drilling through the dense distal fragment. Passage of the pin into the proximal fragment is less difficult. It should be done carefully until the medial cortex is reached. The protruding end of the pin is then cut off well below the skin posteriorly. We have not found it necessary to bend the end of the pin. An example of correct intramedullary pinning of a midclavicular fracture is illustrated in Figure 9-36. Figure 9-37 shows examples of poor fixation technique.

POSTOPERATIVE CARE

The shoulder is immobilized by means of a figure-of-eight sling or a modified shoulder spica. The patient should be specifically cautioned *not* to elevate the arm or hand above the horizontal until union is firm. Excessive use of the shoulder in elevation or abduction may encourage outward migration of the pin, or possible bending of the pin. The pin is usually removed 6 to 8 weeks after surgery, or after the clavicle shows healing on radiographs.

COMPLICATIONS

It is important to emphasize again that the only migration of the pin, using this technique, is outward. It will not migrate inward, if the medial cortex is not entered.

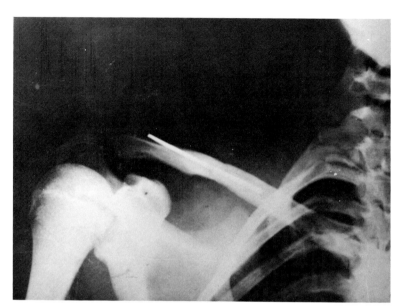

Fig. 9-36. An example of correct pinning of a midthird fracture of the clavicle. Note that the medial cortex of the clavicle is not perforated.

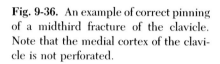

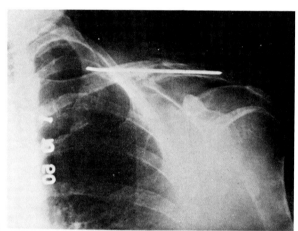

A

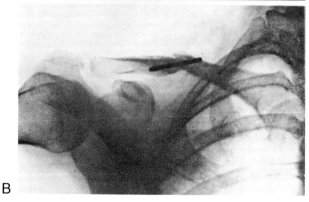

B

Fig. 9-37. Two examples of poor internal fixation techniques. (**A**) The pin has penetrated the medial cortex; this is dangerous. (**B**) A pin that is too short.

Outward migration is less likely to occur if the pin is threaded; however, the smooth fluted-end pin is safer and stronger.

We do not recommend introducing the pin from the cortex of the proximal fragment out through the distal fragment because, having perforated the cortex of the proximal clavicle, the pin may migrate medially into the mediastinum or lung, instead of outward. Kremens and Glauser[3] reported a patient in whom two Steinmann pins were inserted across the fracture in the middle portion of the clavicle. One pin perforated the cortex of the medial fragment and was expectorated by the patient 1 month after insertion.

SUMMARY

Due to the high incidence of clavicular fractures, the orthopaedic surgeon and the patient should be grateful to nature for giving the clavicle such strong healing potential. With closed treatment, nonunion rarely occurs. Our primary aim in the treatment of clavicular fractures is to give the patient sufficient immobilization and reasonable comfort during the first few weeks after injury. Figure-of-eight immobilization must be watched very carefully; if the strap slips laterally, it will increase the deformity of the fracture. A very comfortable, effective, and secure method of closed treatment is the half-shoulder spica, as demonstrated.

REFERENCES

1. Gardner E: The embryology of the clavicle. Clin Orthop 58:9, 1968
2. Jupiter JB, Leffert RD: Non-union of the clavicle: surgical management and associated complications. J Bone Joint Surgery 1986
3. Kremens, Glauser F: Unusual sequela following pinning of medial clavicular fracture. Am J Roentgenol 74:1066, 1956
4. Neer CS II: Nonunion of the clavicle. JAMA 172:1006, 1960
5. Neer CS II: Fractures of the distal third of the clavicle. Clin Orthop 58:43, 1968
6. Rockwood CA, Green DP: Fractures in Adults, 2nd ed J.B. Lippincott, Philadelphia, 1984
7. Rowe CR: Shoulder girdle injuries. p. 254. In Cave EF (ed): Fractures and Other Injuries. Yearbook Medical Publishers, Chicago, 1958
8. Rowe CR: An atlas of anatomy and treatment of mid-clavicular fractures. Clin Orthop 58:29, 1968

The Scapula

Carter R. Rowe

Of 1603 injuries to the shoulder girdle reported in our series in 1958,[7] 55 percent involved fractures of the middle third of the scapula and glenoid fossa, 8 percent involved the lower third, and 23 percent involved the upper third of the scapula (Figure 9-38). The majority of the patients were between 40 and 60 years of age; 32 percent were in their 50s. This is consistent with a report of 40 scapular fractures reported by Wilber and Evans [8] in 1977.

EXTENT OF INJURY

Fractures of the body of the scapula were the result, as a rule, of a severe trauma: 71 percent of the patients also had other associated injuries. Forty-five percent had fractured other bones, including the ribs, sternum, and spine (Fig. 9-39). Pneumothorax and subcutaneous emphysema were present in 3 percent (Fig. 9-40), and brachial plexus injuries in 4 percent. Other dislocations of the shoulder girdle occurred in 19 percent.

DIAGNOSIS

A careful evaluation of the lungs, ribs, spine, and upper extremity is essential. The patient usually supports the arm close to the body and avoids motion of the shoulder. Local scapular pain is present on palpation. Initial radiograms should consist of a large film including the lung field and shoulder girdle as well as oblique views of the scapula. Smaller spot films may be used as indicated.

TREATMENT

In general, the majority of fractures of the body of the scapula heal readily and respond satisfactorily to conservative measures.

Fractures of the Body

Fractures of the flat surface of the scapula are treated with rest, ice, and support. Usually after 3 weeks the patient has regained motion and is experi-

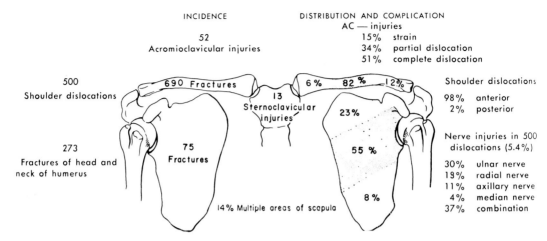

INCIDENCE

DISTRIBUTION AND COMPLICATION
AC — injuries

52
Acromioclavicular injuries

15%   strain
34%   partial dislocation
51%   complete dislocation

500
Shoulder dislocations

690 Fractures   6 %   82 %   12%

13
Sternoclavicular
injuries

23%

Shoulder dislocations

98%   anterior
2%   posterior

273
Fractures of head and
neck of humerus

75
Fractures

55 %

Nerve injuries in 500
dislocations (5.4%)

30%   ulnar nerve
19%   radial nerve
11%   axillary nerve
4%   median nerve
37%   combination

8 %

14% Multiple areas of scapula

Fig. 9-38. Analysis of 1,603 shoulder-girdle injuries, showing the number and distribution of fractures and dislocations.

encing much less pain. Oblique views should be taken to rule out angulation of the fracture on the rib surface, because, occasionally, bony irregularity may result in impingement against the rib cage. In these instances, a decision to explore the scapula surgically should be withheld until healing has taken place; the majority will improve with gentle pendulum exercises (see Fig. 9-39). This has been the experience of Bateman[1] and Rockwood.[6] Should the irregularity persist, surgical removal of the subscapular bony, or fibrous tissue mass, can be carried out successfully.

Fractures of the Coracoid

This is a very difficult bone to fracture, as evidenced by its rare occurrence. A direct blow or a sudden strong muscle pull of the arm flexors could cause a fracture of the process.[1,6] Conceivably, a violent anterior dislocation of the shoulder could fracture the coracoid at its base. The few fractures we have seen have responded to closed treatment. However, open repair would be very easy if it became necessary. We have seen several old nonunions on routine shoulder films, none of which seemed to account for the patient's problem or needed surgical stabilization.

Fractures of the Spine of the Scapula and Acromion

Displaced fractures of the acromion in which there is interference with the motion of the humeral head require manipulation or open elevation and internal fixation (Fig. 9-41). Open reduction is also indicated in the widely displaced fracture illustrated in Figure 9-42. A linear fracture of the acromion may be mistaken for an unfused acromial epiphysis. When in doubt, a film of the opposite shoulder should be taken. Liberson[4] and Neer[5] stress the importance of careful investigation to rule out unfused acromial epiphysis.

Fractures of the Glenoid Fossa and Neck of the Scapula

This is the most important category and deserves classification. There are, in general, two classes:

1. Fractures of the glenoid *not* associated with dislocations
2. Fractures of the glenoid associated with recurrent dislocations

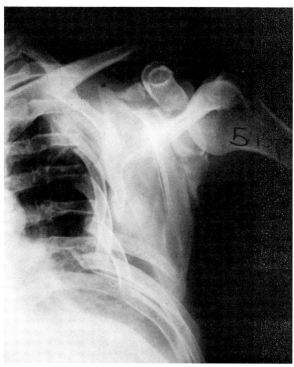

A

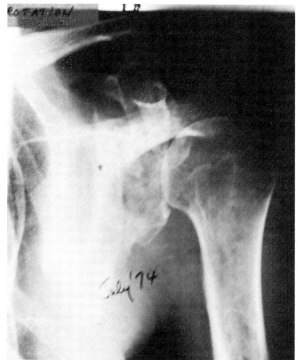

B

Fig. 9-39. (A) Comminuted fracture of the scapula with extensive compression fractures of the chest wall. (B) Excellent response to conservative treatment. (C) The patient 6 months after injury, with filling in of chest wall.

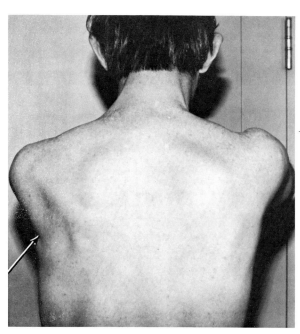

C

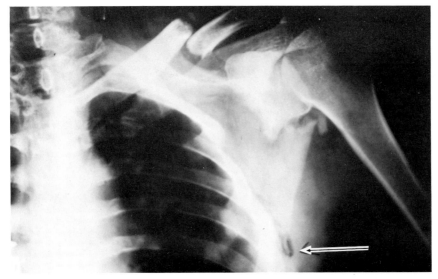

A

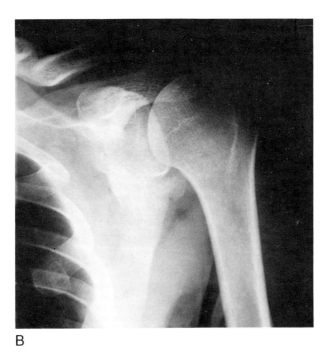

B

Fig. 9-40. (A) The presence of subcutaneous emphysema should be identified in fractures of the scapula (see arrow). **(B)** Conservative treatment gave a very good result.

FRACTURES OF THE GLENOID NOT ASSOCIATED WITH DISLOCATION OF THE HUMERAL HEAD

These can be classified into two types.

Type I

Undisplaced stellate fractures usually respond very well to conservative measures.

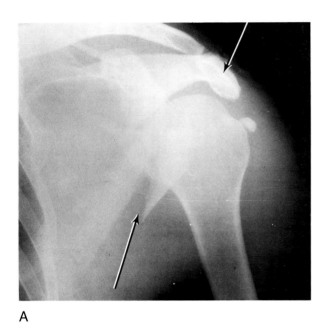

A

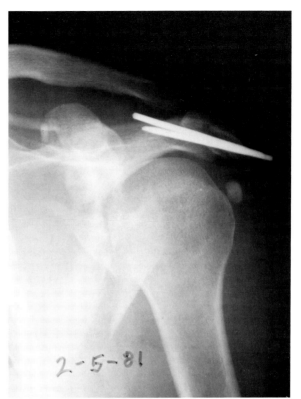

B

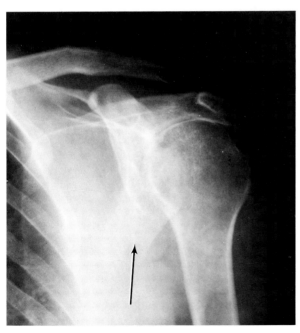

C

Fig. 9-41. (**A**) A severely comminuted fracture of the glenoid fossa with a depressed acromial fracture as a result of a motorcycle accident. (**B**) Postoperative reduction of the acromion. (**C**) Six months later molding of the glenoid is apparent. This patient is back at work with 75 percent of his shoulder motion, and is happy and grateful.

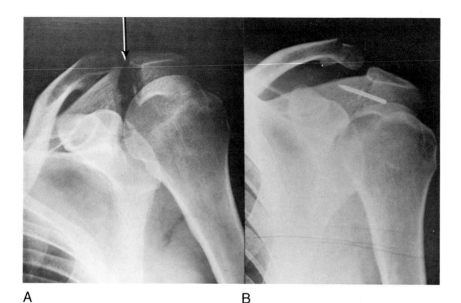

A   B

Fig. 9-42. (**A** and **B**) A displaced fracture of the junction of the spine and acromion treated with internal fixation.

Type II

These are displaced fracture of the glenoid fossa. As a rule, if the space between the fragments is less than 0.5 cm it will most likely fill in and function well (Fig. 9-43). The young man shown in Figure 9-43 injured his shoulder playing hockey. He was referred to us for open reduction, which we considered. However, since his shoulder was stable, we decided on conservative treatment and early pendulum exercises. He has progressed with a stable asymptomatic shoulder. If the opening is extensive, and the fragments in a condition to accept internal fixation, open reduction should be considered. The fragments in Figure 9-44 were favorable for internal fixation with an anterior approach. The severe separation in Figure 9-45 was closed by open reduction without internal fixation, through a posterior approach.

Type III

Severe comminuted shattered fractures of the glenoid usually respond poorly to open reduction because the fragments are too small for internal fixation. In Figure 9-39, the severely shattered fracture of the glenoid was associated with a depressed fracture of the acromion. The acromial fracture was reduced and stabilized with a pin. The patient began very gentle pendulum exercises as soon as tolerated with support

to the shoulder for 2 months. At 3 years, we were pleasantly surprised with his satisfactory result. With gentle motion, the fragments of the glenoid molded to the humeral head, united, and have caused no traumatic incidence to the humeral head. The patient had an acceptable range of motion and was very happy. Because the shoulder is not a weight-bearing joint, it will accept more disturbance of its articular surface than would a hip, knee, or ankle.

FRACTURES OF THE GLENOID RIM ASSOCIATED WITH DISLOCATION OF THE SHOULDER (see Chap. 6)

Of 116 patients operated on for recurrent dislocations of the shoulder, 51 (44 percent) experienced fractures of the rim of the glenoid.[7] Of these 51 dislocations, 18 (35 percent) involved one-sixth of the glenoid rim, 26 (51 percent) involved one-quarter of the glenoid rim, and 7 (14 percent) involved one-third of the glenoid rim. In the majority of these, fractured fragments were displaced and enmeshed in the capsule. It was not necessary to isolate the fracture and reduce it to the glenoid rim, as this would have left an irregular surface and a source of irritation to the shoulder. The capsule was repaired back to the rim of the glenoid with only 2 percent recurrence. The fractured fragments were either resected or left in

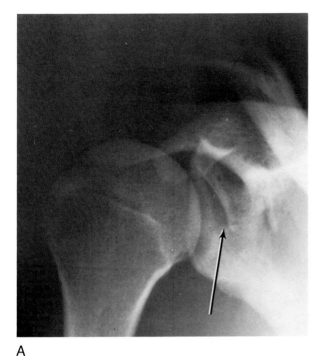

A

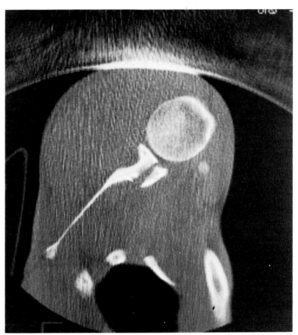

B

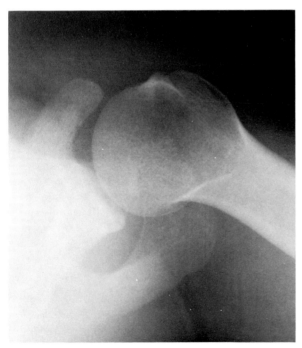

C

Fig. 9-43. (A) Initial views of the fracture of the anterior glenoid (hockey accident) in a 17-year-old boy. The question was whether open reduction should be carried out. **(B)** A CAT scan gave us additional information. Because his shoulder was stable, we chose conservative treatment and early guided pendulum exercises. **(C)** The boy has a stable, strong, painless shoulder as a result of conservative treatment.

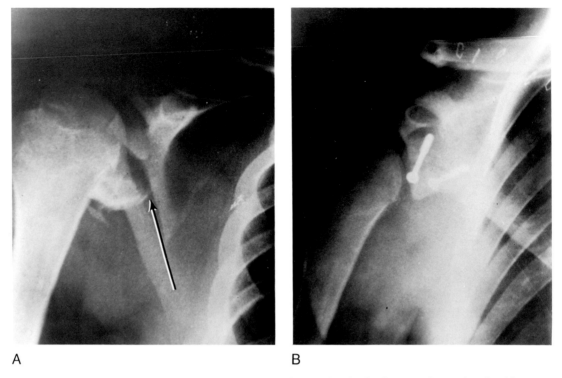

A   B

Fig. 9-44. (**A** and **B**) An anterior inferior fracture as the result of a hockey accident. The shoulder was unstable and open reduction was carried out with internal fixation, with a good result.

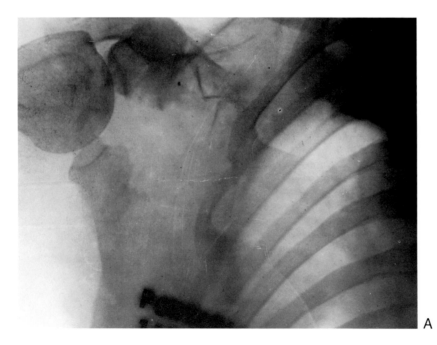

Fig. 9-45. (**A** and **B**) This severe splitting of the glenoid fossa was closed by open reduction from a posterior approach without internal fixation. (*Figure continues.*)

A

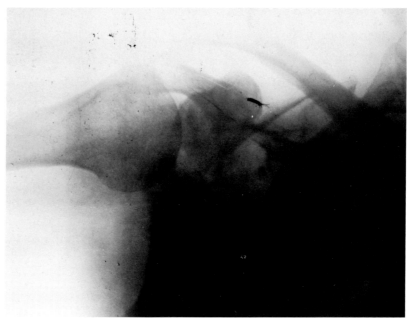

Fig. 9-45 *(Continued).*

B

the repaired capsule. Kummel[3] in 1970 reported the Swedish experience with 200 cases of glenoid fracture to which the reader is referred. Also, the experience of DePalma is significant.[2]

REFERENCES

1. Bateman JE: The Shoulder and Neck, 2nd ed. W.B. Saunders, Philadelphia, 1978

2. DePalma AF: Surgery of the Shoulder, 3rd ed. J.B. Lippincott, Philadelphia, 1983

3. Kummel BM: Fracture of the glenoid causing chronic dislocation of the shoulder. Clin Orthop 69:189, 1970

4. Liberson F: Os acromiale, contested anomaly. J Bone Joint Surg 19:683, 1937

5. Neer CS II: Nonunion of the clavicle. JAMA 172:1006, 1960

6. Rockwood CA, Green DP: Fractures in Adults, 2nd ed. J.B. Lippincott, Philadelphia, 1984

7. Rowe CR: Shoulder girdle injuries p. 254. In Cave EF (ed): Fractures and Other Injuries. Yearbook Medical Publishers, Chicago, 1958

8. Wilber MC, Evans, EB: Fractures of the scapula—an analysis of 40 cases. J Bone Joint Surg 59A:358, 1977

Fractures and Dislocations About the Shoulder in Children

10

Mark C. Gebhardt

Injuries to the shoulder girdle in children are uncommon compared to other injuries in childhood, and to shoulder trauma in adults. Several types of injuries unique to patients with open physes and which differ from those in the adult years will be the focus of this chapter. Epiphyseal separations of the proximal humeral physis, medial and distal clavicle, and greenstick fractures do not present after skeletal maturity, whereas glenohumeral and acromioclavicular dislocations are exceedingly rare in children. The patterns and management of these latter injuries do not differ from that covered in chapters on these conditions in adults.

It is helpful to categorize fractures and dislocations about the pediatric shoulder by age group and type of injury (Table 10-1). Neonatal injuries are defined as those in children less than 1 year age group and include fractures of the clavicle and proximal humeral physis. Fractures in the older age group include those in patients from 1 year through skeletal maturity: fractures of the scapula, clavicle, proximal humeral physis and metaphysis, and dislocations of the shoulder, and acromioclavicular and sternoclavicular joints. Finally it is important to recognize certain "special" types of fractures such as pathologic fractures, stress fractures, sports injuries, and those due to child abuse.

INCIDENCE

Statistics dealing with the exact incidence of pediatric fractures about the shoulder are difficult to derive; however, several large series from Sweden do address the question. Horak and Nilsson[52] studied the incidence of proximal humerus fractures and noted that this was primarily an injury of the osteoporotic elderly woman, with only a small percentage of proximal humerus fractures occurring in children. Another study from the same city[60] evaluated 8,682 fractures in children 15 years of age or younger. Although fractures of the forearm and hand accounted for nearly half of pediatric fractures, the clavicle was the next most frequently fractured bone (8.1 percent), whereas fractures of the proximal humerus were relatively uncommon (2.2 percent). This latter figure concurs with that of Neer,[91] who found that proximal humeral fractures accounted for 3 percent of pediatric fracture patterns. It is difficult to arrive at current statistics, but it is evident from earlier studies that birth fractures are uncommon; they occur in 0.025 to 3.5 percent of live births.[3,26,35,52,60,73,121] This figure is higher in complicated deliveries. A report by Snedecor stated that 6 percent of their breech deliveries

Table 10-1. Classification of Childhood Shoulder Girdle Injuries

I. Neonatal injuries (less than 1 year of age)
    Fractures of the clavicle
    Fractures of the proximal humeral physis
II. Fractures in older children (from 1 year to skeletal maturity)
    Fractures of the clavicle
    Fractures of the scapula
    Fractures of the proximal humeral physis and metaphysis
III. Dislocations
    Glenohumeral joint
    Acromioclavicular joint
    Sternoclavicular joint
IV. Special injuries
    Pathologic fractures
    Sports-related injuries
    Battered child syndrome

had radiographic evidence of fracture of a long bone at the seventh day of life. The vast majority of neonatal fractures are clavicle fractures (80 to 90 percent); the humerus accounts for most of the remainder.[23,26,60,73,118]

NEONATAL FRACTURES

Fractures in the newborn, as mentioned above, are largely confined to the clavicle and humerus, with the femur being the next most frequently injured bone. Most occur at the time of delivery, usually associated with some difficulty in the delivery. The incidence of clavicle fractures, 3 to 7 per 1,000 term deliveries,[23,49,73,118] is higher in vertex deliveries, whereas other long bone fractures occur more commonly in breech deliveries.[118,124] The fracture rate does not appear to be higher in premature births.[35,73] Birth fractures are more frequent in male than female babies, are usually unilateral, and the right side is affected approximately 60 percent of the time.[127] There does not appear to be a higher incidence in large babies or in mothers with contracted pelves. Fractures are less common in spontaneous deliveries than in those requiring version or other obstetric maneuvers.[73]

Before we discuss fractures of the clavicle, it is appropriate to review briefly the embryology and anatomy of this bone.[37,68,87,100] The clavicle (along with the mandible) is the first bone of the skeleton to appear in the human embryo, beginning at about the fifth postovulatory week (12 to 18 mm in crown–rump length). It forms by intramembranous ossification and subsequently cartilaginous growth centers develop at each end. Most of the longitudinal growth comes from the medial end, which develops a secondary ossification center in the adolescent years (11 years in girls; 14 years in boys). This center fuses with the body of the bone by 21 to 25 years of age. The lateral end generally has no secondary ossification center. The clavicle develops a double curve: convex anteriorly in the medial end and posteriorly in the lateral third. The clavicle is the only bone in the upper extremity that articulates with the axial skeleton through a synovial joint and contributes significantly to the stability of the shoulder girdle. The sternoclavicular joint has a meniscus present from birth. The clavicle acts as a rigid base for muscular attachments and increases the power of the arm–trunk mechanism. It also serves as protection for the major vessels at the base of the neck.[1,69,87]

Fractures of the Clavicle

Fractures of the clavicle can occur as the shoulder passes through the maternal pelvis.[73] The anterior clavicle is most frequently injured as it becomes compressed against the symphysis pubis, but occasionally the obstetrician's fingers can cause the injury.[73] The fracture is almost always a greenstick type at the junction of the middle and lateral thirds of the clavicle.[8,35,73] No relationship to maternal pelvis size, size of the baby, or difficulty in delivery has been established in clavicle fractures.[35] They occur even in premature births and there is a higher incidence in multiparous deliveries.[35] A relationship between fractured clavicles and calcium homeostasis has been demonstrated.[7]

These fractures are often not recognized by the physician and parent.[35,78] The baby may be irritable and have a mild temperature elevation, but there are usually few external signs of trauma initially.[73] Occasionally crepitation at the fracture site or failure to move the affected extremity ("pseudoparalysis") will be observed. Obstetrical palsy is checked for by testing the deep tendon reflexes and observing withdrawal from unpleasant stimuli. Frequently, however, the first clinical sign is a palpable callus 1 to 2 weeks following the injury or the appearance of the fracture on a radiograph.[26,78]

These are benign injuries and will usually heal without difficulty. There are no reported long-term sequelae. Radiographs obtained on the seventh day of life show abundant callus formation and remodeling of the fracture takes place over the ensuing year. Treatment is seldom necessary: a figure-of-eight splint may be applied but is cumbersome in a neonate. The arm may be splinted to the chest with an elastic bandage[129] or by pinning the pajama sleeve across the chest if the baby experiences any discomfort or deformity.[73] Parents should be warned to handle and position the child carefully.

Proximal Humeral Epiphyseal Separations

These are the second most common type of shoulder injury to occur in the newborn and can at times be very difficult to differentiate from a joint infection, brachial plexus palsy, or the very rare shoulder dislocation.[21,25,46,59,66] It is helpful to remember that the proximal humerus develops from three secondary centers of ossification.[38,39,98,101] The major one appears between 4 to 6 months, whereas the greater and lesser tuberosity centers appear at 3 and 5 years, respectively. The three centers coalesce around the age of 7 years and fuse to the humeral shaft between the ages of 20 to 22 years. Also of importance in discussing injuries to this region is the fact that 80 percent of the longitudinal growth of the humerus occurs from this growth center.[47]

Most injuries are classified as type I in the Salter-Harris classification.[119] Dameron[27,28] has studied the mechanism of these injuries in cadavers and noted that the posteromedial periosteum is considerably stronger than the anterolateral periosteum in this region. He postulated that an extension–adduction force displaces the metaphysis anterior and lateral to the biceps tendon through this relatively weak periosteum. The epiphysis becomes flexed, abducted, and slightly externally rotated by the pull of the external rotators, whereas the metaphysis and shaft is pulled anteriorly and medially by the pectoralis major.

Clinically these injuries can be extremely difficult to detect.[16,64,121] The arm is usually held motionless, and attempts at passive motion are painful to the new-

born. The arm is held in extension and external rotation, and tenderness and swelling are noted on physical examination. A low-grade temperature elevation may be noted. The neurologic examination is extremely difficult to ascertain, making the distinction from a brachial plexus palsy impossible at times. The two injuries may coexist on occasion.[44] Because the neonatal secondary ossification center is not ossified, interpretation of radiographs is difficult. Many reports of "congenital dislocation" of the shoulder probably were epiphyseal separations. Arthrography will usually settle the issue by outlining the epiphysis in the shoulder joint and demonstrating the fracture line more clearly.[44] It also affords the opportunity to aspirate the joint for culture if infection is a possibility. Fractures missed at birth show perimetaphyseal ossification on radiographs by about 2 weeks following the injury due to the periosteal stripping and new bone formation[44,73,91] (Fig. 10-1). The epiphysis on the involved side may appear earlier and be larger than the unaffected side.[44]

Reduction, if necessary, is achieved by gentle traction, slight external rotation, abduction, and flexion of the distal fragment. Anatomical reduction is not necessary because of the tremendous remodeling potential of this area[44] (Fig. 10-1B). A simple Velpeau dressing is sufficient immobilization. The fractures unite at 3 to 4 weeks and there are few long-term sequelae. Madsen[73] noted that unreduced fractures can result in late shortening and rotational deformities despite the great remodeling potential, so it is generally thought necessary to reduce the displaced fractures. There are reports of exaggerated retroversion of the proximal humerus, with an internal rotation contracture requiring humeral osteotomy or soft tissue release,[121] but in the author's experience this is extremely rare.

FRACTURES IN OLDER CHILDREN

Clavicle

The clavicle is the most frequently fractured bone in the body in children. An analysis of 690 fractures (of all ages) of the clavicle showed that the majority of (82 percent) occurred in the middle third, usually

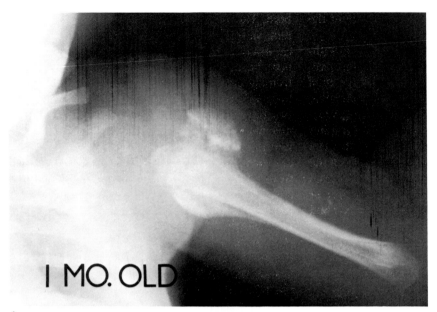

I MO. OLD

A

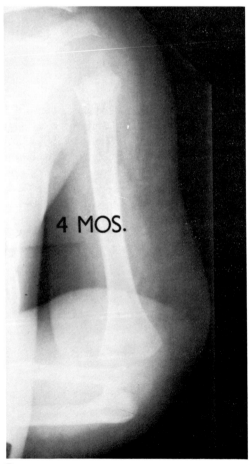

4 MOS.

B

Fig. 10-1. (A) This 1-month-old baby had an unrecognized Salter-Harris type I fracture of the proximal humerus at birth. At 1 month the callus about the fracture site is obvious. (B) By 4 months the proximal humerus has almost completely remodeled and the secondary ossification center is present.

at the junction of the middle and lateral thirds.[115] The development and anatomy of the clavicle have been outlined above, but it is important to consider that among the functions of the clavicle is protection of the subclavian vessels and brachial plexus. The clavicle also serves as a prop to hold the scapula away from the body, a bony framework for muscle origins and insertions, and a means of transmitting the supporting force of the trapezius muscle to the scapula through the coracoclavicular ligaments.[1,69,87]

The injury is usually due to a fall on the outstretched arm or, less often, a direct blow to the bone.[111,115,129] The ligamentous attachments of the outer and inner clavicle provide some protection, which explains the low incidence of fracture in these locations. In the older child the fractures are usually complete, although greenstick fractures are also present. Tachdjian[129] has divided pediatric clavicular fractures into three categories (based on Allman[3]):

1. Fractures at the junction of the middle and lateral thirds
2. Fracture of the lateral third
3. Fracture of the medial third

Shaft fractures of the clavicle are quite common and present with pain, local swelling, and tenderness at the fracture site. In complete fractures crepitus is often present and the fracture deformity is usually visible. The shoulder and lateral clavicle may appear drooped due to the weight of the arm, and the medial clavicle is displaced superiorly and posteriorly by the insertion of the sternocleidomastoid muscle. The patient usually holds the arm to the side of the body, supporting it with the uninjured upper limb; there may be a torticollis with the head tilted toward the injured side due to spasm of the sternocleidomastoid muscle. Careful attention to the neurologic and vascular exam is mandatory, because, although rare, injury to the brachial plexus or underlying blood vessels may occur.[53,84,104,131] Posteriorly bowed greenstick fractures can compress the subclavian vein and lead to venous congestion despite adequate perfusion of the arm.[85]

The radiographic findings are usually obvious, and it is important to look carefully for less apparent associated injuries on the film. An oblique film (lordic) will indicate the degree of anteroposterior displacement of the fractured fragments of the clavicle.[115] Greenstick and undisplaced fractures can be harder to detect and, on occasion, plastic bowing may occur.[4,15] It is important to remember that congenital pseudarthrosis of the clavicle may mimic a nondisplaced fracture in the very young child. The latter is usually right sided and there is no associated pain or tenderness. On radiographs the congenital pseudarthrosis shows a characteristic radiolucency with smooth bony ends at the site of deformity and no evidence of callus formation.[129]

Treatment centers on providing comfort for the patient. Children under 6 years of age seldom need reduction because of their tremendous remodeling potential and can be immobilized in a figure-of-eight bandage for 3 to 4 weeks (Fig. 10-2). For children of this age it is easiest to construct the bandage out of stockinette and felt padding, since "off the shelf" commercial bandages often fit poorly. Parents are instructed to tighten the dressing periodically if it loosens and to lift the child by the waist instead of the arms. Care should be taken to avoid skin irritation or compression of the axillary vessels by too tight a dressing. A sling in addition to the bandage may relieve the associated torticollis. In the older child with significant displacement, an attempt at reduction may be necessary.[129] Reduction is accomplished by elevation and backward extension of the shoulder after some relaxation and pain control are achieved with sedative medications or a hematoma block with local

anesthesia. This can be achieved by placing the child supine on a table with a bolster between the shoulders and allowing the arms to fall backwards by gravity. Alternatively, the child may be sitting while the physician gently pulls the shoulders backwards and upwards with a bolster on his or her knee between the scapulae. An anatomical reduction is not required since nonunion is extremely uncommon[12,75,88,95,130] and malunion is inconsequential. The position can be maintained by a commercial figure-of-eight bandage or a modified half-shoulder spica.[115] It is important to prevent the clavicular strap from sliding laterally when using a figure-of-eight bandage, because it then produces a downward pull on the shoulder and increases the deformity. Healing is usually complete by 6 weeks in this age group. This treatment protocol is usually successful; however, there is a case report by Jablon et al.[54] of a 13-year-old girl with an irreducible clavicular fracture due to perforation of the trapezius by the posteriorly displaced medial fragment. An open reduction without internal fixation was performed to reduce the possibility of skin and subclavian vessel damage by the fracture ends.

Open fractures of the clavicle are extremely rare and the treatment principles are similar to other open fractures.[67] Internal fixation is usually not required after debridement.[111] The only absolute indication for open reduction and internal fixation of a clavicle fracture in a child is injury to the subclavian or axillary vessels,[129] which may occur from the sharp bony ends of the fracture segment. An enlarging supraclavicular hematoma is usually present. Prompt surgical action is needed because these injuries may be fatal if not recognized and treated promptly.[85,104]

The majority of clavicle fractures heal without sequelae, but it is important to warn the parents that a "bump" of callus will be present initially (Fig. 10-2A). It usually remodels by 9 to 12 months (Fig. 10-2B). Overriding and shortening of the clavicle are not uncommon after complete fractures, but this is seldom a clinical problem. Nonunion is distinctly rare in children.[75,88,95,138] It is important to observe the healing process for at least 6 months before accepting the occurrence of nonunion. Given enough time, almost all clavicular shaft fractures will heal, with the reported incidence of nonunion being 0.1 to 1.9 percent (all ages).[74] The usual cause of nonunion is interposition of soft tissues (usually trapezius) between the fracture ends. Attempts at open reduction to achieve

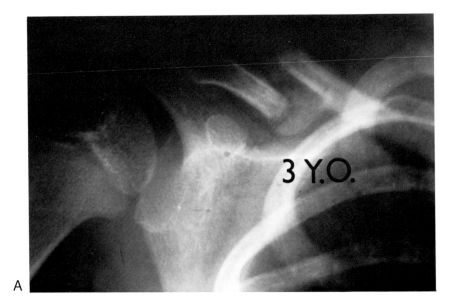

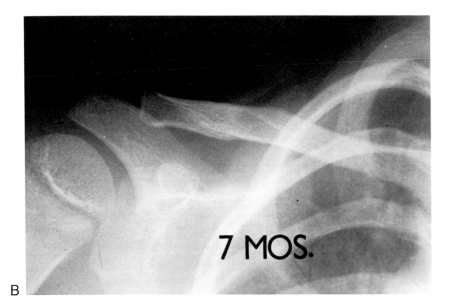

Fig. 10-2. (A) This 3-year-old child sustained a displaced fracture of the midclavicle that was allowed to heal in the position shown. Callous formation is evident 2 weeks following the injury. **(B)** By 7 months the clavicle has almost completely remodeled.

union are hazardous, because of both the adjacent vascular anatomy and the potential for intramedullary fixation devices to migrate.[141] A recent report by Manske[74] included two adolescent patients treated for nonunion by compression plating and iliac crest bone grafting. There were no noted complications and the patients achieved union. This method has been successful at our institution, and avoids the risk of metal migration.[41]

Other complications are much rarer and include vascular injury[85,104] and delayed compression of the brachial plexus due to excessive callus formation. This lesion is a neurapraxia and usually responds to decompression of the nerves and removal of callus.[84]

Fractures of the Lateral Clavicle

There has been considerable confusion in the literature regarding lateral clavicle fractures, although when the growth and development of the bone are remembered, the fracture patterns are quite straightforward.[37] As mentioned in the previous sections, the clavicle is formed by membranous bone formation early in the embryologic sequence.[100] Subsequently a cartilaginous epiphysis develops at the lateral end, which contributes to 20 to 30 percent of the longitudinal growth of the bone.[39,97,100] A secondary growth center does not usually appear, but the distal clavicular cartilaginous epiphysis persists into the early third decade or longer.[97] The acromioclavicular ligaments attach to the perichondrium and periosteum of the distal clavicle and, in other regions of the immature skeleton, form a stronger bond than the adjacent metaphyseal–physeal junction. Thus, as in other injuries in children, a sprain of the acromioclavicular joint is distinctly rare; a similar mechanism produces a fracture, either through the distal clavicular metaphysis or through the growth plate. The strong conoid and trapezoid ligaments remain attached to the inferior perichondrium and periosteum, and the clavicle "dislocates" through a superior slit in the periosteal tube (Fig. 10-3). The acromioclavicular joint itself remains intact. Such a sequence has been referred to in the literature as a "pseudodislocation,"[34] referring to the fact that it is really a fracture or growth plate injury occurring in a child and mimicking the adult acromioclavicular dislocation (Fig. 10-4).

The injury may occur at any time from birth through skeletal maturity,[97] although beyond the ages of 13 and 16,[32,109,110,111] true acromioclavicular joint dislocations predominate. The mechanisms include birth trauma, child abuse, falls, and vehicular accidents that produce a direct blow to the shoulder region. The usual patient is an active young teenager who has fallen from his or her bicycle or has been injured in sports and has pain and tenderness over the acromioclavicular joint. The pain is aggravated by movement of the shoulder. Swelling over the joint is present and the shoulder may droop inferiorly. In severe injuries, the medial clavicle is displaced superiorly and posteriorly, occasionally becoming trapped in the trapezius.

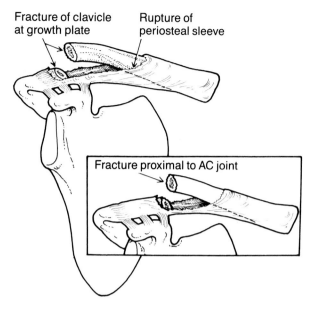

Fracture of clavicle at growth plate

Rupture of periosteal sleeve

Fracture proximal to AC joint

Fig. 10-3. Diagram of the fractures of the distal clavicle that can mimic acromioclavicular joint dislocations. Note that these are either epiphyseal separation injuries or fractures through the distal clavicle (inset), but the coracoclavicular ligaments remain intact.

The early radiographic findings may be minimal, especially if the injury is a physeal (Salter-Harris type I) injury. Stress roentgenograms of the joint with comparison views as well as oblique[89] and lordotic views may be helpful. If the fracture is through the distal metaphysis, the diagnosis is usually evident, whereas a high index of suspicion and knowledge of the pathophysiology of childhood injuries are necessary to recognize the physeal fractures (Fig. 10-4A). Computed tomography scans may be helpful in locating metaphyseal fractures. As the fracture heals, the periosteal tube fills in with bone, which becomes evident on the radiograph by 10 to 14 days[110,111] (Fig. 10-4B). In unreduced fractures this leads to union of the fracture by 3 to 6 weeks, and subsequent remodeling of the superiorly displaced medial clavicular segment (Fig. 10-4C). An incomplete remodeling process has probably led to the erroneous diagnosis of duplication of the clavicle and medial notch and spurs at the coracoclavicular ligaments as developmental anomalies rather than traumatic injuries.[97]

Neer classified injuries to the lateral clavicle into

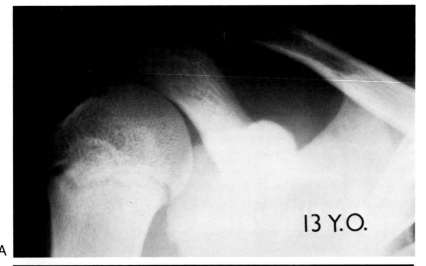

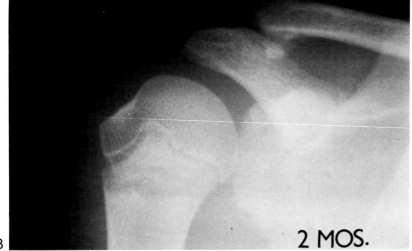

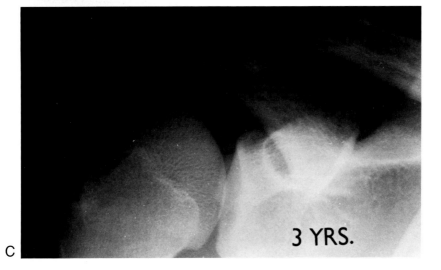

Fig. 10-4. (**A**) This 13-year-old boy sustained a shoulder injury playing football and was believed to have an "AC separation." He was treated in a Kenny-Howard type of sling. (**B**) Two months after injury callous formation is evident in the area of the intact periosteal tube, indicating that this was actually an epiphyseal separation with a tear in the periosteal tube. (**C**) At 3 years the distal clavicle has remodeled.

two categories depending on the status of the coracoclavicular ligaments.[89] In type I injuries the ligaments remain attached to both the medial and lateral fracture fragments, so little displacement is permitted. In type II injuries the ligaments are avulsed from the medial fragment, allowing the medial clavicle to displace superiorly. In children, this classification system does not apply because of the attachments of the ligaments to the periosteal tube. Rockwood[111] presents a complex classification of injuries to the distal clavicle. He describes two major injuries: fractures of the lateral clavicle and acromioclavicular "joint" injuries. The latter implies that the coracoclavicular ligaments remain intact, whereas the acromioclavicular ligaments are disrupted. He describes six types of acromioclavicular joint injuries.

The author prefers to classify injuries to this joint in children more simply. In skeletally immature patients, an injury that would produce an acromioclavicular dislocation in adults either produces a distal clavicular fracture (much more frequently) or a true joint dislocation (extremely rare below the age of 16). The fractures are either Salter-Harris type I or II injuries to the physeal plate or metaphyseal fractures of the distal clavicle (Fig. 10-3). The actual fracture pattern may vary with the extent of the injury, but the coraclavicular ligaments remain attached to the periosteal tube. A variation is the coracoid avulsion fracture, in which the ligaments remain intact but there is an avulsion of the coracoid epiphysis.[86,93]

Treatment considerations have also led to controversy in the literature.[17,32,34,110,111] Falstie-Jensen and Mikkelson[34] reported on two cases of this fracture pattern and recommended operative repair of the periosteal tube and temporary fixation of the acromioclavicular joint with a Kirschner wire. Rockwood[110,111] recommends nonoperative treatment, stating that remodeling will occur as described above and that adequate functional results occur once the fracture has united. He reserves operative treatment for his type IV injury in which the medial clavicle is trapped in the fibers of the trapezius muscle and cannot be reduced by closed means. Eidman et al.[32] reported on 25 children less than 16 years of age all of whom were treated surgically. They confirmed that a true acromioclavicular dislocation is rare below the age of 13 and recommended conservative treatment for this age group. Injuries in children above this age were likely to be adult-type injuries

for which Eidman et al. recommended surgical repair. Ogden[97] noted good results with either nonoperative treatment or cross-pinning of the joint, although one patient treated by closed methods required trimming of a distal clavicular "duplication" that failed to remodel.

It seems reasonable to treat the non- or minimally displaced fractures in a sling for comfort and to attempt to reduce the displaced ones. A sling that supports the arm and provides downward compression on the medial clavicle, such as the Kenny-Howard sling, may be used to hold the reduction until callus formation is evident at 2 to 3 weeks. This approach requires close monitering of the patient for displacement of the reduction and skin irritation from the sling. For extremely unstable injuries, open reduction and suture of the periosteal tube may be necessary to maintain the reduction. An alternative is closed reduction and fixation with a percutaneous pin, but the reader is cautioned about the potential catastrophic dangers of pin migration. Eidman et al.[32] noted two cases of asymptomatic arthritis of the acromioclavicular joint from pinning. Irreducible fractures may require operative reduction to free the clavicle from the trapezius if it is thought that the displacement is significant enough to prevent union. For true AC joint dislocations, operative intervention is rarely warranted, and then only if the clavicle tents the skin.[108,112] The reader is referred to Chapter 8 for further details.

Fractures of the Medial End of the Clavicle

These are distinctly rare, accounting for only 6 percent of clavicular fractures in Rowe's series.[115] True fractures in this area are easy to diagnose and treat but much confusion has centered on the distinction between epiphyseal fractures and true dislocations in children. Again, it is helpful to review the embryology and anatomy of this area.[11,37] A cartilaginous growth area develops at the medial clavicle and most of the longitudinal growth of the clavicle is from this center. A secondary growth center develops at the medial end from 15 to 18 years of age, which fuses by the 25th year. The sternoclavicular joint is the only diarthrodial articulation between the upper extremity and the axial skeleton,[111] and this joint develops a meniscal cartilage that is present at birth. The meniscus is either complete (discoid) or incomplete (meniscoid)[30,100] and is attached around its periphery to the sternoclavicular capsule/ligament complex.[100] These attachments are quite strong, making physeal disruption more likely than ligamentous disruption prior to epiphyseal closure. There is no direct attachment of the meniscus to either the clavicular epiphysis or sternum.[100] The meniscus acts as a buffer to the stresses placed upon the incongruent opposing surfaces of the medial clavicle and the sternum.[30] This arrangement allows considerable motion through 3° of freedom at this joint[30] and it functions similarly to a ball-and-socket articulation.[111] The ligamentous structures about the joint contribute to its stability, and the most important of these is the costoclavicular or rhomboid ligament which arises from the superior medial portion of the first rib and runs obliquely upward, laterally, and backward to insert into the costal tuberosity of the undersurface of the medial clavicle.[30]

The mechanism of injury to the medial clavicle is from an indirect blow such as a fall on the shoulder or the "piling on" injury in football, which drives the clavicle inward and upward.[111,129] If the force is directed from posterolaterally, the displacement will be posterior; if from the anterolateral shoulder, it will lead to anterior displacement.[111] Occasionally, direct violence to the medial clavicle area may be the cause of this injury.[29] In adults a similar mechanism leads to a sternoclavicular dislocation, but in children a fracture of the medial clavicle or a Salter-Harris type I or II epiphyseal separation is much more likely (Fig. 10-5). The latter may mimic a true dislocation clinically and radiographically and has led to confusion in the literature. At least two of the cases described by Simurda[125] and all of the cases in Elting's[33] report appear to have been epiphyseal separations rather than true dislocations.

Nondisplaced fractures of the medial clavicle cause little deformity and present with localized pain and tenderness. Anteriorly displaced epiphyseal separations are painful on attempts at shoulder motion and demonstrate local swelling, tenderness, and a visible prominence of the displaced clavicular metaphysis. *Posteriorly* displaced separations can be life-threatening, cause all of the problems associated with posterior sternoclavicular dislocations, and have prompted numerous reports in the literature.[40,43,48,57,62,63,80,92,102,120,122,128,132] These problems include venous con-

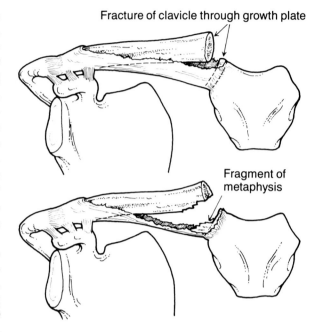

Fig. 10-5. Diagram of the childhood sternoclavicular injury. Note that this is usually an epiphyseal separation (Salter-Harris type I or II) rather than a true dislocation.

gestion in the neck, difficulty in breathing, a choking sensation, difficulty in swallowing, and decreased circulation to the arm.[40,43] The patient may present in a full state of shock and have a pneumothorax. The prominence of the medial clavicle is absent and a depression medial to the sternoclavicular joint may be appreciated.[114]

These injuries occur in all ages from infancy[136] to the time of closure of the epiphyseal plate, but are most commonly seen in adolescents.[29,33,125] The radiographs may be difficult to interpret (Fig. 10-6) and lordotic views are mandatory. Rockwood has described a 40° cephalic tilt view in which anterior displacements display the medial clavicle superior to the uninjured side; in posterior displacements it is inferior to the normal side.[109,111] It is difficult to identify an epiphyseal separation without tomographic views even after the appearance of the secondary ossification center.[69] The computed tomogram has helped considerably with the diagnosis of this injury (Fig. 10-7).[31] It easily differentiates anterior from posterior displacements[65] and can distinguish Salter-Harris type I from type II injuries. It is also helpful in assessing the adequacy of the reduction.

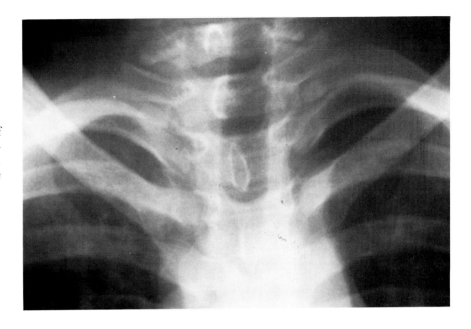

Fig. 10-6. Plane radiographs of a 14-year-old girl with a sterno-clavicular injury on the right. It is difficult to appreciate the injury.

Treatment of nondisplaced medial clavicular fractures consists of splinting the patient with a sling for comfort until the fracture heals. Epiphyseal separations are treated with an attempt at closed reduction which is usually successful in anterior displacements.[43] Manual pressure on the prominent anteriorly displaced metaphyseal end of the clavicle with concurrent abduction, mild extension, and traction on the arm will usually lead to reduction. An audible or plapable clunk is appreciated at the point of reduction and this usually signals a stable situation. Immobilization in a Valpaeu sling is all that is necessary, although a figure-of-eight splint may be added.[13] Because this is a growth plate fracture, healing is usually rapid. Closed reduction is occasionally unsuccessful, however, and operative reduction may be in-

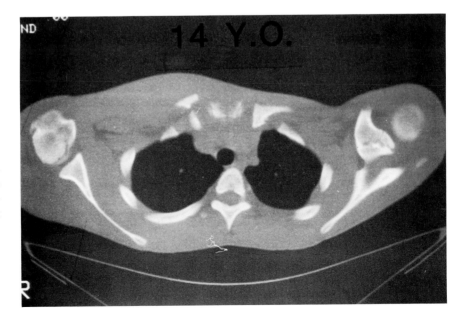

Fig. 10-7. A computed tomography scan of the same child demonstrates the injury nicely and suggests that there has been an epiphyseal separation on the right because the secondary ossification center remains juxtaposed to the manubrium (*arrow*). Note the soft tissue swelling.

dicated.[29,33,102] The metaphysis of the medial clavicle is displaced from a rent in the periosteal tube; once it has been restored back to its anatomical location, suture of the periosteum may provide stability. On occasion, instability will require fixation but extreme caution should be taken when inserting Kirschner wires in this location because of the close proximity of the great vessels. Pin migration has led to several reports of deaths and near deaths from pins migrating into the pulmonary artery, innominate artery, aorta, and pericardium.[22,111] On occasion, chronic instability of the sternoclavicular joint is encountered as a late sequela of this injury (Ehrlich, M.G., personal communication). The patient is able to sublux voluntarily and reduce the medial clavicle with respect to the sternum. This is an asymptomatic condition that does not usually require operative intervention.

Posterior displacements demand reduction and an attempt at closed reduction is warranted (see Chap. 8). If signs of vascular compromise are present, it is wise to alert the cardiovascular team (and have them present in the operating room) because there are reports of sudden death from massive hemorrhage during closed reduction of posterior dislocations. As in the adult injury, a towel clip carefully placed around the medial metaphysis of the bone aids in reduction. Retraction of the shoulders with caudal traction on the arm while the patient is supported by an interscapular bolster has been suggested.[18] At times closed reduction is not possible and operative means are needed.[16,29,33,42,125] The medial clavicle may be displaced posterior to the sternum, but the epiphysis, meniscus, and joint remain intact. The warnings mentioned for anterior displacements apply. Ligament reconstruction for the rare chronic dislocation in athletic (older) children has been described.[13,70,71]

Scapula

Fractures of the scapula in children (as well as in adults) are rare injuries but are problematic because they are usually caused by violent injuries and are often difficult to detect on initial examination. Scapular injuries occurred in only 4.7 percent of the 1,603 injuries to the shoulder girdle in Rowe's series[116] (see Chap. 9). Fourteen percent of these injuries had multiple sites of fracture within the scapula, attesting to the severity of the injury. The author is unaware of any large series of fractures of the scapula in children.

The scapula develops by endochondral and membranous bone formation.[99] An initial primary ossification center begins in the body of the scapula centered slightly towards the glenoid. Ogden[99] proposes that the vertebral border of the scapula acts as the "proximal" epiphyseal center, whereas the growth centers of the glenoid, acromion, and coracoid act as the "distal" center. The shape of the scapula is largely determined in utero, the length being approximately one and one-half times that of the width. At least seven secondary growth centers appear during the development of the scapula, the importance of which become evident when one attempts to differentiate these from fractures. Fortunately, most of the secondary ossification centers are bilaterally symmetrical. The ossification center for the coracoid appears between 15 and 18 months[129] (as early as 3 months according to Ogden,[102] and a bipolar growth plate develops at its base between the coracoid process and the body of the scapula. Secondary ossification centers subsequently appear at the epiphysis of the acromion (two) at 14 to 16 years; they coalesce at 19 years of age and usually fuse to the scapular spine by the 22nd or 25th year. Other secondary centers appear at the vertebral border of the scapula, inferior tip of the scapula, tip of the acromion, and inferior glenoid rim. These appear in late adolescence and usually fuse in the early 20s.[99]

A classification of pediatric scapular fractures has been proposed in Tachdjian's text[129] and a similar one is presented in Weber's book.[135] The fractures can be divided into those of the body, glenoid, acromion, coracoid,[142] and scapular neck. The fracture types may appear multiply in the same patient and can be easily overlooked. True anteroposterior and lateral views of the scapula are necessary as well as axillary views and obliques. A 30° lordotic view may be helpful for detecting coracoid fractures. Plain or computed tomograms are helpful in detecting fractures and in determining their extent, especially with regard to the glenoid articular surface.

The mechanism of injury is usually violent trauma, most frequently from motor vehicle accidents or falls.[79,129,137] Associated injuries to the chest and shoulder girdle are common, and the patients are frequently multiple trauma victims with severe injuries to the chest, head, or abdomen. This may make the detection of scapular injuries difficult, especially in patients with obtundation from cerebral injuries. Obviously, life-saving measures must assume importance over the treatment of these fractures. In an alert patient, pain with motion of the arm, swelling, tenderness, and crepitus over the fracture are often present. Careful attention must be paid to the neurovascular status, because brachial plexus injuries and subclavian or axillary vessel injury may be associated with scapular fractures.

Fractures of the body are usually comminuted and minimally displaced because of the stabilizing effect of the surrounding musculature. Operative reduction is seldom necessary; a sling for 3 to 4 weeks and motion exercises when the patient is comfortable are usually all that is required.

Fractures of the neck of the scapula are usually vertical from the suprascapular notch to the axillary border of the scapula. Nondisplaced fractures are of little consequence and may be treated with a sling and pendulum exercises, but more severe injuries may be displaced and associated with injuries to the acromioclavicular or coracoclavicular ligaments. The glenohumeral joint ligaments remain intact, and the weight of the upper extremity may pull the lateral fracture fragment inferiorly. A fracture lateral to the coracoid process may also displace. Severely displaced fractures may require reduction either by lateral skeletal traction through an olecranon pin or, in rare instances, operative reduction. Hardegger et al.[45] recommend interfragmentary compression and buttress plating of significantly displaced fractures, but his series was largely composed of adults. There are no references to surgical treatment in the pediatric orthopaedic literature.

Fractures of the glenoid may occur due to a compression force of the humeral head on the glenoid from a direct blow or fall on the arm or may be associated with shoulder dislocation. Opinion is divided regarding treatment. Most authors recommend nonoperative treatment and early motion exercises when the patient is comfortable, usually about 2 to 3 weeks following the injury. However, operative reduction should be considered if there are large fracture fragments displaced more than 1 cm. Such displacement can lead to glenohumeral joint instability. Although reasonable results have been reported with operative treatment in adult glenoid fractures,[45] complications are present and some authors warn that poor range of motion may result. Stellate comminuted

fractures are probably best managed by skeletal traction and early motion.

Fractures of the acromion lateral to the coracoacromial ligaments are usually due to a direct blow and are undisplaced. Symptomatic treatment with a sling is all that is necessary. One should be careful not to mistake a linear fracture of the acromion for an unfused acromial epiphysis. If in doubt, the opposite shoulder should be examined radiographically.

Fractures of the coracoid are rare but may mimic acromioclavicular joint dislocation. Montgomery and Loyd[86] reported two cases of avulsions through the epiphysis of the coracoid process in association with acromioclavicular injuries. If the injury is recognized, it can probably be managed nonoperatively.[129]

Avulsion injuries due to violent muscular contractions may occur, but they are uncommon in children.[50] Dislocation of the scapula from the thoracic wall is extremely rare in children.

Proximal Humerus

Fractures of the proximal humerus in older children are uncommon injuries and are greatly outnumbered by fractures of the supracondylar area of the humerus.[51,52,60,91,140] The majority of these are relatively easily treated because of the tremendous remodeling potential at this site, which contributes 80 percent of the longitudinal growth of the bone[47,55] and because the deltoid muscle masks even moderately severe bony deformity. The limitations of range of motion are seldom of functional significance in malunited fractures. Nevertheless, these fractures can be serious injuries and present challenging treatment dilemmas to the treating orthopaedic surgeon.

After the newborn period, childhood fractures of the proximal humerus occur with greatest frequency in the 11- to 15-year age group.[113] Fractures in boys greatly outnumber those in girls except in geographical areas where horseback riding is popular among girls.[60] Hohl[51] has estimated that upper humeral fractures constitute only 0.45 percent of all fractures in childhood, but if only epiphyseal fractures are considered, the figure is 3 to 6.7 percent.[91,105] Peterson,[105] in a study from the Mayo Clinic, found that epiphyseal fractures of the proximal humerus represented the fourth most common epiphyseal fracture, following fractures of the distal radius, distal tibia, and phalanges of the hand.

The embryology of the proximal humerus has been reviewed above, but it should be recalled that the secondary ossification center of the proximal humerus appears by the 6th month and is usually not present radiographically at birth.[38,39,98,101] The greater and lesser tuberosity secondary centers appear at approximately 3 to 5 years, respectively, and coalesce by age 7. Fusion of the epiphysis with the metaphysis does not occur until 18 to 22 years of age. There is some histologic evidence to suggest that these centers appear earlier than would be predicted by radiographs, and that fusion between the greater tuberosity and humeral head may begin toward the end of the 1st year of life.[101] Nuances of the radiographic appearances of these ossification centers at various stages of development may lead to the need for comparison radiographs to assess fracture anatomy.

It is helpful to classify fractures of the proximal humerus into two groups: true physeal separations and fractures of the proximal humeral metaphysis. Although theoretically any pattern is possible, in practice only Salter-Harris types I and II fractures are encountered.[111] In younger children, type I epiphyseal separations predominate, whereas in older children a type II injury is more common. There has been only one report of a fracture–dislocation in a child;[93] similarly, fractures of the humerus, radius, and ulna in the same extremity are rare, and the majority of the humerus fractures in this instance are supracondylar fractures.[106]

The mechanism of epiphyseal separations has been well described by Dameron.[27] Based upon anatomical studies in stillborns, he noted the cone-shaped epiphyseal plate with its base inferiorly and its apex situated slightly medially and posteriorly. The irregular shape of growth plate produced an interlocking of the epiphysis that adds to the stability of the proximal humerus.[19] The posterior periosteum is stronger than that anteriorly, and thus a fall on the outstretched arm with the extremity held in adduction, extension, and internal rotation forces the metaphysis to displace through the relatively weak anterior periosteal sleeve (Fig. 10-8). The final position of unstable fractures is determined by the muscle pull. The epiphysis is held in flexion, abduction, and external rotation by the teres minor, infraspinatus, supraspinatus, and subscapularis. The pectoralis major, latissi-

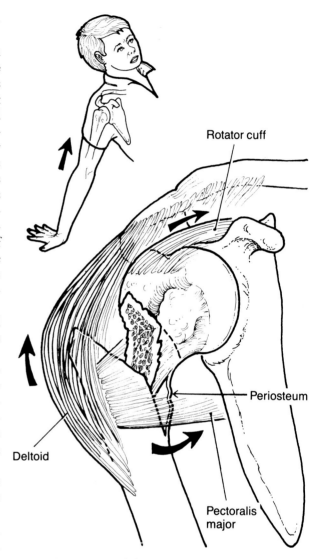

Rotator cuff

Periosteum

Deltoid

Pectoralis major

Fig. 10-8. Diagram of the mechanisms of epiphyseal fractures of the proximal humerus.

mus dorsi, and teres major hold the metaphyseal fragment anteriorly, medially, and upward. Another mechanism thought by Neer and Horowitz[91] to operate more frequently is a direct blow to the shoulder causing a posterolateral shearing force that adducts the humeral shaft and displaces it forward. In children below the age of 5 the fracture line propagates through the entire growth plate producing a type I injury (Fig. 10-9). In the older child (11 to 15 years) the fracture line enters the metaphysis leaving a posteromedial metaphyseal fragment with the epiphysis

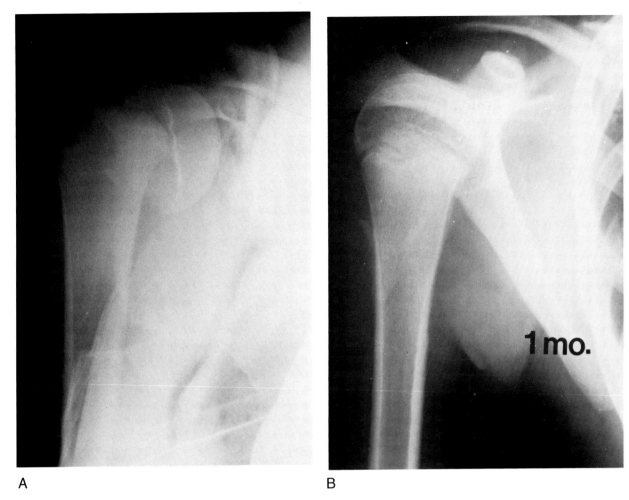

A   B

Fig. 10-9. **(A)** Type I epiphyseal separation of the proximal humerus in an 8-year-old boy. **(B)** The separation was reduced by closed means and was found to be stable. He was managed in a Velpeau dressing and the fracture is nearly healed by 1 month.

and producing a type II fracture (Fig. 10-10).[101] Other mechanisms for this fracture have also been proposed and discussed by Williams.[139]

The clinical presentation is pain and swelling in the shoulder area with varying amounts of ecchymosis and warmth. The arm is shortened and, if the fracture is markedly displaced, the arm is held in extension and abduction. A palpable prominence may be noted in the axilla anteriorly. The hematoma may be quite large, and it is usually not possible to elicit crepitus because the patient resists efforts to move the arm. A careful neurologic examination should be carried out to check for signs of nerve injury.

The treatment varies with the severity of the frac-

ture and the age of the patients but, in most instances, is nonoperative.[58] In patients less than 5 to 6 years of age, most of whom have Salter-Harris type I injuries, reduction by gentle longitudinal traction or by traction, flexion, and abduction usually is sufficient. An anatomical reduction is not necessary because of the remodeling potential and growth disturbance is unusual. For fractures in older children (primarily type II injuries) Neer and Horowitz[91] have developed a grading system for the amount of displacement of proximal humeral epiphyseal separations:

Grade I: less than 5 mm displacement
Grade II: displaced to ⅓ the width of the shaft

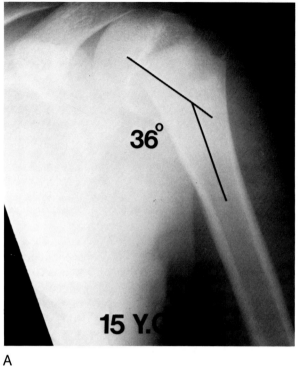

A

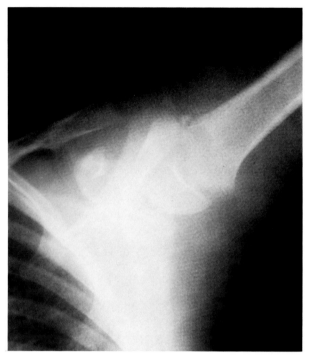

B

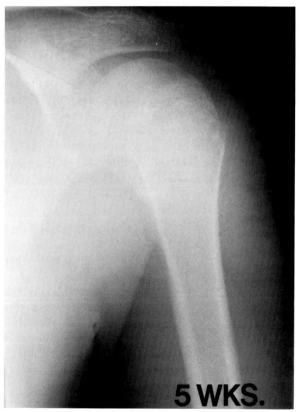

C

Fig. 10-10. (**A**) This 15-year-old boy fell while playing and sustained a Salter-Harris type II fracture of the proximal humerus. The initial angulation was 36°. (**B**) Closed reduction was accomplished, but the fracture was unstable and he was immobilized in the "salute" position in a shoulder spica. (**C**) At 5 weeks the reduction is maintained and the fracture has essentially healed.

Grade III: displaced to ⅔ the width of the shaft
Grade IV: displacement greater than ⅔ the width of the bone or complete displacement

They believe that grade I and II displacements lead to few late complications and shortening in only 9 percent of fractures and, therefore, gentle manipulative reduction will suffice. The more severe grade III and IV may need closed reduction or, on occasion, an operative procedure. The indications for reduction are not clear, however, and there is a marked variation in the amount of angulation considered to be "acceptable" in the literature. The range of motion possible at the glenohumeral joint, the ability of the deltoid to mask even severe bony angulation, and the tremendous remodeling potential make it possible to accept rather severe amounts of angulation.[6,58] Some authors recommend reduction for as little as 20° of angulation,[111,125,133] whereas others have documented complete remodeling with up to 60° of angulation.[6,77,126] The reader will have to decide, but a good rule of thumb is to consider an attempt at reduction if the angulation exceeds 35° (Fig. 10-11).

The reduction procedure can either be carried out in the emergency ward with sedation and a hematoma block[111] or with general anesthesia. The former is probably preferable, but it is often difficult to achieve adequate pain relief. A general anesthetic may be preferred and aids in getting relaxation, but there is a danger of causing unrecognized damage to the neurovascular bundle during the manipulation with the patient asleep. It is also more difficult to apply a shoulder spica (should it be necessary) with the patient anesthetized.

The reduction is achieved by traction, flexion, and abduction to about 90° and correction of rotation. Because it is difficult to control the proximal fragment, the reduction process may be difficult, especially in severely displaced fractures. Tachdjian[129] has suggested placing a percutaneous pin under sterile technique into the proximal fragment temporarily to gain a hold on the epiphyseal fragment in difficult reductions. A sensation of reduction may not be appreciated by the surgeon, and it may not be possible to achieve an anatomical reduction. The latter is not required because of the tremendous remodeling potential of this area, but guidelines for acceptability of the reduction are difficult to find. Some authors recommend accepting no more than 20° to 35° of angulation,[111,133]

whereas others contend that up to 60° will remodel and leave the patient with an acceptable functional and cosmetic result.[6,77,126] Achieving apposition of 50 percent or more is usually sufficient in the completely displaced fractures.[91] Rarely, it may not be possible to attain a "satisfactory" reduction, due to an infolding of the periosteum into the fracture site or entrapment of the long head of the biceps tendon between the fracture fragments.[133] The frequency of the latter occurrence has probably been overemphasized and most authors find that open reduction is seldom necessary, even for severe displacements.[14,20,24,28,36,77,91,94,123,126]

Once reduction has been achieved, an assessment of stability must be made.[139] The image intensifier is helpful for this step, and the reduction is checked as the arm is slowly brought back down to the patient's side. If the reduction is maintained, the fracture can be managed in a Velpeau bandage with padding in the axilla.[123] Caution must be exerted, however, as the reduction may be slowly lost in the first few days after reduction. Follow-up radiographs must be made and the patient warned of the possibility of needing further reductive procedures. On occasion, the fracture is very unstable at the start and for these patients a shoulder spica is used.[14,91,123] As mentioned it is difficult to apply this with the patient asleep, and the options are to apply the body portion of the cast before the patient is anesthetized or to place the patient in traction for a brief period after reduction, and then apply the cast. The arm must usually be held in forward flexion, abduction, and medial rotation (the so-called "salute" position).[60,111,123] An alternative is the "Statue of Liberty"[51,107] position, which allows more forward flexion (and external rotation if necessary), but this position is more dangerous relative to the neurovascular status[51] and more cumbersome for the patient. The fractures usually unite solidly by 6 weeks, but are stable much sooner than this. It is recommended that the patient in a cast be brought out of abduction by about 3 weeks, because deltoid muscle contractures can develop with prolonged immobilization in the abducted position. Range[107] has suggested percutaneous pinning for these unstable fractures, which seems to be an attractive alternative, but the author has no experience with this technique.

Traction (skin or skeletal) is another alternative for obtaining or maintaining reduction.[111,129] It is occa-

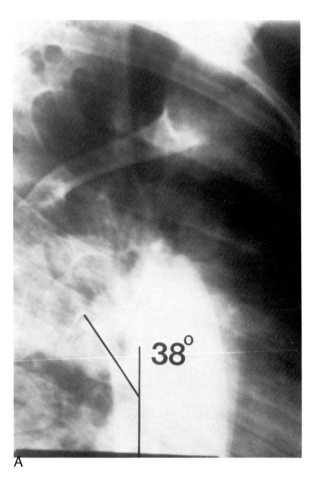

A

sionally possible to achieve reduction slowly with a period of overhead traction, and this avoids the chance of neurologic injury during manipulation. Traction is also an attractive means to hold an unstable fracture, because the fracture usually becomes "sticky" in a very short period of time (7 to 10 days) and then the arm can slowly be brought down to the side and immobilized in a Velpeau dressing without the need for spica casting. The major disadvantage to this form of treatment is the length of hospital stay required, the cost of which may prohibit the use of traction except in unusual cases. A hanging cast is an ambulatory form of traction recommended by some authors, however, it requires that the child sleep upright and the initial discomfort is usually too great for one to recommend this form of treatment for children.[123]

The results of treatment are generally good even if moderate amounts of angulation are accepted.[123] Several studies show that moderate amounts of shortening do persist following treatment, probably due to injury of the growth plate and residual angulation.[2,14] Neer and Horowitz[91] noted, however, that shortening could occur even in minimally displaced injuries. In their study of 89 patients they noted shortening of 1 to 3 cm in 9 percent of grade I and II injuries and in 33 percent of their grade IV

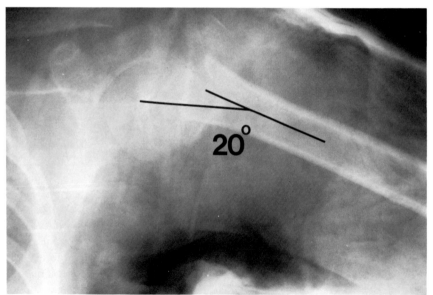

B

Fig. 10-11. (A) This patient sustained a displaced Salter-Harris type II of the proximal humerus with 38° of angulation. (B) It was possible to reduce this to 20° and he was placed into a shoulder spica. (*Figure continues.*)

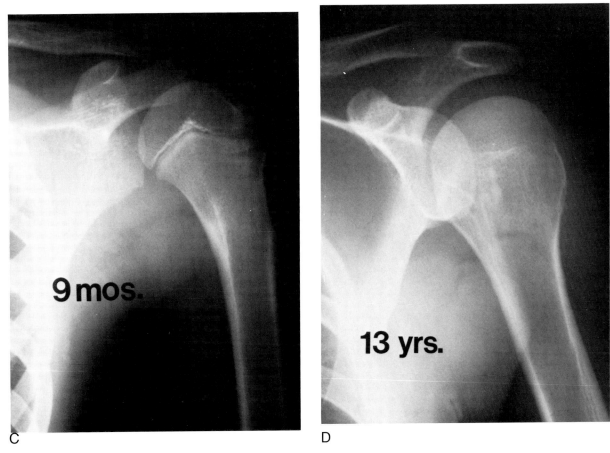

Fig. 10-11 *(Continued)*. **(C)** By 9 months there is considerable remodeling. **(D)** Thirteen years following the injury, there has been complete remodeling of the fracture site.

injuries. Of interest was that no permanent shortening occurred in patients under 11 years of age, presumably because of the tremendous remodeling potential of this age group. In no instance was the shortening a functional problem, and this finding has been confirmed by others.[10] Nilsson and Svarthom[94] studied the results of proximal humerus fractures in 44 children under 17 years of age, most of whom were treated by closed means. They noted shortening of 1 to 2 cm in two cases. There was only one poor functional result and this occurred in a patient treated operatively. The displacement observed at the end of initial treatment disappeared by the time of follow-up (7.8 years in this series). They concluded that open reduction was associated with muscle atrophy and weakness and should be avoided. Hohl[51] analyzed a series of 15 patients, of whom had types III and IV,

and concluded that there was no pressing need to achieve anatomical reduction. Closed reduction and casting or traction was recommended, but even in those where the reduction was lost, a residual palpable deformity anteriorly was the only untoward result. Most of the remodeling of the deformity occurred in the first 9 months following fracture. Most authors agree that there is seldom an indication for open reduction of fractures of the proximal humeral growth plate[58,123] and, in fact, the results of operated cases are worse than those treated closed. The potential of creating an unappealing scar, the risks of anesthesia and infection, and the chance of redisplacement make open reduction an unattractive alternative for all but the exceptional case (e.g., those rare ones with biceps entrapped in the fracture site)[133] or in open fractures.

Fractures of the proximal humeral metaphysis are

relatively less common than epiphyseal injuries, but occur in the same age groups. The clinical presentation is exactly the same as for the epiphyseal plate injuries. Greenstick or minimally displaced fractures can be treated symptomatically in a sling of Velpeau for 3 to 4 weeks and union is rapidly evident on radiographs. Displaced fractures with angulation and some apposition can be reduced closed to improve the angulation, but the same principles apply as for epiphyseal injuries. The deltoid masks even moderately severe angulation and the range of motion of the glenohumeral joint precludes any functional loss of

movement. Completely displaced fractures are very difficult to reduce anatomically because applied traction is dissipated in the glenohumeral joint, and the strong muscles about the shoulder are difficult to overcome (Fig. 10-12). An attempt may be made with muscle relaxation under general anesthesia and, if successful, the reduction can be maintained in a coaptation splint or with skin or skeletal traction until the fracture becomes "sticky." Apposition of the fracture fragments is not required and bayonette apposition, if properly aligned, may be accepted. Residual disability is unusual regardless of the amount of angulation or displacement: there is seldom an indication for open reduction.[77]

Dislocations

Children are much more likely to sustain a fracture through a growth plate rather than dislocate a joint, but dislocations do occur on occasion.[5,114,117,140] The distinction between an acromioclavicular dislocation and an epiphyseal injury has been made in a previous section. The true acromioclavicular dislocation, when it occurs (usually in a patient over the age of 13 to 16 years), is managed similarly to the same injury in an adult, and the reader is referred to Chapter 7. It is unclear whether true dislocations of the sternoclavicular joint occur in children but, again, the management is identical to that in the adult. Glenohumeral joint dislocations and their treatment[9,91] are well cov-

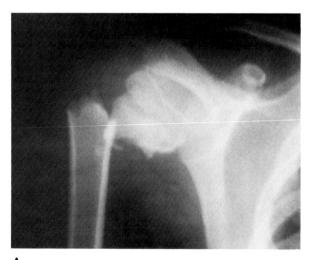

A

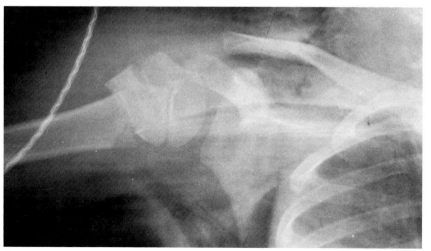

B

Fig. 10-12. (A) A completely displaced proximal humeral metaphyseal fracture in a child with multisystem trauma. (Courtesy of John B. Emans, M.D., Children's Hospital, Boston, MA.) **(B)** An attempt at reduction and skeletal traction yielded good alignment. (*Figure continues.*)

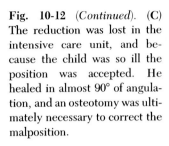

Fig. 10-12 *(Continued)*. **(C)** The reduction was lost in the intensive care unit, and because the child was so ill the position was accepted. He healed in almost 90° of angulation, and an osteotomy was ultimately necessary to correct the malposition.

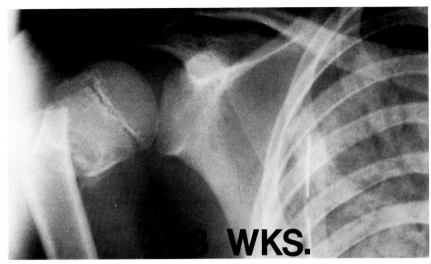

C

ered in Chapter 6, where the high incidence of redislocation in children was pointed out.[72,90,116,121,134] Children may present with atraumatic dislocations of the shoulder in patients with Ehlers-Danlos disease and other connective tissue diseases[111] and voluntary and habitual dislocations.[61,76,117]

OTHER INJURIES

The principles of diagnosis and management of traumatic injuries about the shoulder in children have been presented, but it must be remembered that in dealing with patients who cannot always provide a complete, accurate history, nontraumatic entities may also be present or mimic fractures. The proximal humerus is a common site for certain bone tumors that may present as pathologic fractures. At times the underlying process may be difficult to appreciate, so a high index of suspicion must be maintained, especially if the magnitude of the insult is not severe. The benign lesions that commonly appear in this location in children are the unicameral bone cyst (Fig. 10-13), fibrous cortical defect, nonossifying fibroma, chondroblastoma, and eosinophilic granuloma, although almost any bone tumor can occur in this site. More details about these lesions are provided in

Chapter 19. In general, if the radiograph shows a benign-appearing lesion, it is best to allow the fracture to heal prior to dealing with the tumor. Occasionally, as in some unicameral bone cysts, the stimulus of the fracture will lead to healing of the lesion. In addition, it is difficult to deal properly with the bony defect created by the tumor if a fracture is present.

It is crucial to remember that the proximal humerus is the third most common site for osteosarcomas and that not all osteosarcomas are blastic. The pain of a malignant tumor may initially be ascribed to trauma (children are always falling!), thus delaying the diagnosis. If in doubt, always obtain a radiograph. Remember that the presence of a fracture can mask the underlying malignant process if the radiograph is interpreted casually, and the orthopaedist can be lulled into treating the fracture while ignoring the underlying tumor.

Fractures of the proximal humerus may occur commonly in battered or abused children.[56,81,96,129,141] This occurs mostly in infants and children less than 3 years of age. The best way of making the diagnosis is to be alert to the possibility. A careful history of the traumatic event must be obtained, and any discrepancy between the magnitude of the injury and the stated mechanism must be noted. A history of prior fractures should be ascertained and attention paid to the social setting. Although more common in families with young parents and in poorer socioeconomic settings, the syndrome is by no means absent

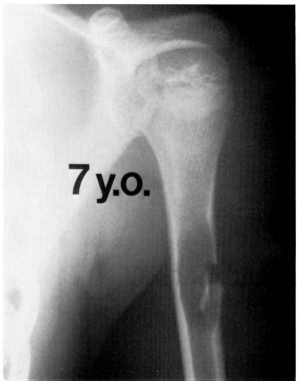

A

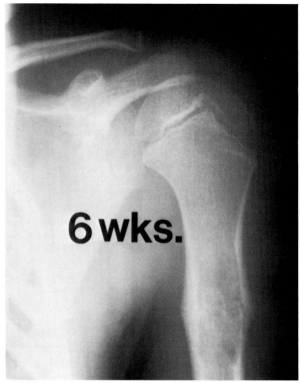

B

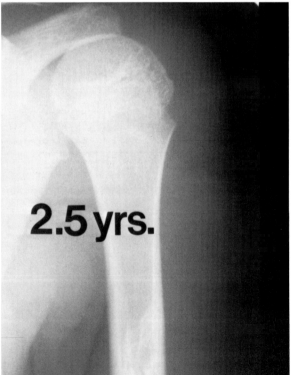

C

Fig. 10-13. (**A**) A 7-year-old boy with a pathologic fracture through a solitary bone cyst of the humerus. (**B**) Sometimes a fracture of the cyst may stimulate healing. (**C**) Two and a half years following the injury the fracture and the cyst have healed.

in well-to-do families. Most hospitals have teams of social workers and physicians knowledgeable in this area to aid the orthopaedist in properly identifying children who are subjects of such abuse. On physical examination other signs of trauma may be present such as cigarette burns, bruises, blunt abdominal trauma, and, in severe cases, subdural hematomas. Radiographs may show multiple fractures at various stages of repair. Metaphyseal fractures and physeal injuries are most common, but spiral and transverse fractures may also be present. Posterior rib fractures are a common manifestation. The amount of soft tissue swelling and bruising may be so great as to mimic a septic process in the shoulder joint (Fig. 10-14). The

differential diagnosis includes osteogenesis imperfecta, congenital indifference to pain, nutritional disturbances such as scurvy, and Caffey's disease (infantile cortical hyperostosis). The importance of recognizing the battering syndrome cannot be overemphasized: treatment of the fracture is routine; treatment of the child and family is much more complex, and missed diagnoses can lead to unnecessary permanent injury or even death of the child.

On occasion, metabolic diseases can present radiographic findings that mimic fracture. In patients with renal osteodystrophy, epiphyseal widening can occur and on occasion slippage of the epiphysis develops (the latter is much more common about the hip, how-

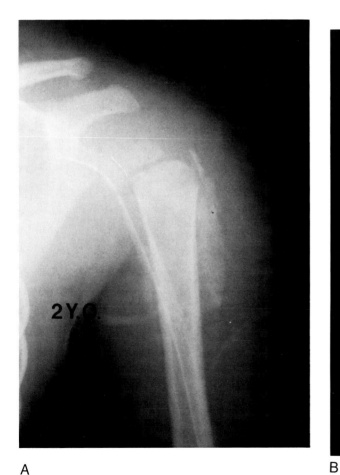

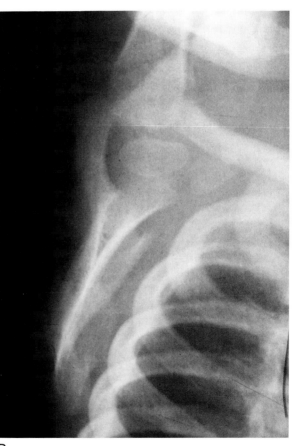

A   B

Fig. 10-14. **(A)** This 2-year-old boy with a fever and massive swelling of his proximal humerus was believed to have a septic shoulder joint or osteomyelitis. Cultures from aspiration and drainage of the joint were sterile. **(B)** It was subsequently noted that the child had other fractures of varying ages, such as the fractures of the scapula and proximal humerus seen here. (*Figure continues.*)

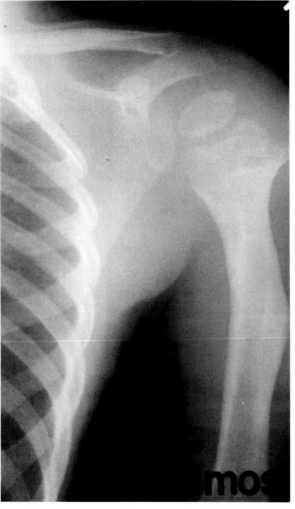

C

Fig. 10-14 *(Continued).* **(C)** In addition to receiving fracture care, a social worker was assigned to his case. By 8 months the fractures have healed but not quite completely remodeled. There was some residual shortening of the humerus, presumably due to direct injury to the growth plate.

ever). The Looser's transformation zone or umbauzonen of rickets may be seen on the axillary border of the scapula; the clinical setting and diffuse osteopenia are usually sufficiently apparent to exclude the possibility of fracture.

Stress fractures are uncommon in the proximal humerus, but have been reported in children participating in Little League pitching.[19] The stresses generated during throwing are severe and predispose to

injury. This overuse syndrome presents in young teenagers with pain and inability to perform the sport. The radiographs show a widened epiphyseal plate, suggesting an epiphyseal separation as the pathologic basis for this syndrome. It is relieved with rest.

Swimmers and pitchers may also develop impingement syndromes similar to those in adults due to impingement of the rotator cuff between the humeral head and the coracoacromial ligament or acromion.[82,83,89] It is unusual for this to occur before the age of 10 years. Tenderness is concentrated to the rotator cuff and may be accentuated by pressure over the coracoacromial ligament. Radiographs may show some calcifications in the cuff area in older children but are usually normal. Acute treatment is with anti-inflammatory medication and subsequent shoulder-girdle-strengthening exercises. Division of the ligament may infrequently be necessary. Overuse may also produce contractures about the shoulder with loss of internal rotation with the shoulder in 90° of abduction and increased external rotation.[82,83] It is thought that a tight posterior capsule can lead to anterior subluxation. Response to physical therapy that emphasizes resisted internal rotation and improving range of motion is rewarding.

REFERENCES

1. Abbott LC, Lucas DB: The function of the clavicle. Its surgical significance. Ann Surg 140:583, 1954
2. Aitken AP: End results of fracture of the proximal humeral epiphysis. J Bone Joint Surg 18:1036, 1936
3. Allman FL: Fractures and ligamentous injuries of the clavicle and its articulation. J Bone Joint Surg 49A:774, 1967
4. Angle CR: Congenital bowing and angulation of long bones. Pediatrics 13:257, 1954
5. Asher MA: Dislocations of the upper extremity in children. Orthop Clin North Am 7:583, 1976
6. Aufranc OE, Jones WN, Butler JE: Epiphyseal fracture of the proximal humerus. JAMA 213:1476, 1970
7. Bagnoli F, et al: Calcitonin and parathyroid hormone in newborn infants with fracture of the clavicle. Calcif Tissue Int 36:357, 1984
8. Balata A, Olzai MG, Porcu A et al: Fracture of the clavicle in the newborn. Riv Ital Ped, 1980
9. Bankart ASB: An operation for recurrent dislocation

(subluxation) of the sternoclavicular joint. Br J Surg 26:320, 1938

10. Baxter ME, McIntyre W, Wiley J: Fractures of the proximal humeral epiphysis. Orthop Trans 9:506, 1985

11. Bearn JG: Direct observations on the function of the capsule of the sternoclavicular support. J Anat 101:159, 1967

12. Blount WP: Fractures in Children. Williams and Wilkins, Baltimore, 1955

13. Booth CM, Roper BA: Chronic dislocation of the sternoclavicular joint. Clin Orthop 140:17, 1979

14. Bourdillon JF: Fracture-separation of the proximal epiphysis of the humerus. J Bone Joint Surg 32B:35, 1950

15. Bowen AD: Plastic bowing of the clavicle in children. J Bone Joint Surg 65A:403, 1983

16. Brooks AL, Henning GD: Injury to the proximal clavicular epiphysis. J Bone Joint Surg 54A:1347, 1972

17. Browne JE et al: Acromioclavicular joint dislocations: comparative results following operative treatment with and without primary distal clavisectomy. Am J Sports Med 5:258, 1977

18. Buckfield CT, Castle ME: Acute traumatic dislocation of the clavicle. J Bone Joint Surg 66A:379, 1984

19. Cahill BR, Tullos HS, Fain RH: Little league shoulder. J Sports Med, 2:150, 1974

20. Campbell J: Fracture-separation of the proximal humeral epiphysis. J Bone Joint Surg 59A:262, 1977

21. Chung MK, Nissenbaum MM: Congenital and developmental defects of the shoulder. Orthop Clin North Am 6:381, 1975

22. Clark RL, Milgram JW, Yawn DH: Fatal aortic perforation and cardiac tamponade due to a Kirschner wire migrating from the right sternocalvicular joint. South Med J 67:316, 1974

23. Cohen AW, Otto SR: Obstetrical clavicular fractures: a three year analysis. J Reprod Med 25:119, 1980

24. Conwell EH: Fractures of the surgical neck and epiphyseal separations of the upper end of humerus. J Bone Joint Surg 8:508, 1926

25. Cozen L: Congenital dislocation of the shoulder and other anomalies. Arch Surg 35:956, 1937

26. Cumming WA: Neonatal skeletal fractures. Birth trauma or child abuse? J Can Assoc Radiol 30:30, 1979

27. Dameron TB, Reibel DB: Fractures involving the proximal humeral epiphyseal plate. J Bone Joint Surg 51A:289, 1969

28. Dameron TB, Rockwood CA: Fractures and dislocations of the shoulder. p. 577. In Rockwood, Wilkins, King: Fractures in Children. J.B. Lippincott, Philadelphia, 1984

29. Denham RH, Dingley AF: Epiphyseal separation of the medial clavicle. J Bone Joint Surg 49A:1179, 1967

30. DePalma AF: The role of the disks of the sternoclavicular and the acromioclavicular joints. Clin Orthop 13:222, 1959

31. Destouet JM, Gilula LA, Murphy WA, Sagel SS: Computed tomography of the sternoclavicular joint and sternum. Radiology 138:123, 1981

32. Eidman DK, Siff SJ, Tullos HS: Acromioclavicular lesions in children. Am J Sports Med 9:150, 1981

33. Elting JJ: Retrosternal dislocations of the clavicle. Arch Surg 104:35, 1972

34. Falstie-Jensen S, Mikkelsen P: Pseudodislocation of the acromioclavicular joint. J Bone Joint Surg 64B:368, 1982

35. Farkas R, Levine S: X-ray incidence of fractured clavicle in vertex presentation. Am J Obstet Gynecol 59:204, 1950

36. Fraser RL, Haliburton RA, Barber JR: Displaced epiphyseal fractures of the proximal humerus. Can J Surg 10:427, 1967

37. Gardner E: The embryology of the clavicle. Clin Orthop 58:9, 1968

38. Gardner E, Gray DJ: Prenatal development of the human shoulder and acromioclavicular joints. Am J Anat 92:219, 1953

39. Gray DJ, Gardner E: The prenatal development of the human humerus. Am J Anat 124:431, 1969

40. Greenlee DP: Posterior dislocation of the sternal end of the clavicle. JAMA 125:426, 1944

41. Gumley GJ, Jupiter JJ: Clavicle non-union—a review of management and presentation of a stable bone graft. Orthop Trans 9:29, 1985

42. Gunther WA: Posterior dislocation of the clavicle. J Bone Joint Surg 31A:878, 1949

43. Hadesman W, Trotter D, Ibrahim K: Consultation corner. A little help from your friends. Orthopaedics 5:603, 1982

44. Halburton RA, Barber JR, Fraser RL: Pseudodislocation: an unusual birth injury. Can J Surg 10:455, 1967

45. Hardegger FH, Simpson LA, Weber BG: The operative treatment of scapular fractures. J Bone Joint Surg 66B:725, 1984

46. Heck CC: Anterior dislocation of the glenohumeral joint in a child. J Trauma 21:174, 1981

47. Hedstrom O: Growth stimulation of long bones after fracture or similar trauma. A clinical and experimental study. Acta Orthop Scand Suppl 122:7, 1969

48. Heinig CF: Retrosternal dislocation of the clavicle: early recognition, x-ray diagnosis and management. J Bone Joint Surg 50A:830, 1968

49. Hensinger RN, Jones ET: Neonatal Orthopaedics. Grune & Stratton, New York, 1981

50. Heyse-Moore GH, Stoker DJ: Avulsion fractures of the scapula. Skel Radiol 9:27, 1982

51. Hohl JC: Fractures of the humerus in children. Orthop Clin North Am 7:557, 1976

52. Horak J, Nilsson BE: Epidemiology of fracture of the upper end of the humerus. Clin Orthop Rel Res 112:251, 1975

53. Howard FM, Shafer SJ: Injuries to the clavicle with neurovascular complications: a study of fourteen cases. J Bone Joint Surg 47A:1335, 1965

54. Jablon M Sutker A, Post M: Irreducible fractures of the middle-end of the clavicle. J Bone Joint Surg 61A:296, 1979

55. Jeffrey CC: Fracture separation of the upper humeral epiphysis. Surg Gynecol Obstet 96:205, 1953

56. Kempe CH, Silverman FN, Steele BF et al: The battered-child syndrome. JAMA 251:3288, 1984

57. Kennedy JC: Retrosternal dislocation of the clavicle. J Bone Joint Surg 31B:74, 1949

58. Kohler R, Trillaud JM: Fracture and fracture separation of the proximal humerus in children: report of 136 cases. J Pediatr Orthop 3:326, 1983

59. Kuhn D, Rosman M: Traumatic, nonparalytic dislocation of the shoulder in a newborn infant. J Pediatr Orthop 4:121, 1984

60. Landin LA: Fracture patterns in children. Acta Orthop Scand Suppl 202:1, 1983

61. Lawhon SM, Peoples, AB, MacEwen GD: Voluntary dislocation of the shoulder. J Pediatr Orthop 2:590, 1982

62. Lee FA, Gwinn JL: Retrosternal dislocation of the clavicle. Radiology 110:631, 1974

63. Lemire L, Rosman M: Sternoclavicular epiphyseal separation with adjacent clavicular fracture. J Pediatr Orthop 4:118, 1984

64. Lemperg R, Liliequist B: Dislocation of the proximal epiphysis of the humerus in newborns. Report of two cases and discussion of diagnostic criteria. Acta Pediatr Scand 59:377, 1970

65. Levisohn EM, Bunnell WP, Yuan HA: Computed tomography in the diagnosis of dislocations of the sternoclavicular joint. Clin Orthop 140:12, 1979

66. Lichtbalu PO: Shoulder dislocation in the infant. Case report and discussion. J Fla Med Assoc 64:313, 1977

67. Lindseth RE, DeRosa GP: Fractures in children. General consideration and treatment of open fractures. Pediatr Clin North Am 22:465, 1975

68. Ljunggren AE: Clavicular function. Acta Orthop Scand 50:261, 1979

69. Lourie AA: Tomography in the diagnosis of posterior dislocation of the sterno-clavicular joint. Acta Orthop Scand 51:579, 1980

70. Lowman CL: Operative correction of old sternoclavicular dislocation. J Bone Joint Surg 10:740, 1928

71. Lunseth PA, Chapman KW, Frankel VH: Surgical treatment of chronic dislocation of the sterno-clavicular joint. J Bone Joint Surg 57B:193, 1975

72. Lyne DE: Traumatic shoulder dislocation in children with open epiphyses. J Pediatr Orthop 2:446, 1982

73. Madsen ET: Fractures of the extremities in the newborn. Acta Obstet Gynaecol Scand 34:41, 1955

74. Manske DJ, Szabo RM: The operative treatment of mid-shaft clavicular non-unions. J Bone Joint Surg 67A:1367, 1985

75. Marsh HO, Hazarian E: Pseudarthrosis of the clavicle. J Bone Joint Surg 52B:793, 1970

76. May VR, Jr: Posterior dislocation of the shoulder: habitual, traumatic and obstetrical. Orthop Clin North Am 11:271, 1980

77. McBride EO, Sisler J: Fractures of the proximal humeral epiphysis and juxta-epiphyseal humeral shaft. Clin Orthop 38:143, 1965

78. McClelland CQ, Heiple KG: Fractures in the first year of life. A diagnostic dilemma. Am J Dis Child 136:26, 1982

79. McGahan JP, Rab GT, Dublin A: Fractures of the scapula. J Trauma 20:880, 1980

80. McKenzie JMM: Retrosternal dislocation of the clavicle. A report of two cases. J Bone Joint Surg 45B:138, 1961

81. Merten DF, Kirks DR, Ruderman RJ: Occult humeral epiphyseal fracture in battered infants. Pediatr Radiol 10:151, 1981

82. Michele LJ: Overuse injuries in children's sports: the growth factor. Orthop Clin North Am 14:337, 1983

83. Michele LJ, Smith AD: Sports injuries in children. p. 9. In Current Problems in Pediatrics. Year Book Medical Publishers, Chicago, 1982

84. Miller DS, Boswick JA: Lesions of the brachial plexus associated with fractures of the clavicle. Clin Orthop 64:144, 1969

85. Mital M, Aufranc OE: Venous occulsion following greenstick fracture of the clavicle. JAMA 206:1301, 1968

86. Montgomery SP, Loyd D: Avulsion fracture of the coracoid epiphysis with acromioclavicular separation. J Bone Joint Surg 59A:963, 1977

87. Moseley HF: The clavicle: its anatomy and function. Clin Orthop 58:17, 1968

88. Beer CS II: Fractures of the distal third of the clavicle. Clin Orthop 58:43, 1968

89. Neer CS II: Nonunion of the clavicle. JAMA 172:1006, 1968

90. Neer CS II, Foster CR: Inferior capsular shift for involuntary inferior and multidirectional instability of the shoulder. J Bone Joint Surg 62A:897, 1980

91. Neer CS II, Horwicz BS: Fractures of the proximal humeral epiphyseal plate. Clin Orthop 41:24, 1965

92. Nettles JL, Linscheid RL: Sternoclavicular dislocations. J Trauma 8:158, 1968

93. Nicastro JF, Adair DM: Fracture–dislocation of the shoulder in a 32-month-old child. J Pediatr Orthop 2:427, 1982

94. Nilsson S, Svartholm F: Fracture of the upper end of the humerus in children. A follow-up of 44 cases. Acta Chir Scand 130:433, 1965

95. Nogi J, Heckman JD, Hakala M, Sweet DE: Nonunion of the clavicle in a child. A case report. Clin Orthop 110:19, 1975

96. O'Neill JA, Jr., Meacham WF, Griffin PP, Sawyers JL: Patterns of injury in the battered child syndrome. J Trauma 13:332, 1973

97. Ogden JA: Skeletal Injury in the Child. Lea & Febiger, Philadelphia, 1982

98. Ogden JA: Radiology of postnatal skeletal development. VII. The scapula. Skel Radiol 9:157, 1983

99. Ogden JA: Distal clavicular physeal injury. Clin Orthop 188:68, 1984

100. Ogden JA, Conlogue CJ, Bronson ML: Radiology of postnatal skeletal development. III. The clavicle. Skel Radiol 4:196, 1979

101. Ogden JA, Conlogue GJ, Jensen P: Radiology of postnatal skeletal development: the proximal humerus. Skel Radiol 2:153, 1978

102. Omer GE: Osteotomy of the clavicle in surgical reduction of anterior sternoclavicular dislocation. J Trauma 7:584, 1967

103. Paterson DC: Retrosternal dislocation of the clavicle. J Bone Joint Surg 43B:90, 1961

104. Penn I: The vascular complications of fractures of the clavicle. J Trauma 4:819, 1964

105. Peterson CA, Peterson HA: Analysis of the incidence of injuries to the epiphyseal growth plate. J Trauma 12:275, 1972

106. Pierce RO, Hodurski DF: Fractures of the humerus, radius and ulna in the same extremity. J Trauma 19:182, 1979

107. Rang M: Children's Fractures. J.B. Lippincott, Philadelphia, 1983

108. Rauschning W, Nordesjo LO, Nirdgren B et al: Resection arthroplasty for repair of complete acromioclavicular separations. Arch Orthop Trauma Surg 97:161, 1980

109. Rockwood CA: Subluxations and dislocations about the shoulder. p. 577. In Rockwood, CA, Jr., Wilkins KE, King RE (eds): Fractures in Adults, J.B. Lippincott, Philadelphia, 1984

110. Rockwood CA, Jr.: Fracture of the outer clavicle in children and adults. J Bone Joint Surg 64B:642, 1982

111. Rockwood CA, Jr., Wilkins KE, King RE: Fractures in Children. J.B. Lippincott, Philadelphia, 1984

112. Roper BA, Levack B: The surgical treatment of acromioclavicular dislocations. J Bone Joint Surg 64B:597, 1982

113. Rose SH, Melton LJ, Morrey BF et al: Epidemiologic features of humeral fractures. Clin Orthop 168:24, 1982

114. Rowe CR: An atlas of anatomy and treatment of midclavicular fractures. Clin Orthop 58:29, 1968

115. Rowe CR: Fractures of the scapula. Surg Clin North Am 43:1565, 1963

116. Rowe CR: Prognosis in dislocation of the shoulder. J Bone Joint Surg 38A:957, 1956

117. Rowe CR, Pierce DS, Clark JG: Voluntary dislocation of the shoulder. J Bone Joint Surg 55A:445, 1973

118. Rubin A: Birth injuries: incidence, mechanism and end result. Obstet Gynecol 23:218, 1964

119. Salter RB, Harris WR: Injuries involving the epiphyseal plate. J Bone Surg 45A:587, 1963

120. Salvatore JE: Sternoclavicular joint dislocation. Clin Orthop 58:51, 1968

121. Scaglietti O: The obstetrical shoulder trauma. Surg Gynecol Obstet 66:868, 1938

122. Selesnick FH, Jablon M, Frank C, Post M: Retrosternal dislocation of the clavicle. J Bone Joint Surg 66A:297, 1984

123. Sherk HH, Probst C: Fractures of the proximal humeral epiphysis. Orthop Clin North Am 6:401, 1975

124. Shulman BH, Terhune CB: Epiphyseal injuries in breech delivery. Pediatrics, 8:693, 1951

125. Simurda MA: Retrosternal dislocation of the clavicle: a report of four cases and a method of repair. Can J Surg 11:487, 1968

126. Smith FM: Fracture–separation of the proximal humeral epiphysis. Am J Surg 91:627, 1956

127. Snedecor ST, Wilson HB: Some obstetrical injuries to the long bones. J Bone Joint Surg 31A:378, 1949

128. Stein AH: Retrosternal dislocation of the clavicle. J Bone Joint Surg 39A:656, 1957

129. Tachdjian MO: Pediatric Orthopaedics. W.B. Saunders, Philadelphia, 1972

130. Taylor AR: Non-union of fractures of the clavicle: a review of thirty-one cases. J Bone Joint Surg 51B:568, 1969

131. Tse DHW, Slabaugh PB, Carlson PA: Injury to the axillary artery by a closed fracture of the clavicle. J Bone Joint Surg 62A:1372, 1980

132. Tyler HDD, Sturrock WDS, Callow FMC: Retrosternal dislocation of the clavicle. J Bone Joint Surg 45B:132, 1963

133. Visser JD, Reitberg M: Interposition of the tendon of the long head of biceps in fracture separation of the proximal humeral epiphysis. Netherlands J Surg 32:12, 1980

134. Wagner KT, Jr., Lyne ED: Adolescent traumatic dislocations of the shoulder with open epiphyses. J Pediatr Orthop 3:61, 1983

135. Weber BG, Brunner C, Freuler F: Treatment of Fractures in Children and Adolescents. Springer-Verlag, Berlin, 1980

136. Wheeler ME, Laaveg SJ, Sprague BL: S-C joint disruption in an infant. Clin Orthop 139:68, 1979

137. Wilbur MC, Evans EB: Fractures of the scapula. An analysis of forty cases and a review of the literature. J Bone Joint Surg 59A:358, 1977

138. Wilkins R, Johnston RM: Ununited fractures of the clavicle. J Bone Joint Surg 65A:773, 1983

139. Williams DJ: The mechanisms producing fracture-separations of the proximal humeral epiphysis. J Bone Joint Surg 63B:102, 1981

140. Wilson JC: Fractures and dislocations in children. Pediatr Clin North Am 14:659, 1967

141. Zenni EJ, Krieg JK, Rosen MJ: Open reduction and internal fixation of clavicle fractures. J Bone Joint Surg 63A:147, 1981

142. Zilberman Z, Rejouitzky R: Fracture of the coracoid process of the clavicle. Injury 13:203, 1981

Shoulder Injuries in Sports

11

Bertram Zarins
Chadwick C. Prodromos

The shoulder joint is commonly injured in sports. A recent study of athletic injuries incurred in 22 sports at two colleges disclosed that 7.5 percent of injuries involved the shoulder. Only the knee and ankle had higher rates of injury.[49]

The purposes of this chapter are to describe types of shoulder injuries commonly sustained in different sports and to review the changing picture of physical therapy with its specific indications to each sport. The amount of information available on shoulder injuries in each sport varies. Some sports, such as baseball, have been studied extensively. In other sports, only clinical impressions and anecdotal information are available.

The shoulder can be injured as a result of acute trauma or from chronic overuse or misuse. Overuse injuries that result from repetitive shoulder action, such as throwing or swimming, will be discussed. Detailed information regarding the diagnosis and treatment of the specific injuries can also be found in the chapters in this book that deal with each anatomic part.

BASEBALL

A wide spectrum of shoulder problems afflict baseball players, especially pitchers. "Injuries to the throwing arm" has been the subject of three national conferences sponsored by the United States Olympic Committee and United States Baseball Federation, the proceedings of which have been published in a book bearing this title.[115] To properly understand how to prevent overuse injuries due to throwing, it is important to understand the throwing motion. One can then advise the pitcher on correct body mechanics and techniques. Using the correct throwing motion and proper body mechanics are the most important aspects in preventing overuse injuries to the shoulder.

The most common shoulder injuries incurred in baseball are rotator cuff lesions and the impingement syndrome, anterior glenohumeral subluxation, glenoid labrum tears, acromioclavicular joint injuries, posterior shoulder instability, proximal humeral physeal separations, neurovascular syndromes, suprascapular nerve entrapment, and other lesions.[115]

The Pitching Mechanism

The pitching mechanism has been studied by several investigators[5,6,28,37,57] and is well described by Jobe[53] and McLeod.[68]

The pitching motion can be divided into five phases[68]:

1. Wind-up
2. Cocking
3. Acceleration
4. Release and deceleration
5. Follow-through

THE WIND-UP

The wind-up phase (Fig. 11-1A) begins with an initial balance stance phase. This phase takes place in slow motion. Both feet are planted on the ground. The opposite leg is cocked and the ball is removed from the glove.

COCKING

The contralateral leg is planted directly in front of the body and the pelvis is rotated internally (Fig. 11-1B). The pitching shoulder is abducted to 90 degrees and the humerus is externally rotated to 160°. This places the anterior shoulder capsule under tension. The deltoid, supraspinatus, infraspinatus, and teres minor muscles undergo forceful contraction. The ball is not moved forward during this phase but the shoulder and chest advance forward.

ACCELERATION

When the forward movement of the chest and shoulders stops, the acceleration phase (Fig. 11-1C) of the ball begins. The body is brought forward and the arm follows behind it. The latissimus dorsi, pectoralis major, and teres major muscles contract. High valgus stress is applied to the elbow as the arm whips forward. The ball is accelerated from 0 to 80 mi/h in approximately 80 msec. The energy that was developed by the body moving forward is transferred to the arm to accelerate the humerus. The internal rotator muscles contract forcefully. Three posterior rotator cuff muscles (supraspinatus, infraspinatus, and teres minor) contract forcefully for a short duration to impart deceleration forces to the horizontal adduction movement of the humerus.

RELEASE AND DECELERATION

The deceleration forces (Fig. 11-1D) are approximately twice as strong as acceleration forces. Ball release occurs over an approximately 8 to 10 msec interval. At the moment of ball release the ball has been accelerated to achieve maximum velocity. At this time, arm motion must be quickly decelerated to prevent the humeral head from subluxating. The rotator cuff and deltoid muscles contract. Peak deceleration torques are as high as 300 in lb at ball release.

At the beginning of the deceleration phase, the humerus is internally rotating quickly as the elbow is rapidly extending. Considerable forearm pronation results and high forces are transferred across the elbow to decelerate the forearm.

FOLLOW-THROUGH

During this phase, the body moves forward with the arm (Fig. 11-1E). This reduces distraction forces across the shoulder and reduces tension on the rotator cuff muscles. Planting the opposite leg is an important factor; this helps the pitcher maintain balance during the smooth transition from violent deceleration forces to recovery.

The motions of the shoulder during throwing different types of pitches are very similar. Atwater[6] has demonstrated that the amount of shoulder abduction remains approximately the same during overhead throwing, three quarters, or sidearm delivery. The difference occurs in the amount of body lean.

The force acting across the shoulder joint varies with different pitches, however. The fast ball requires less deceleration force than the curve ball or slider, and is, therefore, less traumatic. The curve ball requires the highest deceleration velocities, even though it is thrown at a slower speed.

Adaptive Changes

The dominant arm of a pitcher undergoes adaptive changes that should be recognized and distinguished from pathologic lesions. The muscles as well as bones undergo hypertrophy.[111] The throwing shoulder has significantly increased external rotation and decreased internal rotation compared to the nondominant shoulder. Excess external rotation is so commonly seen in pitchers that, if it is not present, it is a sign of injury.[3,57,70]

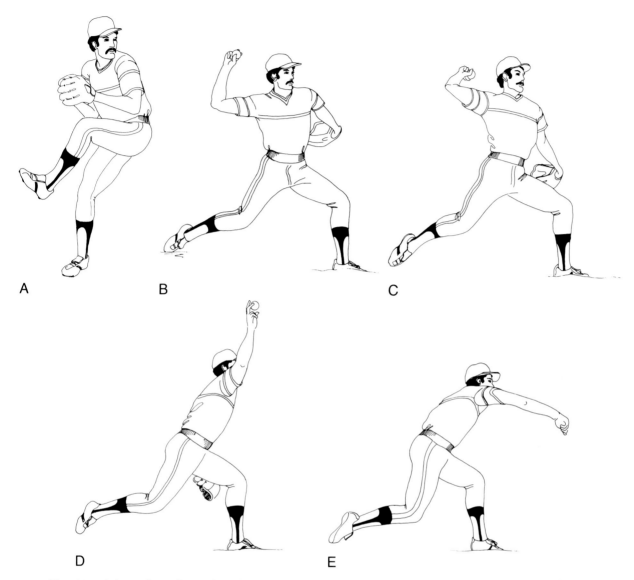

Fig. 11-1. (**A**) Wind-up phase of pitching motion. (**B**) Cocking phase. (**C**) Acceleration phase. (**D**) Release and deceleration phase. (**E**) Follow-through phase. (McLeod W: The pitching mechanism. p. 22. In Zarins R, Andrews JR, Carson W (eds): Injuries to the Throwing Arm, WB Saunders, Philadelphia, 1985. Reprinted with permission from WB Saunders, Co.)

Rotator Cuff Injury and Impingement Syndrome

The rotator cuff and capsule function to stabilize the humeral head in the glenoid cavity during shoulder motions. If the rotator cuff is injured or the capsule redundant from overstretching and the extrinsic forces on it are too great, the humeral head may subluxate or impinge against the acromial arch or the coracoid process. Impingement is less if the supraspinatus muscle sufficiently depresses the head of the humerus. This depressing action prevents the greater tuberosity from hitting against the coracoacromial arch. Whether impingement is the primary event causing rotator cuff tendinitis or whether impingement occurs secondary to rotator cuff disease is unproven. In all likelihood, both mechanisms of injury can occur.

The commonest symptom of rotator cuff pathology is pain located in the front of the shoulder. Pain is worse during the acceleration and follow-through phases. Impingement usually is aggravated by putting the shoulder in a position of 80 to 120° abduction, slight forward flexion, and internal rotation. It is relieved by abducting the shoulder in a position of external rotation. A pitcher who fixes his scapula by contracting his muscles theoretically exposes his shoulder more to impingement than the pitcher who allows his scapula to glide freely along the chest wall during pitching.

Subdeltoid or subacromial bursal adhesions have been reported to be a cause of anterior shoulder pain in baseball players.[76] In this condition, the investigators reproduced symptoms by abducting the shoulder and externally rotating the humerus to a cock-up position. At surgery, they found an inflamed bursa overlying a normal rotator cuff and long head of biceps tendon.

As the rotator cuff and biceps tendon are commonly the sites of degenerative tears,[10,40] treatment should include correction of abnormal throwing mechanics[37,53] as well as appropriate conservative or surgical therapy.[52] Variable prognoses for effective return to baseball pitching have been reported.[48,109]

Anterior Glenohumeral Subluxation

When the shoulder goes into extreme external rotation while in a position of 90° abduction (the cocking phase of the pitching motion) (Fig. 11-1B) an anteriorly directed force is exerted upon the anterior shoulder capsule by the humeral head. Repetitive force, as noted, can stretch the anterior capsule and result in anterior shoulder subluxation.[17] The athlete feels transient pain and disability when his arm is in this overhead position. This clinical syndrome has been referred to as the "dead arm syndrome."[94] The athlete has difficulty throwing forcefully, swimming and serving in tennis (see Ch. 7).

Physical examination shows a positive apprehension sign. Subluxation can be reproduced by pushing forward on the humeral head while the arm is abducted and externally rotated. Radiographs are usually normal. Arthrotomography occasionally demonstrates a torn anterior glenoid labrum. Arthroscopy may reveal a torn anterior glenoid labrum, a Bankart lesion, or an overstretched capsule.

It is common to overstretch the anterior capsule and to develop a sore shoulder in pitchers. Jobe[51] postulated that the pitcher who has this condition may be "opening up" too soon and dropping his elbow when pitching; the pitcher could be turning his trunk rapidly and dragging the arm behind it, levering the humeral head forward. Another secondary lesion we have noted in patients with the "dead arm" syndrome is an increase in the opening between the subscapularis and supraspinatus tendons extending out over the head of the humerus[94] (see Ch. 7).

Glenoid Labrum Tears

The anterior glenoid labrum can tear as the humeral head slides over the anterior glenoid rim. This can occur in anterior glenohumeral dislocation.[7,93] Glenoid labrum tears can also occur with recurrent anterior shoulder subluxation.[18,86,94] Glenoid labrum tears have also been reported to occur in stable shoulders, especially in throwing athletes.[2,82]

It appears that two types of glenoid labrum tears occur most commonly: the circumferential (vertical longitudinal) tear or the "flap" or radial tear (see Fig. 5-24, Ch. 5). Circumferential tears of the anterior glenoid labrum at the glenoid rim (Bankart lesion) usually occur in unstable shoulders. Various grades of severity can occur ranging from tearing of the labrum itself to avulsion of the capsule from the anterior glenoid rim to fracture of the anterior glenoid.[94]

Pappas has reported on 16 patients who had symptomatic tears of the glenoid labrum and no apparent shoulder instability.[82] Shoulder arthrotomy and resection of the torn labrum relieved symptoms in these patients. Andrews and Carson[2] reported similar findings and results following arthroscopic resection of torn glenoid labra.

The patient who has a torn glenoid labrum usually complains of a painful clicking or snapping of the shoulder as the arm goes into the abducted externally rotated position. The torn labrum itself can cause symptoms, analogous to symptoms caused by meniscus tears in knees.[114] In patients who have stable shoulders, it is probable that tension of the biceps tendon pulls on the anterior labrum when the arm is overhead. In the same shoulder position, symptoms can also be due to anterior glenohumeral subluxation.

New Developments in Rehabilitation of the Pitching Arm

An important development in recent years is the re-evaluation of the techniques of conditioning or restoring function of the shoulder. Instead of "routine" exercises to strengthen the shoulder muscles, the program should be *specific* for each sport.

The technique for improving shoulder function of a pitcher and a football player, for example, differ considerably. The pitcher needs an agile rhythmic whip to his arm and should not strive to develop excessive muscle bulk. This is in contrast to weight lifters and most football players whose aim is to develop muscle strength. The same conditioning program that is used by the football player to increase his muscle mass would probably be deleterious to the baseball pitcher. It would cause the pitcher to "guide" the ball, and destroy his variety of pitches, his accuracy, and variations of speed. A "muscle bound" shoulder does not have the speed and accuracy needed by a pitcher, a fencer, or, in many instances, the tennis player.

Whereas, the football player and weight lifter would gain by strenuous weight lifting and resistive exercises, the pitcher might lose function. The pitcher would do best with appropriate stretching exercises of his shoulder to maintain a range of motions and the rhythmic function of the shoulder required for accuracy and speed. Specific attention should be given to coordination of body and arm movements. Each shoulder motion should have a coordinated body movement.

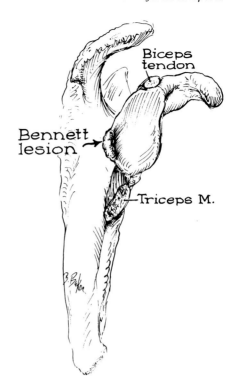

Fig. 11-2. Bennett lesion with ossification posterior inferior glenoid rim. (Barnes OA, Tullos HS: An analysis of 100 symptomatic baseball players. Am J Sports Med 6:62, © 1978. American Orthopaedic Society for Sports Medicine)

POSTERIOR GLENOID RIM LESIONS

Posterior shoulder pain in a baseball player can be caused by a lesion on the posterior inferior border of the glenoid fossa.[11,61] The posterior capsule syndrome was responsible for shoulder symptoms in 24 of 46 symptomatic baseball players.[8] Symptoms can develop suddenly or gradually. Pain typically occurs when the athlete is throwing hard, and can be reproduced by positioning the arm into abduction-external rotation as well as adduction-internal rotation (i.e., both the cocking and follow-through phases of throwing). Upon examination, tenderness can be found in the region of the posterior glenoid rim. Bennett described the pathologic lesions to be hypertrophy of the capsule and ossification at the posterior inferior glenoid fossa ("Bennett Lesion") (Fig. 11-2).[8,11] The lesion can cause irritation of the axillary nerve and referred pain to the deltoid muscle region. In contrast to Bennett's early report,[12] success has been reported following surgical excision of the Bennett lesion in professional baseball players.[61]

Posterior shoulder pain can also be caused by anterior glenohumeral subluxation. This condition should be kept in mind when examining the shoulder of a throwing athlete.

Proximal Humeral Physeal Separation

Proximal humeral physeal separation can occur in skeletally immature baseball players,[1,22,39,59] especially in a boy between the ages of 11 and 15 years who has been pitching extensively. Symptoms are pain and inability to throw hard. Radiographs typically demonstrate physeal widening but can also show demineralization, fragmentation, accelerated growth, and metaphyseal and diaphyseal new bone growth. Treatment includes temporary cessation of pitching. A good prognosis has been reported with 6 weeks rest without immobilization. Physeal closure at maturity should bring an end to disability from this overuse injury.

Biceps Tendon Subluxation

Subluxation of the tendon of the long head of biceps brachii muscle out of the bicipital groove has been reported to be a cause of shoulder pain in throwing athletes.[8,78] O'Donoghue[78] stated that the biceps tendon can ride up over the lesser tuberosity when the arm goes into external rotation and abduction if the transverse humeral ligament is lax. Peterson[84]

found medial displacement of the biceps tendon to occur only in connection with full thickness rupture of the supraspinatus tendon in 5 shoulders in an autopsy dissection study of 77 subjects.

Examination reveals tenderness over the bicipital groove. The tendon can be subluxated from the groove by extending the elbow and shoulder with the forearm pronated or by flexing the elbow against resistance, abducting the arm 90°, then, rotating the arm externally and internally.[78] Hitchcock and Bechtol[43] have demonstrated variation in the angle of the medial wall of the bicipital groove (Fig. 11-3). Radiographic studies can be used to diagnose a shallower than normal bicipital groove.[79] Conservative treatment usually improves symptoms but tenodesis of the tendon of the long head of biceps may be indicated.[78]

Tendinitis (Other Than Rotator Cuff)

Tendinitis can affect the pectoralis major and latissimus dorsi tendons near their insertions in the humerus.[8] The latissimus dorsi hypertrophies in the throwing arm of pitchers.[57] Rupture of this tendon has been reported in a baseball player.[8]

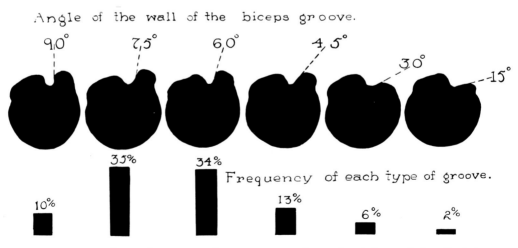

Fig. 11-3. Variation in bicipital groove configuration. Note the angle of the medial wall of the groove. (Hitchcock HH, Bectal CO: Painful shoulder. J Bone Joint Surg 30A:267, 1948.)

Acromioclavicular Joint

The acromioclavicular joint can be injured from a direct blow, such as from falling on the shoulder. Barnes and Tullos[8] reported a 12 percent incidence in baseball players. The acromioclavicular joint can also be the site of chronic injury. This is usually symptomatic in the follow-through phase of the throwing motion and when the arm is adducted (see Chapter 8).

Neurovascular Syndromes

The thoracic outlet syndrome has caused symptoms in baseball players.[105] The diagnosis may be difficult to make, because the physical findings in this condition are similar to the signs of anterior shoulder subluxation (i.e., pain that can be reproduced by externally rotating the abducted shoulder).

Axillary artery occlusion has been reported to occur as the result of pressure on the artery by the pectoralis minor tendon. Occlusion occurred during the hyperabduction cocking phase of the throwing motion in a baseball player.[111] The patient was treated with vascular bypass surgery.

Subclavian vein thrombosis in a college shortstop was reported by Wright and Lipscomb.[113] The patient complained of a sudden onset of swelling and numbness in the arm. The patient was treated by elective transaxial resection of the first rib and division of the scalenus anticus muscle.

BASKETBALL

Injuries to the shoulder comprise only 3 percent of all injuries in professional basketball players.[4,42] Eighty-eight percent of these injuries were contusions and muscle strains. Falls can cause shoulder contusions or acromioclavicular joint injuries.

Overuse syndromes of the shoulder have not been reported to occur in basketball, despite the fact that playing basketball requires repetitive overhead shoulder use. The probable reason is that the shoulder motion used to play basketball is forward elevation (which occurs in the frontal plane). The shoulder is not abducted (in the sagittal plane) as it is in the throwing motion. Hyperextension of the arm during a "lay-up" (i.e., abduction and external rotation) would predispose the shoulder to anterior subluxation or dislocation.

DANCE

The shoulder is not frequently injured in dance. Only 3 of 114 injuries sustained by professional ballet dancers were found to involve the shoulder.[58] Shoulder injuries were not mentioned in three other studies of injuries from dance.[92,95,108] We have seen chronic pain develop in the scapulothoracic joint from isolated shoulder motions used in dance. The emphasis of lean rather than bulky muscles and on grace rather than power of arm movement probably contribute to this low incidence of shoulder complaints.

When the arm is abducted as in the second dance position or flexed forward as in the third, the shoulder is in a position of neutral or slight external rotation. Thus, extreme internal rotation of the shoulder that occurs during the follow-through motion of throwing or in swimming is not present in usual dance motions.

DIVING

Competitive divers are prone to two types of shoulder injuries. Both are caused by improper water entry. Chronic shoulder pain can be caused by use of the "flat entry" technique (Fig. 11-4).[56] This technique is designed to decrease trauma to the head and cervical spine caused by water entry. It also results in less "splash" and higher scores in diving competition. The "flat entry," however, has been implicated in causing chronic shoulder pain in divers. The mechanism can be anterior shoulder subluxation or rotator cuff injury. Injuries are said to occur from this technique in young divers who have inadequately developed shoulder strength.[56]

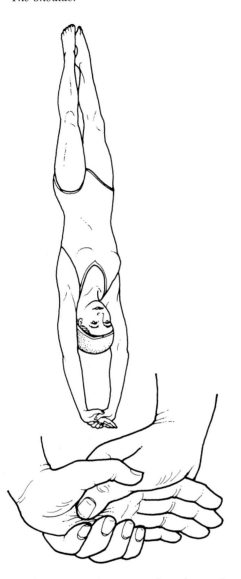

Fig. 11-4. Flat entry technique used in diving that can cause chronic shoulder injury. (Redrawn from Kimball RJ, Carter RL, Schneider RC: Competitive diving injuries. p. 205. In Schneider RC, Kennedy JC, Plant ML (eds): Sports Injuries. Williams & Wilkins, Baltimore, © 1985, The Williams & Wilkins Co.)

The second shoulder injury from diving is anterior glenohumeral dislocation. This unusual injury also occurs at water entry. It is a result of the diver not clasping his hands before entry. The shoulder can be forcefully hyperextended upon water entry and anterior dislocation results. This injury can occur in dives off the 10 meter tower.[56]

FOOTBALL

Falls onto the shoulder are common in football. The shoulder is the point of impact in most tackling and blocking plays in this collision sport. Therefore, it is not surprising that the shoulder girdle is frequently injured in football. The frequency of shoulder injury was found to be second only to the knee in one study of injuries to professional football players.[97] In studies of injuries in high school and college football, shoulder injuries were found to be high in frequency with only the knee and ankle joint more commonly injured.[24,31,80] The National Football League has reported an increase in shoulder injuries from 3.7 to 5.4 percent in 1976 to 1979, to 9 to 11 percent in 1980 to 1982.[73]

The most common shoulder injuries that occur in football are contusions, acromioclavicular joint injuries, brachial plexus injuries, contusions, rotator cuff tears and muscle strains, glenohumeral instability, traumatic myositis ossificans, and clavicle fracture.[99]

Acromioclavicular Joint in Football

In a study of 164 acromioclavicular joint injuries in athletes, Cox[30] found that 67 (41 percent) had occurred in football. Injuries from wrestling and lacross were next in frequency, with 13 percent and 12 percent respectively.

Brachial Plexus Injury

A "burner" or "stinger" is a sudden sharp, burning pain that radiates from the shoulder to the arm and hand. It is caused by a blow that tilts the head and neck to the side and depresses the shoulder (Fig. 11-5). The burning paresthesia usually lasts several

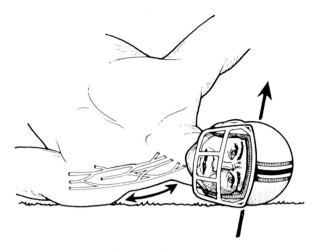

Fig. 11-5. Mechanism of brachial plexus injury.

Contusions

The "shoulder pointer" is an injury to the soft tissues covering the acromion and tip of the shoulder caused by a direct blow. It is analogous to iliac crest contusion or "hip pointer."

Posterior Shoulder Instability

A fall on an internally rotated adducted arm can cause the shoulder to dislocate or subluxate posteriorly (Fig. 11-6). A direct blow to the shoulder can also result in posterior shoulder subluxation. The cause of recurrent posterior shoulder subluxation in 8 out of 19 patients with this diagnosis was direct trauma sustained in football.[77] The patient who has posterior shoulder subluxation typically has pain when he performs shoulder motions that require ad-

seconds and is followed by arm and hand weakness that can last 1 or 2 minutes. The injury is an excess stretching of the brachial plexus[89] and should be distinguished from injury to the cervical spine nerve roots.[71,90] If the brachial plexus has been stretched, the nerves innervating the biceps, deltoid, supraspinatus, or infraspinatus muscles are usually involved.[89] In cervical spine nerve root injuries C5 is usually involved.

If the pain lasts more than a few seconds and if the neck and upper extremity do not return to normal within 1 or 2 minutes, one should assume that the cervical spine or brachial plexus has been injured until proven otherwise.[9] The patient should have a thorough neurologic examination and radiographs of the cervical spine. If preliminary films are negative, lateral views in full flexion and extension should be taken if the patient can actively move the head and neck in these directions.

Rotator Cuff Injuries

The supraspinatus tendon can tear from sudden forceful eccentric overload, such as in blocking with the arm. Stress failure can also occur, but this is due to repetitive force overload such as from weight lifting. If the rotator cuff is torn during play, weight lifting will aggravate symptoms.

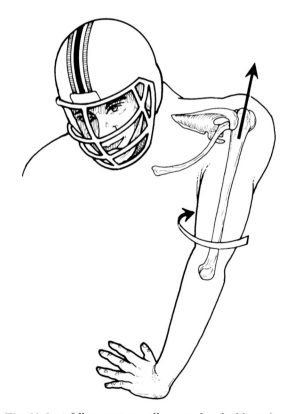

Fig. 11-6. A fall on an internally rotated and adducted arm can result in posterior shoulder dislocation.

duction and internal rotation. Symptoms are usually aggravated during the follow-through phase of throwing or serving in tennis.

Anterior Shoulder Instability

Improper tackling in which the athlete has his arm too far out from the body is a common cause of anterior shoulder dislocation or subluxation (Fig. 11-7). Arm motions of abduction/external rotation and hyperextension are common in football and can result in anterior shoulder instability.

Traumatic Myositis Ossificans

Repetitive contusion of the lateral arm just below the shoulder pad can cause traumatic myositis ossificans. This is called "blocker's exostosis" or "tackler's exostosis."[47] Clinical presentation is pain, a palpable mass, and a flexion contraction of the elbow.

GOLF

The golf swing can be broken down into three components: take-away, impact, and follow-through. The take-away position consists of lining up with the ball and moving the club to the top of the backswing.

During the impact phase, a golfer strikes the ball. More injuries occur during this phase than in any other phase. During follow-through, the club is decelerated as it completes the circle.

Excessive muscle strength is not required to play golf. Although strengthening and conditioning program is important, it must be specific. Excessive or improper weight-lifting or resistance training can cause muscles to tighten with loss of the rhythmic coordination of the arm, as well as injury to the shoulder per se (see Weight Lifting).

In a study of injuries to professional golfers, McCarroll and Gioe[63,64] found that injuries to the left wrist, low back, left shoulder, and left thumb were the most frequent injured body parts. The left shoulder was more commonly injured than the right. Shoulder impingement syndrome has also been reported to occur frequently from golf.[83]

GYMNASTICS

Gymnastics causes acute traumatic injuries as well as overuse syndromes. In a 5-year study of 70 elite women gymnasts, there were 66 major injuries.[101] Forty-five were classified as a traumatic injury and 21 were reportedly caused by repetitive stress. It appears that experienced gymnasts are more likely to experience stress failure and inexperienced gymnasts are more likely to sustain an acute injury.[33] In

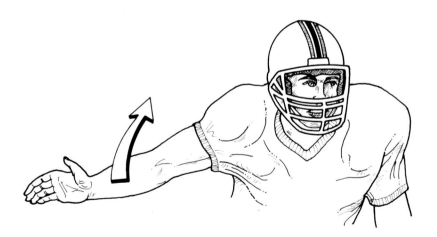

Fig. 11-7. Improper tackling in football can dislocate the shoulder anteriorly. The arm is too far out to the side.

a clinical and radiologic study of nine Olympic caliber gymnasts, the "gymnasts shoulder" was described. The three gymnasts who had been active in this sport for more than 10 years showed acromioclavicular degenerative changes and osteochondral bodies at the glenohumeral joint.[98]

Supraspinatus Tendinitis

The supraspinatus muscle is an extremely important functional unit of the gymnast shoulder. Supraspinatus tendinitis is the most common shoulder problem found in a 5-year study of women's gymnastic injuries.[102] The most common injury was the ankle sprain. Jackson[48] also reported subacromial impingement causing pain in gymnasts.

ICE HOCKEY

Injuries to the head, scalp, face, or eye have been reported to comprise more than 50 percent of all injuries sustained in ice hockey.[14,41,44,106] Most of these studies were carried out before the widespread use of helmets and face masks, which are now mandatory in amateur hockey in the United States. The next most frequently injured area is the leg and upper extremity, each having approximately 20 percent of the total number of injuries. The percentage of injuries that involve the shoulder has been reported to be between 8 and 22 percent.[14,41,44,106] The rate of injuries is directly related to the competitive level of hockey being played. Younger players sustained fewer injuries than older players.

Most shoulder injuries incurred by ice hockey players are acute traumatic injuries. Overuse injuries are uncommon because the arm is seldom used in the overhead position. The most common shoulder injuries are acromioclavicular separation and anterior glenohumeral dislocation or subluxation. Less frequent injuries are contusions, brachial plexus injuries, and traumatic osteolysis of the distal clavicle.

Acromioclavicular Joint and Clavicle

Direct trauma to the shoulder is the cause of most acromioclavicular joint injuries in hockey. This commonly occurs when checking an opponent or "hitting the boards." Indirect force can be transmitted by falling on the elbow or hand. In a study of clavicle injuries in hockey, Norfray et al.[75] found that 46 percent (33 of 77) of professional players had radiographic abnormalities of the clavicle. Acute acromioclavicular joints were most common in professional players, and acute clavicle fractures were most common in amateur players. Post-traumatic changes of the distal end of the clavicle were seen in the professional players. Radiographic abnormalities include widening of the acromioclavicular joint, ununited fracture fragments, exuberant callus, and distal clavicle osteolysis. The authors theorize that newly designed shoulder pads could possibly decrease clavicle injuries caused by direct trauma, but that pads cannot prevent injuries to the clavicle that occur from indirect trauma.

Glenohumeral Joint

In a study of elite ice hockey players in Sweden, Hovelius[45] found the incidence of primary or recurrent glenohumeral dislocation to be 8 percent. More than 90 percent of players greater than 20 years-old had recurrence of dislocation following the initial dislocation. The frequency diminished with increasing age. Hovelius found that the duration of immobilization following the first episode of dislocation did not appear to be related to the subsequent recurrence rate.

Hovelius further reported that the left shoulder is dominant in 80 percent of ice hockey players. Instability of the left shoulder, therefore, causes greater functional impairment and more commonly requires surgical repair. Eighty percent of hockey players use the left grip in which the right hand is on top of the stick and the left hand half way down the shaft. In shooting the puck, the left shoulder is abducted and externally rotated, while the right shoulder functions as a support. The left grip player is, therefore, more likely to dislocate his shoulder when he shoots. Thirty of 32 players who had surgical repair for recurrent shoulder dislocation were able to continue playing ice hockey. Only one-third of players who had recurrent shoulder instability, not treated by surgery, were still able to continue playing ice hockey.

Traumatic Osteolysis of Distal Clavicle

Traumatic osteolysis of the distal end of the clavicle has been reported to occur following acute traumatic injury in sports, including hockey.[75] Cahill[23] found that 45 of 46 men with osteolysis os the distal clavicle lifted weights as part of their physical conditioning. It seems that repetitive weight lifting by hockey players is a more likely cause of this condition than traumatic injury (see Weight Lifting).

MARTIAL ARTS

In a large survey of injuries sustained from the martial arts, the shoulder was involved in 7 percent of all injuries.[16] This placed it seventh in incidence, with injuries to the finger/hand, thigh/leg, foot/toes, trunk, arm/forearm, and ankle occurring more commonly. Injuries to the shoulder most commonly were contusions, sprains, dislocations, lacerations, and fractures, in descending order of frequency.

The frequency of shoulder injury from martial arts is related to the style used.[15,16,112] A study of injuries from judo reported that 44 percent of all injuries involved the shoulder.[112] Acromioclavicular joint or clavicle injuries occur because of improper landing techniques. Osteolysis of the distal clavicle was reported in two judo players after falls.[81] In aikido the shoulder roll is used frequently and acromioclavicular separations are commonly seen. In studies of injuries from karate, the shoulder was not mentioned as a site of injury.[66,67,104] A possible explanation for these differences in incidence is that judo uses leverage to throw the opponent to the ground whereas karate utilizes punching motions with hand or foot.

We have seen several overuse injuries of the shoulder from karate. These appeared to have been caused by the throwing motion with the empty hand. The deceleration of the upper limb is more rapid if no object is held than if a heavy object is thrown. The probable reason is that very rapid acceleration of the limb can be achieved, if no object is being thrown.

PACK PALSY

A compression syndrome affecting nerves about the shoulder has been reported to occur in backpackers,[29] which is referred to as "pack palsy." The brachial plexus or peripheral nerves can be affected. Commonly involved peripheral nerves include the accessory nerve, suprascapular nerve, and long thoracic nerve. The patient complains of weakness of the arm and shoulder without an obvious cause. Atrophy about the shoulder girdle and arm can be seen, as well as winging of the scapula. A careful neurologic examination must be carried out. Electrodiagnostic tests should be performed to confirm the diagnosis except in transient palsies. Viral neuropathies may mimic "pack palsy" and should be ruled out.

Treatment consists of having the patient modify pack carrying technique to eliminate the backpack as a source of nerve compression. During recovery, it is particularly important to avoid further trauma to the brachial plexus or nerves that innervate the shoulder girdle. Thus, heavy weight lifting with an outstretched arm should be *avoided*, as should routine therapeutic resistive exercise programs. In some patients trapezius or deltoid muscle weakness can result in mild acromioclavicular separation or inferior humeral head sag. A sling can be useful for these patients to support the upper extremity while muscle tone is returning. The prognosis is good, with an almost 90 percent recovery rate within 3 months if proper treatment guidelines are followed.

RACKETBALL/SQUASH

Shoulder injuries have been reported to account for approximately 5 percent of all injuries incurred while playing squash.[13] The acromioclavicular joint is a common site of injury because of impact of the shoulder against the wall.

Because the overhead motion is not frequently used in racketball and squash, chronic shoulder overuse symptoms are uncommon in these sports. Several studies of subacromial impingement syndrome in athletes do not report this condition in racketball or squash players[40,48,83] despite the large number of people who participate in these sports. Because of the low forces to which the shoulder is subjected in racketball and squash, these sports can be prescribed as alternative activities for tennis players who have chronic shoulder disorders such as rotator cuff tears. Although racketball and squash strokes differ from tennis motions, there are enough similarities to allow the experienced tennis player to rapidly develop skill in these sports.

SHOOTING

Stress fracture of the coracoid process has been referred to as "trap shooter's" shoulder.[19,96] The mechanism is postulated to be repetitive direct trauma, as well as indirect trauma due to muscle pull. Stress fracture should be distinguished from acute coracoid fracture, which can occur from other sports.[62]

SNOW SKIING (ALPINE)

Approximately 15 percent of all downhill ski injuries involve the shoulder.[107] The shoulder is the second most common site of upper extremity injury, the thumb being the most common.[25,72] The most common types of shoulder injuries in skiing are glenohumeral dislocation, greater tuberosity fracture, acromioclavicular separation, clavicle fracture, humeral shaft fracture, scapular fracture, and miscellaneous shoulder sprains. It has been reported that upper extremity injuries are relatively more common than

lower extremity injuries in expert skiers compared to beginner and intermediate skiers.[32,107]

Glenohumeral dislocations comprise approximately 10 percent of upper extremity injuries in skiing.[72] Mogan and Davis[72] postulate that the ski pole is often responsible for the dislocation by one of two mechanisms: the ski pole basket can catch on vegetation extending the arm and dislocating the shoulder, or the pole can be planted during a forward fall forcing the shoulder into abduction and external rotation. A functional orthosis has been designed for skiers who have recurrent anterior shoulder dislocation.[69]

SWIMMING

Chronic shoulder pain is the most common musculoskeletal problem in competitive swimmers.[54,55] "Swimmer's shoulder" is a term coined by Kennedy and Hawkins[54] to describe the chronic overuse syndrome of shoulder pain that occurs in approximately 3 percent of long-distance swimmers. A survey of 150 competitive swimmers ages 11 and 12 revealed complaints of shoulder pain in 10 percent.[1] The incidence of shoulder pain in highly competitive swimmers has been reported to be as high as 50 percent.[36,88] Several pathophysiologic conditions can cause "swimmer's shoulder."

The four competitive swimming styles are freestyle, backstroke, butterfly, and breaststroke. The freestyle (Fig. 11-8), backstroke (Fig. 11-9), and butterfly (Fig. 11-10) use very similar shoulder motions: adduction, internal rotation, abduction, and external rotation.[88] Richardson et al. found that 92 percent of competitive swimmers who had shoulder pain swam one of these strokes in competition.

Subacromial Impingement and Supraspinatus Tendinitis

Rathburn and MacNab[87] studied the microvascular pattern of the rotator cuff using injection of a microopaque substance into the subclavian artery. They found that the vessels supplying an area of supraspinatus tendon did not fill when the arm was *adducted*.

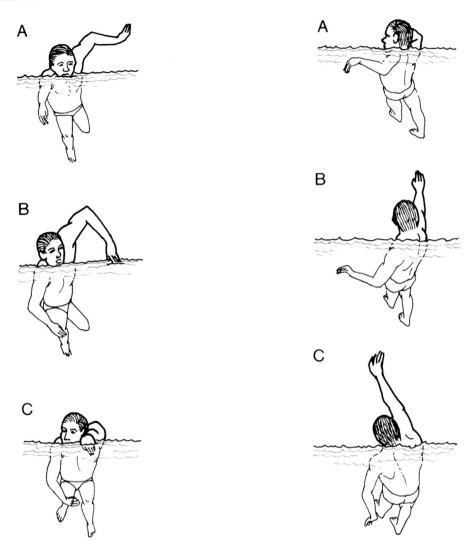

Fig. 11-8. Freestyle swimming stroke. For the right arm, note three stages: (**A**) hand entry, (**B**) midpull-through, and (**C**) end of pull-through. For the left arm, note three stages: (**A**) elbow lift, (**B**) midrecovery, and (**C**) hand entry. (Redrawn from Richardson AB, Jobe FM, Collins HR: The shoulder in competitive swimming. Am J Sports Med 8:159, © 1980, American Orthopaedic Society for Sports Medicine.)

Fig. 11-9. Backstroke. For the right arm, three stages are: (**A**) hand lift, (**B**) midrecovery, and (**C**) hand entry. For the left arm, three stages are: (**A**) hand entry, (**B**) midpull-through and (**C**) end of pull-through. (Redrawn from Richardson AB, Jobe FM, Collins HR: The shoulder in competitive swimming. Am J Sports Med 8:159, © 1980, American Orthopaedic Society for Sports Medicine.)

They postulated that there is a "wringing out" effect with adduction and a zone of avascularity that may be responsible for degenerative changes in the rotator cuff. This mechanism is in contrast to the explanation offered by Neer for the "impingement" syndrome.[74] Neer theorized that repetitive mechanical impinge-

ment of the supraspinatus tendon against the coracoacromial ligament and inferior surface of anterior acromion caused chronic injury. It is reasonable that both mechanisms occur.

The freestyle and butterfly strokes use motions that rely upon the function of the supraspinatus and biceps

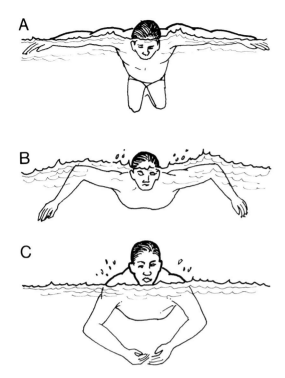

Fig. 11-10. Butterfly stroke. Three stages are shown: (**A**) midrecovery, (**B**) midpull-through, and (**C**) end of pull-through. (Redrawn from Richardson AB, Jobe FM, Collins HR: The shoulder in competitive swimming. Am J Sports Med 8:159, © 1980, American Orthopaedic Society for Sports Medicine.)

muscle functions.[55] Swimmers who have supraspinatus tendinitis and subacromial impingement usually complain of pain in the anterior or lateral aspect of the shoulder. Pain is felt in the follow-through and/or recovery phase of the stroke in all.[88] Pain is usually on the dominant or breathing side. When the pain is present in both shoulders the patient usually is a butterfly swimmer. Swimmers who are at increased risk to develop "swimmer's shoulder" are (1) high caliber swimmers; (2) butterfly, freestyle, and backstroke swimmers; (3) sprinters, as opposed to long-distance swimmers; and (4) swimmers who use hand paddles as part of their training program.[55,88]

Physical examination of the swimmer who has impingement symptoms reveals tenderness over the greater tuberosity and pain with shoulder abduction that is aggravated by internally rotating the arm, especially against resistance. The skeletally immature patient is usually tender over the coracoid and/or acro-

mial apophyses. Radiographic findings can include (1) "mound atrophy" on an anteroposterior film taken with the shoulder in external rotation; (2) subacromial spurring on a 15° caudad anteroposterior film; and (3) a coracoid cyst or spur seen on the axillary view.

Preswimming stretching has been reported to decrease the incidence of shoulder pain in competitive swimmers.[27,36] Proper swimming biomechanics are also important in preventing overuse syndromes. These include varying of the breathing side, keeping arm recovery high, attaining adequate body lift in the butterfly, achieving good body roll in the freestyle, and avoiding excessive internal rotation at the beginning of arm recovery,[36,46,88] as the rotator cuff is jammed under the acromial arch in this position. Developing good strength of the shoulder external rotator muscles may also be important.[36] In patients who continue to have impingement symptoms despite a conservative treatment program, resection of the coracoacromial ligament may be helpful.[26]

Anterior Subluxation

Anterior subluxation of the humeral head is most common in backstrokers. The swimmer experiences a feeling of apprehension when reaching backward over his head to do the flip turn because the arm is in a position of elevation and external rotation at this time (Fig. 11-11)[54] and the rotator cuff glides up the arm, leaving only the capsule to stabilize the head. This condition has been termed "apprehension shoulder" by Kennedy and Hawkins.[54] Subluxation can be surgically corrected with the Bankart procedure or anterior shoulder capsulorrhaphy.[94]

Posterior Subluxation

Fowler examined 188 competitive swimmers in 1982, 54 percent of whom had shoulder pain.[36] Fifty-four percent had posterior humeral subluxation. However, a control group of nonswimming athletes of similar age had a 52 percent incidence of posterior instability that may be physiologic for complete range of motion in the active athlete. Although no clear causal relationship has been demonstrated between posterior subluxation and shoulder pain, instability

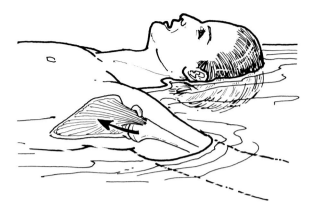

Fig. 11-11. Shoulder motion of extreme external rotation in the overhead position that can cause shoulder symptoms in backstroke swimmers. (Redrawn from Kennedy JC, Craig AB Jr, Schneider RC, et al: Swimming. p. 376. In Schneider RC, Kennedy JC, Plant ML (eds): Sports Injuries. Williams & Wilkins, Baltimore, © 1985, The Williams & Wilkins Co.)

in all directions should be identified in swimmers who have shoulder symptoms.

TENNIS

The term "tennis shoulder" has been coined by Priest and Nagel to describe a characteristic postural change in the dominant arm of tennis players.[85] Although there is a normal lowering of the dominant shoulder, in tennis players, the lowering of the shoulder is accentuated with an apparent lengthening of the upper extremity. The reasonable explanation of this asymmetry is (1) shoulder depression secondary to elongation of the shoulder suspensory muscles by the serving motion and (2) depression of the shoulder by the weight of the hypertrophied arm. Shoulder depression was seen in more than 50 percent of a group of world class players.[85] Theoretically this shoulder depression may produce or exacerbate rotator cuff symptoms, may produce a functional compensatory scoliosis, or may predispose to the development of thoracic outlet syndrome.

Subacromial impingement symptoms are common in tennis players.[40,83] A common cause of persistent shoulder and elbow (the "tennis" elbow) pain, is the "arm player" (usually a beginner) who strokes the ball with this arm extended, without proper leg or body motion. The "arm" player exerts maximum strain on his shoulder, whereas the experienced player uses his legs, with a good body turn and elbow dropped to lessen the strain on the shoulder.

Shoulder pain in tennis is most often felt during the overhead stroke or serve. The backhand stroke is next most common to cause symptoms because the arm is extended and the follow-through motion abducts the shoulder. The two handed backstroke helps to eliminate the strain of a backhand return.

Serratus anterior muscle paralysis is an uncommon problem that can occur in tennis players as well as other athletes.[38] The patient has scapular winging that usually clears in 1 to 14 months.

WEIGHT LIFTING

Weight lifting with the upper extremities applies tremendous forces across the shoulder joint. Both acute and chronic injuries can occur. These include subacromial impingement symptoms, rotator cuff pathology, distal clavicle osteolysis, other acromioclavicular joint disorders, glenohumeral dislocation or subluxation, and pectoralis major muscle rupture. Overall, the incidence of shoulder injury among weight lifters is reported to be low.[20]

Distal Clavicle Osteolysis

Distal clavicle osteolysis has been described in weight lifters and athletes who lift heavy weights for exercise.[21,23] There was no history of acute trauma in these reported patients. Other reports, however, have attributed osteolysis to acute injury.[50,75] The diagnosis of distal clavicle osteolysis can be made by nucleotide scan or radiography. The presumed cause of osteolysis is excessive repeated compression of the distal clavicle against the acromion. Conservative treatment includes nonsteroidal anti-inflammatory medication and modification of weight-lifting routines. In patients who continue to have pain despite conservative treatment, distal clavicle excision can be helpful.

Glenohumeral Dislocation

Glenohumeral dislocation can be caused by overhead weight lifting exercises if the weight drops behind the coronal plane of the body. This is dramatically illustrated in the Olympic weight lifter (Fig. 11-12) who had his hands placed widely on the bar and allowed the weight to move posterior to his shoulders.

Glenoid Labrum Tear

The anterior superior glenoid labrum can tear from overhead weight lifting in the absence of recognizable shoulder subluxation or dislocation. The mechanism appears to be related to holding the grip too widely on the bar and dropping the bar behind the head (Fig. 11-13). The strain on the shoulder is increased in the sitting position, which eliminates the mechanical adjustment of the body. This mechanism is similar to that causing anterior dislocation.

Pectoralis Major Tendon Rupture

Pectoralis major tendon rupture can occur during the bench press of weight lifting.[65,110] The tendon rupture can be partial or complete. Nonoperative treatment usually results in satisfactory function for activities of daily life. However, surgery can be considered if the patient wishes to return to heavy weight lifting. A differential diagnosis should be made from congenital absence of the pectoralis major muscle.

Subacromial Impingement and Rotator Cuff Injury

Weight lifting causes overload of the rotator cuff. This can result in acute or chronic failure, especially of the supraspinatus tendon. The bench press and pushup exercises are especially stressful to the subacromial joint. Weight lifting exercises as pointed out performed in a sitting position of 90° shoulder abduction also tend to overload the rotator cuff and cause stress failure.

WRESTLING

The shoulder is the second most commonly injured body part in wrestling. The knee is most commonly injured joint.[34,35,103] Shoulder injuries account for about 16 percent of all wrestling injuries. Injuries to the acromioclavicular, sternoclavicular, and glenohumeral joints are most prevalent.

Acromioclavicular Joint Injury

Approximately one-fourth of shoulder injuries from wrestling are acromioclavicular separations.[102] The injury usually occurs during a "takedown."[35] Acromioclavicular separations occur less frequently in Greco-Roman wrestling. Good quality mats have been shown to decrease the frequency of this injury.

Sternoclavicular Joint Injury

Wrestling is the sport with the highest incidence of sternoclavicular joint injury accounting for 15 to 20 percent of shoulder injuries from wrestling.[34,35,60] The mechanism of injury is forced adduction of the arm across the chest as the wrestler falls to the mat and is rolled by the weight of his opponent (Fig. 11-14).

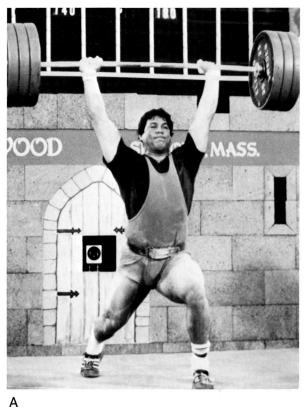

A

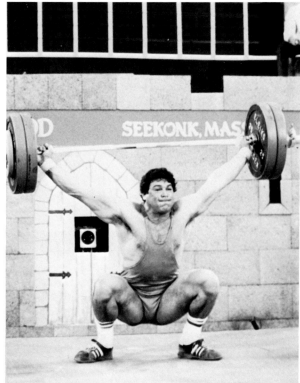

B

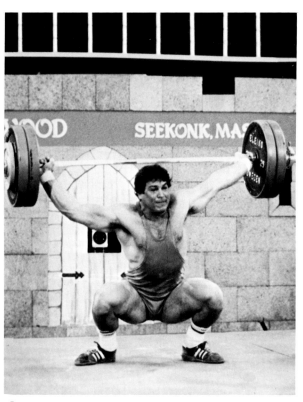

C

Fig. 11-12. Olympic caliber weight lifter during national competition. He has no history of prior shoulder problem. (**A**) Clean and jerk movement with direct overhead grip. This was an uneventful lift. Note position of arms on bar. (**B**) Snatch technique in same competition. Note wide hand grip and movement of the overhead weight behind the coronal plane. At this moment, the right shoulder is beginning to dislocate in an anterior and inferior direction. Note slight bulge in right axilla (at corner of black marking on door). (**C**) The right shoulder continues to dislocate. The right arm is dropping and moving posteriorly. Note that the weight bar is now in a lower position than in Figure 11-12B and has dropped behind his head. This patient fractured his anterior inferior glenoid rim (Bankart lesion, grade IV) and posterior superior humeral head (Hill-Sachs lesion, severe) during this lift. He then developed recurrent anterior shoulder subluxation and was unable to lift weights overhead. A Bankart repair was performed 7 months following injury. At the time of this writing, 3 years following surgery, the patient has resumed lifting weights competitively and has no recurrence of instability. (Photographs courtesy of Bruce Klemens, Clifton, New Jersey.)

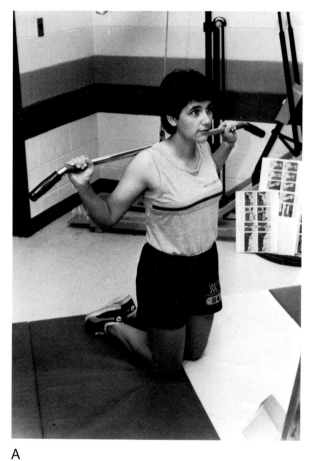

A

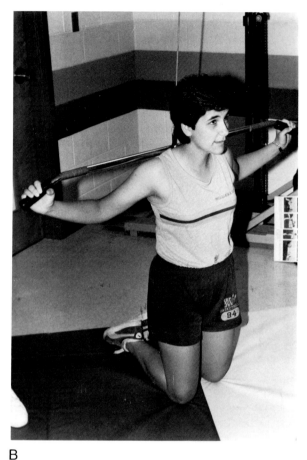

B

Fig. 11-13. College varsity golfer who tore the anterosuperior glenoid labrum in her right shoulder using this weight lifting machine. (See Figure 5-24 in Chapter 5 for arthroscopic view of torn labrum.) (**A**) Correct placement of hands on the bar. (**B**) The patient is demonstrating the wide grip that caused her injury. (Photographs courtesy of Lawrence I. Anson.)

Fig. 11-14. Mechanism of sternoclavicular joint injury: forced adduction of arm across chest while being rolled by weight of opponent.

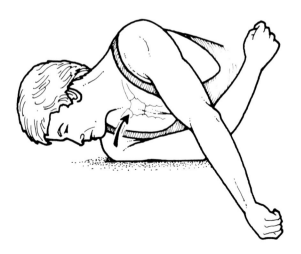

Glenohumeral Subluxation and Dislocation

Glenohumeral sprains are common in wrestlers, accounting for 14 percent of shoulder injuries.[35] Dislocation is less frequent.[180]

WATER POLO

Water polo players have a high incidence of shoulder injury. Data on the 1982 United States national team disclosed a 36 percent incidence of rotator cuff tendinitis and a 2 percent incidence of acromioclavicular joint degeneration.[91] The rotator cuff symptoms were usually not severe and did not cause the athlete to miss competition. The high incidence of impingement-type symptoms may relate to water polo players regimens of training in both swimming and throwing. Anterior glenohumeral dislocations have been estimated to occur with a frequency of 1 to 2 percent.[91] The usual mechanism of injury is an opposing player striking the arm causing forced abduction and external rotation. Suprascapular nerve paralysis has also been reported in water polo players.[91]

REFERENCES

1. Adams JE: Bone injuries in very young athletes. Clin Ortho Rel Res 58:129, 1968
2. Andrews JR, Carson W: The arthroscopic treatment of glenoid labrum tears in the throwing athlete. Ortho Trans 8:44, 1984
3. Andrews JR, Gillogly S: Physical examination of the shoulder in throwing athletes. p. 5. In Zarins B, Andrews JR, Carson W (ed): Injuries to the Throwing Arm. WB Saunders, Philadelphia, 1985
4. Apple DF, O'Toole J, Annis C: Professional basketball injuries. Phys Sports Med 10:81, 1982
5. Atwater AE: Biomechanical analysis of different pitches delivered from the windup and stretch positions. Med Sci Sports 9:49, 1977
6. Atwater AE: Biomechanics of overarm throwing movements and of throwing injuries. Exercise Sport Sci Rev 7:43, 1979
7. Bankart ASB: Recurrent or habitual dislocation of the shoulder joint. Br Med J 2:1132, 1923
8. Barnes DA, Tullos HS: An analysis of 100 symptomatic baseball players. Am J Sports Med 6:62, 1978
9. Bateman JE: Nerve injuries about the shoulder in sports. J Bone Joint Surg 49A:785, 1967
10. Bateman JE: Cuff tears in athletes. Symposium on Sports Medicine. Orthop Clin North Am, 4:721, 1973
11. Bennett GE: Shoulder and elbow lesions of the professional baseball pitcher. JAMA 117:510, 1941
12. Bennett GE: Shoulder and elbow lesions distinctive of baseball players. Ann Surg 126:107, 1947
13. Berson BL, Passoff TL, Nagelberg S, Thornton J: Injury patterns in squash players. Am J Sports Med 6:323, 1978
14. Biener K, Muller P: Ice hockey accidents. (Unpublished data.)
15. Birrer R, Birrer C, Son DS, Stone D: Injuries in tae kwon do. Phys Sports Med 9:97, 1981
16. Birrer RB, Birrer CD: Martial arts injuries. Phys Sports Med 10:103, 1982
17. Blazina ME: Shoulder injuries in athletics. J Am Coll Health Assoc 15:143, 1966
18. Blazina ME, Satzman JS: Recurrent anterior subluxation of the shoulder in athletics—A distinct entity. Proceedings of the American Academy of Orthopaedic Surgeons. J Bone J Surg 51A:1037, 1969
19. Boyer DW: Trapshooter's shoulder: stress fracture of the coracoid process. J Bone Joint Surg 57A:862, 1975
20. Brady TA, Cahill BR, Bodnar LM: Weight training-related injuries in the high school athlete. Am J Sports Med 10:1, 1982
21. Brunet ME, Reynolds MC, Cook SD, Brown TW: Atraumatic osteolysis of the distal clavicle: Histologic evidence of synovial pathogenesis. Orthopedics 9:557, 1986
22. Cahill BR, Tullos HS, Fain RH: Little league shoulder. J Sports Med 2:150, 1974
23. Cahill BR: Osteolysis of the distal part of the clavicle in male athletes. J Bone Joint Surg 64A:1053, 1982
24. Canale ST, Cantler ED, Sisk TD, Freeman BL: A chronicle of injuries of an American intercollegiate football team. Am J Sports Med 9:384, 1981
25. Carr D, Johnson RJ, Pope MH: Upper extremity injuries in skiing. Am J Sports Med 9:378, 1981
26. Ciullo J: Adolescent swimmer's shoulder. Orthop Trans VII:171, 1983
27. Clancy WG (ed): Symposium: shoulder problems in overhead-overuse sports. Am J Sports Med 7:138, 1979

28. Collins HR, Lund D: Baseball Injuries. p. 64. In Schneider RC, Kennedy JC, Plant ML (eds): Sports Injuries. Williams & Wilkins, Baltimore, 1985

29. Corkill G, Lieberman JS, Taylor RG: Pack palsy in backpackers. West J Med 132:569, 1980

30. Cox JS: The fate of the acromioclavicular joint in athletic injuries. Am J Sports Med 9:50, 1981

31. Culpepper MI, Neimann KM: High school football injuries in Birmingham, Alabama. So Med J 76:873, 1983

32. Davis MW, Litman T, Drill FE, Mueller JK: Ski Injuries. J Trauma 17:802, 1977

33. Dzioba RB: Gymnastics. p. 139. In Schneider RC, Kennedy JC, Plant ML (eds): Sports Injuries. Williams & Wilkins, Baltimore, 1985

34. Estwanik JJ, Bergfeld J, Canty T: Report of injuries sustained during the United States Olympic wrestling trials. Am J Sports Med 6:335, 1978

35. Estwanik JJ, Bergfeld JA, Collins HR, Hall R: Injuries in interscholastic wrestling. Physician Sports Med 8:111, 1980

36. Fowler P: Shoulder pain in highly competitive swimmers. Orthop Trans VII:170, 1983

37. Gainor BJ, Piotrowski G, Puhl et al: The throw: biomechanics and acute injury. Am J Sports Med 8:114, 1980

38. Gregg JR, Laborsky D, Harty M et al: Serratus anterior paralysis in the young athlete. J Bone Joint Surg 61A:825, 1979

39. Hansen NM: Epiphyseal changes in the proximal humerus of an adolescent baseball pitcher. Am J Sports Med 10:380, 1982

40. Hawkins RJ, Kennedy JC: Impingement syndrome in athletes. Am J Sports Med 8:151, 1980

41. Hayes D: Hockey injuries: How, why, where, and when? Phys Sports Med 3:61, 1975

42. Henry JH, Lareau B, Neigut D: The injury rate in professional basketball. Am J Sports Med 10:16, 1982

43. Hitchcock HH, Bechtol CO: Painful shoulder. J Bone Joint Surg 30A:267, 1948

44. Hornof Z, Napravnik C: Analysis of various accident rate factors in ice hockey. Med Sci in Sports 5:283, 1973

45. Hovelius L: Shoulder dislocation in Swedish ice hockey players. Am J Sports Med 6:373, 1978

46. Hunter LY, Andrews JR, Clancy WG, Funk J: Common orthopaedic problems of female athletes. AAOS Instructional Course Lectures. pp. 126–151, 1982

47. Huss CD, Puhl JJ: Myositis ossificans of the upper arm. Am J Sports Med 8:419, 1980

48. Jackson DW: Chronic rotator cuff impingement in the throwing athlete. Am J Sports Med 4:231, 1976

49. Jackson DS, Furman WK, Berson BL: Patterns of injuries in college athletes: A retrospective study of injuries sustained in intercollegiate athletics in two colleges over a two-year period. Mt Sinai J of Med 47:423, 1980

50. Jacobs P: Post-traumatic osteolysis of the outer end of the clavicle. J Bone Joint Surg 46B:705, 1964

51. Jobe FW: Thrower problems. Symposium: Shoulder Problems in Overhead-Overuse Sports. Am J Sports Med 7:139, 1979

52. Jobe FW, Jobe CM: Painful athletic injuries of the shoulder. Clin Ortho Rel Res 173:117, 1983

53. Jobe FW, et al: An EMG analysis of the shoulder in throwing and pitching. Am J Sports Med 11:3, 1983

54. Kennedy JC, Hawkins RJ: Swimmer's Shoulder. Phys Sports Med 2:35, 1974

55. Kennedy JC, Hawkins MD, Krissoff WB: Orthopaedic manifestations of swimming. Am J Sports Med 6:309, 1978

56. Kimball RJ, Carter RL, Schneider RC: Competitive diving injuries. p. 192. In Schneider RC, Kennedy JC, Plant ML (eds): Sports Injuries, Mechanisms Prevention and Treatment. Williams & Wilkins, Baltimore, 1985

57. King JW, Brelsford HJ, Tullos HS: Analysis of the pitching arm of the professional baseball pitcher. Clin Ortho Rel Res 67:116, 1979

58. Klemp P, Learmonth ID: Hypermobility and injuries in a professional ballet company. Br J Sports Med 18:143, 1984

59. Lipscomb AB: Baseball pitching injuries in growing athletes. J Sports Med 3:25, 1975

60. Lok V, Yuceturk G: Injuries of wrestling. J Sports Med 2:324, 1974

61. Lombardo SJ, Jobe FW, Kerlan RK, et al: Posterior shoulder lesions in throwing athletes. A J Sports Med 5:106, 1977

62. Mariani PP: Isolated Fracture of the coracoid process in an athlete. Am J Sports Med 8:129, 1980

63. McCarroll JR, Gioe TT: Professional golfers and the price they pay. Phys Sports Med 10:64, 1982

64. McCarroll JR: Golf: Common injuries from a supposedly benign activity. J Musculoskeletal Med 3:9, 1986

65. McEntire JE, Hess WE, Coleman SS: Rupture of the pectoralis major muscle. J Bone Joint Surg 54A:1040, 1972

66. McLatchie GR, Davies JE, Caulley JH: Injuries in karate—A case for medical control. J Trauma 20:956, 1980

67. McLatchie G: Karate and karate injuries. Br J Sports Med 17:131, 1983

68. McLeod WD: The pitching mechanism. p. 22. In Zarins B, Andrews JR, Carson W (eds): Injuries to the Throwing Arm. WB Saunders, Philadelphia, 1985

69. Metheny JA: Skiing orthosis for recurrent shoulder dislocation. Am J Sports Med 12:82, 1984

70. Micheli LJ: Overuse injuries in children's sports: the growth factor. Ortho Clin North Am 14:337, 1983

71. Micheli L: Pediatric and Adolescent Sports Medicine. Little, Brown, Boston, 1984, p. 78

72. Mogan JV, Davis PH: Upper extremity injuries in skiing. Clin Sports Med 1:295, 1982

73. National Football League statistics

74. Neer CS: Anterior acromioplasty for chronic impingement syndrome in the shoulder. J Bone Joint Surg 54A:41, 1972

75. Norfray JF, Tremaine MJ, Groves HC, Bachman DC: The clavicle in hockey. Am J Sports Med 5:275, 1977

76. Norwood LA, DelPizzo W, Jobe FW, Kerlan RK: Anterior shoulder pain in baseball pitchers. Am J Sports Med 6:103, 1978

77. Norwood LA, Terry GC: Shoulder posterior subluxation. Am J Sports Med 12:25, 1984

78. O'Donoghue DH: Subluxing biceps tendon in the athlete. J Sports Med 1:20, 1973

79. O'Donoghue DH: Treatment of Injuries to Athletes. WB Saunders, Philadelphia, 1976, p. 203

80. Olson OC: The Spokane study: high school football injuries. Phys Sports Med 7:75, 1979

81. Orava S, Virtanen K, Holopainen YVO: Posttraumatic osteolysis of the distal ends of the clavicle. Ann Chir Gyn p. 83, 1984

82. Pappas AM, Goss TP, Kleinman PK: Symptomatic shoulder instability due to lesions of the glenoid labrum. Am J Sports Med 11:279, 1983

83. Penny JN, Welsh RP: Shoulder impingement syndromes in athletes and their surgical management. Am J Sports Med 9:11, 1981

84. Petersson CJ: Spontaneous medial dislocation of the tendon of the long biceps brachii. An anatomic study of prevalence and pathomechanics. Clin Ortho Rel Res 211:224, 1986

85. Priest JD, Nagel DA: Tennis shoulder. Am J Sports Med 4:28, 1976

86. Protzman RR: Anterior instability of the shoulder. J Bone Joint Surg 62A:909, 1980

87. Rathbun JB, MacNab I: The microvascular pattern of the rotator cuff. J Bone Joint Surg 52B:540, 1970

88. Richardson AB, Jobe FW, Collins HR: The shoulder in competitive swimming. Am J Sports Med 8:159, 1980

89. Robertson WC, Eichman PL, Clancy WG: Upper trunk brachial plexopathy in football players. JAMA 241:1480, 1979

90. Rockett FX: Observations on the "Burner" traumatic cervical radiculopathy. Clin Ortho Rel Res 164:18, 1982

91. Rollins J, Puffer JC, Whiting WC, et al: Water polo injuries to the upper extremity. p. 311. In Zarins B, Andrews JR, Carson W (eds): Injuries to the Throwing Arm. WB Saunders, Philadelphia, 1985

92. Rovere GD, Web LX, Cristina AG, Vogel JM: Musculoskeletal injuries in theatrical dance students. Am J Sports Med 11:195, 1983

93. Rowe CR, Patel D, Southmayd W. The Bankart procedure. A long-term end result study. J Bone Joint Surg 60A:1, 1978

94. Rowe CR, Zarins B. Recurrent transient subluxation of the shoulder. J Bone Joint Surg 63A:863, 1981

95. Sammarco GJ: Diagnosis and treatment in dancers. Clin Ortho Rel Res 187:176, 1984

96. Sandrock AR: Another sports fatigue fracture. Radiology 117:274, 1975

97. Shields CL, Zomar VD: Analysis of professional football injuries. Cont Orthop 4:90, 1982

98. Silvij S, Nocini S: Clinical and radiological aspects of gymnast's shoulder. J Sports Med 2:49, 1982

99. Slocum DB: The mechanics of common football injuries. JAMA 170:1640, 1959

100. Snook GA: The injury problem in wrestling. Am J Sports Med 4:184, 1976

101. Snook GA: Injuries in women's gymnastics. Am J Sports Med 7:242, 1979

102. Snook GA: A survey of wrestling injuries. Am J Sports Med 8:450, 1980

103. Snook GA: Injuries in intercollegiate wrestling. Am J Sports Med 10:142, 1982

104. Stricevic MV, Patel MR, Okazaki T, Swain BK: Karate: historical perspective and injuries sustained in national and international tournament competitions. Am J Sports Med 11:320, 1983

105. Strukel RJ, Garrick JG: Thoracic outlet compression in athletes. Am J Sports Med 6:35, 1978

106. Sutherland GW: Fire on ice. Am J Sports Med 4:264, 1976

107. Tapper EM: Ski injuries from 1939 to 1976: the Sun Valley experience. Am J Sports Med 6:114, 1978

108. Teitz CC: Sports medicine concerns in dance and gymnastics. Ped Clin North Am 29:1399, 1982

109. Tibone E: Shoulder impingement syndrome in athletes treated with an anterior acromioplasty. Orthopaedic Transactions, J Bone Joint Surg VII:483, 1983

110. Tietjen R: Closed injuries of the pectoralis major muscle. J Trauma 20:262, 1980

111. Tullos HS, Erwin WD, Woods GW et al. Unusual lesions of the pitching arm. Clin Ortho Rel Res 88:169, 1972

112. Watanabe R: Injuries from judo commonly involve upper extremities. Sports Med Orthop News p. 29, 1984

113. Wright RS, Lipscomb AB: Acute occlusion of the subclavian vein in an athlete: Diagnosis etiology and surgical management. J Sports Med 2:343, 1975
114. Zarins B, Rowe CR: Current concepts in the diagnosis and treatment of shoulder instability in athletes. Med Science Sports Exer 16:444, 1984
115. Zarins B, Andrews JR, Carson W: Injuries to the Throwing Arm. WB Saunders, Philadelphia, 1985

Nerve Injuries About the Shoulder

12

Robert D. Leffert

The function of the human shoulder joint complex is intrinsically paradoxical, since it is not only the most mobile joint in the body but must also provide a stable base from which to place the hand specifically in space. These diverse functions are accomplished on a skeletal framework of three anatomical joints: the glenohumeral, sternoclavicular, and acromioclavicular, and one "functional" joint, the scapulothoracic interval. The muscles that bring about this complex, coordinated movement extend not only between the scapula and humerus to cross what is normally considered the "shoulder joint," but also from the head, chest, and thorax to be inserted on the scapula and humerus. Although a detailed discussion of the kinesiology of the shoulder is beyond the scope of this chapter, the reader is referred to the writings of Inman and co-workers,[25] Steindler,[65] Saha,[56,57] Codman,[11] and Jacqueline Perry in Chapter 1 of this book, for both anatomical and historical background.

Crucial to the understanding of the effect of nerve injuries upon shoulder function is the realization that the muscles do not act independently of each other. Although economy and wishful thinking would have us believe otherwise, it is not possible to substitute surgically for the loss of voluntary control, even in one plane, by the transfer of a single muscle, due to the complex nature of the force couples responsible for normal motion.[19,49,58,59]

Whereas it would appear obvious that nerve injuries can cause disability about the shoulder, it should also be appreciated that injury to the bones and joints of the shoulder joint complex may indirectly result in nerve injury and further disability. Finally, the static and dynamic effects of posture, particularly with reference to the relationship between the scapula, the ribcage, and the regional neurovascular structures must be considered not only acutely but also in the context of the chronic effects on nerves, vessels, and soft tissues themselves.

The neural structures to be considered in this chapter are as follows:

Spinal accessory nerve
Long thoracic nerve
Brachial plexus
Suprascapular nerve
Axillary nerve
Thoracic outlet and its relationship to the shoulder

SPINAL ACCESSORY NERVE

Anatomy

The spinal accessory nerve is actually not a peripheral but a cranial nerve, despite the fact that it has its origins in the upper five or six cervical segments. These fibers enter the skull through the foramen magnum with the spinal cord and then exit through the jugular foramen to enter the neck. The nerve enters the deep surface of the sternomastoid muscle, about 5 cm below the tip of the mastoid process, and appears in the posterior triangle of the neck at the midpoint of the posterior border of the sternomastoid. It is extremely superficially placed and overlies the levator scapulae muscle immediately beneath the deep fascia, where it is quite vulnerable to injury by unwary prospectors for masses felt in the posterior triangle.[40,48,69,70] Its path is oblique and posterolaterally directed to the anterior border of the trapezius muscle 2 to 3 fingerbreadths above the clavicle. The nerve then crosses the medial angle of the scapula to supply the trapezius muscle on its deep surface, to which it is adherent. In some specimens, an external, more laterally placed branch of the nerve may be observed crossing the posterior triangle. The contribution to the innervation of the trapezius by cervical nerves 3 and 4 has been the subject of debate, since in some animals the cervical fibers are sensory only, whereas in humans some of them may be motor. However, most patients with lacerations of the spinal accessory nerve has little or no control of the trapezius muscle.

Mechanism of Injury

The spinal accessory nerve may be injured by direct contusion, although this is rare and not likely to be an isolated phenomenon that spares the subjacent brachial plexus.

Traction lesions may elongate the spinal accessory nerve sufficiently to cause paresis or even paralysis of the trapezius muscle. They may occur in conjunction with brachial plexus injury, as the head and shoulder are forced apart while the neck is laterally deviated, or they may accompany subluxation or dislocation of either the sternoclavicular or acromioclavicular joints[51] (Fig. 12-1). In this situation, early attention may be confined to the skeletal injury. Only after the patient continues to experience significant difficulty with abduction of the arm does it become apparent that there is a lack of trapezius function. The lesion may recover spontaneously, although I

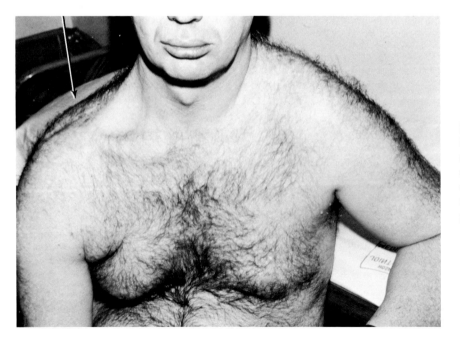

Fig. 12-1. This patient had been struck on the scapula by a rotating gun emplacement aboard ship 10 years previously. Note the dislocated sternoclavicular joint and total atrophy of the right trapezius.

have observed three patients in the last 20 years who have had permanent paralysis as a result of this combination.

Lacerations of the spinal accessory nerve are, unfortunately, all too commonly incurred during the course of surgical procedures performed in the posterior triangle of the neck[40,48,69,70] (Fig. 12-2). Usually, the procedure is a node biopsy done under local anesthesia by a surgeon who encounters significant bleeding, or who does an extremely thorough exploration because of an inability to find a definitive mass. The patient usually experiences a great deal of pain during the course of the procedure, and pain persists in the immediate postoperative period. It is often accompa-

nied by numbness over the adjacent skin of the neck and ear lobe because of injury to the greater auricular and lesser occipital nerves. Often it takes several days for the patient realize his or her inability to abduct the arm because of weakness, and sometimes weeks and months before the true nature of the lesion is appreciated. If the trapezius weakness is partial under such circumstances, the lesion should be treated expectantly. However, if the biopsy specimen includes nerve tissue or the palsy is complete, these patients should, in my opinion, have their spinal accessory nerves explored before 3 months if there is no evidence of voluntary activity on EMG examination.

In addition to the iatrogenic and inadvertent surgi-

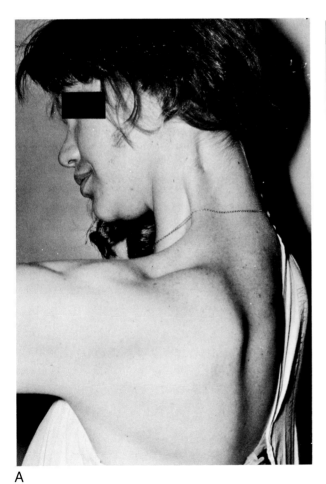

A

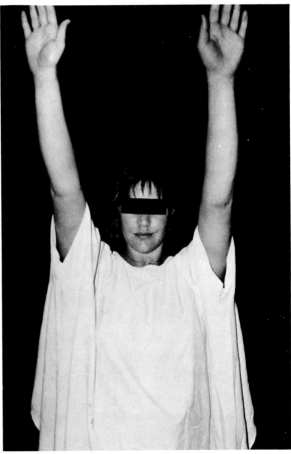

B

Fig. 12-2. **(A)** Paralysis of the trapezius following removal of a benign node from the posterior triangle of the neck. **(B)** Following scapular stabilization, the patient has excellent motion and no pain even though her trapezius is still paralyzed.

cal transections of the spinal accessory nerve, in some patients there is a need to sacrifice the nerve during the course of a radical neck dissection. Clearly, that decision must be left to the operating surgeon, but in some cases the nerve may be spared without influencing the possible recurrence of the tumor.[55] The difference to the patient in terms of function is enormous, so that this point should be considered prior to such surgery.

Rarely, the spinal accessory nerve may be the site of isolated spontaneous palsy.[16]

The disability that results from loss of function of the trapezius due to a spinal accessory nerve lesion is accounted for by the loss of the major suspensory muscle of the scapula and shoulder joint complex. Even though the levator scapulae and rhomboid muscles are presumably intact, they cannot prevent the weight of the limb from causing the scapula to displace laterally and anteriorly and rotating so that the acromion is inferior. Winging of the scapula from the chest wall results. In addition to the weakness and inability either to abduct or forward flex above the horizontal, there is significant pain due to the chronic strain on those muscles that must now attempt to maintain the position of the shoulder girdle. Discomfort is very often felt in the region of the insertion of the levator scapulae on the medial angle of the scapula and along the vertebral border. There may, in addition, be secondary effects on the subacromial arch and rotator cuff, which is no longer protected by the ability of the scapula to rotate during motion, or by the production of a thoracic outlet compression with paresthesias along the medial aspect of the arm into the little and ring fingers.

Diagnosis

It should be possible, on the basis of physical examination, to make a diagnosis of trapezius palsy, although obviously it may not be appreciated if the patient is not examined from behind. If the examiner is not sure whether the paralysis is complete or partial and there is a question of whether the weakness is caused by denervation, an EMG examination or a series of them at monthly intervals may be extremely helpful.

Treatment

Although it might be comforting to wait much longer than 3 months to "see whether the nerve will come back" after what was presumably an open injury, the degree of scarring that can supervene with the passage of time can make neurologic reconstruction extremely difficult or impossible. For those patients who have suffered severe traction injuries in addition to the laceration, repair may not be possible. However, a relatively short lesion, such as might be sustained either accidentally in the operating room or elsewhere from a knife wound, might be reparable with the usual techniques of nerve mobilization if the gap is small enough. If the gap cannot be closed without tension, a nerve graft is indicated.[20]

During the time that the fate of the nerve is unknown, the acute symptoms of pain from overstretch may be alleviated by use of a sling or the use of a pelvic support orthosis, such as the "gunslinger splint."

For those patients in whom recovery of the function of the spinal accessory nerve is not expected, function will be significantly compromised and the patient must then decide whether to accept the status quo or to attempt relief by stabilizing the scapula to the chest wall. Although theoretically only one-third of the total arc of elevation of 180° is accounted for by scapulothoracic motion, patients whose scapulae have been fixed to the ribs in a functional position can achieve more than 120° of elevation by means of hypermobility in the glenohumeral joint.

A number of methods of scapular stabilization have been reported. In the operation of Dewar and Harris,[14] a tendon transfer of the levator scapulae to the acromion is done in an attempt to duplicate the function of the upper trapezius. Fascia lata grafts from the vertebral spines to the medial aspect of the scapula provide the stability of the middle and lower parts of the muscle. This procedure is rarely performed today, although if only the upper trapezius has been lost (a rare situation), the transfer laterally of the levator scapulae may work quite well.

For patients in whom it is desired, stabilization of the scapula may be accomplished either with or without arthrodesis. Although the procedure is conceptually quite simple, a number of technical factors must be considered. The procedure as described by

Ketenjian[26] can produce excellent results. I have used both fascia lata and Dacron artificial ligaments. I now no longer use the latter material because of late failure in the second to third years in 4 of 14 patients, with resultant loss of fixation. The procedure may give excellent results, but should not be done on patients who are elderly and who have osteoporotic bone, lest fracture of the ribs cause loss of fixation (Fig. 12-3).

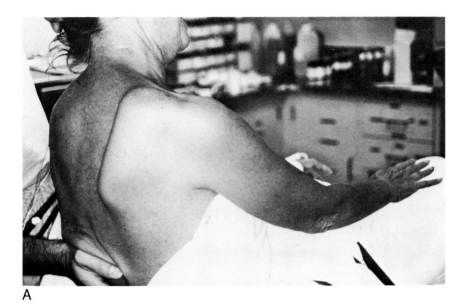

A

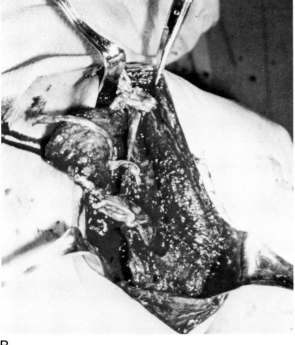

B

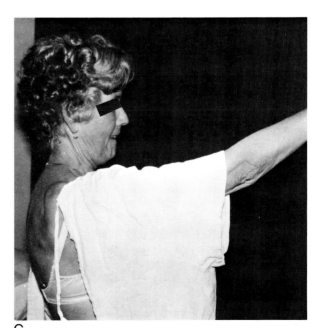

C

Fig. 12-3. (**A**) A node biopsy had resulted in paralysis of the right trapezius in this 57-year-old woman. She is unable to elevate her arm without severe pain. (**B**) Operative photograph of scapular stabilization. (**C**) She can now elevate the arm to 110° without pain.

Salvage of this procedure may be obtained, however, by arthrodesis of the scapula to the ribcage, which is a more extensive procedure, and which in my hands has required the use of a brace or cast in addition to internal fixation with wire and bone graft (Fig. 12-4).

Loss of suspension may be obviated by partial fusion, using a large hole in the inferior angle of the scapula through which one rib is rejoined after osteotomy. This technique was described by Spira[61] (Fig. 12-5).

Finally, the Eden-Lange procedure,[29] as has been recently favorably reported by Bigliani,[2] should be considered as an alternative to scapular stabilization. The levator scapulae is transferred laterally, as are the rhomboids. Active function is said to be quite good with relief of pain and winging of the scapula.

LONG THORACIC NERVE

The long thoracic nerve has a rather enigmatic quality, as it is rarely seen in orthopaedic practice. Paralysis of the serratus anterior can occur in a variety of situations, many of which are nontraumatic.[23,24] These include the sequelae of viral illnesses or innoculations, particularly tetanus toxoid. Long thoracic palsy may occur as an isolated idiopathic entity or as a part of a more generalized brachial neuritis or Paget-Schroeder syndrome. Some patients have experienced long thoracic nerve palsy following bed rest. Figure 12-6 illustrates such a case.

Trauma may produce injury to the nerve in several different ways. Industrial situations involving repetitive use of the shoulder have been reported as a cause.[50,60] Stretch injury, either between the head and shoulder or with abduction of the arm, have been seen as causative, and I have seen a number of gymnasts as well as other athletes who have had this condition. Although open wounds rarely cause isolated long thoracic palsy, the nerve may be injured during surgery. It has been reported as a complication of general anesthesia as well.[50,60] However, specific surgical procedures in the anatomical region of the nerve, such as radical mastectomy, may be responsible. Other operative procedures in the axilla, including first rib

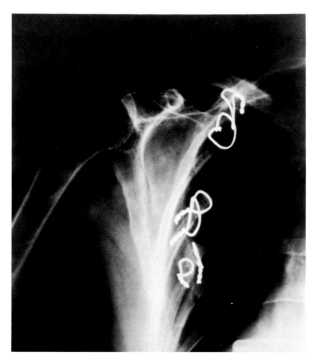

Fig. 12-4. Radiograph of scapulothoracic fusion showing wire fixation and bone graft.

resection and transaxillary sympathectomy, may be followed by serratus palsy.

The long thoracic nerve arises from root collaterals of the C5, C6, and C7 spinal nerves. It has a variable distribution that may include passage of the nerve through the middle scalene muscle or along the posterior border, where it crosses the first rib and then is angulated over the second rib. It then proceeds vertically applied to the digitations of the serratus anterior on the chest wall.

The disability from paralysis of the serratus anterior results from its absence in the force couple with the trapezius that rotates the lower angle of the scapula outward and forward when the arm is elevated. Instability at rest may be observed, although in some patients it may not be apparent to the examiner, even though the patient will complain of difficulty from pressure due to the back of a hard chair. The deformity becomes very apparent on forward elevation of the arm because only the trapezius remains for rotation of the scapula, which wings markedly. In addition to weakness and inability to elevate the arm more than 130° to 140°, patients will complain of pain as

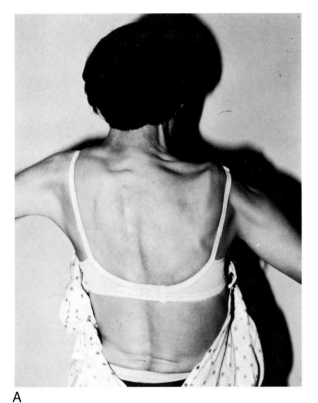

A

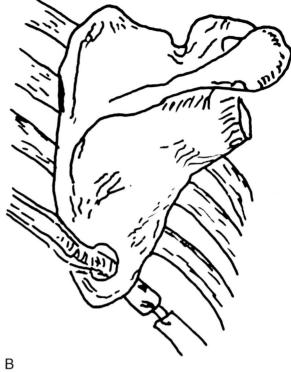

B

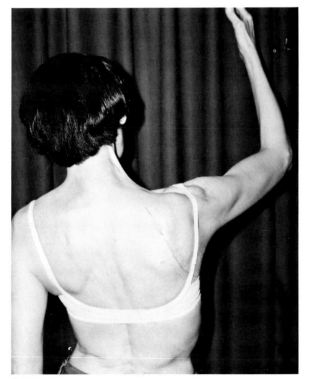

C

Fig. 12-5. (A) This patient had undergone a radical neck dissection for thyroid cancer. The spinal accessory nerve had been sacrificed and she had a very painful shoulder that was without function. **(B)** Diagram of the operative procedure. The fascial suspension is not shown. (Spira E: The treatment of dropped shoulder—a new operative technique. J Bone Joint Surg 30A(1):229, 1948.) **(C)** The postoperative result.

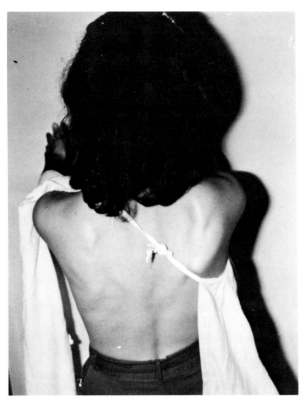

Fig. 12-6. This patient, who is a physical therapist, was hospitalized for inflammatory bowel disease for 10 days. When she was discharged from the hospital, she noted severe shoulder pain. There was total serratus palsy, which persisted for a year, following which she had total recovery.

adjacent muscles attempt unsuccessfully to compensate for the muscle imbalance.

The prognosis for recovery will, of course, depend on the specific nature of the mechanism of injury and the nerve lesion produced. The majority of idiopathic serratus palsies do recover spontaneously, although they may take as long as a year to show significant improvement. In my experience, if a patient shows no clinical or EMG evidence of recovery by 12 months, it is unlikely that the muscle will become functional.

Regular clinical and EMG examinations are necessary, usually at 4- to 6-week intervals, until evidence of recovery is present, at which point, the need for electrodiagnosis is lessened and physical therapy in the form of exercise can then be of some benefit.

The experience with bracing for this condition has been very mixed. Attempts to "hold the shoulder back" by means of cowhorn braces or pressure pads are usually not well tolerated by patients, who soon discard the appliances. For some patients in whom pain in the shoulder from scapular ptosis is a consideration, the use of the pelvic support orthosis (Fig. 12-7) has been successful.

The surgical experience with repair of the long thoracic nerve has not been well documented and I have no personal experience with it. However, a neurorrhaphy would appear to be indicated in the event that a localized lesion can be identified or is documented at surgery.

Reconstructive surgery for symptomatic paralysis of the serratus anterior muscle will depend on the patient's needs. Some patients are able to adapt to the disability, particularly if it involves the nondominant extremity. For those who want to attempt greater stability of their scapulae, a number of alternatives can provide very satisfying results. The ones with which I have the most experience are the use

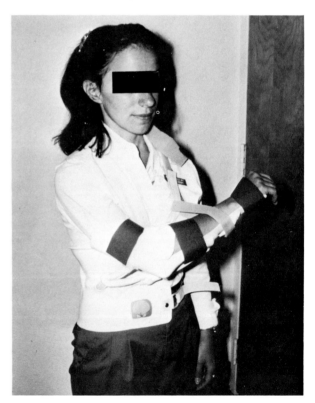

Fig. 12-7. Pelvic support, or "gunslinger" splint.

of the pectoralis minor, as suggested by Chavez[8] and Rapp[53] (Fig. 12-8), and the pectoralis major.[37] The teres major and rhomboids[22] may also be used in tendon transfer.

BRACHIAL PLEXUS

Injuries to the brachial plexus may not result in only significant disability about the shoulder girdle, but because the nerves are encompassed within its anatomical boundaries, the nerve injuries themselves may be significantly determined by the nature of the musculoskeletal injury.[32] In the spectrum of injuries, the clavicle forms an anatomical landmark that is useful in formulating a prognosis once the mechanism of injury is understood. In general, brachial plexus injuries that occur above the level of the clavicle, referred to as supraclavicular, are usually the result of traction resulting from falls that either depress the shoulder or deviate the head and neck away from it so that traction–elongation of the nerves occurs. If the clavicle fractures, the allowable excursion of the shoulder girdle, and subsequently the nerves, will be greater than if the clavicle were intact. Therefore, this type of injury is correspondingly worse than without the fracture. In some cases there may be direct injury to the nerves by the fracture fragments being driven inward, but these are comparatively unusual. It is more common for subclavicular injury to result from hypertrophic callus in situations where a persistent nonunion has narrowed the retroclavicular space or there has been a malunion with the same result.

Injuries to the brachial plexus may result from fractures and fracture–dislocations in the region of the shoulder, usually involving the glenohumeral joint, but fractures of the humerus and scapula may also damage the nerves. In general, these may be differentiated as infraclavicular injuries by the absence of signs of supraclavicular injury, including a Horner's syndrome; evidence of injury to supraclavicular branches, such as the suprascapular nerve; the presence of a swelling; or hematoma within the supraclavicular fossa. The prognosis for the infraclavicular brachial plexus injury is considerably better than for those above the clavicle or those that extend from above to below it.[30] The mechanism of injury is such that the plexus is stretched or compressed by the humeral head or by fracture fragments. If we assume that a sharp fragment has not transected the nerves, the result will either be a neurapraxia, with prompt resolution of the problem, or axonotmesis, with gradual recovery at approximately the rate of 2.5 cm of nerve growth per month. The treatment is, in most cases, expectant, with maintenance of range of motion and appropriate use of exercise and orthoses. Recovery may take as long as 2 years in patients in whom a profound deficit exists. The intrinsic muscles in the hand may not recover completely, while most of the long extrinsic muscles have an excellent prognosis. The axillary nerve is discussed below.

Open Wounds

Fortunately, open wounds are unusual in civilian situations, but they may occur as the result of either gunshot wounds or stab wounds, and may be accompanied by life-threatening hemorrhage or pulmonary collapse.[47] It is important to differentiate the wounding mechanism because of the very significant differences in prognosis. Most sharp wounds, such as might be produced by a knife, can be presumed to have caused a neurotmesis or complete division of the nerve rather than a contusion or axonotmesis that is responsible for the neural deficit. In these cases, if we assume that the deficit is of the upper or intermediate trunk, repair with microsurgical techniques is indicated.[41,46] However, unless there is a concomitant vascular emergency, the operative procedure may be delayed until the patient's condition is stable and an appropriate operating team is in attendance. In children, one may attempt to repair all elements of the brachial plexus, since there is a possibility of recovery; in adults the outflow of the lower trunk has a dismal record of recovery.

Gunshot wounds rarely produce complete deficits in the brachial plexus; if they are initially complete, they usually become incomplete rather quickly. Because of the concussive effect of the shock wave generated by a missile passing through the tissues, much of the apparent deficit will have been caused by momentary deformation of the nerves without transection. Therefore, one should not assume that surgery is necessary to repair a neurotmesis. For the most

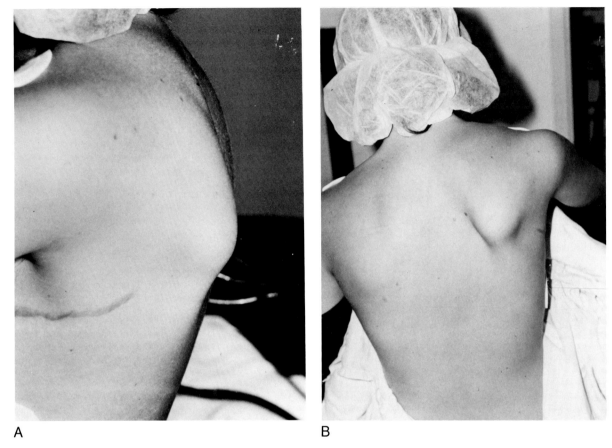

Fig. 12-8. **(A)** Serratus palsy resulting from nerve injury at the time of transaxillary first rib resection. **(B)** Posterior view of same patient. The scapular winging was incapacitating. (*Figure continues.*)

part, these lesions should be treated expectantly. Finally, if a deficit exists in the upper limb that can be either tolerated by the patient or substituted for by peripheral reconstruction, this might be considered as an alternative to direct attack on the plexus, particularly if sensibility in the important parts of the limb is intact. Therefore, tendon transfer may be an alternative to further surgery on the plexus.

Closed Traction Injuries

For those patients who have fallen from a motorcycle, or whose head and shoulder have been stretched forcibly apart and have a significant neurologic deficit in the upper limb, one may presume that a supraclavicular traction injury to the brachial plexus has occurred. There may be a head injury accompanying this lesion, particularly in a cyclist not wearing a safety helmet, and this may obscure identification of the nerve injury. The history is, therefore, of importance, as is a reliable assessment of the initial neurologic deficit if the patient is not seen immediately following trauma. The subsequent course of recovery or lack thereof should also be documented.

Physical examination should begin with a search for a Horner's syndrome. If present, this is a poor prognostic sign that indicates probable avulsion of the first thoracic nerve root. The neck is examined for range of motion and for the presence of a soft swelling over the plexus in cases of recent injury, or the nodularity of neuroma formation in older injuries. If the patient has a flail–anesthetic arm, eliciting a Tinel's sign by tapping over the brachial plexus at

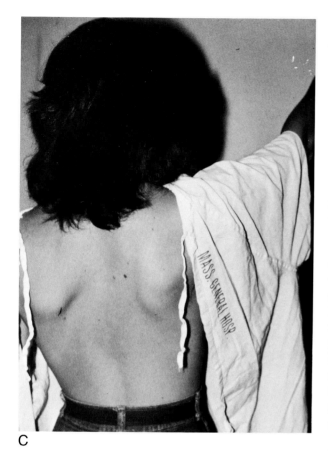

C

Fig. 12-8 *(Continued).* **(C)** Following pectoralis minor transfer, the winging was corrected.

the root of the neck will indicate that at least some of the roots have not been avulsed from the cord, although they may be ruptured distally.[13] This differentiation is the most important and to which all of the further investigative studies are directed. Clearly, if the nerve roots have been avulsed from the cord, there is no hope of spontaneous recovery and no surgical manipulation will effectively alter the prognosis. A distal or infraganglionic lesion, if it is an axonotmesis or lesion in continuity, may recover spontaneously with time. However, if it is a neurotmesis (completely divided) involving the upper or intermediate trunks or their distribution, a graft to overcome the deficits may produce significant functional improvement. Therefore, it is important to not only perform an accurate manual muscle test and sensory evaluation, but also, assuming there is paralysis and sensory loss,

to do a myelogram 1 month from the time of injury.[44,45,71]

We use water-soluble contrast material, metrizamide, with computed tomographic (CT) imaging to demonstrate the presence or absence of pseudomeningoceles (dye pouches where the meninges have been torn), or the nerve roots themselves (Figs. 12-9, 12-10). Plain radiographs of the cervical spine may demonstrate avulsion fractures of the transverse processes, which are the equivalent of finding a pseudomeningocele. However, neither finding is a completely reliable prognostic sign and both should be considered as presumptive evidence of root avulsion.[21]

The evaluation may be completed by the use of electrodiagnostic studies involving both EMG and determination of nerve conduction velocity.[3] The EMG should include the cervical paravertebral muscles. Because they are innervated by the posterior primary rami of the same spinal segments that provide the nerves to the brachial plexus, if they are found to be denervated, root avulsion may be presumed.[5] The demonstration of intact sensory nerve conduction in the absence of motor nerve conduction for the same nerve is indicative of supraganglionic avulsion of the nerve root and has a poor prognosis.

The treatment of the patient with a brachial plexus injury includes all modalities of therapy directed towards maintenance of range of motion in the joints, as well as their support and protection. In patients who have protective sensibility in the hand, dynamic splints may be used to augment function while one is waiting for recovery.

The surgical treatment of brachial plexus injuries involves both neurologic and peripheral reconstruction. All of this surgery is palliative in a sense, since none of it can completely restore the preinjury status quo. Nevertheless, the surgeon should be prepared to use any of these means or combinations thereof in an attempt to provide as much function as possible.[6,7,9,27,30,32,39,63,64] It would be most unlikely for a traction injury to be amenable to direct suture. Usually autogenous nerve grafts will be necessary; the sural nerves are most often used. The results are best for restoration of elbow flexion, although some function may be achieved about the shoulder and considerably less below the wrist and in the hand. Nevertheless, for the patient with a flail–anesthetic arm there is no alternative to neurologic reconstruc-

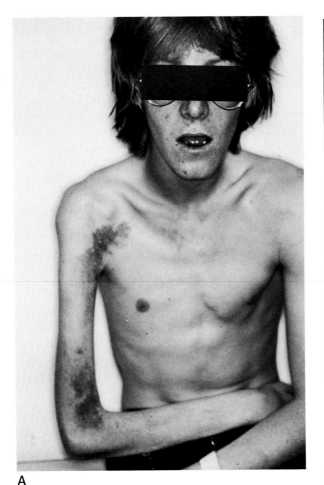

A

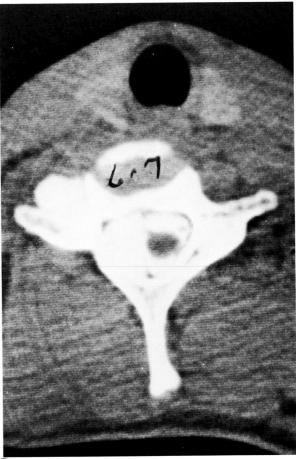

B

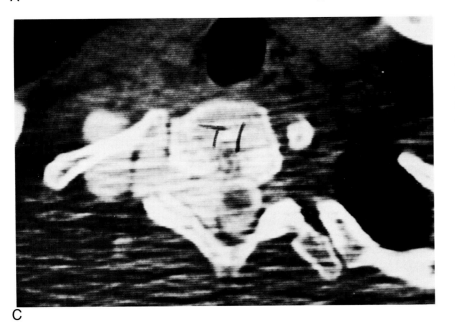

C

Fig. 12-9. (A) A 15-year-old with severe traction injury to the brachial plexus following a fall from a motorcycle. He has a flail–anesthetic arm. (Leffert RD: Brachial Plexus Injuries. Churchill Livingstone, New York, 1985.) (B) A CT scan of metrizamide myelogram showing pseudomeningocele at C7 causing deviation of the spinal cord. (C) Extravasation and large pseudomeningocele at T1.

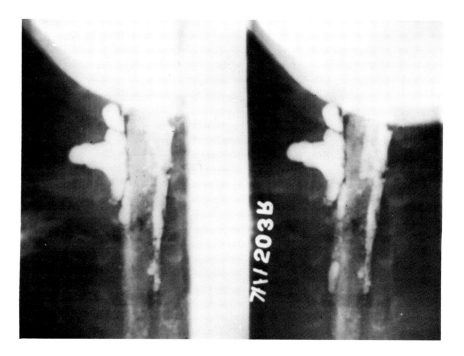

Fig. 12-10. A conventional myelogram with Pantopaque showing meningoceles at C7, C8, and T1.

tion, assuming there has not been root avulsion.[41,46]

For patients with partial lesions, many of the same techniques of peripheral reconstruction are indicated as were employed for the polio patient. Arthrodeses about the shoulder for those with a totally flail shoulder, and multiple tendon transfers for those in whom partial function is preserved, can significantly enhance the use of the limb (Fig. 12-11). Elbow flexion may be restored by transfer of the pectoralis major[9] (Fig. 12-12) or by proximal advancement of the flexor–pronator muscles in the Steindler flexorplasty.[27,39] Rarely is triceps transfer for elbow flexion indicated, but it may be helpful if there is no alternative.[7] The standard techniques of tendon transfer and arthrodesis about the hand may be used for the patient with brachial plexus palsy.

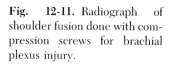
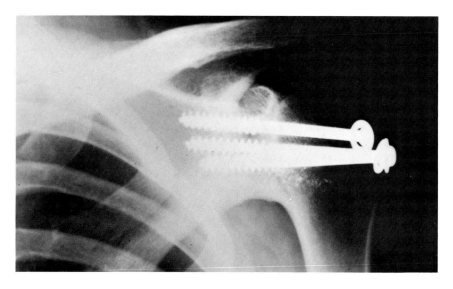

Fig. 12-11. Radiograph of shoulder fusion done with compression screws for brachial plexus injury.

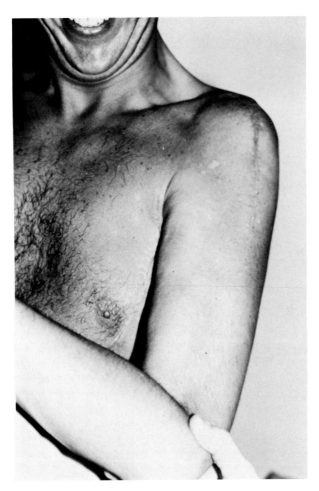

Fig. 12-12. This patient not only has good elbow flexion following pectoral transfer, but is very pleased with the restoration of the bulk of the arm following the operation.

In some cases, where the limb cannot be salvaged, amputation may be performed to rid the patient of a useless encumbrance. For patients in whom the scapular motors, trapezius, and serratus are intact, an arthrodesis of the shoulder combined with an above-elbow amputation and prosthetic fitting may be of some benefit. For patients in whom proprioception at the elbow is preserved in an otherwise insensate limb, the elbow may be saved and a below-elbow ablation done. In some patients, amputations of this type may indeed be the best rehabilitative procedure, although the incidence of amputation has markedly diminished since microsurgical reconstruction of the plexus has become more common.

SUPRASCAPULAR NERVE

The suprascapular nerve arises from the upper trunk of the brachial plexus at the confluence of C5 and C6 and derives most of its fibers from C5. It is the only branch of the upper trunk and is directed posteriorly and laterally beneath the trapezius to the upper border of the scapula, medial to the base of the coracoid process where it goes beneath the superior transverse scapular ligament to pass through the suprascapular notch. The suprascapular artery, which accompanies the nerve, passes above the ligament. The nerve then goes beneath the supraspinatus, which it supplies, and around the lateral border of the spine of the scapula to supply the infraspinatus.

Because of the anatomical confinements and relative fixation of the suprascapular nerve within the notch of the scapula, there is a predisposition to compression and irritation or traction lesions of the nerve with either forceful depression of the shoulder or repetitive movements.[10,28] These can eventuate in pain, with marked weakness of lateral rotation of the humerus, and the clinical complex may be mistaken for rotator cuff pathology.[15] The differential diagnosis may be aided by means of EMG examination as well as arthrography, the latter being indicated when there are other signs of subacromial impingement.

The suprascapular nerve may also be injured by blunt trauma to the supraclavicular fossa, but this is unusual as an isolated event that spares the adjacent upper trunk of the brachial plexus. Nevertheless, it has been observed. Chronic compression from malunited or ununited clavicular fractures may also affect the suprascapular nerve in its most proximal portion (Fig. 12-13).

The surgical treatment of established suprascapular nerve compression within the notch of the scapula involves dissection through the fibers of the trapezius muscle. They are split horizontally with care taken to avoid the medial aspect of the muscle for fear of transecting the spinal accessory nerve. Although the

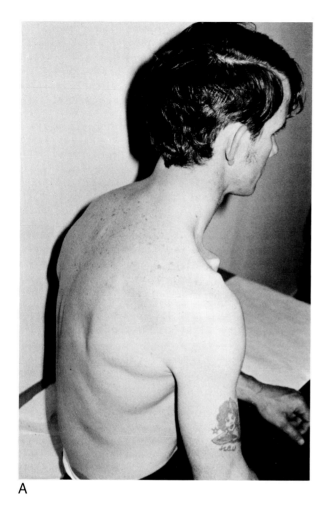
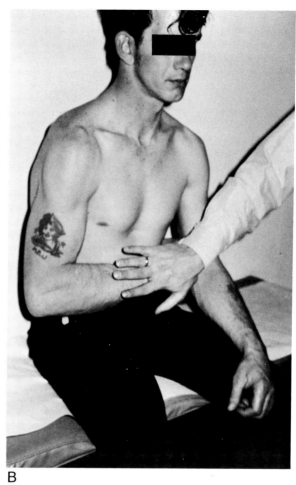

A   B

Fig. 12-13. (A and **B**).** This patient with malunited clavicular fracture had atrophy and weakness of the lateral rotators of the humerus due to suprascapular nerve compression.

operation would appear to be simple from a technical point of view, it requires meticulous dissection and hemostasis to allow adequate inspection of the area of compression. The suprascapular artery must be retracted or ligated, since it lies immediately over the ligament bridging the notch and covering the nerve. The ligament is carefully incised while protecting the subjacent nerve, the appearance of which is often disappointing in its normality. Nevertheless, on a number of occasions I have observed rather normal looking nerves at decompression, followed by very rapid recovery of function of the involved muscles and relief of discomfort.

In patients in whom the loss of suprascapular nerve function has occurred either as a result of birth injury to the plexus or injury later on, the power of lateral rotation and, to a certain degree, elevation of the arm may be augmented by means of a tendon transfer as first described by L'Episcopo in 1934 and 1939.[35,36]

The procedure uses both the latissimus dorsi and teres major, which are medial rotators, to produce lateral rotation by rerouting them around the humerus posterolaterally. They can be attached to bone or to the triceps origin. If, as in the case of Erb's palsy, there is a medial rotation contracture of the shoulder, that must be released prior to the tendon transfer. The results have been extremely gratifying, both in children and adults, and the transfer may be included in the multiple tendon transfers, such as are usually required for a paretic shoulder.

AXILLARY NERVE

The axillary nerve is the smaller of the two terminal divisions of the posterior cord of the brachial plexus and is supplied by the fifth and sixth cervical nerves. It descends on the subscapularis muscle behind the axillary artery and at the lower border of the subscapularis, where it proceeds posteriorly through the quadrangular space just beneath the glenohumeral joint capsule. Upon emerging from the quadrangular space, it is beneath the deltoid with the teres minor above and the teres major below. The nerve then divides into its two terminal divisions. A branch to the teres minor is given off usually as the nerve comes through the quadrangular space. Its medial division supplies the posterior portion of the deltoid and becomes cutaneous to supply the skin of the lateral aspect of the arm over the deltoid. The lateral or anterior division, along with the circumflex humeral artery, comes around the surgical neck of the humerus and is subfascially applied to the deep surface of the deltoid muscle to supply the middle and anterior deltoids. The nerve is located approximately 5 cm inferior to the acromion, an important consideration in surgical incisions.

Because the axillary nerve is immediately inferior to the capsule of the shoulder joint, it may be injured by dislocations or fracture–dislocations of the humerus or surgical neck fractures.[42,43] In addition, operations on the inferior capsule are potentially hazardous to the nerve. Further, as the nerve crosses anterolaterally to supply the major portion of the deltoid muscle it is at risk of being injured by any muscle-splitting incision that is prolonged more than 5 cm inferior to the acromion (Fig. 12-14).

Paralysis of the deltoid does not always result in inability to abduct the arm since a variable amount of abduction may be effected by trick and supplementary motions, including rotation of the scapula and contraction of the rotator cuff and long head of the

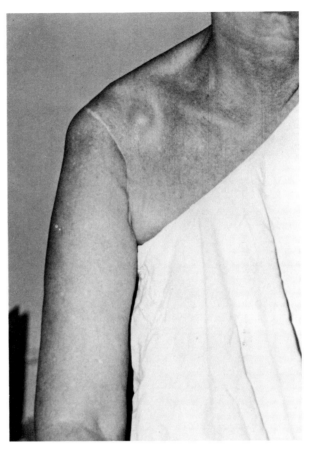

Fig. 12-14. A misplaced deltopectoral groove incision in this patient's deltoid denervated the entire anterior muscle medial to the incision.

biceps.[62] (Fig. 12-15). The clavicular pectoralis major is also involved in producing this movement.

As has been previously indicated, the axillary nerve is at great risk of injury from direct compression or traction by the humeral head in cases of dislocation. Although Leffert and Seddon[33] in 1965 found little or no recovery in six isolated stretch lesions of the axillary nerve caused by injuries in the region of the shoulder joint and stated that the prognosis for recovery in this situation was extremely poor, I believe that this statement ought be reevaluated in the light of a number of factors.

The first of these is that it is not at all rare to find evidence of axillary nerve injury by sensory testing in patients seen under emergency conditions with dislocations of the shoulder. Yet very few of these

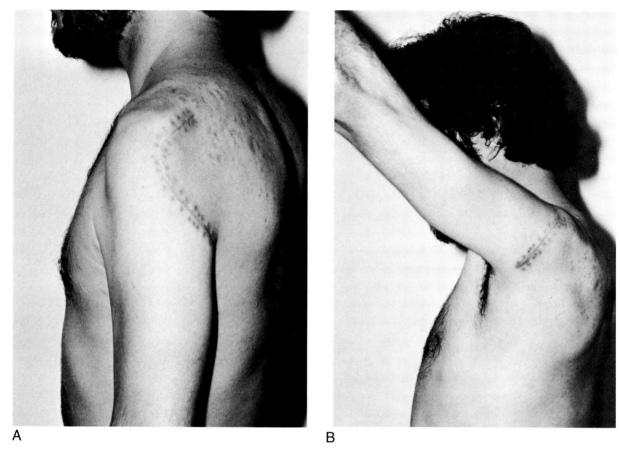

A

B

Fig. 12-15. (A) This patient was documented at surgery to have an irrevocably damaged axillary nerve and no functioning deltoid. **(B)** He is able to achieve elevation of his arm by means of adjacent muscles.

go on to experience permanent paralysis. Second, the statistical validity of the statement made by Sir Herbert and myself in 1965 is questionable since our patients came from the Nerve Injury Centre at Oxford and the Royal National Orthopaedic Hospital, both of which they attended because they had clinically apparent nerve injuries. I am convinced that many patients who had nerve injuries at the time of their dislocations were never seen for the nerve injuries because either the lesions were not initially detected or they had essentially resolved by the time the acute period of the dislocation had passed.

Watson-Jones[67,68] noted 15 cases of axillary palsy and dislocation of the shoulder over a 5-year period. Ten recovered spontaneously within 6 months, three between 6 and 12 months, and two remained permanently paralyzed.

The question of intervention in closed injuries with reference to its timing remains problematical. The nerve may require extensive surgical exposure.[52] A recent excellent monograph by Coene,[12] which analyzes the cases operated upon in the clinic of Dr. Narakas in Lausanne, has detailed analysis of these patients. This author advocated operation when there was no sign of recovery of the axillary nerve 3 to 4 months after trauma and indicated that further delay usually worsened the ultimate prognosis of nerve reconstruction. The follow-up for axillary nerve reconstruction and neurolysis after 1 year revealed good results—at least M4 in 60 percent of 54 patients—and what was characterized as an acceptable result—at least M3—in over 70 percent.

For those patients in whom the deltoid cannot be restored, there are a variety of options. Arthrodesis of the shoulder has remained the benchmark and is discussed in Chapter 16. If the serratus anterior and trapezius are intact, a stable and strong shoulder girdle can be obtained to move the arm within a restricted range. The reader is referred to Chapter 16 for further discussion.

For patients in whom partial function of the deltoid remains, usually the anterior or anterior and middle portions have been paralyzed. This may represent either a failure of complete regeneration by a closed injury or sequelae of a misplaced surgical incision or one following an accident that transected the axillary nerve. A variety of muscle transfers can be done,[18,49] including a rotational transfer of the deltoid. In this the entire muscle is detached and then rotated anteriorly on its neurovascular pedicle, so that the intact posterior deltoid occupies the former position of the middle deltoid.[18] Transfer of the long head of the biceps to the acromion and shift of the clavicular pectoralis major laterally can further enhance function.[19] Although numerous attempts have been made to use the trapezius muscle to substitute for both the paralyzed deltoid and rotator cuff,[1,38] this procedure has not enjoyed continuing popularity and use because it attempts to substitute a single muscle or part thereof for an extremely complex function. In addition, it adversely affects the function of the trapezius so that it may not be available for moving an arthrodesis of the shoulder, should that be required as a salvage procedure.

RELATIONSHIP BETWEEN DISORDERS OF THE SHOULDER JOINT COMPLEX AND THE THORACIC OUTLET

Patients who have disorders of the shoulder girdle from various causes may, even after seemingly successful surgical treatment of these entities, continue to complain of vague paresthesias and pain in the upper extremity. The entity of "dead arm syndrome" has been well described by Rowe and Zarins[54] as a concomitant of anterior subluxation of the glenohumeral joint. A subsequent analysis of another group of patients with anterior subluxation by Leffert and

Gumley[34] advances the thesis that the neurologic complaints of these patients are a manifestation of thoracic outlet syndrome. With correction of the instability of the glenohumeral joint and muscle reeducation, it has been possible to influence positively the postural ptosis of the scapula that resulted from pain and disuse and essentially to relieve the symptoms of thoracic outlet compression in the majority of cases. The coexistence of shoulder pathology and thoracic outlet compression resulting from it is not rare and may explain the continued symptoms in patients who ought otherwise to have been completely relieved of them.[31]

REFERENCES

1. Bateman JE: The Shoulder and Environs. C.V. Mosby, St. Louis, 1954
2. Bigliani L, Perez-Sanz J: Treatment of trapezius muscle paralysis with levator scapula and rhomboid muscle transfer. Ortho Trans 8:92, 1984
3. Bonney G, Gilliat RW: Sensory nerve conduction after traction lesion of the brachial plexus. Proc R Soc Med 51:365, 1958
4. Brooks DM: Open wounds of the brachial plexus. In Seddon HJ (ed): Peripheral Nerve Injuries. Her Majesty's Stationery Office, London, 1954
5. Bufalini C, Pescatori G: Posterior cervical electromyography in the diagnosis and prognosis of brachial plexus injuries. J Bone Joint Surg 51B:627, 1969
6. Bunnell S: Restoring flexion to the paralytic elbow, J Bone Joint Surg 33A:566, 1951
7. Carroll RE: Restoration of flexor power to the flail elbow by transplantation of the triceps tendon. Surg Gynecol Obstet 93:685, 1952
8. Chaves JP: Pectoralis minor transplant for paralysis of the serratus anterior. J Bone Joint Surg 33B:228, 1951
9. Clark JMP: Reconstruction of biceps brachii by pectoral muscle transplantation. Br J Surg 34:180, 1946
10. Clein LJ: Suprascapular entrapment neuropathy. J Neurosurg 43:337, 1975
11. Codman EA: The Shoulder. G. Miller, Brooklyn, 1934
12. Coene LNJEM: Axillary Nerve Lesions and Associated Injuries. Privately printed by deKempenaer, Oegstgeest, Holland, 1985
13. Copeland S, Landi A: Value of the Tinel sign in brachial plexus lesions. Ann R Coll Surg 61:470, 1979
14. Dewar FP, Hawes RI: Restoration of function of the

shoulder following paralysis of the trapezius by fascial sling fixation and transplantation of the levator scapulae. Ann Surg 132:1111, 1950

15. Drez D: Suprascapular neuropathy in the differential diagnosis of rotator cuff injuries. Am J Sports Med 4:43, 1976

16. Eisen A, Bertrand G: Isolated accessory nerve palsy of spontaneous origin. Arch Neurol 27:496, 1972

17. Haas SL: The treatment of permanent paralysis of the deltoid muscle. JAMA 104:99, 1935

18. Harmon PH: Anterior transplantation of the posterior deltoid for shoulder palsy and dislocation in poliomyelitis. Surg Gynecol Obstet 84:117, 1947

19. Harmon PH: Surgical reconstruction of the paralytic shoulder by multiple muscle transplantation. J Bone Joint Surg 32A:583, 1950

20. Harris HH, Dickey JR: Nerve grafting to restore function of the trapezius muscle after radical neck dissection. Ann Otolaryngol 74:880, 1965

21. Heon M: Myelogram: a questionable aid in diagnosis and prognosis in avulsion of brachial plexus components by traction injuries. Conn Med 29:260, 1965

22. Herzmark MH: Traumatic paralysis of the serratus anterior relieved by transplantation of the rhomboid. J Bone Joint Surg 33A:235, 1951

23. Horowitz MT, Tocantins LM: An anatomic study of the role of the long thoracic nerve and the related scapular bursae in the pathogenesis of local paralysis of the serratus anterior muscle. Anat Rec 71:375, 1938

24. Horowitz T: Isolated paralysis of the serratus anterior muscle. Orthopaedics 1:100, 1959

25. Inman U, Saunders M, Abbott C: Observations on the function of the shoulder joint. J Bone Joint Surg 26A:1, 1944

26. Ketenjian AY: Scapulocostal stabilization for scapular winging in fascioscapulohumeral muscular dystrophy. J Bone Joint Surg 60A:476, 1978

27. Kettelkamp DB, Larson CB: Evaluation of the Steindler flexorplasty. J Bone Joint Surg 45A:513, 1963

28. Kopell HP, Thompson WAL: Peripheral Entrapment Neuropathies. Williams and Wilkins, Baltimore, 1963

29. Lange M: Orthopaedisch–Chirurgische Opeerationsleh. JF Borgmann, Munchen, 1951

30. Leffert RD: Reconstruction of the shoulder and elbow following brachial plexus injury. In Omer GE, Spinner M (eds): Management of Peripheral Nerve Problems. W.B. Saunders, Philadelphia, 1980

31. Leffert RD: Thoracic outlet syndrome and the shoulder. In Jobe F (ed): Clinics in Sports Medicine. Symposium on Injuries to the Shoulder in the Athlete. W.B. Saunders, Philadelphia, 1983

32. Leffert RD: Brachial Plexus Injuries. Churchill Livingstone, New York, 1985

33. Leffert RD, Seddon H: Infraclavicular brachial plexus injuries. J Bone Joint Surg 47B:9, 1965

34. Leffert RD, Gumley G: Dead arm syndrome is thoracic outlet syndrome Ortho Trans 9:44, 1985

35. L'Episcopo JB: Tendon transplantation in obstetrical paralysis. Am J Surg 25:122, 1934

36. L'Episcopo JB: Restoration of muscle balance in the treatment of obstetrical paralysis. NY State J Med 39:357, 1939

37. Marmon L, Bechtel CO: Paralysis of the serratus anterior due to electric shock relieved by transplantation of the pectoralis major muscle. A case report. J Bone Joint Surg 45A:156, 1963

38. Mayer L: Transplantation of the trapezius for paralysis of the abductors of the arm. J Bone Joint Surg 9:412, 1927

39. Mayer L, Green W: Experiences with the Steindler flexorplasty at the elbow. J Bone Joint Surg 36A:775, 1954

40. Mead S: Posterior triangle operations and trapezius paralysis. Arch Surg 64:752, 1952

41. Millesi H: Surgical management of brachial plexus injuries. J Hand Surg 2(5):367, 1977

42. Milton GW: Mechanism of circumflex and other nerve injuries in dislocations of the shoulder and the possible mechanisms of nerve injuries during reduction of dislocation. Aust NZ Surg 23:25, 1953

43. Milton GW: The circumflex nerve and dislocation of the shoulder. Br J Phys Med 17:136, 1954

44. Murphey F, Hartung W, Kirklin JW: Myelographic demonstration of avulsing injuries of the brachial plexus. Am J Roentgenol 58:102, 1947

45. Murphey F, Kirklin JW: Myelographic demonstration of avulsion injuries of the nerve roots of the brachial plexus—a method of determining the point of injury and the possibility of repair. Clin Neurosurg 20:18, 1972

46. Narakas A: Brachial plexus injury. Orthop Clin North Am 12(2):303, 1981

47. Nelson KG, Jolly PC, Thomas PA: Brachial plexus injuries associated with missile wounds of the chest. J Trauma 8(2):268, 1968

48. Norden A: Peripheral injuries to the spinal accessory nerve. Acta Chir Scand 94:515, 1946

49. Ober FR: Transplantation to Improve the Function of the Shoulder Joint and Extensor Function of the Elbow Joint. Am Acad of Orthopaedic Surgeons Instructional Course Lecture, Vol. 2. J.W. Edwards, Ann Arbor, 1944

50. Overpeck DO, Ghormley RK: Paralysis of the serratus magnus muscle caused by lesions of the long thoracic nerve. JAMA 114:1994, 1940

51. Patterson WR: Inferior dislocation of the distal end of

the clavicle. A case report. J Bone Joint Surg 49:1184, 1967

52. Petrucci FS, Morelli A, Raimondi PL: Axillary nerve injuries—21 cases treated by nerve graft and neurolysis. J Hand Surg 7(3):271, 1982

53. Rapp IH: Serratus anterior paralysis treated by transplantation of the pectoralis muscle. J Bone Joint Surg 36A:852, 1954

54. Rowe CR, Zarins B: Recurrent transient subluxation of the shoulder. J Bone Joint Surg 63A:863, 1981

55. Roy PH, Beahrs OH: Spinal accessory nerve in radical neck dissection. Am J Surg 118:800, 1969

56. Saha AK: Theory of Shoulder Mechanism. Charles C. Thomas, Springfield, Ill, 1961

57. Saha AK: Surgery of the paralyzed and flail shoulder. Acta Orthop Scand Suppl 79, 1962

58. Schottstaedt ER, Larsen LJ, Bost FC: The surgical reconstruction of the upper extremity paralyzed by poliomyelitis. J Bone Joint Surg 40A:633, 1958

59. Schottstaedt ER, Larsen LJ, Bost FC: Complete muscle transplantation. J Bone Joint Surg 40A:633, 1958

60. Skillern PG: Serratus magnus palsy with proposal of a new operation for intractable cases. Ann Surg 57:909, 1913

61. Spira E: The treatment of dropped shoulder—a new operative technique. J Bone Joint Surg 30A(1):229 1948

62. Staples OS, Watkins AL: Full active abduction in traumatic paralysis of the deltoid. J Bone Joint Surg 25(1):85, 1943

63. Steindler A: Orthopaedic operations. Charles C. Thomas, Springfield, Ill, 1940

64. Steindler A: Reconstruction of the poliomyelitic upper extremity. Bull Hosp Joint Dis 15:21, 1951

65. Steindler A: Kinesiology of the Human Body Under Normal and Pathological Conditions. Charles C. Thomas, Springfield, Ill, 1955

66. Thorek M: Compression paralysis of the long thoracic nerve following an abdominal operation. With report of case. Am J Surg 40:26, 1926

67. Watson-Jones R: Fracture in the region of the shoulder joint. Proc R Soc Med 29:1058, 1930

68. Watson-Jones R: In Wilson JN (ed): Fractures and Joint Injuries. Churchill Livingstone, Edinburgh, 1976

69. Woodhall B: Operative injury to the accessory nerve in the posterior cervical triangle. Arch Surg 74:122, 1951

70. Woodhall B: Trapezius paralysis following minor surgical procedures in the posterior cervical triangle. Ann Surg 136:375, 1952

71. Yeoman PM: Cervical myelography in traction injuries of the brachial plexus. J Bone Joint Surg 50B:25, 1968

Shoulder Problems in Children 13

Michael G. Ehrlich

SPRENGEL'S DEFORMITY

Certainly, the most common of the congenital shoulder problems seen by the pediatric orthopaedist is Sprengel's deformity.[11]

Clinical Presentation

Oddly enough, while this may be very dramatic in its presentation, the diagnosis is often missed. In some cases, the deformity is only detected when the patient is abducting both arms simultaneously, and one does not seem to go as high (Fig. 13-1). Often this will not be noticed until the child is in a gym class and is 7 or 8 years old. The reason for missing the lack of abduction is that the loss is usually only about 60°, and when a child is reaching on that side, he or she tilts his body to compensate (Fig. 13-2). This is certainly missed by the parents, usually by the pediatrician and even frequently by the orthopedist. It would also not be difficult to understand why the diagnosis is often confused with an Erb's palsy with limited shoulder abduction. However, the patient with Erb's palsy should have full passive abduction, but even that is sometimes lost after a few years. Also, the Erb's palsy patient occasionally develop ra-

dial head subluxation. One might think that a patient has a Sprengel's deformity simply because another, apparently congenital, anomaly such as radial head subluxation is present.

Bilateral Sprengel's deformity is even harder to diagnose, since, as with congenital hip dislocation, the asymmetry factor is not available to help with the diagnosis. This may appear as a "short neck," and it is often associated with Klippel-Feil syndrome or fusion of the cervical vertebrae. Similarly, the unilateral Sprengel's deformity is often misinterpreted as a congenital scoliosis, because of fullness in the shoulder region (Fig. 13-3). It is often also associated with congenital scoliosis, a factor requiring consideration when discussing treatment. As anecdotal comments on the subject of diagnosis, we have seen the son of the Chief of Surgery in one major hospital who did not have the diagnosis made until he was high school age. Similarly, recently we saw a patient with Sprengel's deformity who had seen another orthopedist for probable chondrosarcoma.

The diagnostic clues most helpful are fullness in the posterior clavicular area, limited abduction of the shoulder, an abnormal shape to the scapula, asymmetry of scapula height on the radiograph, and, occasionally, the presence of an omovertebral bone. To understand why these anomalies are present, one should know something of the cause of the deformity.

455

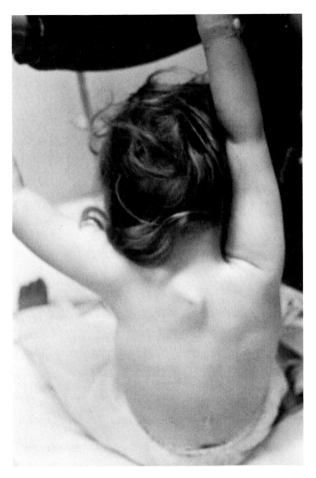

Fig. 13-1. Limited abduction of left shoulder in Sprengel's deformity. Scapula becomes prominent on abduction.

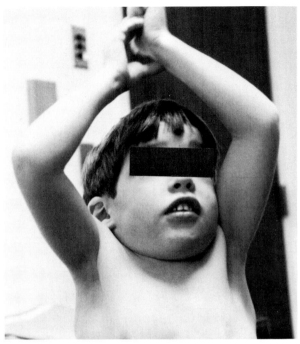

Fig. 13-2. Limited abduction of right shoulder could easily be missed as patient tilts body to compensate (Sprengel's deformity).

Embryologic Basis of Clinical Appearance

The fetal scapula differentiates between the fourth and sixth cervical vertebrae at about 5 weeks of age.[6] Between the ninth and twelfth weeks, it descends to its adult location, between the second, and seventh ribs. The scapula also retains its fetal shape, wherein the horizontal diameter is relatively greater than the vertical height. The elevated scapulae generally appear to be smaller than those of the opposite side. Cavendish has suggested that the scapula muscles may occasionally be absent or hypoplastic.[2] This was particularly true of the pectoralis major (5 cases out of 100); with 3 cases involving the trapezius and the

rhomboids, 3 with the serratus anterior and 2 with the latissimus dorsi. Grogan et al.[5] suggest in their recent work that the absence of the serratus anterior may contribute to winging and clinical deformity. However, I have not noticed this in my patients preoperatively. Early on, when I did not make a major effort to reattach the serratus anterior, I did see postoperative winging. That has not been a problem in recent years, leading me to wonder if the muscle hypoplasia is really of great significance.

The very definite deformities, in addition to those mentioned, include a rotation or tilting of the scapula, so that the inferior angle is medial and superior and the glenoid tilts so that it faces down. In about 25 percent of the cases there is a connection from the superior angle of the scapula to the cervical spine. This is called an omovertebral connection, and can represent bone or soft tissue (cartilage or fibrous tissue)[1] (Fig. 13-4).

Sprengel's deformity frequently implies a host of other anomalies. At the Massachusetts General Hos-

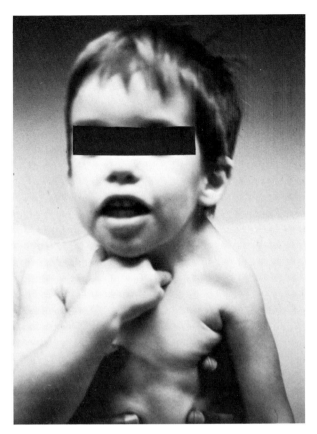

Fig. 13-3. Fullness in the shoulder area can be mistaken for a high thoracic scoliosis. However, a scoliosis may be present as well as a Sprengel's deformity.

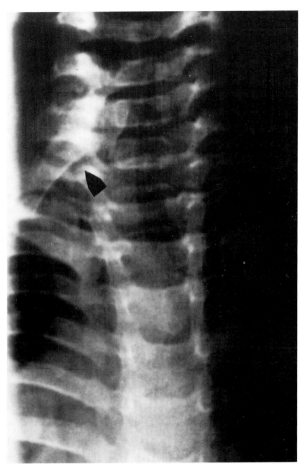

Fig. 13-4. Omovertebral bone (arrow) on radiograph, attaching to cervical spine.

pital, we often see it as part of Goldenhar's syndrome, or oculoauriculovertebral dysplasia, a condition often associated with retention of primitive branchial clefts, or manifest as an accessory auricular appendage, incomplete formation of the external ear, underdevelopment of the maxilla and mandible, and segmental defects of the cervical spine.[17]

However, in one reported series of 100 cases,[2] 98 had other anomalies. These included 39 cases of scoliosis, 28 cases of spina bifida (including 3 diastometamyeliae), 25 rib anomalies, 20 Klippel-Feil syndromes, 14 abnormal musculatures, 4 torticollis, and multiple other single anomalies ranging from club feet to dislocated hips. The most important feature of this is the need to sort out the contribution of the scoliosis to the deformity in the neck region. Fam-

ilies may be unhappy if the scapula is operated upon but the high shoulder still remains because of a cervical–high thoracic scoliosis.

Treatment

As in everything else in orthopaedics, there is some controversy as to the need for treatment and the best type of treatment available. Within the last 20 years, well known orthopaedists have suggested that surgical intervention does not offer much in the way of functional or cosmetic improvement.[10]

However, the pendulum has swung so that it is generally agreed today that one can make significant improvements in both cosmesis and function, providing the caveats suggested above are followed. In cases of severe deformity, particularly when there is a scoliosis to the same side, the improvement may not be as dramatic as desired. Furthermore, because of the abnormal shape of the scapula, it will never be completely normal, even in a mild case (Fig. 13-5). Also, as pointed out, many patients with a mild Sprengel's deformity will not even notice the limited abduction or the postsurgical gain. In Carson's series, where the range of motion was carefully measured, the average patient gained 29°. However, those patients with less than 120° abduction preoperatively gained an average of 50°. In the same series, 82 percent of the patients indicated that they were satisfied with the surgical results. The objections were to postoperative winging that had been mildly present preoperatively and to which I alluded previously and to unsightly scar formation. Similarly, in Cavendish's operated patients, most improved by one or two grades cosmetically (on a scale of cosmetic deformity that he devised). Therefore, today I think there is general agreement that most patients would benefit from surgical intervention,[11,13] except perhaps those with the most mild conditions. This latter group should be evaluated because their condition can progress. Range-of-motion exercises do not do much to alter the function of these patients, so nonsurgical treatment is really nontreatment.

The question is therefore, what form of surgical intervention is called for. Surgical intervention, by and large, involves three main features. These include transplantation of the scapula inferiorly, resection of the prominent supraspinous bump, and release of the omovertebral bone or fibrous band. Jeannopoulos[7] originally suggested that the operation be done in patients between ages 2 or 3 and 5. The group from Emory and Scottish Rite suggested that age 7 or 8 is the upper limit, and generally I ascribe to this.[1] The reason is due to fear that lowering of the scapula after that age, when there is reduced flexibility of the nerve trunks, will cause compression of the nerves between the clavicle and the first rib and result in a brachial plexus palsy.[3,12] Robinson et al. and Chung and Farahvar both suggested that morcellation (grinding up) or osteotomy of the middle third of the clavicle might prevent this. With patients below the age of 2 or 3, there is fear that the structures are not strong enough for adequate suture purchase. Also, the advantage of not doing it in patients who are too old is that there is always a certain amount of remodeling. I have not found the operation to be technically difficult at age 2, and find that the younger the patient, the better the result.

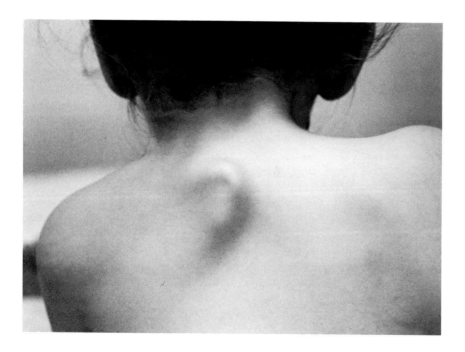

Fig. 13-5. Preoperative Sprengel's deformity. The scapula has an abnormal shape, so that even after surgery it will not look completely normal.

After the age of 7 or 8, therefore, the operative procedure of choice is just resection of the supraspinous portion of the scapula, and of the omovertebral bone. If there is just a fibrous band, it would not require resection, only release. Some people believe that this is the most important part of the operation, from a functional and cosmetic viewpoint, and therefore it certainly is worth doing in the older patient (Fig. 13-6). Carson et al.[1] had also suggested that by adding morcellation or osteotomy of the middle one-third of the clavicle, transplantation could be performed satisfactorily in the older patient. However, in reviewing their figures, the maximum lowering in surgery after age 7 was 1.6 cm and the rest averaged only 0.6 cm. I would suggest that most of that difference, being so slight, may only have been caused by rotating the scapula. I therefore would still have

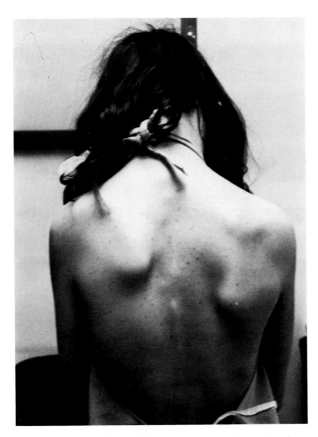

Fig. 13-6. In an older child who had resection only of supraspinous part of scapula, the neck/shoulder line looks good and she will look normal with clothes on. However, her scapulae are at markedly different levels.

reservations about lowering the scapula significantly in older patients.

The classic operation for Sprengel's deformity was Schrock's.[14] This involved resection of the supraspinous portion of the scapula and subperiosteal stripping of the entire bone, which is anchored inferiorly to a rib. That has the problem of recurrence of deformity, especially when the bone grows back into the resected supraspinous portion.[7,8] Therefore, the operations done today rely on extraperiosteal dissection of the supraspinous portion, followed by resection of it. Then they involve transplantation of the scapula, which requires release of the omovertebral bone and the medial and deep tethers of the scapula. Carson and his group thought that the Woodward procedure was probably the best today. This involves release of the muscles along the spinous process, as well as extraperiosteal resection of the supraspinous portion.[16] Grogan et al. agreed and did not routinely incorporate osteotomy of the clavicle.[5] Both groups agree that there is an advantage to a midline approach. Also they believe that this is a more physiological operation than the procedure described by Green[4] because, in the latter, wires are used to pull the scapula down. In the Woodward procedure, the muscle aponeurosis, which is stripped from the spine, is reattached lower down.

There is more support in Europe for Konig's operation, which is essentially similar.[9] As recently described by Wilkinson and Campbell, it involves osteotomy of the medial border of the scapula. This accomplishes the same thing as the Woodward procedure.[15]

My personal preference is for a modification of the original Green procedure.[4] The Green operation involved moving the muscles off their scapula attachments and reattaching them back to the scapula, which is held at a lower level by a spring-attached wire. While I keep to the Green procedure in removing the muscles, I reattach the scapula into a pocket of the latissimus dorsi. This is coupled with extraperiosteal dissection of the supraspinous portion of the scapula and then removal of the supraspinous part. It seems more logical to make the skin incision over the scapula, rather than over the spine as in the Woodward procedure, since it is necessary to be quite far lateral to reach the suprascapular notch (Fig. 13-7). That point represents the limit of resection of the supraspinous portion, which, from a cosmetic point

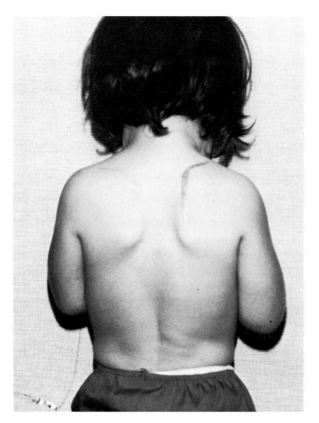

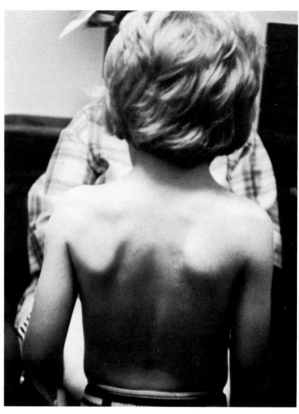

Fig. 13-7. Bilateral Sprengel's deformity after surgery. The scar on the right is fresh but the scar on the left has already blanched; these scars, plus the one in Figure 13-8, are not unsightly.

Fig. 13-8. Compare this to Figure 13-7. The right scapula has been lowered to the same level as the opposite side by the modified Green procedure. The cosmetic appearance is excellent.

of view, is probably the most helpful part of the operation. I have not found the scars more objectionable than the midline scars (Fig. 13-8).

In doing the operation, one peels the trapezius off the spine of the scapula with cutting current (Fig. 13-9A). This exposes the deep layer of muscles, especially the supraspinatus. Then we elevate the latter two-thirds of the supraspinatus of the scapula extraperiosteally. The trapezius is retracted to expose the omovertebral connection, which is severed (Fig. 13-9B). The rhomboids and levator are tagged and separated from their scapular attachments.

The scapula is then lifted with a rake retractor, exposing the subscapularis and the strong fibers of the serratus anterior. The subscapularis is also elevated extraperiosteally where it is opposite the supraspinatus (Fig. 13-9C). The serratus fibers are

marked and cut. Unless they are released the scapula does not move, and unless they are carefully reattached, the scapula wings.

We then bluntly dissect with the Cushing elevator along the top of the scapula, until the elevator comes into the edge of the suprascapular notch. Then, while the elevator is used to protect the nerve and vessels in the notch, the supraspinous portion of the scapula and its periosteum are removed up to the notch with a bone cutter (Fig. 13-9D). A pocket is made in the lattisimus dorsi and the scapula is pulled into this (Fig. 13-9E). The serratus is reattached higher up on the scapula (Fig. 13-9F) and then the other muscles are also reattached higher up. The scapula is sutured to the muscle and fascia of the latissimus pocket (Fig. 13-9G.)

OTHER MOVEMENT DISORDERS OF THE SHOULDER

Besides the limited motion of the shoulder produced by Sprengel's deformity, shoulder motion in the child or adolescent can be limited by muscle weakness. The two most common conditions seen by the pediatric orthopedist are facioscapulohumeral dystrophy and Erb's palsy.

Facioscapulohumeral Dystrophy

Facioscapulohumeral dystrophy generally occurs in children of either sex, and usually several years later than Duchenne's dystrophy. It is typical to see this present in the preteen years or during adolesence.[21] The patients that I see usually come in because of winging of the scapula. In the differential diagnosis, one has to consider polio and isolated damage to the long thoracic nerve.[20] Early on, they will not complain that much about shoulder weakness because they use compensatory motions. Many of these adolescents are even able to continue playing basketball. The deltoid and the rotator cuff seem to function fairly well during the adolescent years; the problem occurs more in the trapezius–serratus-type muscles. The face is usually involved, and often asymmetrically.[22] One boy said he had noticed difficulty blowing out his birthday candles for years.

The disease has an autosomal dominant form of inheritance. It is not unusual for a parent who brings in a child to have the condition, since it is not severe enough to preclude having children.

The diagnosis is made by the characteristic muscle pattern of involvement. The face, shoulder, and humeral muscles are affected. The involvement is asymmetrical and the progression quite slow. Often one shoulder will wing, and then the other will become involved several years later.[22] The EMGs may show recruitment phenomena and low voltage. There are no fibrillation patterns or giant potentials. The muscles sampled for biopsy should be at least grade III in strength. Use of weaker muscles may only show areas of fibrosis. The biopsy shows findings characteristic of a dystrophy, although one is unable to distinguish which type of dystrophy.[22]

Treatment by an orthopedist can be very effective.

One is able to improve both appearance and function by scapulothoracic fusion or stabilization.[18–20] The approach is with the same incision used for the Sprengel's operation, along the medial border of the scapula. The trapezius is raised from the spine and reflected craniad. Then the levators and rhomboids are removed from the medial border and the subscapularis is elevated subperiosteally. We usually resect the portion of this muscle, otherwise it will interfere with the bony union. Then three ribs are exposed subperiosteally, and their surface as well as the undersurface of the scapula roughened with a Hall air drill. Three 18-gauge wires are placed under the ribs (just as one would do with Luque wires) and brought through the scapula and tied down (Fig. 13-10). The scapula, except on its edge, is tissue-paper thin, and not given to debridement with a gouge. Cancellous bone graft from the ilium is placed between the scapula and the ribs. Postoperative immobilization consists of a Rowe sling for 3 months. We always add a plaster velpeau, otherwise adolescents will remove their slings. In the third month, gentle range-of-motion exercises are allowed, mostly for the elbow. The improvement in function and appearance is usually dramatic, and patients always return for the procedure on the opposite side (Fig. 13-11).

Erb's Palsy

Another reason for inability to abduct the shoulder, besides Sprengel's deformity and facioscapulohumeral dystrophy, is Erb's palsy. In Chapter 12, Dr. Leffert goes into great detail on brachial plexus injuries. However, we thought it appropriate to make some mention of treatment in children. Most of the children that we see are quite young and generally make an excellent recovery. That obviously is not because we are treating it better, but because of the greater awareness among obstetricians as to the precipitating causes. In a report from New York Hospital, the incidence declined from 1.56 per 1000 live births in 1938 to 0.38 per 1000, a fourfold decline by 1962.[23] The most important causative factors are a breech presentation and increased birth weight, both of which may suggest the diagnosis.[23] As we noted earlier, one common source of confusion in patients with limited shoulder abduction is the involvement of the elbow. In making the diagnosis, the treating physician

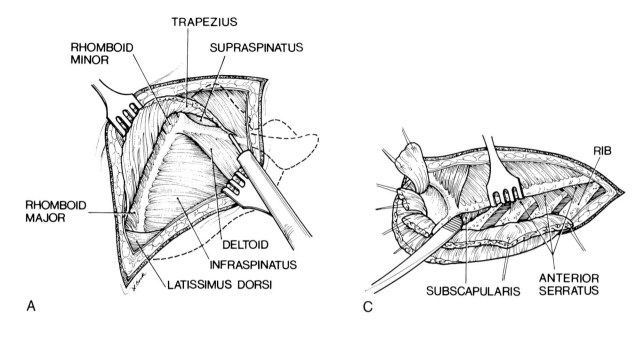

A

C

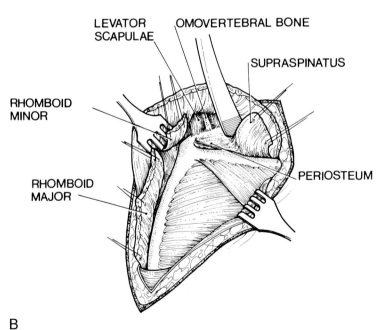

B

Fig. 13-9. (A) Elevation of the trapezius off the spine of the scapula exposes all the deep muscles. (B) The supraspinatus is elevated extraperiosteally. The omovertebral bone is severed. (C) The subscapularis is elevated and the serratus is tagged and released. (*Figure continues.*)

is likely to mistake an Erb's palsy for some other congenital lesion because of subluxation of the radial head. These deformities occur in as many as one-third of the patients with the palsy, and we have not yet found a good way to prevent them.[24]

Therefore, we have parents put young children through a range-of-motion program. For flaccid paralysis, once a day is sufficient. We generally stress elbow flexion and extension, and abduction and external rotation of the shoulder. Splinting in abduction

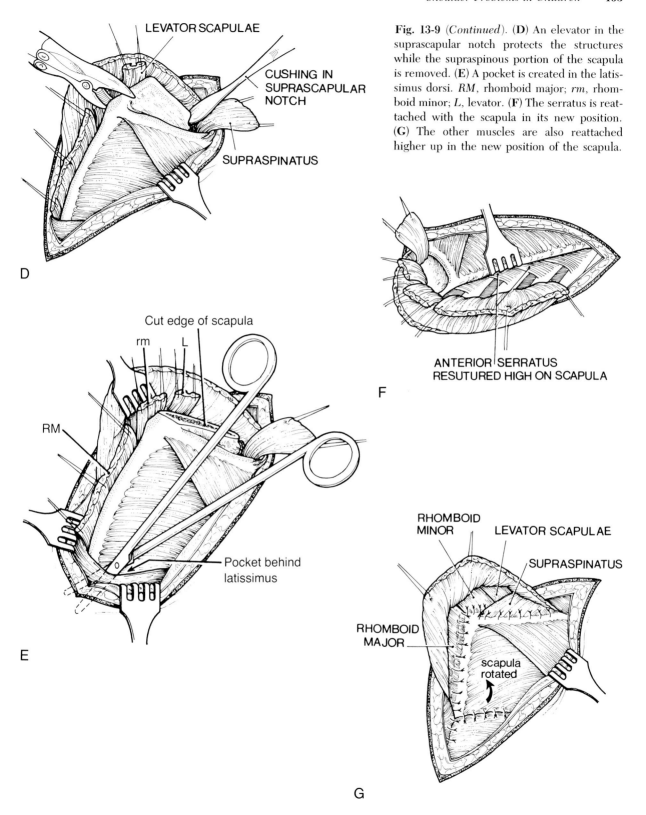

LEVATOR SCAPULAE

CUSHING IN SUPRASCAPULAR NOTCH

SUPRASPINATUS

D

Fig. 13-9 (*Continued*). (**D**) An elevator in the suprascapular notch protects the structures while the supraspinous portion of the scapula is removed. (**E**) A pocket is created in the latissimus dorsi. *RM*, rhomboid major; *rm*, rhomboid minor; *L*, levator. (**F**) The serratus is reattached with the scapula in its new position. (**G**) The other muscles are also reattached higher up in the new position of the scapula.

Cut edge of scapula

rm   L

RM

Pocket behind latissimus

E

ANTERIOR SERRATUS RESUTURED HIGH ON SCAPULA

F

RHOMBOID MINOR   LEVATOR SCAPULAE

SUPRASPINATUS

RHOMBOID MAJOR

scapula rotated

G

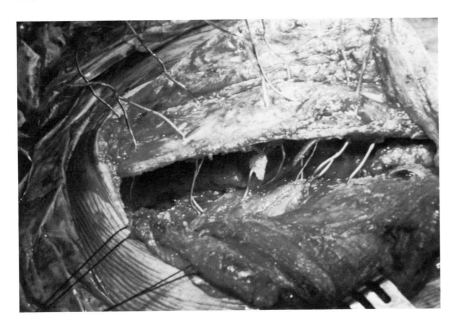

Fig. 13-10. Surgical photograph of wires around the ribs going through scapula.

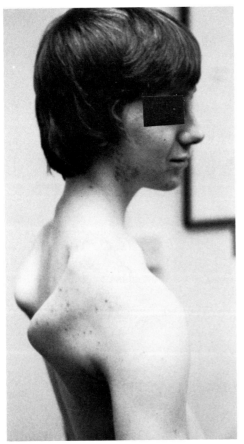

A

B

Fig. 13-11. (**A**) Frontal view of patient with facioscapulohumeral dystrophy. He is unable to abduct greater than 60°. Note that he uses all the accessory muscles, causing an unsightly bulge around the shoulders. (**B**) Lateral view of same patient with severe winging. (*Figure continues*)

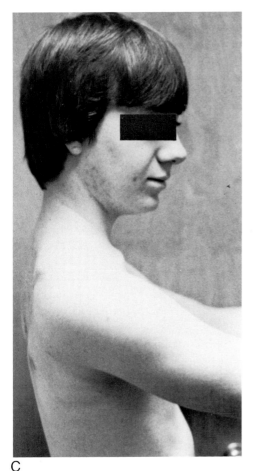

C

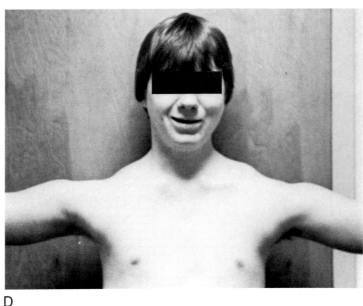

D

Fig. 13-11 (*Continued*). (**C**) Lateral view postoperatively shows winging corrected. (**D**) Frontal view postoperatively. He can now abduct to 90° and no longer has to use the accessory muscles.

is no longer used, since it tended towards abduction contractures.[26] One common complaint among parents is that the treating physicians do not follow up on the deformity, once a certain stage of initial improvement is reached. Many of the patients make dramatic gains during the first 18 months while the nerve function is recovering. However, they are then usually not followed up with annual visits. It is not uncommon, in our experience, to find them left with enough muscle imbalance that they develop internal rotation contractures as a relatively late event, at about 6 or 7 years old. The incidence of complete recovery ranges between 7 and 13 percent.[23,28]

The contraindications to tendon transfers generally around the shoulder are reduced sensation and function in the hand and weakness of the deltoids (usually less than grade II or III), and weakness of the muscles

to be transferred: the latissimus dorsi and teres major (less than grade IV).[25]

The operative procedure we perform is essentially the Green modification of the Sever-L'Episcopo procedure as described by Tachdjian.[27] It involves lengthening the subscapularis and the pectoralis major anteriorly, and then transfering the teres major and latissimus dorsi as a single unit posteriorly to act as an external rotator. The patients and parents are generally very satisfied with the surgical results, but it is important to stress that strengthening exercises must be kept up through the period of growth. I generally immobilize the patients in a shoulder spica for 4 weeks, but do not use any other form of immobilization afterwards (Fig. 13-12).

For those children 10 years old or older, soft tissue transfers may not be enough. If 30° or 40° of external

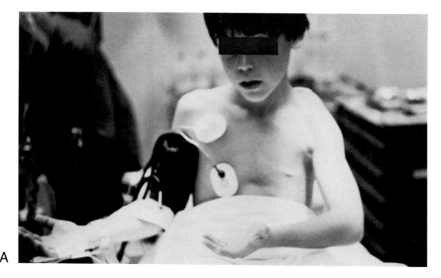

A

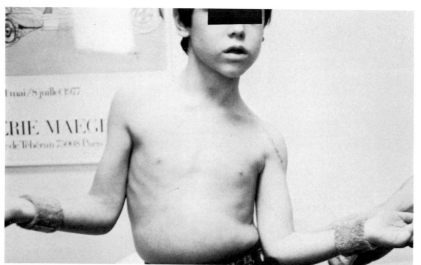

B

Fig. 13-12. (A) Patient with Erb's palsy preoperatively. He has an internal rotation contracture and no active external rotation. **(B)** Postoperatively he has good external rotation, but has to hold his arm in an unusual position to permit the transferred muscles to function. **(C)** Excellent external rotation and abduction with shoulder flexed.

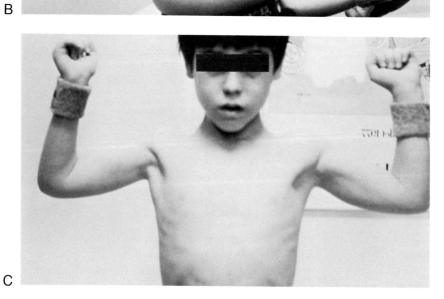

C

466

rotation are not achieved after the soft tissue release, usually a derotational osteotomy is added, which is held with a compression plate. Opening of the capsule is generally discouraged, as it may later lead to dislocation of the shoulder.

It is wise to stress to the parents that the operation does not restore a completely normal shoulder. The patients seem to have to abduct the shoulder slightly to bring the new external rotators in a position where they have enough mechanical advantage to function. It is not difficult to retrain them in their new role, but it is important to reemphasize the importance of keeping up strength so that the muscles do not become overpulled. After the initial 6 months, when everything is functioning well, I encourage the children to do the exercises once or twice per week, and evaluate them on a 6-monthly basis to ensure some degree of compliance.

SEPTIC ARTHRITIS AND OSTEOMYELITIS

Clearly one of the most difficult diagnoses to make in an infant is septic arthritis of the shoulder. Along with osteomyelitis of the proximal humerus, this often also presents as a motion disorder. It is important to realize that this may be mistaken for a neurologic disorder, trauma, or be missed completely.

Clinical Presentation

We have seen septic arthritis occur in infants as early as 7 days of age. The patient always has a temperature elevation, and pseudoparalysis (or pain in the older child) is the most characteristic feature. When stimulated the child may move the hand or elbow, but never the shoulder. The onset may be dramatic or insidious. In one case a neurologist was not consulted for several days because the referring physician thought there was an Erb's palsy. Another case was evaluated in the hospital for several days and treated for a *Hemophilus* meningitis. The treating physicians thought the patient had a spastic hemiparesis because he did not move his arm or leg on one

side. It turned out that both the shoulder and hip joints were septic. The confusing aspect is that many of the children with shoulder joint involvement are already under treatment for a septic process elsewhere. Previous antibiotic therapy may mask the temperature, due to the excellent diffusion of most antibiotics into the joint. However, the child will continue not to move the shoulder. One reliable guide under these circumstances will be the continued elevation of the erythrocyte sedimentation rate (ESR).

In our experience, technetium 99 diphosphonate scanning is very helpful with osteomyelitis, but not too helpful with septic arthritis of the shoulder. In the latter case, it may appear as a blush, or one may see nothing. Sometimes a scan with gallium 67, which localizes to the lysosomes of white cells, may be more helpful. The diagonosis, however, is most strongly suggested by widening of the distance between the humeral head and the glenoid on the radiograph. The definitive diagnosis is made by aspirating the joint. In septic arthritis, there are usually in the neighborhood of 100,000 white blood cells (WBC/mm^3, most of which are polymorphonuclear leukocytes. The joint fluid protein is in the range of over 4 g, and the mucin clot is poor. The sugar is low compared to the serum. It is important to bear in mind that similar findings can be found in a joint involved with juvenile rheumatoid arthritis, (JRA) although the sugar is usually not as low, and the WBC level may be closer to 30,000/mm^3. However, I have seen JRA fluid levels of 100,000/mm^3 and certainly one can have an elevated temperature and ESR in JRA. Also, the test for antinuclear antibody and rheumatoid factor may be negative in JRA. Therefore, use of a Gram stain is extremely important.

Treatment

It is generally accepted in orthopaedics that if there is a significant amount of purulence, it should be drained. However, surgical drainage is not always necessary. The shoulder is easily accessible, and a large-bore needle can be placed anteriorly, lateral to the coracoid process. The antibiotic level in the joint closely approaches the serum level for the commonly used antibiotics, so antibiotics do not have to be instilled in the joint directly. The purulent fluid, however, has to be removed. Therefore, perhaps twice the first day or two, and daily for a few days thereafter, the joint should be aspirated and then irrigated with saline until clear. If the patient is not improving clinically, and if the fluid remains purulent after a couple of days, the joint should definitely be opened. In fact, if there is no contraindication to surgery, and particularly if the organism is *Staphylococcus aureus*, we open the joint primarily.

The most common infecting organism in children is *S. aureus*.[30] In the first year of life, however, *Hemophilus* influenzae is a common culprit. Therefore, if the offending organism has not been identified, one would start treatment with a penicillinase-resistant antibiotic such as oxacillin, and an antibiotic that the *H. influenzae* is not resistant to, such as cefamandole. If the cultures come back indicating sensitivity to ampicillin for *H. influenzae*, obviously this is preferable. In the first month of life any organism can be involved, so it becomes extremely important to determine the offending organism.

The entire humeral head is made of cartilage at birth, and the enzymes of the WBCs (the granulocyte elastase) destroys the proteoglycans of the cartilage and can irreparably damage the head. Therefore, it is of greatest importance to make the diagnosis early and initiate treatment rapidly.[29,30] Osteomyelitis of the proximal humerus is less of a problem in infants because the bones tend to undergo remodeling, and it is rare to see chronic osteomyelitis after an infantile infection. Older children can develop chronic osteomyelitis, but because of the excellent vascular supply to the bones in the shoulder, we usually do not have the same problems with chronic osteomyelitis that we see in the tibia. We usually treat acute osteomyelitis for 4 weeks, and chronic osteomyelitis for at least 6 weeks. Most centers agree that a minimum of 1 to 2 weeks intravenous antibiotics is necessary. After that, the substitution of oral antibiotics is a matter of dispute.[31] Some centers have suggested that oral antibiotics be used only if the organism has been isolated and one can obtain serum levels of the antibiotic to match against sensitivities. We do not believe that is always necessary, but strongly believe that only patients with the most conscientious families should be allowed out of the hospital on an early oral regimen. The risks are too great to allow latitude in taking the medication. Previous studies over many years showed that inadequate courses of antibiotics, gener-

ally under 3 weeks, usually led to recurrence of the osteomyelitis.

CONGENITAL PSEUDARTHROSIS OF THE CLAVICLE

Among the many shoulder disorders that occur in children, one relatively uncommon one that is still subject to considerable controversy is congenital pseudarthrosis of the clavicle. Previous workers ascribed the lesion to failure of union of two separate growth centers of the clavicle, with failure of fusion of the masses at the seventh week of prenatal development.[37] The multiple ossification center theory was questioned because some workers found only a solitary center for the clavicle. The controversy may have arisen because there apparently are two centers of condensed mesenchyme appearing at the 6 weeks or 18 mm embryo stages. Then there is a rapid ossification and fusion of these two centers by the 23 mm stage. Next there is resorption of the mesenchymal ossification mass, periosteal vascular invasion, and the rest of the bone is formed by endochondral ossification.[33] It may be that the pseudarthrosis is formed by local interference or failure of the blood vessels to enter the mesenchymal mass.[38] It is now considered to be related, in some way, to abnormal pressure exerted by the great vessels as they leave the aorta. For this reason most of the pseudarthroses are localized to the right side. Lloyd-Roberts et al.[35] have suggested that the reason for the right-sided involvement is pressure of the subclavian artery on the developing clavicle. It arises higher than its counterpart on the left and remains closer to the clavicle. It is further suggested that the addition of a cervical rib, or more higher-riding ribs on that side, tend to force the vessels even closer. In 3 reported series 59 of 60 patients had the lesion on the right.[32,34,36]

There is also an association between congenital pseudarthrosis of the clavicle and neurofibromatosis. Some authors claim that if the ends of the pseudarthrosis are really tapered to a point, that suggests neurofibromatosis as a possible cause.

We have recently found a child with bilateral

pseudarthroses of the clavicle, which has apparently been reported previously. We did not note any abnormal vascular pattern with this child, and it becomes difficult to reconcile the vascular theory with the bilateral pseudarthroses. The vascular theorists contend that the bilateral cases may represent bilaterally elevated rib cases, or cervical ribs forcing the subclavian against the bone, or may in fact represent cases of cleidocranial dysostosis.[35] Most children present with a painless bump in the clavicular region. The lump is usually in the midclavicular area and is generally unaccompanied by other abnormalities. The radiograph usually shows a bulbous appearance and the medial half usually protrudes upwards.[36] It is generally not difficult to distinguish this from a fracture.

The latter has callus formation after a short time; it is painful and is accompanied by pseudoparalysis in the young child.

The debate stems from whether or not surgical intervention is called for. There is some question as to whether this is painful in later life, but certainly the teenagers whom I have seen do not complain about pain or restriction of function (Fig. 13-13). Owen reviewed 33 patients from 70 surgeons, and found some cases of aching around the shoulder after exercise, but admitted that the disability was never serious.[36] The indications for surgery are therefore, essentially, cosmetic. We offer the choice between a scar and at least two operations (plating and bone grafting and later plate removal), and a bump. Most parents choose the latter.

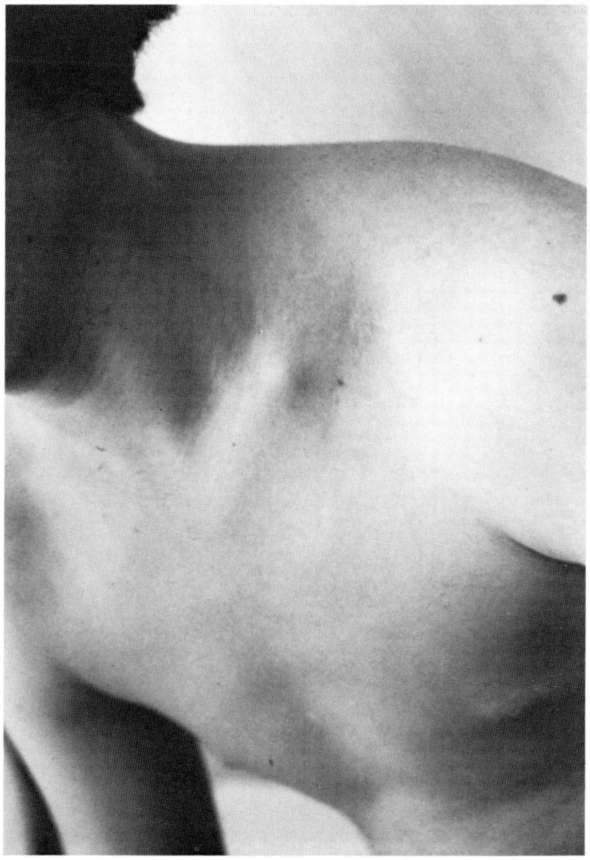

Fig. 13-13. Prominence seen in patient with congenital pseudarthrosis of the clavicle. This patient is asymptomatic. Is the bump worse than a scar?

REFERENCES

Sprengel's Deformity

1. Carson WG, Lovell WW, Whitesides TE: Congenital elevation of the scapula: surgical correction by the Woodward procedure. J Bone Joint Surg 63A:1199, 1981
2. Cavendish ME: Congenital elevation of the scapula. J Bone Joint Surg 54B:395, 1972
3. Chung SMK, Farahvar H: Surgery of the clavicle in Sprengel's deformity. Clin Orthop 116:138, 1976
4. Green WT: The surgical correction of congenital elevation of the scapula (Sprengel's deformity). J Bone Joint Surg 39A:1439, 1957
5. Grogan DP, Stanley EA, Bobechko WP: The congenital undescended scapula. J Bone Joint Surg 65B:598, 1983
6. Horowitz AE: Congenital elevation of the scapula: Sprengel's deformity. J Bone Joint Surg 34A:260, 1982
7. Jeannopoulos CL: Congenital elevation of the scapula. J Bone Joint Surg 34A:883, 1952
8. Jeannopoulous CL: Observations on congenital elevation of the scapula. Clin Orthop 20:132, 1961
9. Konig F. Eine neue Operation des angeborenen Schulterblatthochstandes. Beitr Klin Chir 94:530, 1914
10. Mercier W, Duthie RN: Orthopaedic Surgery, 6th ed. Edward Arnold, London, 1964
11. Pinsky HA, Pizzutillo PD, MacEven GD: Congenital elevation of the scapula. Orthop Trans 4:288, 1980

12. Robinson RA, Braun RM, Mack P, Zadek R: The surgical importance of the clavicular component of Sprengel's deformity. J Bone Joint Surg 49A:1481, 1967 (abst)

13. Ross DM, Cruess RL: The surgical correction of congenital elevation of the scapula. A review of seventy-seven cases. Clin Orthop 125:17, 1977

14. Schrock RD: Congenital elevation of the scapula. J Bone Joint Surg 8:207, 1926

15. Wilkinson JA, Campbell D: Scapular osteotomy for Sprengel's shoulder. J Bone Joint Surg 62B:486, 1980

16. Woodward JW: Congenital elevation of the scapula. Correction by release and transplantation of muscle origins. A preliminary report. J Bone Joint Surg 43A:219, 1961

17. Wynne-Davies R: Heritable Disorders in Orthopaedic Practice. Blackwell, Oxford, 1973

Facioscapulohumeral Dystrophy

18. Bunch WH: Scapulo-thoracic fusion for shoulder stabilization in muscular dystrophy. Minn Med 56:391, 1973

19. Copeland SA, Howard RC: Thoracoscapular fusion for facioscapulohumeral dystrophy. J Bone Joint Surg 60B:547, 1978

20. Ketenjian AY: Scapulocostal stabilization for scapular winging in facioscapulohumeral muscular dystrophy. J Bone Joint Surg 69A:476, 1978

21. Merritt HH: A Textbook of Neurology. Lea and Febiger, Philadelphia, 1959

22. Vignos PJ: Diagnosis of progressive muscular dystrophy. J Bone Joint Dis 49A:1212, 1967

Erb's Palsy

23. Adler JB, Patterson RL: Erb's palsy. Long-term results of treatment in eighty-eight cases. J Bone Joint Surg 49A:1052, 1967

24. Aitken J: Deformity of the elbow joint as a sequel to Erb's obstetrical paralysis. J Bone Joint Surg 34B:352, 1952

25. Hofer MM, Wickenden R, Roper B: Brachial plexus birth palsies. J Bone Joint Surg 60A:691, 1978

26. Milgram JE: Discussion of the Paper by L'Episcopo JB: Restoration of muscle balance in the treatment of obstetrical paralysis. NY State J Med 39:357, 1939

27. Tachdjian MO: Pediatric Orthopaedics. W.B. Saunders, Philadelphia, 1972

28. Wickstrom J: Birth injuries of the brachial plexus. Treatment of defects in the shoulder. Clin Orthop 23:187, 1962

Osteomyelitis and Septic Arthritis

29. Curtiss PH, Jr.: The pathophysiology of joint infections. Clin Orthop 96:129, 1973

30. Lunseth PA, Heiple KG: Prognosis in septic arthritis of the hip in children. Clin Orthop 139:81, 1979

31. Nelson JD, Howard JB, Shelton S: Oral antibiotic therapy for skeletal infections of children. I. Antibiotic concentrations in suppurative synovial fluid. J Pediatr 92:131, 1975

Congenital Pseudarthrosis of the Clavicle

32. Alldred AJ: Congenital pseudarthrosis of the clavicle. J Bone Joint Surg 45B:312, 1963

33. Anderson H: Histochemistry and development of the human shoulder and acromioclavicular joints with particular reference to the early development of the clavicle. Acta Anat 55:124, 1963

34. Gibson DA, Carroll N: Congenital pseudarthrosis of the clavicle. J Bone Joint Surg 52B:629, 1970

35. Lloyd-Roberts, GC, Apley AG, Owen R: Reflections upon the aetiology of congenital pseudarthrosis of the clavicle. J Bone Joint Surg 57B:24, 1975

36. Owen R: Congenital pseudarthrosis of the clavicle. J Bone Joint Surg 52B:644, 1970

37. O'Rahilly R: p. 10 In Frantz CH (ed): Normal and Abnormal Embryological Development. National Research Council Publication, 1479, Washington, D.C.

38. Wall JJ: Congenital pseudarthrosis of the clavicle. J Bone Joint Surg 52A:1003, 1970

Arthritis of the Shoulder

14

John A. Mills

Inflammatory diseases of the glenohumeral joint are difficult to evaluate clinically and often hard to distinguish from other disorders of the joint because of the indiscriminate involvement of the rotator cuff. Dysfunction of the rotator cuff mechanism, which serves both supporting and operating functions, occurs in almost any painful shoulder, with the result that different diseases produce similar symptoms and signs.[4,14] A detailed examination of the shoulder may provide clues to the nature of the primary problem but often the evaluation requires radiographic and other laboratory studies to be more specifically diagnostic.[3] The examination of the shoulder joint has been described in detail in Chapter 4 and will not be reconsidered here except as it pertains to certain specific diseases.

The glenohumeral joint is affected in most forms of arthritis, either those involving predominantly the peripheral or the axial (rhizomelic) joints. The commonly encountered rheumatic diseases of the shoulder in their order of prevalence are seronegative spondyloarthropathies, seropositive (classic) rheumatoid arthritis, pseudogout, gout, Reiter's syndrome, juvenile arthritis, ankylosing spondylitis, and hemochromatosis. It is often difficult to detect signs of inflammation or to be sure that the process is inflammatory. Tenderness over the coracoid process is very suggestive of inflammatory joint disease; it is not commonly elicited in primary rotator cuff or other noninflammatory disorders.

Pain at rest or on the slightest motion rarely occurs in rheumatoid arthritis and the seronegative rheumatoid variants. Such extreme sensitivity to joint motion may indicate septic arthritis, gout, a severe injury, or a tumor that involves the articular bone.

One of the few signs that helps to differentiate between inflammatory conditions and degenerative disorders of the shoulder is pain on passive motion, either rotation or flexion, that does not involve abduction. However, because of the stabilizing function of the rotator cuff, it may be difficult to obtain full relaxation. If that can be done (by bending forward), full rotation is usually obtained in degenerative disorders but an inflamed capsule will cause pain and give the sensation of gradual resistance as the joint is moved from the neutral position.

When treatment is problematic and the diagnosis of inflammatory joint disease is not certain, the analysis of synovial fluid may be helpful. A synovial leukocyte count above 10,000/mm^3 with a predominance of neutrophils points strongly to a rheumatoid disorder if infection- and crystal-induced synovitis can be excluded. A clearly positive serum test for rheumatoid factor adds weight to the diagnosis of rheumatoid arthritis but low titers are frequently misleading.

RHEUMATOID ARTHRITIS

Stiffness and pain in the shoulders are frequent early manifestations of rheumatoid arthritis.[8] However, in the classic seropositive form of the disease, chronic disabling involvement usually does not occur until late in its course.[6] Passive and active shoulder motion remains relatively satisfactory although rotator cuff dysfunction may allow superior subluxation of the humerus and acromiohumeral impingement. Once this occurs, trauma to the supraspinatus tendon is inevitable.[19] Synovitis of the adjacent acromioclavicular joint may also damage the tendon. In some patients, capsular damage allows anterior subluxation of the humeral head, especially if the glenoid labrum is eroded. A common problem in patients with chronic synovitis is rupture of the long head of the biceps. The event may be acute with pain and a hematoma, or insidious, going unnoticed until a bulge in the biceps is observed.

Bone erosion in the rheumatoid shoulder may be slight even when the articular cartilage is extensively damaged. Erosions, when present, usually begin in the region of the greater tuberosity (Fig. 14-1). However, chronic arthritis, especially cases that begin in childhood, may completely destroy the humeral head, leaving the shaft of the humerus articulating under the acromion or coracoid process.

As noted previously, patients with rheumatoid arthritis of the glenohumeral joint usually do not develop large effusions. In a few cases, often in joints that are not very painful, voluminous effusions can occur. The synovial fluid is opalescent and may contain cholesterol crystals. The pathogenesis of this condition is not understood. Rupture of the shoulder capsule is another rare occurrence that can be locally asymptomatic but result in diffuse edema of the arm and sometimes pain similar to the "pseudothrombophlebitis" syndrome caused by a ruptured Baker's cyst of the knee.[7]

An acute arthritis that affects older individuals and involves the shoulders, and often the wrists accompanied by puffy edema of the hands and forearms, has been described as rheumatoid arthritis of the elderly. It seems to run a course of 4 to 6 months, during which it can be very disabling. About one-half of the

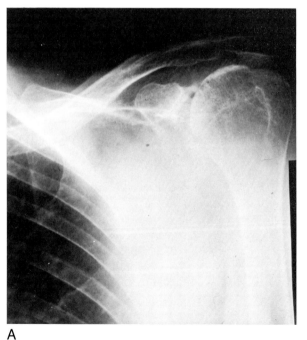
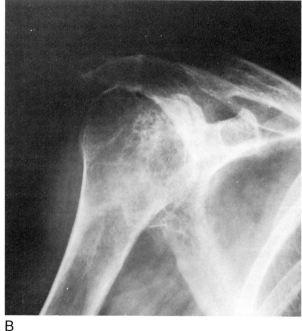

A   B

Fig. 14-1. Rheumatoid arthritis. (**A**) Erosion beginning at greater tuberosity. (**B**) Advanced destruction of shoulder joint.

patients respond to a nonsteroidal anti-inflammatory drug. Those who do not often require low-dose glucocorticoid therapy for at least several months. Patients with this syndrome do not have rheumatoid factor in the serum. The erythrocyte sedimentation rate (ESR) is usually elevated and some patients turn out to have giant cell arthritis. Others may have the shoulder–hand syndrome.

JUVENILE RHEUMATOID ARTHRITIS

The various forms of juvenile rheumatoid arthritis commonly involve the shoulders although not usually early in the disease.[2] The shoulder is more likely to be affected in juvenile spondylitis or the polyarticular rather than the pauciarticular form.

The diagnosis of juvenile chronic arthritis depends heavily on exclusion. In cases of isolated shoulder arthritis in children, tuberculosis, osteonecrosis (often due to sickle cell disease), and tumor are at least as common as juvenile rheumatoid arthritis. In the systemic onset form of juvenile rheumatoid arthritis, widely referred to as Still's disease, a characteristic fever and rash occur. Joint pain may be severe but is usually episodic. Juvenile ankylosing spondylitis is a disease of adolescent boys. Early in the disease, the diagnosis is largely made on the family history, since diagnostic radiographic changes may not appear for 2 to 4 years. Rheumatoid factor is found in less than 10 percent of children with arthritis. Children who are seropositive tend to have a severe adultlike course in which destructive shoulder involvement is common.[16]

Although the management of chronic arthritis in children does not differ in principle from that in adults (and is discussed in a later section), the use of corticosteroid, either intraarticularly or systemically, should be avoided even more strongly. Probably because children pay less attention to painful joints and tend to work (or play) around them, restricted motion accompanied by severe shoulder girdle atrophy is a frequent consequence of neglected shoulder arthritis. Joints so affected can be very difficult to mobilize and constant attention is necessary to prevent joint contractures.

Children with juvenile rheumatoid arthritis, particularly the pauciarticular form, must have thorough eye examinations at least four times per year to detect the presence of an iridocyclitis that is usually asymptomatic and can have severe consequences.

SERONEGATIVE SPONDYLOARTHROPATHIES

The axial joints, including the shoulders, are usually affected both earlier and to a greater extent in the seronegative "rheumatoid variants" than in classic seropositive disease. These disorders, now called seronegative spondyloarthropathies, include psoriatic arthritis, the polyarthritis that occurs in patients with inflammatory bowel disease, and ankylosing spondylitis. Although these tend to be less severe as a group than classic rheumatoid arthritis, rapidly destructive shoulder arthritis can occur, especially in patients with the psoriatic form. Sometimes the psoriasis is so mild as to escape detection unless carefully sought. Occasionally it does not appear until years after the onset of arthritis.

In ankylosing spondylitis, hip and shoulder arthritis usually follows clinically obvious spine involvement. In some cases, particularly in younger patients, shoulder arthritis is a presenting feature and a frozen shoulder may result from the progressive loss of articular cartilage. There may be few signs of inflammation in the shoulder. A radiograph of the sacroiliac joint can be diagnostic in seronegative polyarthritis and should be obtained when one of those diseases is suspected.

REITER'S SYNDROME

Reiter's syndrome is grouped with the seronegative spondyloarthropathies. Its onset is associated with urethral infection or bacterial enterocolitis.[13] Sporadic cases usually follow sexually acquired urethritis, *Clamydia trachomatis* being the agent in about 50 percent of these. The syndrome presents as an acute arthritis often accompanied by conjunctivitis. The shoulder is less commonly affected than the ankle, subtalar, and knee joints. Heel pain due to inflammation at the origin of the plantar ligament or the Achilles insertion is present in almost half of the patients. While the majority have a limited course with spontaneous recovery after a few weeks or months, some have a chronic arthritis and are more likely to have shoulder involvement. The features of the arthritis resemble those of psoriatic arthritis; indeed, a distinctive skin eruption, keratoderma blennhoragicum, which is histologically similar to pustular psoriasis, occurs in 25 percent of chronic cases.

CRYSTAL-INDUCED SYNOVITIS

The intraarticular presence of at least three different kinds of crystals can produce an arthritis. These are urate, calcium pyrophosphate, and calcium phosphate dihydrate. Any of the three can affect the shoulder.

Gout

Since only a minor fraction of individuals with hyperuricemia develop gout, the diagnosis cannot be made on the basis of the serum urate level alone. In suspected cases of crystal-induced synovitis, the diagnosis should be established by demonstrating the crystals in synovial fluid.[17] The shoulder is rarely affected early in the course of gout but it is sometimes the presenting joint in postoperative flares and in postmenopausal women, who may have a subacute polyarticular onset of the disease. It also presents as an acute subacromial bursitis or a rotator cuff syndrome. In large joints, gout can cause fever occasionally as high as 102° to 103°F with a moderate leukocytosis. In such cases, arthrocentesis to rule out septic arthritis is essential.

The radiographic features of gouty arthritis are those of juxtaarticular tophi: sharply outlined erosions, often with sharp spike-like bone margins, and less osteopenia than is associated with rheumatoid arthritis. Slightly radiopaque tophi are seen occasion-

ally in the periarticular soft tissue. However, the radiographic differential diagnosis can be very difficult.

Pseudogout

Pseudogout occurs more commonly in the shoulder than gout. It may be an acute or a chronic destructive process. Chondrocalcinosis is evident in about 50 percent of cases when high-quality radiographs are examined carefully (Fig. 14-2). Almost always diagnostic pleomorphic, positively birefringent, calcium pyrophosphate dihydrate crystals can be identified in synovial fluid. In contrast to gout, pseudogout affects men and women about equally. It may be polyarticular. In such cases, hyperparathyroidism or hemochromatosis should be ruled out by appropriate blood tests.

The Milwaukee Shoulder

The third form of crystal-induced synovitis, sometimes called apatite gout occurs most commonly in

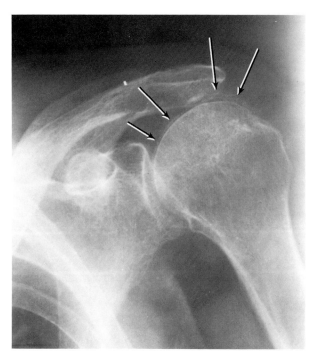

Fig. 14-2. Chondrocalcinosis. Fine linear calcium deposits in articular cartilage (arrows).

the shoulder, where it has been named the Milwaukee shoulder.[11] The majority of patients with this disorder are elderly women. Chronic but relatively mild discomfort and a large boggy effusion are the usual findings. The synovial fluid is characteristically noninflammatory with leukocyte counts less than 1,000/mm^3, predominantly mononuclear cells. The diagnosis depends on the demonstration of basic calcium phosphate crystals of several types, often accompanied by particulate collagen fragments. Both of these are too small to be identified by light microscopy but the presence of calcium crystals often can be shown by staining them with alizarin red R. This stain is not specific for apatite and will reveal other calcium salts as well.[17]

The majority of patients with the Milwaukee shoulder have severe rotator cuff pathology and some degree of joint instability. Calcium deposits of uncertain composition are often identified in the periarticular soft tissues and chondrocalcinosis may be present.

Large and relatively asymptomatic knee and shoulder effusions have been described in patients on long-term hemodialysis for renal failure. Crystals of various calcium salts, including apatite and oxalate, have been identified in the synovial fluid.

OTHER CONNECTIVE TISSUE DISEASES

The shoulder joint is not commonly involved in other inflammatory disorders of connective tissue such as lupus erythematosus or the various forms of systemic arteritis. However, arthritis involving the shoulders and other joints occurs in about 20 percent of cases of Wegener's granulomatosis. Migratory polyarthritis is characteristic of rheumatic fever and Henoch–Schonlein purpura. The shoulder may be affected in either disease. Shoulder involvement was noted by Sydenham in his classic description of rheumatic fever.

The synovial fluid in the arthritis of lupus erythematosus usually contains less than 10,000 leukocytes/mm^3 and often a preponderance of mononuclear cells. In the other systemic diseases of connective tissue, including rheumatic fever, the synovial fluid is similar to that of rheumatoid arthritis. It should be noted that early or acute arthritis, whether rheumatoid or other, may not have the synovial fluid composition characteristic of the more established cases. That often leads to some diagnostic uncertainty.

Polymyalgia rheumatica is a disease of unknown cause in which the cardinal manifestation is arthralgia and myalgia involving the shoulder and pelvic girdles. Several groups of investigators have shown, by means of radionuclide scans, that a low-grade arthritis of axial joints may be responsible for the symptoms.[12] Only rarely is any abnormality evident by physical examination of the joint itself, although often joint motion is limited by pain. In a few cases, evidence of mild synovitis also has been found by synovial fluid analysis.

OSTEOARTHRITIS

Primary degenerative joint disease of the shoulder is rare. In almost all cases there is a history of trauma, often with resultant rotator cuff injury. Diseases that affect articular cartilage such as hemochromatosis, ochronosis, and primary chondrocalcinosis can lead to severe cartilage degeneration. In patients with syringomyelia, neuropathic changes often develop in the shoulder and will lead ultimately to all of the features of a Charcot joint; a relatively painless joint with radiographic evidence of severe destructive and hypertrophic bone reaction.

NONINFLAMMATORY SYNOVIAL REACTIONS

Proliferation of the synovium of unknown cause results in two distinct disorders that occasionally affect the shoulder.

Pigmented Villonodular Synovitis

The first of these reactions is pigmented villonodular synovitis (PVNS).[10] Tendon sheaths, especially in the hands and feet, are more commonly involved than is articular synovium, in which case it is often referred to as a giant cell tumor of tendon sheath. The *shoulder joint is rarely involved:* there are less than 1 in 200 cases from the literature. The synovium is characterized by hypertrophy, with the subsynovial connective tissue showing proliferation of fibroblasts, infiltration by mononuclear cells, and the presence of many multinucleate giant cells. Microvascular proliferation is also prominent together with erythrocyte extravasation and the phagocytosis of hematogenous pigment that gives the disorder its name.

Symptoms caused by PVNS include relatively painless joint swelling and limitation of motion caused by mechanical factors. Synovial fluid examination reveals low to moderate numbers of neutrophils and mononuclear phagocytes, many of which contain hemosiderin. The diagnosis can be confirmed by arthrography or arthroscopy. It is characteristically a disorder of young adults.

Treatment of PVNS involves as complete a synovectomy as possible to reduce the likelihood of recurrence. The disorder is currently thought not to be neoplastic and radiation therapy is not recommended either for initial treatment or to prevent recurrence.

Osteochondromatosis

The second presumably reactive proliferative disorder of the synovium is osteochondromatosis. As with PVNS, symptoms are caused by mechanical interference with joint motion due to the presence of numerous areas of synovial proliferation and intraarticular loose bodies.[15] Hypertrophy of the synovial connective tissue with focal cartilaginous metaplasia appears to be the primary event. Pedunculated projections of the lining become separated as loose bodies. Some of the metaplastic cartilage usually calcifies and the resulting focal intraarticular calcifications allow easy roentgenographic diagnosis. In cases where the calcifications are not seen, arthrographic or arthroscopic diagnosis is needed. The synovial fluid is noninflammatory and is characteristically viscous. This and the presence of the loose bodies makes arthrocentesis difficult.

Osteochondromatosis, like PVNS, is treated by synovectomy, although simple removal of the loose bodies by arthroscopy or arthrotomy may produce long-lasting benefit.

NONRHEUMATIC DISEASES

Hemarthrosis

The shoulder joint is a relatively frequent site of intraarticular hemorrhage. Underlying causes include hemophilia and other hematologic disorders,[9] anticoagulant therapy, trauma, and spontaneous intraarticular hemorrhage that occurs in the elderly. The acute onset of severe pain and swelling is characteristic and will usually lead to a diagnostic arthrocentesis. Probably as a result of partial coagulation with subsequent mechanical or enzymatic lysis, the blood aspirated is defibrinated and does not reclot in the syringe or test tube.

Tensely swollen or very painful joints should be aspirated and wrapped with a bandage. Hemorrhage rarely recurs except in patients with hemophilia. Hemarthrosis in a patient with hemophilia should be treated by immobilization and ice packs until sufficient factor VIII can be given to allow safe arthrocentesis. Prevention of trauma and careful monitoring of plasma factor VIII levels are important to reduce the risk of chronic hemophilic arthropathy.

A recurrent hemarthrosis in a patient without hemophilia may indicate the presence of a synovial hemangioma or other tumor. Villonodular synovitis occasionally causes frankly hemorrhagic joint fluid.

Osteonecrosis

Osteonecrosis can occur spontaneously in patients with systemic lupus erythematosus but is much more common in any patient who has been treated with synthetic adrenocorticoid drugs in moderate to high doses for at least several months.[21] The hip is affected far more commonly than the shoulder. Affected shoulders are variably painful. Severe discomfort may be felt at rest and lying on the shoulder is almost always painful, but the passive range of motion is maintained until focal collapse of the articular cortex and deformity of the humeral head produce a frozen shoulder.

When osteonecrosis is suspected, a bone scan will be abnormal well before the revascularization process results in characteristic radiographic changes. The earliest radiographic sign is a thin radiolucent line immediately below the subchondral cortex of the humeral head (Fig. 14-3).

polyarticular disorders that fail to respond to other antirheumatic therapy may be treated with cytotoxic drugs such as methotrexate, azathioprine, cyclophosphamide. The first of these is currently preferred. In contrast to the other cytotoxic drugs, methotrexate induces a rapid response and seems to be effective only as long as it is administered weekly. It is given in a once weekly dose of 7.5 to 15 mg, either as a single intramuscular injection or orally in three divided doses 6 hours apart. It is probably the safest of the three cytotoxic agents. *Close hematologic monitoring is mandatory in the use of all these agents.* There are numerous other potential side effects that require the patient and physician to be fully informed.

Gout

Once the acute arthritis of gout has been treated with anti-inflammatory drugs, management of the hyperuricemia should be undertaken. If it is the first attack, which is unlikely in the shoulder, and the serum urate level is less than 9 or 10 mg/dl, many authorities recommend waiting until attacks begin to occur more regularly, which, in some cases, can be years. This is reasonable because the control of hyperuricemia can be effectively obtained at almost any stage by the use of allopurinol. Treatment should be started with 100 mg orally per day and the dose increased in 100 mg increments, at 2-weekly intervals, until the serum urate level is 5 mg/dl or less. In most cases, a 300 mg/day dose is sufficient.

Allopurinol is a relatively frequent cause of hypersensitivity reactions and in such cases the uricosuric drugs, probenecid or sulfinpyrazone must be used. When those drugs are employed, it is important to ensure an increased fluid intake, and, when the urine uric acid exceeds 800 mg per day, alkalinization of the urine to prevent uric acid stone formation. An anti-inflammatory drug should be continued in a prophylactic dosage at least until the serum urate level has been kept in the normal range for 3 to 6 months. This is because paradoxic flares of gouty arthritis may occur when allopurinol or uricosuric therapy is initiated. As an alternative to one of the NSAIDs, colchicine 0.6 mg twice daily is often used.

The need to treat acute gouty arthritis when a patient is unable to take food by mouth is a common problem. Colchicine given intravenously at a dosage of 2 mg followed at 6 and 12 hours by additional doses of 1 mg is recommended. The total dosage should not exceed 4 mg in the first 24 hours or 2 mg/day thereafter and it should not be given parenterally for more than 5 days. The usual warnings of toxicity, such as vomiting and diarrhea, rarely occur. Parenteral ACTH or methyprednisolone is a useful alternative to colchicine, but rebound flares are a problem when doses of these agents are tapered.

SURGICAL MANAGEMENT

Few conservative surgical procedures are useful in patients with glenohumeral arthritis. Acromioclavicular arthroplasty for patients with severe arthritis of the acromioclavicular joint or with a tendency to superior subluxation of the humerus but with an intact rotator cuff may delay further damage to the supraspinatus tendon. However, once there is severe rotator cuff destruction, decompression surgery may lead only to further subluxation.

Patients with a severe loss of articular cartilage or erosion of the subchondral bone with disabling pain should be considered for shoulder joint replacement with a Neer or other prosthesis. Unfortunately, the result is likely to be disappointing if the rotator cuff is too damaged to ensure a stable joint.

REFERENCES

1. Anonymous: Intraarticular steroids. Lancet p. 385, 1984
2. Ansell BM: Joint manifestations in children with juvenile chronic polyarthritis. Arthritis Rheum 20:204, 1977
3. Bennett RM: The painful shoulder. Postgrad Med 73:153, 1983
4. Bland JH, Merrit JA, Boushey DR: The painful shoulder. Semin Arthritis Rheum 1:21, 1977
5. Cannon SR: Massive osteolysis. J Bone Joint Surg 68B:24, 1986
6. Curran JF, Ellmann MH, Brown NL: Rheumatologic

aspects of painful conditions affecting the shoulder. Clin Orthop 173:27, 1983

7. deJager P, Fleming A: Shoulder joint rupture and pseudothrombosis in rheumatoid arthritis. Ann Rheum Dis 43:503, 1984

8. Ennevarra K: Painful shoulder joint in rheumatoid arthritis. A clinical and radiological study of 200 cases with special reference to arthrography of the glenohumeral joint. Acta Rheum Scand Suppl 11:1, 1967

9. Epps CH, Jr.: Painful hematologic conditions affecting the shoulder. Clin Orthop 173:38, 1983

10. Granowitz SP, d'Antonia J, Mankin HJ: The pathogenesis and long term end results of pigmented villonodular synovitis. Clin Orthop 114:335, 1976

11. Halverson PB, McCarty DJ, Cheung HS et al: Milwaukee shoulder syndrome. Eleven additional cases with involvement of the knee in seven. Semin Arthritis Rheum 14:36, 1984

12. Healey LA: Long term follow-up of polymyalgis rheumatica. Evidence of synovitis. Semin Arthritis Rheum 13:322, 1984

13. Keat A: Reiter's syndrome and reactive arthritis in perspective. N Engl J Med 309:1606, 1983

14. Kessel L: Clinical Disorders of the Shoulder. Churchill Livingstone, New York, 1982

15. Milgran JW: Synovial chondromatosis: a histopathologic study of 30 cases. J Bone Joint Surg 59:792, 1977

16. Rothschild BM: Severe generalized (Charcot-like) joint destruction in juvenile rheumatoid arthritis. Clin Orthop 75, 1981

17. Schumacher HR: Synovial fluid analysis. In Kelley WN et al (eds): Textbook of Rheumatology, W.B. Saunders, Philadelphia, 1985

18. Vanderbrouke JM, Jadoul M, Maldague B et al: Possible role of dialysis membrane characteristics in amyloid osteoarthropathy. Lancet 1210, 1986

19. Weiss JJ, Thompson GR, Daust N: Rotator cuff tears in rheumatoid arthritis. Arch Intern Med 135:521, 1975

20. Yunis M, Masi AT, Calabtro J et al: Primary fibromyalgia (fibiositis): clinical study of 50 patients with matched normal controls. Semin Arthritis Rheum 11:151, 1981

21. Zizic TM, Hungerford DS, Stevens MB: Ischaemic bone necrosis in SLE. Medicine 59:134, 1980

Total Shoulder Arthroplasty

15

Thomas S. Thornhill
William P. Barrett

HISTORY

The first total shoulder replacement (TSR) is credited to Pean[1] in 1893. He described replacing the proximal humerus in a young man with tuberculosis involving the glenohumeral joint and proximal humerus. In a two-stage procedure, Pean first resected the proximal humerus, which was replaced at a later date with a platinum shaft and hardened rubber ball (Fig. 15-1). The patient experienced pain relief and functional improvement following recovery from his surgery.

In 1955, Neer reported on the use of a metal hemiarthroplasty for articular replacement of the humeral head in 12 patients with acute or chronic fracture–dislocations of the humeral head.[21] The results showed generally good pain relief and functional improvement and served as the prototype for future humeral procedures. Encouraged by early results, he began using the hemiarthroplasty in patients with primary or secondary osteoarthritis of the glenohumeral joint. In 1974, he reported his results in a series of 47 patients.[22] Good or excellent outcomes were noted in 40 of the patients evaluated. One patient underwent resurfacing of the glenoid fossa in an attempt to decrease the occasional excessive excursion of the humeral head on the glenoid fossa. During the 1970s, several authors reported their experience with total shoulder replacements and the various designs ranging from the nonconstrained prosthesis exemplified by the Neer components to the constrained ball and socket design reported by Post.[27]

ANATOMY

The shoulder consists of four articulations: the glenohumeral joint, the acromioclavicular joint, the sternoclavicular joint, and the scapulothoracic articulation. Degenerative or inflammatory arthritis may affect any of the above joints and must be assessed when considering TSR. A detailed anatomical description of the shoulder girdle is beyond the scope of this chapter and is covered in detail in Chapter 1. A brief description of pertinent operative anatomy is reviewed.

The glenohumeral articulation is a minimally constrained joint that allows multiplane motion and has

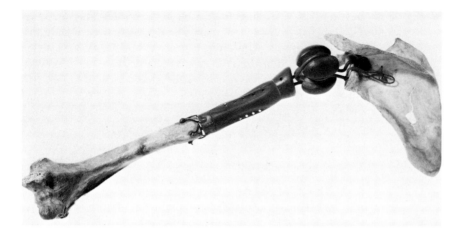

Fig. 15-1. Original prosthesis inserted by Pean in 1893. (Courtesy of the National Museum of American History, Smithsonian Institution.)

minimal static stability. The humeral head represents approximately one-third of an irregular sphere. It is inclined relative to the shaft at an angle of 130° to 150° and retroverted relative to the transcondylar axis of the distal humerus 30° to 40°. The average vertical dimension of the articular surface is 48 mm with the radius of curvature measuring 25 mm. The average transverse dimension is 45 mm with a 22-mm radius of curvature.[29] The glenoid fossa is the articular surface of the scapula, which is relatively flat in its anterior–posterior and superior–inferior dimensions. Its articular surface has a pear-shaped configuration approximately one-fourth the size of the humeral head. The average height is 35 mm and width is 25 mm at its widest portion inferiorly.[29] The glenoid fossa is inclined slightly posterior with respect to the scapular neck.[4,11] The glenoid fossa is functionally deepened by the glenoid labrum, a redundant fold of capsular tissue composed of dense fibrous connective tissue. The outer surface is continuous with the capsule and merges with the periosteum of the scapular neck; the inner surface is covered with synovium and merges with the articular cartilage. Superiorly, the labrum is continuous with the long head of the biceps tendon and serves as the origin of both the superior and inferior glenohumeral ligaments. The capsule of the glenohumeral joint is reinforced anteriorly by the superior, middle, and inferior glenohumeral ligaments. These anterior capsular thickenings provide a degree of static stability to resist anterior and inferior subluxation of the humeral head.

The rotator cuff muscles consisting of the subscapularis, the supraspinatus, infraspinatus, and teres minor serve at least three major functions: rotation of the humerus with respect to the glenoid; dynamic stabilization of the humeral head with respect to the glenoid fossa to resist deforming forces; and compression of the humeral head against the glenoid fossa to provide a secure scapulohumeral link for upper extremity function.[15,19] The subscapularis muscle provides anterior stability to the glenohumeral joint, particularly in the lower ranges of abduction and, along with the pectoralis major and latissimus dorsi muscles, internally rotates the humerus with respect to the glenoid. The infraspinatus and teres minor resist posterior subluxation of the humerus as well as provide at least 80 percent of the power for external rotation.[26] The supraspinatus, along with the tendon of the long head of the biceps, prevents superior instability of the glenohumeral joint. The supraspinatus in concert with the deltoid provides active abduction of the humerus. A functioning rotator cuff, or the ability to restore a functioning rotator cuff, is thus extremely important with respect to the ultimate function of a TSR.

The acromioclavicular joint is a small diarthrodial joint, formed by the articulation of the distal clavicle and acromion. The joint is surrounded by a rather weak capsule reinforced superiorly and inferiorly by the acromioclavicular ligaments. This articulation is further reinforced by the clavicular and acromial attachments of the trapezius and deltoid muscles. The coracoclavicular ligament, comprised of the lateral trapezoid and medial conoid divisions, serves to bind the scapula to the clavicle. This articulation allows gliding and shear-type movements between the distal clavicle and acromion. Rotation and angulation of the distal clavicle occur at the acromioclavicular joint both in abduction and forward flexion of the shoulder. Arthritic conditions involving the glenohumeral joint can involve the acromioclavicular joint and both should be assessed prior to TSR. If significant involvement of the acromioclavicular joint is noted, excision of the distal 2 cm of the clavicle, as described by Weaver and Dunn can be performed without compromising stability of the shoulder complex.[32]

BIOMECHANICS

Kinematics

As stated by Inman et al. in 1944, the motion at the shoulder is the sum of the movement contributed by the synchronous participation of the glenohumeral, sternoclavicular, acromioclavicular, and scapulothoracic joints. The various shoulder motions are defined as follows. Elevation is movement of the humerus away from the side in any plane and is generally measured in degrees from the vertical. Elevation can be subdivided into forward elevation (elevation in the sagittal plane), abduction (elevation in the coronal plane), and elevation in the "plane of the scapula." External and internal rotation refer to rotation of the humerus with respect to the glenoid fossa. Maximum elevation represents the sum of the individual motions at each of the above-mentioned joints.

Glenohumeral Joint

The glenohumeral joint, as previously discussed, sacrifices some stability for its multiplane, near-hemispheric range of motion. Elevation of the humerus to 120° is possible at the glenohumeral joint, at which point bony impingement restricts further elevation at this articulation. Analysis of surface joint motion at the glenohumeral joint for elevation in the plane of the scapula was carried out by Poppen and Walker.[25,26] The primary motion found between the humeral head and the glenoid was rotation. The instant centers of rotation were found to lie within 6.0 ± 2 mm of the center of the humeral head. Along with rotation, a small amount of translation, either superior or inferior, also occurred. From 0° to 30°, and often from 30° to 60°, the humeral head moved upward with respect to the glenoid fossa by approximately 3 mm. With each successive 30° of further elevation, the center of the head changed only 1.0 ± 0.5 mm, indicating almost pure rotation.

Scapulothoracic Articulation

The scapula is attached to the thorax via the acromioclavicular joint, sternoclavicular joint, and various musculotendinous units. Several motions are possible at this articulation, including protraction, retraction, and rotation about an axis perpendicular to its flat surface. Several investigators have evaluated the relationship between glenohumeral and scapulothoracic motion. Different planes of elevation have been utilized which may explain some of the discrepancy in the results. Most studies agree that within the first 0° to 30° of elevation, the glenohumeral to scapulothoracic motion is highly variable. It is also believed that elevation of the humerus to 180° results from glenohumeral motion contributing two-thirds and scapulothoracic motion contributing one-third of the total elevation. Inman estimated that of the 60° of scapular elevation, 20° takes place at the acromioclavicular joint and 40° at the scapulothoracic joint.[15] Inman concluded that the ratio of humeral to scapulothoracic motion was 2:1, as did Saha.[28] Poppen and Walker, evaluating elevation in the plane of the scapula, found a ratio of 1.25:1 for the range of elevation 24° to 120°.[25] However, for the range of motion from 0° to 120°, the ratio of glenohumeral to scapulothoracic motion was also 2:1.

Acromioclavicular and Sternoclavicular Joint

The acromioclavicular joint allows motion about a horizontal axis and, according to Inman, permits 20° of abduction which occurs during the first 30° and last 45° of abduction.[15] Three arcs of motion occur at the sternoclavicular joint: protraction and retraction, elevation and depression, and rotation. Inman stated that with elevation of the arm from 0° to 180°, 40 percent of the clavicular elevation occurred at the sternoclavicular joint.[15] This movement begins early and is nearly complete by 90° of elevation.

Kinetics

The primary motors for elevation and rotation of the humerus are the deltoid and rotator cuff. Contraction of the lateral fibers of the deltoid without the stabilizing effects of the rotator cuff will cause upward migration of the humerus along the axis of the deltoid, but will not produce elevation of the humerus. When the fulcrum of the glenohumeral joint is fixed by the capsule and functioning rotator cuff, contraction of the deltoid results in humeral elevation. The rotator cuff muscles, by virtue of their origins and insertions, act to rotate the humerus and resist displacement by compressing the humeral head into the glenoid.

Forces across the glenohumeral joint were calculated by Poppen and Walker.[26] They found that the resultant force for elevation of the humerus in the scapular plane leads to a maximum of approximately 90 percent of body weight at 90° of abduction. The direction of the resultant force changed from 0° to 150° of elevation, being inferior to the glenoid at 0°, superior to the glenoid from 30° to 60°, and directly into the center of the glenoid beyond 60°. This would imply that from 30° to 60° of elevation the humerus

without a functioning rotator cuff or superior stabilizers could subluxate superiorly.

PROSTHETIC DESIGN

The various commonly used prostheses can be classified, albeit artificially, into nonconstrained, semiconstrained, and constrained devices. A nonconstrained prosthesis replaces both the humeral and glenoid articular surfaces, with stability provided by its soft tissue envelope and functioning rotator cuff. The prototype for the nonconstrained prosthesis is the Neer II System (Fig. 15-2). The Neer humeral component has a radius of curvature similar to that of an intact humerus and is available in two thicknesses to allow proper tensing of the rotator cuff. Several stem lengths and thicknesses are available. The Neer glenoid component has a radius of curvature that matches the prosthetic head and has a keel for anchoring the component in the scapular neck. Gle-

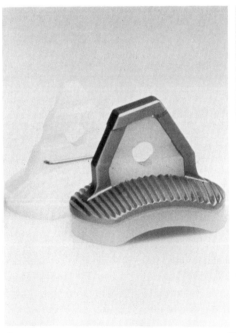
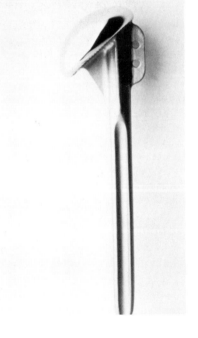

Fig. 15-2. (A) Polyethylene- and metal-backed glenoid components and **(B)** Neer II humeral component. (Courtesy of Orthopaedics Products Division, 3M.)

A   B

noid components are available in either a high-density polyethylene or a metal-backed high-density polyethylene design that is intended to decrease stresses at the bone–cement interface.

A semiconstrained prosthesis provides more stability at the glenohumeral articulation, most often in the form of a more constrained glenoid component. All currently available nonconstrained designs can become semiconstrained by substituting an alternative glenoid design with a superior hood or lip. This is intended to resist the superior subluxation of the humerus during abduction of the shoulder in the absence of a functioning rotator cuff. The benefits of increased constraint must be weighed against the risk of increased interface stresses when one is considering use of a semiconstrained prosthesis.

A constrained prosthesis provides a fixed articulation in the form of a linked ball and socket joint that allows rotation but prevents translation. The Michael Reese prosthesis is typical of such a device (Fig. 15-3). The humeral and glenoid components are joined by a locking ring that allows dislocation of the two components when a certain torque value is exceeded.

However, relocation of the two components requires an open reduction. The stability of a constrained prosthesis greatly increases the stress at the bone–cement interface. To help offset this increased stress on the glenoid side, the glenoid component is anchored to the scapula with a central peg and two screws.

Indications and Contraindications

Pain asosciated with radiographic loss of glenohumeral articular cartilage is the primary indication for TSR (Table 15-1). Pain is generally associated with decreased motion and function. In as much as shoulder function is critically dependent upon soft tissue integrity, shoulder reconstruction should be considered before extensive soft tissue contractures have developed. The loss of articular cartilage and subsequent glenohumeral incongruity has many causes. Osteoarthritis and rheumatoid arthritis are the respective prototypes of noninflammatory and inflammatory disease (Fig. 15-4). Other diagnoses include previous fracture or fracture–dislocation of the humeral head, rotator cuff tear arthropathy, arthritis of recurrent dislocation, inflammatory arthritides, and avascular necrosis of the humeral head if significant glenoid involvement is noted. Most often the above conditions affect both the humeral head and glenoid articular cartilage, necessitating resurfacing of both with a TSR. One notable exception is avascular necrosis, which can affect primarily the humeral head and leave the glenoid relatively intact. In such conditions, resurfacing of the humeral head alone has yielded satisfactory results.[20,24]

Contraindications to TSR include active or recently

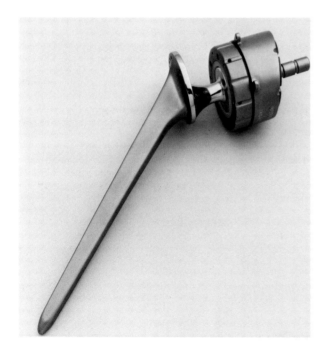

Fig. 15-3. Michael Reese constrained type prosthesis. (Courtesy of the Richards Medical Co.)

Table 15-1. Indications and Contraindications for Total Shoulder Arthroplasty

Indications
  Pain
  Radiographic destruction of glenohumeral joint
  Functional limitation
  Failure to respond to conservative measures
Contraindications
  Recent infection
  Charcot joint
  Inadequate bone stock
  Excessive physical demands
  Inadequate neuromuscular structures

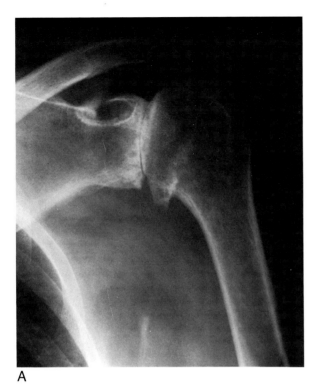

A

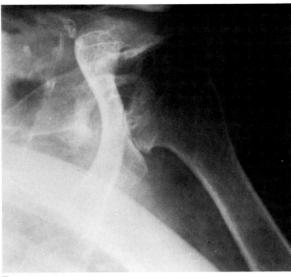

B

Fig. 15-4. (**A**) Osteoarthritic shoulder with periarticular osteophytes and preservation of bone stock. (**B**) Rheumatoid shoulder with loss of subchondral bone from the humeral head.

active infection involving the glenohumeral or contiguous joints, a Charcot joint, and paralysis of the upper extremity musculature involving both the deltoid and rotator cuff musculature (Table 15-1). Paralysis of the deltoid or rotator cuff musculature alone, or a partial paralysis of both, is not an absolute contraindication.[24] A relative contraindication to TSR is inadequate glenoid bone stock, which is sometimes noted in rheumatoid arthritis and would necessitate a hemiarthroplasty.

Specific indications for the various prosthetic designs of TSR are dictated by the integrity of the rotator cuff. The incidence of rotator cuff pathology varies with the underlying diagnosis. In patients with osteoarthritis, Neer et al.[24] reported a 5 percent incidence of full thickness rotator cuff tear, while Cofield[7] reported a 19 percent incidence of full thickness rotator cuff tear. In rheumatoid patients, Neer et al. reported complete thickness tears in 42 percent, most of which were small and readily repaired. Cofield reported a 24 percent incidence of complete tears. Both authors noted that thinning of the rotator cuff is characteristic of moderate or severe rheumatoid arthritis.

Most authors would agree that a nonconstrained resurfacing-type TSR is indicated with an intact rotator cuff or one that can be repaired.[1,3,7,24,30] If the rotator cuff tear is so extensive that a nonfunctional repair is attained, some authors would argue that a semiconstrained system, which in theory provides the stability lost by the nonfunctioning cuff, is indicated.[12,13,16,18] As Post stated, TSR using a constrained prosthesis should be regarded as a salvage operation, used in carefully selected patients[27] (Fig. 15-5).

Surgical Technique

The patient must be positioned to allow access to both the glenoid and humeral surfaces. Moreover, the patient's head must be stabilized and the endotracheal tube protected. A semireclined or "beach chair" position, with the table in moderate Trendelenburg and the foot comfortably flexed, is utilized (Fig. 15-6). The patient is moved to the side of the operative table so that the shoulder can easily be extended for insertion of the humeral component. A towel roll is

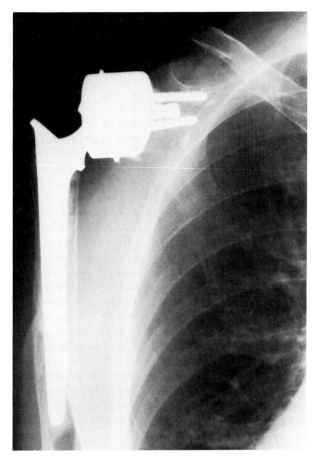

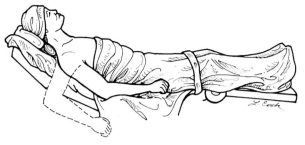

Fig. 15-6. "Beach chair" position for TSR. Patient must be towards the edge of the table to allow flexion/extension of shoulder.

its insertion upon the clavicle. This is important to facilitate retraction of the deltoid and will generally obviate the need for removing its clavicular attachment. It should be noted that the axillary nerve runs anteriorly at the level of the lower border of the subscapularis and all deltoid retraction must be proximal to that level to avoid injury to the nerve. A cobra retractor placed proximally under the deltoid and over the greater tuberosity may be helpful for retraction (Fig. 15-9), but it is advisable to relax this retrac-

Fig. 15-5. Patient treated with constrained prosthesis after previous acromionectomy and severe soft tissue damage.

placed behind the medial border of the scapula to improve access for glenoid component insertion. Care must be taken to avoid the tendency to limit the surgical field during draping. A sterilely covered Mayo stand can provide support for the arm during the procedure.

The skin incision is based just lateral to the coracoid and extends proximally to the clavicle and distally just lateral to the anterior axillary fold (Fig. 15-7). This allows access to the acromioclavicular joint, the anterior acromion, and distally to release the superior portion of the pectoralis tendon if necessary. The incision can be extended distally if a portion of the deltoid insertion must be released. The key to the deltopectoral interval is the cephalic vein (Fig. 15-8); it may be sacrificed or retracted during the procedure. The anterior edge of the deltoid is exposed proximally to

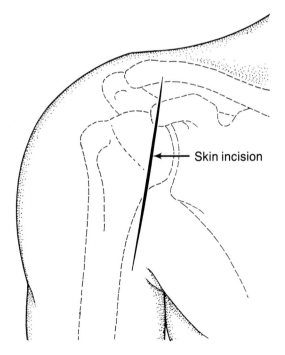

Fig. 15-7. Skin incision for TSR with bony landmarks outlined.

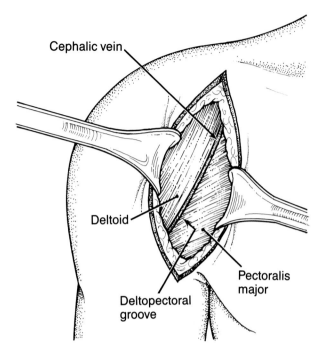

Fig. 15-8. Deltopectoral interval identified by location of the cephalic vein.

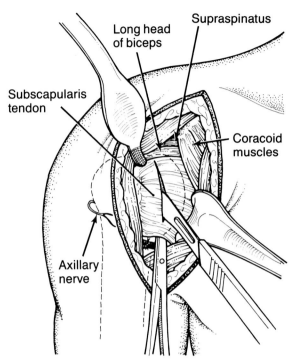

Fig. 15-9. Division of the subscapularis tendon; note clamp in the interval between subscapularis and capsule. Circumflex vessels have been ligated inferiorly, biceps tendon protected superiorly. Note axillary nerve at the level of the subscapularis tendon.

tion several times during surgery to prevent inadvertent nerve injury. The clavipectoral fascia is now identified and divided at the lateral edge of the conjoined tendon, from the vessels of the circumflex humeral system marking the lower border of the subscapularis distally to the coracoacromial ligament proximally.

In rheumatoid patients, the coracoacromial ligament is preserved because it provides a restraint to superior subluxation of the humeral head. In osteoarthritic patients with chronic impingement and/or AC joint arthritis, it may be necessary to divide the coracoacromial ligament as part of an acromioplasty. The conjoined tendon can frequently be retracted medially to expose the anterior edge of the glenoid. The coracoid process may be predrilled and osteotomized or the lateral fibers of the tendon divided to improved access.

The arm is now placed on the padded Mayo stand in a position of slight elevation, abduction, and external rotation. The three vessels from the humeral circumflex system marking the lower border of the subscapularis are identified and ligated. A Kelly clamp

is used to dissect bluntly the interval between the subscapularis tendon and the capsule, at an interval 1 to 2 cm medial to the tendinous insertion on the lesser tuberosity (Fig. 15-9). The superior border of the subscapular is identified by the long head of the biceps tendon crossing to its insertion on the glenoid. Care should be taken to avoid dividing this structure, it is a superior constraint to proximal migration of the humeral head. Before dividing the subscapularis, the corners of the tendon are tagged to allow anatomical restoration of the tendinous unit (leave the medial tags approximately 5 cm long as the subscapularis tendon may retract medially and be difficult to identify during closure). In patients with an internal rotation contracture, the subscapularis tendon can be lengthened by freeing it from the capsule or even performing a Z-plasty (Fig. 15-10). The underlying capsule, particularly in the rheumatoid patient, may be thin and impossible to identify as a separate struc-

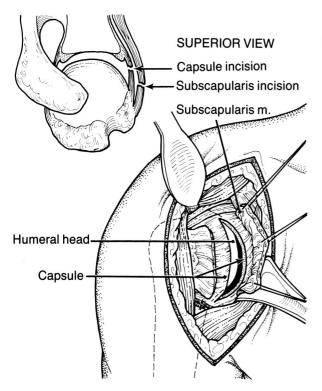

SUPERIOR VIEW

Capsule incision

Subscapularis incision

Subscapularis m.

Humeral head

Capsule

Fig. 15-10. Division of capsule and technique of "Z"-lengthening if necessary.

ture. In this case, the capsule and subscapularis tendon are treated as a single unit.

The arm is now extended and externally rotated to dislocate the humeral head anteriorly. It is frequently necessary at this point to release the inferior capsule and capsular adhesions from the inferior neck of the humerus to facilitate dislocation of the head. A trial humeral component is placed beside the humeral head to determine the level of humeral resection (Fig. 15-11). Care is taken to avoid excessive humeral resection, which could lead to postoperative instability. The humerus is resected so that the humeral component will be placed in approximately 40° of retroversion. The final preferred retroversion will vary from 30° to 45°, depending upon the position of the prosthetic glenoid and will be determined just prior to humeral component insertion.

A humeral head retractor is now placed behind the posterior rim of the glenoid, retracting the humeral shaft laterally and posteriorly (Fig. 15-12). A second retractor is placed over the anterior edge of

the glenoid onto the glenoid neck to retract the conjoined tendon medially. At this point a decision is made concerning glenoid resurfacing, based upon cartilage destruction, patient diagnosis, extent of synovitis, and glenoid bone stock. The initial step in glenoid insertion is to identify the glenoid vault without jeopardizing the subchondral bone. The axis of the glenoid keel can be determined by the longest diameter of the anatomical glenoid (Fig. 15-12). A finger placed upon the glenoid neck anteriorly can help determine the center of the glenoid vault. Glenoid osteophytes and/or bony erosions can distort these anatomical relationships, leading to improper orientation of the component. The vault is entered with a navicular gouge or small curette and then elongated and deepened using a curette or high-speed drill (Fig. 15-13). Care is taken to preserve subchondral bone anteriorly and posteriorly for proper seating of the glenoid. Use a metal-backed glenoid component, as this will distribute the forces more evenly and, at least theoretically, decrease the incidence of loosening. Before cementing, the trial glenoid should be well-seated against

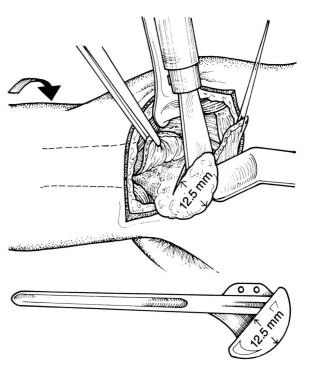

Fig. 15-11. Removal of portion of humeral head that corresponds to the prosthesis.

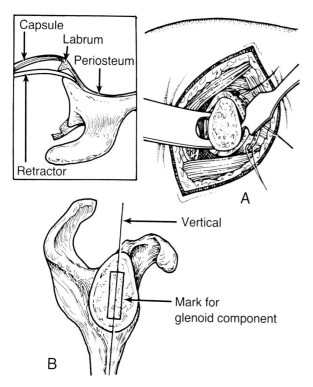

Fig. 15-12. Glenoid exposure with placement of ring retractor posteriorly (**A**) and Homan retractor anteriorly (inset). (**B**) Orientation for placement of glenoid component keel.

the subchondral bone both anteriorly and posteriorly. The glenoid vault is then packed with thrombin-soaked Gelfoam, treated with pulsatile lavage, and thoroughly dried before insertion of methylmethacrylate.

At this point, the shoulder is extended and externally rotated to facilitate insertion of the humeral component. The canal is sounded and then prepared with appropriate reamers (Fig. 15-14). A thin-stem trial component is inserted to determine proper humeral head thickness and humeral retroversion. The shoulder is reduced and carried through a range of motion to examine the congruity between the humeral and glenoid components. Humeral retroversion can be adjusted at this point. Based upon the preoperative radiographic evaluation of the humeral intramedullary shaft, the proper humeral stem size is now determined and the humeral component is inserted in the predetermined amount of retroversion. In cases of poor bone stock or the inability to attain a solid press-

fit application, the humeral component is cemented. Excessive bone is now trimmed from the humeral neck to prevent impingement (Fig. 15-15). The shoulder is reduced and again carried through a range of motion (Fig. 15-16).

The subscapularis tendon is replaced using nonabsorbable sutures. The rotator cuff is carefully examined and then the subacromial adhesions released and mechanical integrity restored. Frequently, small tears anteriorly can be sutured primarily but larger lesions may require proximal advancement of the subscapularis or anterior displacement of the infraspinatus. Small Hemovac drains are placed in the wound and the subcutaneous tissue and skin are closed in a standard fashion.

Postoperative Rehabilitation

A supervised rehabilitation program is critical to the success of TSR. The surgeon must take an active role during this rehabilitation process. Moreover, the operative range of motion must be carefully documented to guide the therapist in limiting the postoperative arc. The guidelines listed in Table 15-2 are adjusted for the individual patient.

The patient is placed in a sling and swathe and kept supine with a pillow behind the ipsilateral elbow until the first postoperative day. At that point, the patient is generally more comfortable in a seated position or ambulating.

Pendulum exercises and supine active assisted forward elevation are begun on the first postoperative day. Active assisted external rotation is limited by the intraoperative range determined after closure of the subscapularis tendon. The patient is gradually taught to do active assisted exercises using the opposite hand, first in the supine position and then against gravity. If the anterior deltoid has not been removed, active exercises both supine and against gravity are begun within the first postoperative week.

The patient is generally discharged on the fifth to seventh postoperative day and all patients have a supervised rehabilitation program to be followed at home. Isometric exercises are begun at 4 to 6 weeks postoperatively. The specific active assisted, active, and isometric exercises are similar to those outlined in published reports.[14]

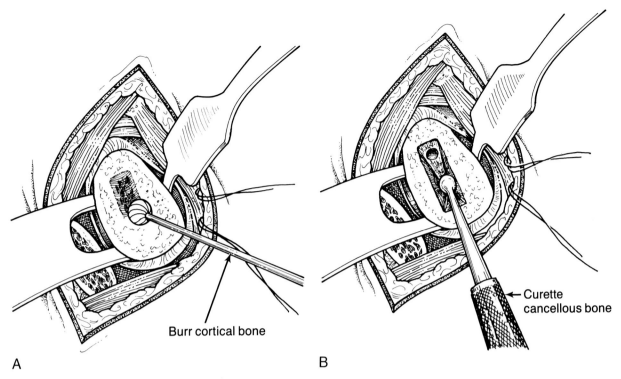

Burr cortical bone

Curette
cancellous bone

A   B

Fig. 15-13. (**A**) Preparation of glenoid component keel hole initially using a burr for the subchondral bone. (**B**) Keel hole is deepened with curettes; remaining subchondral bone preserved.

Drill enters just medial to greater tuberosity

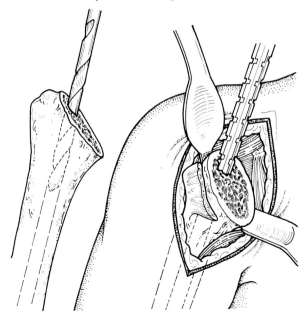

Fig. 15-14. Preparation for humeral shaft with small drill and then humeral reamers.

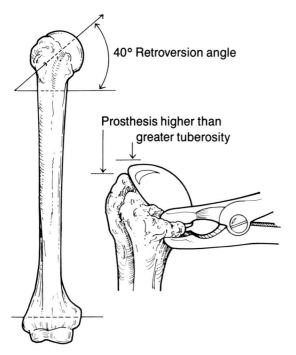

Fig. 15-15. Orientation of humeral head in 40° of retroversion with regard to transcondylar axis of elbow and appropriate head–tuberosity height. Osteophytes are trimmed as necessary.

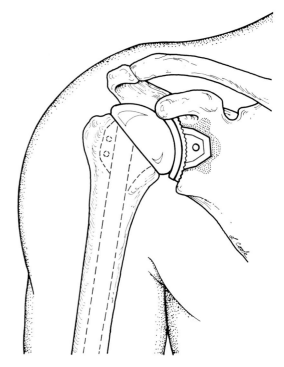

Fig. 15-16. Completed TSR with cemented metal back glenoid component and press-fit humeral component.

Table 15-2. Postoperative Shoulder Rehabilitation

Postop Period	Exercises	Function
Day 1	Pendulum exercises	Sling and swathe × 24 hours after surgery. Ambulate with assistance
Day 2–7	Initiate supine active assisted elevation, external rotation[a] and internal rotation. Progress to sitting exercises. Initiate shoulder pulley exercises. Initiate active exercises as appropriate[b]	Remove sling for exercises and during the day as tolerated. Activity of daily living training by O.T. Sling at night when sleeping. Discharge from hospital.
Day 8–week 6	Continue above. Strengthening exercises for anterior deltoid, external and internal rotators[c]	Sling may be discontinued once patient is comfortable. Continue work on activities of daily living
Week 7	Incorporate ROM and strengthening exercises as a "way of life"	

[a] Amount of external rotation is determined by integrity of subscapularis repair.
[b] Active forward elevation and external rotation withheld for 6 weeks in patients with rotator cuff repair.
[c] Internal rotator strengthening initiated at 6 weeks.

Postoperative Evaluation

Evaluation of results and comparison between various series are greatly simplified if a standardized evaluation form is utilized. The American Shoulder and Elbow Surgeons have proposed a system that evaluates shoulder pain, range of motion, function of the shoulder, and the patient's response with regard to the outcome of surgery. The authors strongly recommend the use of this system when evaluating and reporting results of TSR (see Fig. 20-4).

Results

To date, several studies have been published that detail results of TSR. However, comparison of these studies is limited by the lack of a uniform method of reporting. Comparison of certain variables such as pain relief and improvement in range of motion can be made.

Nonconstrained and Semiconstrained Systems

Neer et al. reported on 192 TSRs evaluated for a minimum of 2 years.[24] The preoperative diagnoses in this group of patients included osteoarthritis, rheumatoid arthritis, history of previous trauma, arthritis of recurrent dislocation, and cuff tear arthropathy. Results were graded excellent if the patient was enthusiastic about the operation, had no significant pain, full use of the shoulder, near normal muscle strength, active elevation of the arm to within 35° of the normal side, and rotation within 90 percent of that of the normal side. Satisfactory results were given to shoulders that had no more than occasional pain or aching with changes in weather, good use of the shoulder for full daily function from the top of the head down, a minimum of 30 percent of normal muscle strength, 90 to 135° of elevation and rotation to 50 percent of that on the normal side. In an unsatisfactory result, none of the above criteria were met. In the patients with osteoarthritis, 90 percent of the results were excellent, 7.5 percent satisfactory, and one patient was placed in a limited goals rehabilitation program. The limited goals classification included patients with massive rotator cuff tears, loss of bone stock, and extensive soft tissue contractures. The average increase in elevation was 77° and in external rotation 50°. Pa-

tients with rheumatoid arthritis had 65 percent excellent results; 28 percent satisfactory, and 7 percent unsatisfactory. The average increase in forward elevation was 57° and in external rotation 60°. In patients with a history of previous trauma, excellent results were obtained in 46 percent of patients, satisfactory in 20 percent, and unsatisfactory in 34 percent of patients. The average increase in forward elevation was 33° and in external rotation 58°. Patients with arthritis of recurrent dislocation had 75 percent excellent results, 17 percent satisfactory, and 8 percent unsatisfactory results. The average increase in forward elevation was 51° and in external rotation 66°.

Thornhill et al. reported the Brigham experience with total shoulder arthroplasty using the Neer I and Neer II systems.[30] They presented the results of 150 TSRs performed in 136 patients. The primary diagnosis was rheumatoid arthritis in 105 patients, osteoarthritis in 27, osteonecrosis in 2, ankylosing spondylitis in 1, and juvenile rheumatoid arthritis in 1 patient. Eighteen percent of the shoulders were noted to have major rotator cuff tears, 41 percent had minor rotator cuff tears and 41 percent had intact rotator cuffs. The minimum follow-up was 12 months, with an average follow-up of 31 months. Significant pain relief was obtained in 91 percent of the patients following TSR. Active elevation in the patients with rheumatoid arthritis averaged 56° prior to surgery and 88° following TSR. In the osteoarthritic patients, active elevation averaged 53° preoperatively and 109° following TSR. The patient response following TSR revealed that 61 percent of the patients felt much better, 32 percent felt better, 3 percent were unchanged, and 3 percent were worse following TSR.

Cofield reported a series of 65 patients who underwent 73 Neer TSRs at the Mayo Clinic with a minimum radiographic follow-up of 2 years.[7] This group included 29 patients with a diagnosis of osteoarthritis, 24 with rheumatoid arthritis, and 12 with a history of previous trauma. In association with TSR, an anterior acromioplasty was performed in 38 patients and a distal clavicle excision in 23 patients. Significant pain relief was obtained in 92 percent of the patients at follow-up. The range of motion in active abduction increased from an average of 76° preoperatively to 120 degrees postoperatively. The postoperative range of motion was thought to be directly related to the integrity and function of the rotator cuff. Those patients who had a normal rotator cuff had active abduction that averaged 143° following surgery. Functional improvement was noted in many of the patients following surgery. For example, 27 patients were unable to comb their hair prior to surgery, whereas 55 were able to do so after surgery. Sixty-seven of the 73 shoulders (90 percent) were considered to be better or much better, 4 shoulders were unchanged, and two were worse following surgery.

Barrett et al. reported on 50 TSRs performed in 44 patients at the University of Washington.[3] The average follow-up was 3.5 years. The diagnoses were osteoarthritis in 33 shoulders, rheumatoid arthritis in 11, and previous trauma in 6 shoulders. Nine patients were noted to have rotator cuff tears, five described as massive (greater than 5 cm in diameter). Significant pain relief was obtained in 94 percent of the patients following TSR. The range of motion in active forward elevation in the patients with osteoarthritis improved from an average of 73° preoperatively to 117° following TSR. In patients with rheumatoid arthritis, the average preoperative elevation was 66° and 100° following TSR. In the group with previous trauma, the average preoperative forward elevation was 67° and this improved to 79° following TSR. Functional improvement in five activities of daily living was analyzed. Fourteen percent of the patients were able to perform these various activities prior to surgery and following TSR 78 percent of the patients were able to perform them. Ninety-two percent of the patients considered that their shoulder was either better or much better following TSR, 8 percent felt their shoulder was the same, none felt it was worse.

Wilde et al.[33] reported on 38 patients who underwent 44 TSRs. The diagnoses were rheumatoid arthritis in 20 shoulders, osteoarthritis in 12, previous trauma in 7, fracture in 2, juvenile rheumatoid arthritis, avascular necrosis, and failed TSR in 1 shoulder each. The average follow-up in this group was 36 months. Significant pain relief was obtained in 92 percent of the patients following TSR. Active elevation of the arm improved in 89 percent of the patients following TSR; the average improvement was 68° External rotation improved in 84 percent of the patients, an average of 40°.

Bade et al. reported the results of total shoulder arthroplasty performed at the Hospital for Special Surgery.[2] Their series included 24 patients who underwent 27 TSRs. Diagnoses were rheumatoid arthritis in 13 patients, osteoarthritis in 3, previous trauma in 3, and avascular necrosis in 5 patients. Significant pain relief was obtained in the majority of patients, with 66 percent of the patients having no pain following surgery and mild pain was present in 33 percent following TSR. Range of motion in active forward flexion improved from an average of 68° prior to surgery to 118° following TSR. Results were based on a 100 point rating system that included evaluation of pain, range of motion, function, and strength. Using this evaluating system, 78 percent of their patients had excellent or good results following TSR.

Clayton et al. reported on 22 shoulders that underwent 3 different types of arthroplasty.[6] Seven shoulders had proximal humeral arthroplasty alone; seven had proximal humeral arthroplasty with a polyethylene subacromial spacer; and eight had a Neer TSR with conventional glenoid component. In this series, 19 had mild or no postoperative pain, 2 had moderate, and 1 had severe postoperative pain. In the TSR group, active forward elevation improved on an average from 73° to 80° in patients with osteoarthritis and 59° to 94° in those with rheumatoid arthritis. External rotation improved from 13° to 70° in patients with osteoarthritis and from 34° to 46° in patients with rheumatoid arthritis. Overall function was rated on a scale from 1 to 100 points, with 100 points being normal function. For the patients with TSR, postoperative functional improvement increased 50 points in patients with osteoarthritis and 41 points in patients with rheumatoid arthritis.

Amstutz et al. reported on their results with the UCLA anatomical total shoulder prosthesis following up 11 patients for an average of 26 months.[1] Diagnoses in this group included osteoarthritis in five patients, rheumatoid arthritis in two, previous trauma in three, and avascular necrosis in one patient. Excellent pain relief was noted in 9 of 11 patients. The average improvement in active forward elevation was 40° and the average improvement for the arc of internal and external rotation was 43°. Functional improvement was noted in 10 of 11 patients.

Cruess gave a preliminary report of 26 Neer-type TSRs with a follow-up of from 6 months to 5 years.[10] Patients in this study had either rheumatoid arthritis or osteoarthritis. Significant pain relief was noted following TSR and the range of motion was satisfactory in all but two patients.

Brumfield et al. reported on 18 patients who underwent 21 TSRs using the Neer II prosthesis.[5] Fifteen patients had rheumatoid arthritis and three patients had osteoarthritis. Significant pain was noted postoperatively. Forward elevation increased from 78° preoperatively to 106° following surgery. External rotation improved from an average of 29° prior to surgery to 45° following TSR.

In a summary of the data for pain relief following TSR from the five largest series using the Neer unconstrained prosthesis, 93 percent of the patients reported significant relief of pain following this procedure (see Fig. 15-17A). In reviewing the results of patients with a diagnosis of rheumatoid arthritis and osteoarthritis with regard to shoulder elevation following TSR, it was noted overall that there was a 50° improvement in shoulder elevation. In those series differentiating postoperative shoulder elevation by diagnosis, it was noted that patients with rheumatoid arthritis had, on an average, a 45° improvement in elevation and patients with a diagnosis of osteoarthritis had a 50° improvement in shoulder elevation following TSR (see Fig. 15-17B).

Several authors have reported their results utilizing a semiconstrained total shoulder prosthesis. Lettin et al. reported their results using the Stanmore total shoulder replacement.[16] Fifty TSRs were performed; 40 patients were presented in the follow-up data. Nine patients underwent excisional arthroplasty, eight for a failed TSR and one for infection; one patient died 1 week postoperatively. Of the 40 patients evaluated, 31 had minimal or no pain following surgery. Six of the 40 had pain with activity and 3 had significant pain following surgery. The average increase in forward elevation was 20°; from 55 to 75°; and 45° in external rotation. Twenty-one of the 40 patients returned to work and 32 of 36 patients questioned felt they were better after the surgery.

Coughlin et al. reported on 15 patients who underwent 16 TSRs that used the semiconstrained Stanmore prosthesis with a minimum 2-year follow-up.[9] The authors noted that 50 percent of the patients had complete relief of pain following surgery. Active forward elevation increased an average of 33°, from 60° to 93° following surgery. The combined arc of external and internal rotation increased from an average of 52° preoperatively to 112° following surgery. Overall, patients were very satisfied with the outcome of their surgery.

Gristina et al. reported their results on 85 TSRs, utilizing the monospherical prosthesis with a follow-up ranging from three to 52 months.[13] The authors noted almost complete relief of pain and a doubling of the preoperative motion in their short-term follow-up.

Faludi and Weiland reported on 12 patients who underwent 13 English-McNab cementless semiconstrained TSRs.[12] Follow-up ranged from 27 to 62 months. Pain relief was achieved in most patients. Active abduction improved from 36° preoperatively to 75° following surgery. External rotation improved from 10° prior to surgery to 25° postoperatively. Function was rated on a scale of 1 to 10 with 10 being normal activities. Overall function improved from 1.8 preoperatively to 5.6 following surgery.

Constrained

Post et al. have presented the largest series of constrained TSRs.[27] They reported on 43 TSRs performed in patients with functionally inadequate rotator cuffs. Prerequisites for their prosthesis included intact glenoid rim and scapular neck, a strong serratus anterior and trapezius muscles to stabilize the scapula, and a strong deltoid muscle. Twenty-two of the 43 TSRs were Series I, which were made of 316 L stainless steel. Twenty-one procedures utilized the Series II, which were made of cobalt-chrome with a larger neck. Pain was measured on a 75-point scale, of the 28 patients who required no postoperative revision of their prosthesis, 21 had excellent pain relief, 4 good, 2 fair, and 1 poor following surgery. Functional improvement in the group not undergoing revision revealed a 60 to 83 percent improvement in overall function when compared to preoperative status.

Radiographic Evaluation

Radiographic evaluation of the TSR should be made preoperatively and in the immediate postoperative period. Follow-up radiographs at 3 to 6 months and then on a yearly basis are usually obtained. Three views of the shoulder are recommended: a 40° posterior-oblique radiograph with internal and external rotation of the humerus and an axillary view (Fig. 15-17). These projections allow good visualization of the glenoid prosthesis–cement–bone interface, as well as the humeral component–cement–bone interface. Radiographs are examined for component position, migration, subsidence, loosening, and radiolucent lines.

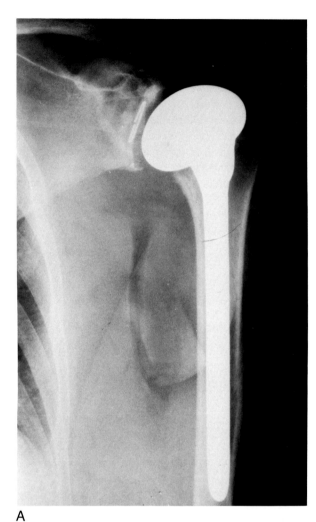

A

In the series reported by Neer et al., 194 shoulders were followed radiographically for an average of 37 months and 30 percent of the glenoids exhibited lucent lines.[24] Ninety-four were present in the early postoperative period and none were progressive. One hundred forty-four humeral components were cemented and 50 were press-fit. One cemented humerus had a lucent line of 4 mm and one press-fit prosthesis had a lucent line of 3 mm. None of the shoulders have been revised for loosening or mechanical failure.

Thornhill et al. reported an 88 percent incidence of radiolucency about the glenoid component.[30] There were complete radiolucent lines about the glenoid component in 32 percent of the shoulders evaluated. Six percent had glenoid lucent lines greater than 2 mm and were considered to be radiographically loose (Fig. 15-18). One-third of the humeral components in the series were cemented and two-thirds utilized a press-fit. There was no evidence of radiographic loosening about the cemented humeral components. In the press-fit group, six humeral stems showed incomplete radiolucencies and six other stems showed some evidence of humeral subsidence (Fig. 15-19). None of these shoulders were symptomatic and further progression of the findings was not noted.

Cofield reported radiographic evidence of loosening of the glenoid component in 8 of 73 total shoulder arthroplasties evaluated.[7] Seven of these patients had a diagnosis of osteoarthritis and one rheumatoid arthritis. All seven patients with osteoarthritis showed

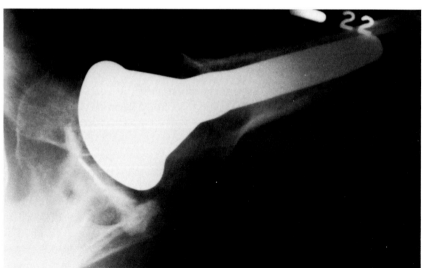

B

Fig. 15-17. (A) An AP Radiograph in the plane of the glenohumeral joint (40° posterior oblique view). (B) Axillary lateral view following TSR.

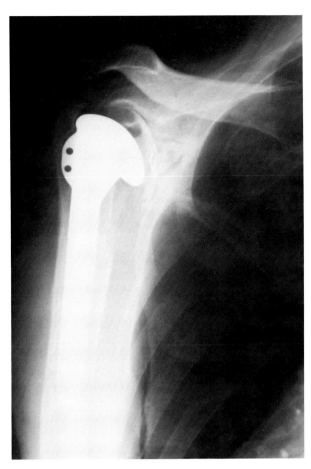

Fig. 15-18. Example of a complete glenoid lucent line, greater than 2 mm in a radiographically loose glenoid component.

a shift in the position of the glenoid component on the scapula. The lucent lines appeared postoperatively and progressed to 1 mm in thickness with none exceeding 1.5 mm in thickness. Three of these patients had been revised at the time of his report and a fourth was under consideration for revision. Of the remaining 65 shoulders, 20 percent had no lucent lines at the glenoid bone–cement interface while 80 percent had lucent lines about the glenoid prosthesis. None of these prostheses showed radiographic evidence of loosening. Seven of the 73 humeral components were cemented and one of these had a 1.5 mm lucent line. None of the humeral components showed radiographic evidence of loosening.

Barrett et al. reported a 74 percent incidence of radiolucent lines about the glenoid component; 38 percent were under the flange and 35 percent about the keel of the prosthesis.[3] Ten percent of the lucent lines were greater than 2.0 mm and three of these four have been revised because of symptomatic loosening. Thirty-five of the 50 humeral components were cemented. There was an 8 percent incidence of incomplete lucent lines about the humeral component, none of these greater than 1 mm.

Wilde et al. reported radiolucent lines about three areas of the glenoid component.[33] Area one, which was around the superior and inferior flange of the glenoid prosthesis, had an 89 percent incidence of radiolucent lines and an average thickness of 1.4 mm. Area two, about the base of the keel of the prosthesis, had a 75 percent incidence of radiolucent lines, 1.1 mm in thickness, and area three, about the tip of the keel, had a 67 percent incidence of radiolucent lines, 1.1 mm in thickness. They noted one loose glenoid component in their series. Press-fit fixation was utilized in 35 of the humeral components, while 9 components were cemented. In the press-fit group, sclerosis developed about the tip of the prosthesis in 44 percent of the patients and sclerosis around the entire stem was noted in 8 percent of patients.

Bade et al. noted a 67 percent incidence of lucent lines about the glenoid component and again most were noted in the early postoperative period and thought to be nonprogressive.[2] One glenoid component had radiolucent lines around the entire prosthesis greater than 2 mm and was thought to be radiographically loose. All but one of the humeral components in their series were cemented. Radiolucent lines were noted about the humeral component in 26 percent of the cases, and in two of these patients the radiolucent lines were greater than 2 mm and considered to be radiographically loose.

Amstutz et al. divided the prosthesis–cement–bone interface into five sections about the glenoid component and noted that 10 of 11 components showed radiolucency in one or more of the five zones.[1] Two of the 11 patients demonstrated progressive widening of the radiolucent zones and concomitant sclerotic bone reaction during the first year following arthroplasty. However, follow-up 2 and 3 years later showed no change in the radiolucent zones and the patients are asymptomatic. There was no evidence of radiographic loosening in any of the 11 humeral components.

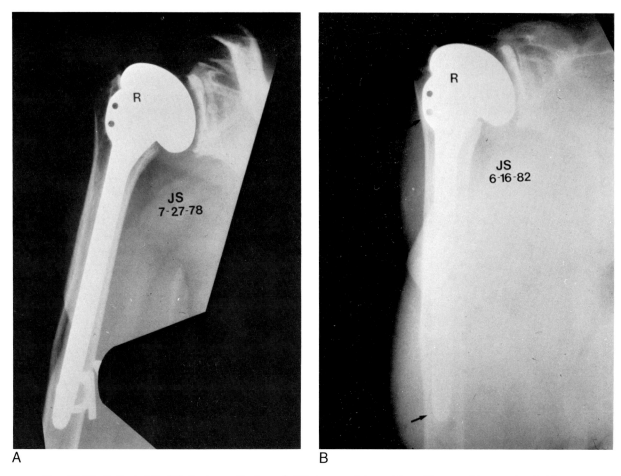

Fig. 15-19. Patient J.S. (**A**) Postoperatively and (**B**) 4 years later with evidence of humeral subsidence (arrows).

Review of the data on glenoid lucent lines as well as loosening of the glenoid component for the unconstrained Neer-type prosthesis reveals a wide range of results. With follow-up ranging from 3 to 4½ years, lucent lines were present at follow-up in between 30 and 89 percent of the glenoids examined (Table 15-3). Radiographic evidence of loosening was present anywhere from 0 to 11 percent at follow-up examina-

Table 15-3. Radiographic Evaluation of Cemented Neer Glenoid Components

	Average Follow-up (yrs)	Shoulders with Glenoid Lucent Lines (%)	Radiographically Loose Glenoid Components (%)
Neer et al.[24]	3.1	30	0
Thornhill et al.[31]	3.6	88	6
Cofield[7]	3.8	82	11
Barrett et al.[3]	3.5	74	10
Wilde et al.[33]	3.0	89	2
Bade et al.[2]	4.5	67	4

tion. The incidence of humeral lucent lines has been significantly lower as seen from the above data. From a radiographic point of view, there has not been an increased incidence of loosening in the cemented versus uncemented groups of components. Thornhill et al. reported six cases of subsidence of the humeral component; however, these were not clinically symptomatic.[30]

The incidence of radiographic and clinical loosening in the semiconstrained series has been higher as would be expected with a more constrained prosthesis. Lettin et al. reported no loosening about the humeral component; however, 10 of 49 patients (16 percent) evaluated had loosening of the glenoid component.[16] In eight of these patients, the glenoid was replaced; however, six of the eight revisions subsequently became loose and required excisional arthroplasty.

Gristina et al., in their short-term follow-up of 85 monospherical TSRs, reported revision for glenoid loosening in 2 cases and revision for loosening of the humeral component in 1 case.[14] Faludi and Weiland reported radiographic follow-up on eight shoulders in which the uncemented English-McNab prosthesis was used.[12] They noted no evidence of humeral or glenoid component loosening.

Post, reporting on the constrained Michael Reese prosthesis, noted a 33 percent incidence of radiolucent lines about the humeral component; one of these patients had progressive widening of the radiolucent zone and obvious loosening by radiographic criteria.[27] There was a 9 percent incidence of radiolucent zones surrounding the glenoid components, with no evidence of radiographic loosening in these reported cases.

Complications

Complications following TSR can be classified into early complications that include errors in surgical technique, violation of important neurovascular structures, humeral or glenoid fracture, malposition of either component, poor soft tissue repair leading to subsequent instability and/or weakness, and perioperative infection. Late complications include infection usually by hematogenous spread, either persistent or recently acquired instability (Fig. 15-20), either atraumatic or traumatic failure of the rotator cuff re-

pair, fracture of the surrounding bone stock (Fig. 15-21), and mechanical failure of the implant. Component loosening is discussed above under the heading of Radiographic Evaluation.

Neer reported 24 complications in the 194 TSRs (12 percent) evaluated.[24] One patient had a postoperative wound infection necessitating removal of the prosthesis. One patient fell from a ladder sustaining a humeral fracture and subsequent rotation of the humeral component in the shaft, causing posterior dislocation. This necessitated revision of the prosthesis. Four patients (2 percent) dislocated the prosthesis, two anteriorly and two posteriorly. All were reduced, closed and immobilized 3 to 6 weeks prior to initiation of physical therapy. Five patients (2.5 percent) sustained rotator cuff tears postoperatively; surgical repair was carried out on two of these patients. There were no cases of mechanical failure of either the humeral or glenoid component reported in his series.

Thornhill et al. reported fracture of the greater tuberosity in three patients, and posterior dislocation of the humeral component in three patients of which two required revision.[30] One patient developed an axillary nerve palsy that resolved. Two shoulders in one patient became septic as a terminal event.

Cofield reported 14 complications in 73 procedures (19 percent).[7] Among these was an intraoperative laceration of the axillary nerve in a multiply operated shoulder. One patient had a large hematoma that required evacuation and one patient had a nonfatal pulmonary embolus. Five patients (7 percent) had recurrent rotator cuff tears. One patient who felt he was worse than prior to surgery was considering further surgery; however, the remaining four, though their function was somewhat limited, had no significant pain and no further surgery was planned. There were no cases of mechanical failure of the components.

Barrett et al. reported a 17 percent incidence of complications following TSR.[3] Intraoperatively, one patient sustained a humeral shaft fracture, one patient a greater tuberosity fracture, and one patient developed an anterior deltoid palsy that did not resolve postoperatively. In the postoperative period, one patient developed posterior subluxation of the humeral head that resolved with rotator cuff strengthening exercises. One patient had persistent impingement syndrome from a high-riding greater tuberosity, one patient sustained a rotator cuff tear in an altercation,

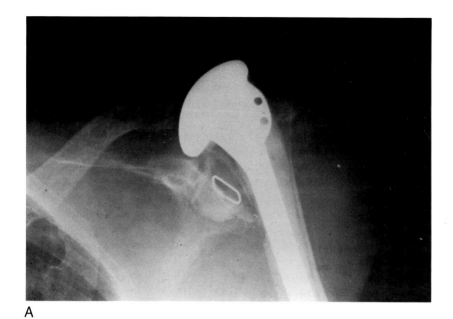

A

B

Fig. 15-20. (A) Anterosuperior dislocation of prosthetic humeral head. (B) Posterior dislocation of prosthetic head on polyethylene glenoid (outlined in black.)

one patient had limitation of external rotation secondary to a mass of cement posterior to the glenoid component, and one patient had malposition of the glenoid and humeral component that blocked adequate rotation of the arm, thus revision surgery was performed. None of the patients developed superficial or deep infections following TSR.

Wilde et al. in their series noted five complications; these included one infection, three anterior dislocations, and one loose glenoid component.[33] Bade et al. reported 17 complications, which included 5 rotator cuff tears, 1 lateral cord neuropraxia that resolved after 6 weeks, 3 loose components, and 2 cases of impingement syndrome.[2]

Table 15-4. Complications following Unconstrained Neer Total Shoulder Arthroplasty: Review of 540 Cases

	Number of Cases	Percent
Infection	2	0.4
Postoperative instability	12	2.2
Postoperative rotator Cuff tear	16	3.0
Fracture of humerus intra/postop	6	1.1
Nerve palsy (axillary, lateral cord)	4	0.7

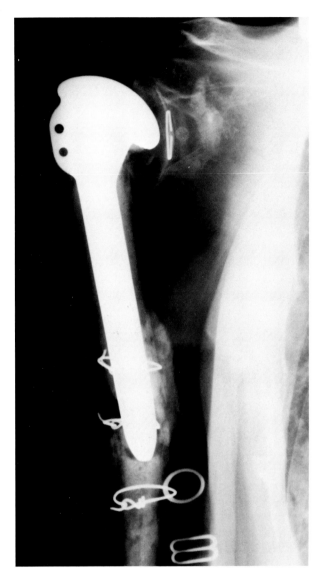

Fig. 15-21. Humeral shaft fracture during TSR, treated with cerclage wiring, and resultant fibrous union.

Review of the complications from the six series utilizing the nonconstrained Neer prosthesis reveals a very low rate of infection postoperatively (Table 15-4). However, it does show a significant incidence of postoperative instability, including anterior, posterior, and superior dislocation. A significant number of patients experienced a rotator cuff tear following TSR, and this often required further surgery to repair the rotator cuff. Fortunately, the incidence of axillary nerve palsy and brachial plexus injury has been ex-

tremely low in the reported series. Other problems that have been encountered during the surgery that are often not reported as complications include extensive resection of the humeral head, which leads to placement of the humeral component inferior to the greater tuberosity, predisposing the patient to postoperative shoulder instability (Fig. 15-22).

Lettin, in his series of patients with the semiconstrained Stanmore prosthesis, reported one infection 15 months after surgery which required excisional arthroplasty.[16] Three patients (7.5 percent) sustained a dislocation of the prosthesis following surgery. Two were reduced closed under general anesthesia; the third continued to dislocate secondary to atrophic shoulder girdle muscles and eventually underwent excisional arthroplasty. Coughlin et al., reporting on the Stanmore prosthesis, noted one case of deep infection requiring excisional arthroplasty and one case of persistent dislocation of the prosthesis which required revision surgery.[9]

Post, using the constrained Michael Reese prosthesis, reported a complication rate of 37 percent.[27] This included 11 revisions of the 22 Series I type prostheses; 3 for dislocation; 6 for breakage of the stem, and 3 for mechanical failure and bending of the neck. Using the Series II component, which was a cobalt–chrome prosthesis with a larger neck, two revisions (10 percent) were required; one for a loose humeral component and one for dislocation of the components. One patient (2 percent) developed an infection around the prosthesis that required an excisional arthroplasty.

Revision

As mentioned in the section dealing with radiographic evaluation and complications, revision arthro-

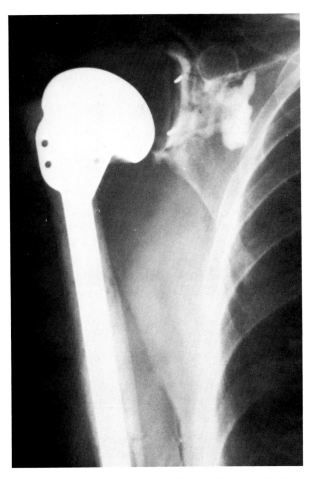

Fig. 15-22. Excessive resection of humeral head and tuberosities resulting in subluxation of humeral prosthesis on the glenoid surface.

plasty is sometimes required and most likely its incidence will increase in the future as longer follow-up accrues. The indications for revision arthroplasty of a TSR are similar to those for other total joint replacements. The most common indications include loosening, mechanical failure of either component, malalignment or malrotation of one or the other component, intra-articular infection with loosening, and soft tissue abnormalities such as deficient or scarred rotator cuff musculature or detachment or scarring of the deltoid. Fortunately, loosening of the humeral component has been an infrequent finding; however, loosening of the glenoid component has occurred with increasing frequency and has necessitated revision arthroplasty

in several cases. Mechanical failure of a nonconstrained prosthesis is very unusual; however, with the more highly constrained prosthesis, breakage of the components and loss of fixation has been observed.[16,23,27] Malalignment of the humeral or glenoid component can occur with incorrect retroversion of the humeral component and abnormal tilting of the glenoid component as causative factors of instability. This is particularly common in patients with significant glenoid bone loss and requires special techniques to augment the glenoid to prevent the improper angulation of its surface. The infection rate as noted above is similar to that for other total joint replacements and, fortunately, is an infrequent problem. Neer and Kirby noted weakening and/or detachment of the anterior deltoid in the majority of their patients seen for revision arthroplasty.[23] Surgical incisions had denervated the anterior deltoid in 5 of their 40 patients.

Technique

Revision arthroplasty of the shoulder is a very demanding procedure and should be undertaken only by those familiar with shoulder surgery. Previous skin incisions can be used; however, the deltopectoral interval is recommended for exposure of the underlying joint. Detachment of the deltoid should be avoided; if previous detachment of the anterior deltoid has occurred this should be repaired. If indicated, anterior acromioplasty should be performed prior to dealing with abnormalities of the rotator cuff. If the rotator cuff is intact, it should be preserved; if it is deficient, repair should take place following removal of the components. Removal of the components, as with other types of total joint arthroplasty, should be performed with preservation of bone stock and in nonseptic cases, removal of sufficient cement to allow proper orientation of the new components. In the case of septic joints, both components as well as all cement should be removed from the humeral cavity as well as the glenoid fossa and scapular neck.

In the case of a septic joint, determination of future reimplantation should be made based on the infecting organism, the quality of the soft tissues, and the quality of the remaining bone stock. In the case of a Gram-positive organism, future reimplantation can be contemplated. We would recommend thorough debridement of the joint following removal of the components and cement, and a course of intravenous antibiotics, ranging from 4 to 6 weeks. At that time, a delayed reimplantation with the appropriate prosthesis can be contemplated. In cases with Gram-negative organisms such as *Pseudomonas*, a resection arthroplasty should be planned and if pain persists following resolution of the infection, attempts at fusion can be made. Fusion in such a joint can be difficult and bone graft with internal fixation as well as external immobilization is required to obtain the best possible results.

In nonseptic cases, whenever possible, revision to a nonconstrained prosthesis is indicated. Neer and Kirby reported a minimum 2-year follow-up on 26 shoulders that underwent prosthetic revision.[23] Eleven shoulders were treated successfully for limited goals activity. The remaining 15 shoulders placed in the regular postoperative physical therapy program yielded 7 excellent results, 3 satisfactory, and 5 unsatisfactory. The unsatisfactory results were because of inadequate active motion due to a weak deltoid and rotator cuff, secondary to scarring from previous surgeries. One of these five shoulders was noted to have persistent pain.

Discussion

The data reviewed in this chapter underscore the efficacy of TSR in the treatment of painful inflammatory and noninflammatory arthritis of the shoulder. Each series reports good pain relief, restoration of function necessary for activities of daily living, and an acceptable early and late complication rate. Clearly the most worrisome aspect has been the high incidence of radiographic glenoid loosening.

Several issues remain unresolved and must be considered. What are the indications for using a more constrained prosthesis? Is there a correlation between superior subluxation of the humerus and the functional result? What are the indications for uncemented application? What are the indications for hemiarthroplasty in glenohumeral arthritis?

It is generally accepted that minimal prosthetic constraint is ideal to prevent transfer of constraining forces to the bony interface. This requires an intact or reconstructable rotator cuff and sufficient neuromuscular function. When possible, rotator cuff lesions should be repaired and a nonconstrained prosthesis utilized. In irreparable cuff lesions, a superior hood or oversized glenoid is necessary to maintain the gle-

nohumeral relationship. The authors believe that anterior and posterior glenoid constraint should be avoided, as there is a normal translation between the humeral head and glenoid with internal and external rotation as the humerus articulates with the glenoid surface, labrum, and capsule. Additional anterior/posterior constraint promotes limited rotation or subluxation/dislocation. A constrained prosthesis is used as a salvage procedure in cases of irreparable soft tissues in patients with low demands and limited goals.

Postoperative superior dislocation of the humeral head is associated with limited motion and decreased function, even though the patient may obtain substantial pain relief.[30] It is the authors' impression that there is a direct correlation between function, strength, and motion with maintenance of the proper glenohumeral articulation. Superior migration may be progressive and eventually will limit the functional result. If maintenance or reconstruction of the superior constraint (rotator cuff, biceps tendon, coracoacromial ligament) is impossible, additional glenoid constraint is necessary.

Recent interest has focused on press-fit and tissue ingrowth methods of fixation. Press-fit fixation of humeral stems is advised in patients with adequate bone stock where initial rigid fixation is obtained. Humeral subsidence has been reported with uncemented components but, to date, no clinical problems have been observed.[30] Addition of a porous surface on the undersurface of the humeral head but not the stem may promote tissue ingrowth while not stress-shielding the proximal humerus. Most currently available glenoid components are intended for use with cement. The major difficulty is the small subchondral surface and relatively empty glenoid vault that limits immediate rigid fixation necessary for an uncemented design. Recent experience with porous surfaces combined with bone screws might provide initial fixation and promote tissue ingrowth. To date, these designs are experimental and do not justify use of TSR in the younger, active patient.

Hemiarthroplasty, when possible, is an attractive alternative to TSR in terms of operative time, ease of exposure, and avoidance of the reported high incidence of radiographic glenoid loosening. In conditions such as osteonecrosis in which the pathology is limited to the humeral head, hemiarthroplasty is the preferred procedure. Moreover, in situations of severe loss of glenoid bone stock precluding glenoid component fixation, a hemiarthroplasty may provide sufficient pain relief for the low-demand patient.

The authors believe, however, that most patients undergoing TSR for inflammatory and noninflammatory arthritis should have the glenoid resurfaced. In the rheumatoid patient with active synovitis, failure to resurface the glenoid may lead to persistent synovitis and progressive erosion, as reported in the knee.[31] Patients with primary osteoarthritis undergoing TSR reported better pain relief when the glenoid was resurfaced.[8,20] An exception to this may be the younger, more active osteoarthritic or hemophilic patient with a relatively spared glenoid in whom the desire to minimize possible late glenoid complications would justify the slightly inferior results of hemiarthroplasty compared with TSR. This situation underscores the need for improvement in glenoid fixation.

In the past decade, major advances in the understanding of shoulder biomechanics, kinematics, and prosthetic designs have been realized. The surgical treatment of glenohumeral disease has greatly improved. The major problems with TSR to resolve in the coming decade are improved glenoid component fixation and sufficient soft tissue reconstruction to allow use of nonconstrained prosthesis in all cases.

REFERENCES

1. Amstutz HC, Sew Hoy AL, Clarke IC: UCLA anatomic total shoulder arthroplasty. Clin Orthop 155:7, 1981
2. Bade HA, Warren RF, Ranawat CS, Inglis AE: Long term results of Neer total shoulder replacement. In Bateman JE, Welsh RP (ed): Surgery of the Shoulder. B.C. Decker and C.V. Mosby, St. Louis, 1984
3. Barrett WP, Jackins SE, Wyss C, Matsen FA III: Total shoulder arthroplasty: the University of Washington experience. Presented at the second open meeting, the American Shoulder and Elbow Surgeons. New Orleans, Louisiana, February 1986
4. Basmajian JV, Bazani FJ: Factors preventing downward dislocation of the abducted shoulder joint. J Bone Joint Surg 41A:1182, 1959
5. Brumfield RN, Schilz J, Flinders BW: Total shoulder replacement arthroplasty: a clinical review of 21 cases. Orthop Trans 5:398, 1981
6. Clayton ML, Ferlic DC, Jeffers PD: Prosthetic arthroplasties of the shoulder. Clin Orthop 164:184, 1982
7. Cofield RH: Total shoulder arthroplasty with the Neer prosthesis. J Bone Joint Surg 66A:899, 1984
8. Cofield RH, Zuckerman JD: Proximal humeral prosthetic replacement in shoulder arthritis. Presented at the second open meeting, the American Shoulder and Elbow Surgeons. New Orleans, Louisiana, February 1986
9. Coughlin MJ, Morris JM, West WF: The semiconstrained total shoulder arthroplasty. J Bone Joint Surg 61A:574, 1979
10. Cruess RL: Shoulder resurfacing according to the method of Neer. J Bone Joint Surg 62B:116, 1980
11. DePalma AF: Surgery of the Shoulder. J.B. Lippincott, Philadelphia, 1983
12. Faludi DD, Weiland AJ: Cementless total shoulder arthroplasty: preliminary experience with thirteen cases. Orthopaedics 6:431, 1983
13. Gristina AG, Webb LX, Carter RE, Romano RL: The monospherical total shoulder. Orthop Trans 9:54, 1985
14. Hughes M, Neer CS II: Glenohumeral joint replacement and post operative rehabilitation. Phys Ther 55:850, 1975
15. Inman VT, Saunders JB, Dec M, Abbott LC: Observations on the function of the shoulder joint. J Bone Joint Surg 26A: 1, 1944
16. Lettin AWF, Copeland SA, Scales JT: The Stanmore total shoulder replacement. J Bone Joint Surg, 64B:47, 1982
17. Lugli T: Artificial shoulder joint by Pean (1893). Clin Orthop 133:215, 1978
18. MacNab I: Total shoulder replacement—a bipolar glenohumeral prosthesis. J Bone Joint Surg 59B:257, 1977
19. Matsen FA III: Biomechanics of the Shoulder. In Basic Biomechanics of the Skeletal System. Philadelphia, Lea and Febiger, 1980
20. Matsen FA III, Barrett WP, Jackins SC: The use of hemiarthroplasty in the treatment of degenerative conditions of the glenohumeral joint. Orthop Trans 7(1):139, 1983
21. Neer CS II: Articular replacement for the humeral head. J Bone Joint Surg 37A:215, 1955
22. Neer CS II: Replacement arthroplasty for glenohumeral osteoarthritis. J Bone Joint Surg 56A:1, 1974
23. Neer CS II, Kirby RM: Revision of humeral head and total shoulder arthroplasties. Clin Orthop 170:189, 1982
24. Neer CS II, Watson KC, Stanton FJ: Recent experience in total shoulder replacement. J Bone Joint Surg 64A:319, 1982
25. Poppen NK, Walker PS: Normal and abnormal motion of the shoulder. J Bone Joint Surg 58A:195, 1976
26. Poppen NK, Walker PS: Forces at the glenohumeral joint in abduction. Clin Orthop 135:165, 1978
27. Post M, Haskell SS, Jablon M: Total shoulder replace-

ment with a constrained prosthesis. J Bone Joint Surg 62A:327, 1980

28. Saha AK: Mechanism of shoulder movements and a plea for the recognition of "zero position" of glenohumeral joint. Clin Orthop 173:3, 1983

29. Sarrafian SK: Gross and functional anatomy of the shoulder. Clin Orthop 173:11, 1983

30. Thornhill TS, Karr MJ, Averill RM, et al: Total shoulder arthroplasty: The Brigham experience. Orthop Trans 7:497, 1983

31. Thornhill TS, Dalziel RW, Sledge CB: Alternatives to arthrodesis for failed total knee arthroplasty. Clin Orthop 170:131, 1982

32. Weaver JK, Dunn HK: Treatment of acromioclavicular injuries, especially complete acromioclavicular separation. J Bone Joint Surg 54A:1187, 1972

33. Wilde AH, Bordon LS, Brems JJ: Experience with the Neer total shoulder replacment. Bateman JE, Welsh RP (eds): Surgery of the Shoulder. B.C. Decker and C.V. Mosby, St. Louis, 1984

Advances in Arthrodesis of the Shoulder

16

Carter R. Rowe
Robert D. Leffert

With the control of tuberculosis and infantile paralysis in the past 50 years, the need for arthrodesis of the shoulder has markedly diminished. However, this technique has rightfully retained an important place in the armamentarium of the shoulder surgeon, since it can provide a strong shoulder for lifting, pushing, pulling, and situations where prosthetic replacements cannot be expected to endure. In fact, the results of arthrodesis of the shoulder do not deteriorate with time, which gives the technique a unique advantage over any prosthesis available today. Also, fusion remains the dependable salvage operation for failed reconstructive surgery.

The indications for arthrodesis of the shoulder may be listed as follows:

1. Traumatic arthritis
2. Deltoid and rotator cuff paralysis (with preservation of the scapulothoracic muscle power)
3. Irreparable rotator cuff rupture with pain and subluxation
4. Traumatic destruction of the joint
5. Unreduced dislocation, in poor position and painful
6. Arthritides
7. Infection with joint destruction (nontuberculous)
8. Brachial plexus injury
9. Chronic extensive posttraumatic and unrelieved adhesions of the joint

Despite the wide applicability of this operation, there continues to be misunderstanding of what a fusion of the shoulder can offer. The popular misconception, even among medical personnel, is that arthrodesis of the shoulder results in an arm fixed to the body with no free motion. In reality, with proper positioning at the arthrodesis site (Fig. 16-1A), the movement in the scapulothoracic "joint" can enable the patient to reach the face, back pocket, anal region, and feet (Fig. 16-1B). In addition, lifting strength is greatly increased with the arm at the side of the body.

As with other surgical techniques, there have also been advances in the past 10 to 15 years in arthrodesis of the shoulder.

OPERATIVE TECHNIQUE

Operative technique has evolved to the use of various forms of internal fixation, which have become standard, although the precise method may differ ac-

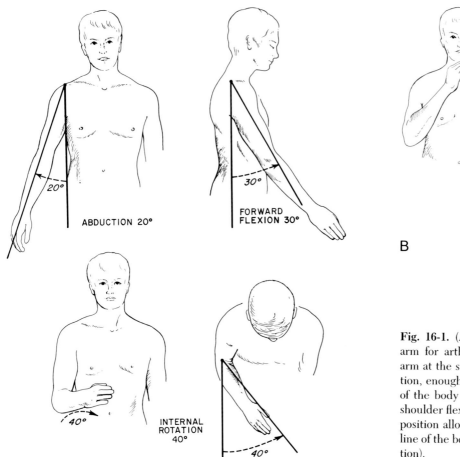

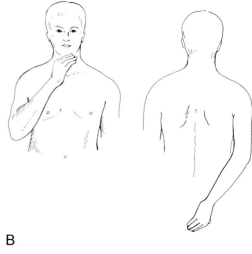

ABDUCTION 20°

FORWARD FLEXION 30°

INTERNAL ROTATION 40°

A

B

Fig. 16-1. (A) The recommended position of the arm for arthrodesis of the shoulder is with the arm at the side of the body, in only 20° of abduction, enough internal rotation to reach the midline of the body and flexion to reach the face (30° of shoulder flexion and 90° of elbow flexion). **(B)** This position allows the patient also to reach the midline of the body posteriorly (a very necessary function).

cording to various surgeons. Carroll,[2] for example, has advocated the use of wire loop fixation, which allows adjustment of the position of the fusion site in the immediate postoperative period. Others have used compression screws or plates and screws. These can eliminate the need for external fixation and long immobilization in a plaster spica, which increases patient acceptance. There is considerably less morbidity both generally and in terms of stiffness of the upper limb, particularly at the elbow.

POSITION OF THE ARM

The position of the arm has been a subject of controversy both for surgeons and patients. In the past, there has been lack of agreement, not just about the

optimal position for fusion but even over the anatomical landmarks used to make the measurements. These have included the relationship between the arm and the trunk, and between the arm and the vertebrae, axillary border, and spine of the scapula. The 1942 study of the Research Committee of the American Orthopaedic Association used the vertebral border of the scapula and recommended 50° of abduction of the shaft of the humerus and 15° to 25° of forward flexion.[6] Rotation was determined with the patient in the supine position and the arm in desired amounts of abduction and flexion, proceeding to rotate externally 25° from that position in which the forearm was vertical. This was defined as the "salute position." It should be noted that since the abducted arm is forward flexed, returning it to the side actually produces a final resting position of internal rotation, whereas the external rotation would persist if there were no forward flexion. The study included only children and adolescents with infantile paralysis in whom no internal fixation was used and in whom, with time, the angle of abduction diminished to some extent.

During the 1960s, Dr. Rowe saw a number of adult patients who were very unhappy following arthrodesis of the shoulder because of muscular strain and winging of the scapula.[7] Figure 16-2 shows a 45-year-old woman whose shoulder had been arthrodesed in 80° of abduction of the arm from the trunk. She was comfortable only when she supported her arm. When her arm was lowered to the side of her body, there was marked winging of the scapula. She had little use of the arm and was in constant pain. Obviously, her shoulder had been arthrodesed in excessive abduction and forward flexion.

Shortly thereafter, another patient, a 45-year-old construction worker, was seen because of "constant pain" following arthrodesis of his shoulder. When his scapula was placed in the neutral position, his arm was in 80° of abduction from the side of his body (Fig. 16-3A). When he lowered his arm, he inclined his body to lessen the strain on his shoulder and the winging of his scapula (Fig. 16-3B). Because of the position of his arm, he had been unable to return to construction work. Both of these patients were greatly improved by osteotomy of the surgical neck of the humerus, which eliminated excessive abduction of the arm.

The choice of a comfortable, functional, and cosmetic position of the arm in shoulder fusion was decided by Dr. Rowe in a patient who was admitted

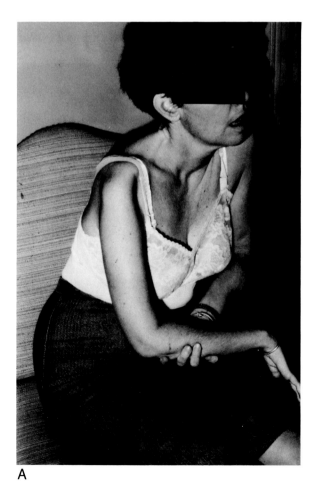
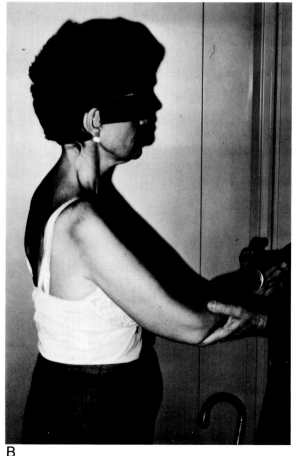

A   B

Fig. 16-2. (A) A 45-year-old woman whose shoulder was arthrodesed in 80° of abduction. When her arm was lowered to the side of her body, there was marked winging of the scapula. (B) She was comfortable only when her arm was supported.

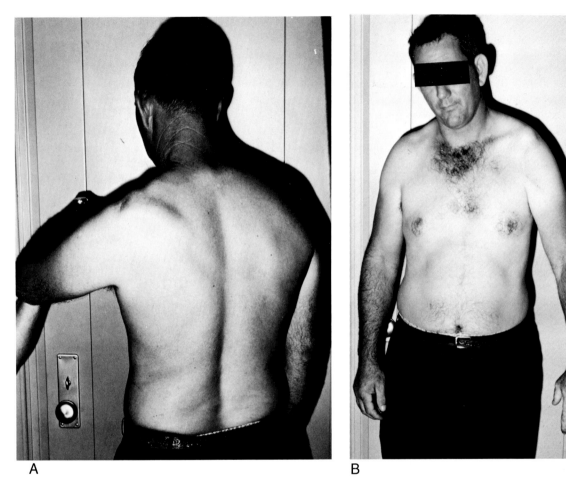

A   B

Fig. 16-3. (**A**) In a 45-year-old construction worker whose shoulder was arthrodesed in 80° of abduction his scapula lay flat only if his arm was abducted. (**B**) When his arm was lowered, he had to incline his body to lessen the discomfort of his winged scapula.

to the Massachusetts General Hospital because of sepsis of his left shoulder following an open reduction for a displaced fracture of the humerus. His arm rested comfortably at his side, although motion was painful. It was decided to debride his septic shoulder and fuse it in the resting position of his arm. At follow-up, the patient's pain was relieved, his arm was in a strong position for lifting, and there was no prominence of his scapula. He could reach his face and head, his pants pocket and the midline of his back. He was very happy with the result, a serendipitous solution for the patient and doctor. Subsequently, we have arthrodesed all shoulders, as demonstrated in Figure 16-1, with the arm in a resting position at

the side of the body in only 20° of abduction, with enough internal rotation for the hand to reach the midline of the body (usually 40° to 45°) and enough forward flexion for the hand to reach the face with flexion of the elbow (usually 30°). When the motion of the scapulothoracic joint is added to this, the patient should be able to reach well above the head, as demonstrated in Figure 16-4F.

The patient in Figure 16-4 was to undergo arthrodesis of both shoulders. The question arose: should one shoulder be arthrodesed in abduction and the other shoulder at the side of the body? The decision was made to arthrodese both shoulders in the same neutral position as described above, with the arms at

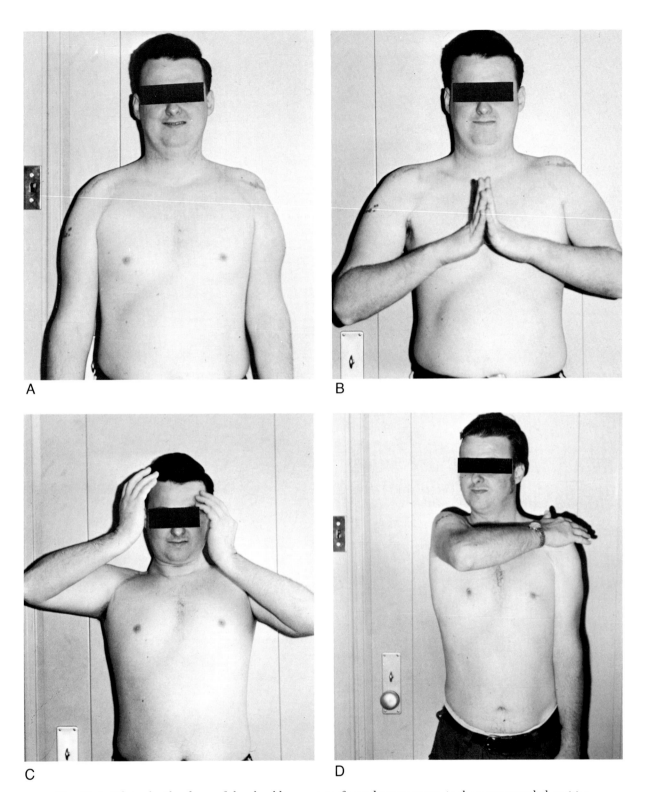

Fig. 16-4. Bilateral arthrodeses of the shoulder were performed a year apart, in the recommended position. (**A**) The patient's arms are comfortable at the side of his body. (**B**) He reaches the midline of his body with ease. (**C**) He reaches his face and head and (**D**) his opposite shoulder. (*Figure continues.*)

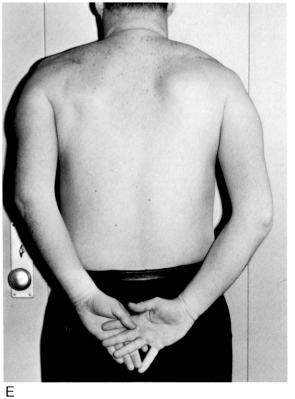

E

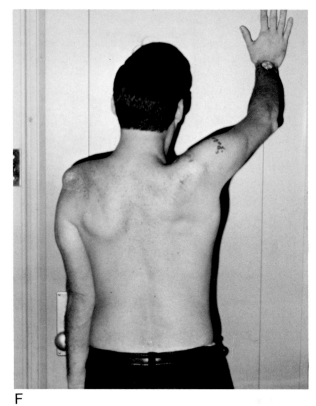

F

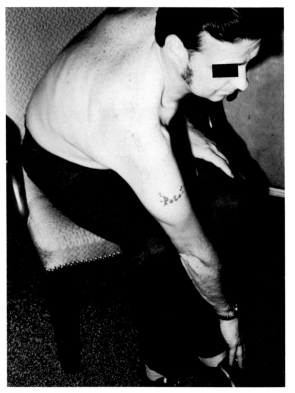

G

Fig. 16-4 (*Continued*). (**E**) He reaches the midline of his back with both arms. (**F**) With scapular motion, he has 135° of elevation. (**G**) He reaches his shoes. He has a full-time job as a bartender and lifts heavy boxes of beverages with no pain.

the side of the body. The outcome has been most successful. The patient functions well as a bartender, is free of pain, has strong shoulders, and is able to lift crates of beer and bottled liquors. He is able to reach his face, well above his head, his shoes, and the front and back of his body with either arm. He has good reasons to be well satisfied with his result.

The patient in Figure 16-5 had her left shoulder fused in 35° from the lateral border of the scapula, or in 15° of abduction from the side of the body. She is satisfied with her shoulder, takes care of her children, and is free of pain.

The problems of excessive abduction of the hu-

merus in shoulder fusion have been illustrated, and are representative of a number of other patients we have examined. Although Cofield and Briggs[3] found there was no statistically significant evidence that shoulders fused in more than 45° of abduction were more painful than those fused in less abduction, these data showed a trend suggesting that there might have been a significant relationship had more patients been available for the studies.

Davis and Cottrell[4] reported their experience with a 50-year-old patient who had intolerable pain following arthrodesis of his shoulder with the humerus at a 75° angle from the side of the body. An osteotomy

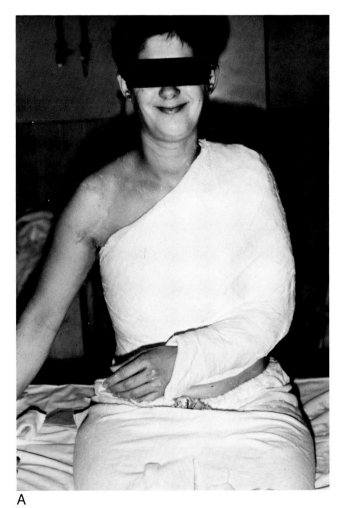

A

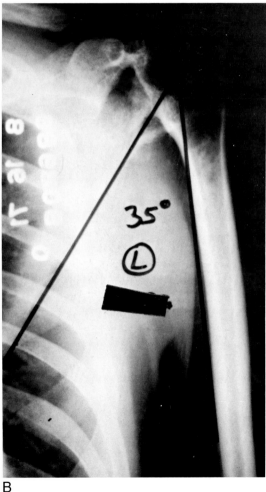

B

Fig. 16-5. (A) This 35-year-old woman had experienced multiple unsuccessful operations of both shoulders because of voluntary dislocations. Her left shoulder was arthrodesed with her arm at the side of her body. She is comfortable in a light shoulder spica postoperately. **(B)** Her shoulder was solidly fused 6 months after surgery, pain-free and strong. She has been followed over the years as a busy happy mother.

was performed to reduce the angle to 25°, which relieved his pain. Bateman also recommended that the abduction angle for fusion in adults be reduced "sufficiently" from 60° to permit the patient to reach the pants pocket and the posterior aspect of the body.[1] DePalma[5] also cautioned that one of the mistakes in the position of arthrodesis is not only excessive abduction but also excessive forward flexion.

On the basis of our clinical experience, as well as that of others, the position of the arm for arthrodesis of the shoulder, as we have described it, is comfortable, with no winging of the scapula, and strong, with a functional range of motion. We quote from DePalma[5]:

> Since Rowe's publication of these findings in 1974, I have reviewed as many of my unsatisfactory results as I could assemble. I found the chief factor for failure was position, especially too much abduction. Now, except in special situations, I strive to attain a fusion with the arm in the position recommended by Rowe.

PREOPERATIVE PLANNING AND DISCUSSION

The essentially permanent nature of the result of arthrodesis makes it essential to discuss the pros and cons of the procedure at length with a patient who is contemplating the operation. While it is difficult for most lay people to comprehend how arthrodesing the shoulder joint can *still allow motion of the shoulder girdle*, an attempt should be made to convey that information in understandable terms. The general hoped-for range of motion and potential for function should be given with the important caveat that each patient is different and that there can be no assurance of the ultimate result. It should be made quite clear to the patient that, although apparent rotation will occur because of the glide of the scapula on the chest wall, no true rotation of the shoulder will be possible, nor will the complete "hands-up" position. Nevertheless, it should be possible for the patient to reach above the horizontal and manage to eat, toilet, and, with some limitations, comb hair. Some patients will find sleeping on the fused side uncomfortable. For patients in whom a generalized arthritis is present or adjacent joints are abnormal,

it must be said that these joints may become involved and consequently some motion may be lost. Furthermore, for people who are extremely physically active, there is a definite danger of fracture of the humerus due to falling, skiing, or playing contact sports. However, it is reasonable that fracture would be less likely to occur with less abduction of the arm. The patient must realize that all conceivable functional needs cannot be totally met by fusion, and some might be compromised for the benefit of others. Individual functional requirements may therefore dictate variations in the position chosen. For example, a patient who has a significant flexion contracture at the elbow will require less forward flexion at the fusion site, to prevent the arm and hand from sticking out in front of the body in an unnatural manner. Patients who have paralytic limbs and who require tendon transfers for restoration of elbow flexion will be aided by increased abduction and forward flexion of the humerus, to facilitate weak elbow flexion. This same group of paralytic patients may also have weakness of the periscapular musculature, particularly the trapezius and serratus anterior, which, if sufficiently severe, will compromise the strength and effective range of motion of the shoulder fusion. It is highly desirable to have a normal trapezius and serratus as a minimum; without these the optimal function of the fusion will simply not be obtained. For patients with diminished musculature, one must carefully decide whether a fusion done under such circumstances will be sufficiently functional to make it worthwhile.

The patient's understanding of what is involved in living with a shoulder fusion can be aided by having more than one discussion, with time between the sessions for formulation of questions. In addition, having the patient meet another patient who has had a fusion is also helpful, although it should be stressed that the surgeon is not contracting to produce an identical result.

ADVANCES IN TECHNIQUE

Utility Incision

Every conceivable operative approach has been employed to perform arthrodesis of the shoulder, with advocates for most of them. Dr. Rowe prefers the anterior–superior approach with the patient semisitting (45°) and the extremity completely draped. The routine utility incision is used, turning down the deltoid osteoperiosteal sleeve from the clavicle and acromion (see Chap. 3). After exposure of the humeral head, the articular cartilage of the head and glenoid is removed. The distal inch of the clavicle is removed. The surgeon holds the arm so that the hand reaches the midline of the body and, with elbow flexion, reaches the face. The humeral head is then osteotomized to face a flat side to the glenoid fossa. The arm in this position will be in approximately 20° of abduction, 30° of forward flexion, and 40° of internal rotation in relation to the side of the body. In this position, the humerus usually makes an angle of 35° with the lateral border of the scapula (Fig. 16-5B). Two 6.5 mm. AO cancellous bone screws or a long vitallium nail are then introduced across the neck of the humerus and the humeral head into the glenoid (Fig. 16-6). Sixteen mm threads will give compression. One nail or screw may be introduced down from the acromion if necessary. The surgeon may osteotomize the acromion and depress it to the humeral

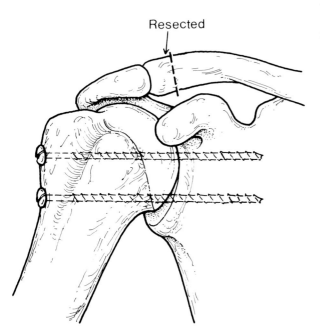

Fig. 16-6. Two AO cancellous bone screws with 16 mm threads are passed through the surgical neck and head to the glenoid, giving firm fixation. The less the abduction of the arm, the more secure the screws will be. Resection of the distal clavicle may aid in elevation.

head, or the head may be displaced upward to meet the acromion. Resection of the distal clavicle may aid in elevation. Bone chips from the distal clavicle are placed around the glenoid head junction.

After closure of the wound, the arm is supported in a reinforced pillow dressing. A light plaster cast is applied a few days later, as shown in Figure 16-5A. This position leaves the arm comfortable, at the side of the body, in a strong position with no winging of the scapula, as shown in Figure 16-4B. Dr. Leffert prefers the posterior approach, which has its specific advantages and indications, and should be carefully reviewed. The position under general anesthesia of lateral decubitus can be maintained either with kidney rests or a "bean bag" and allows for access to the entire shoulder girdle, as well as the iliac crest if it is required as a source of bone graft. The arm on the involved side can be supported on a padded Mayo stand and maintained in the desired position without having to rely on an assistant who will invariably fatigue during the course of the operation. It can be moved as needed for exposure until internal fixation is completed. The draping should allow for visualization and palpation of the vertebral border of the scapula, since this, as well as the chest wall, may be used as a point of reference. Dr. Leffert prefers the vertebral border of the scapula as a reference point for the humeral angle because its position is not altered when the patient is in the side-lying position. In addition, the operator should be aware of the position of the patient's head and neck so that the draped hand can be brought to the level of the mouth on the other side of the drapes prior to finalization of fixation.

Posterior Incision

The posterior incision has several advantages. It is relatively cosmetic, has no neurovascular structures of consequence within its field, and can be done relatively simply with minimal blood loss. It does not interfere with subsequent tendon transfers, if they are needed. It begins and parallels the spine of the scapula, but should be made 1 fingerbreadth inferior to it to avoid adhesion to the bone. It continues laterally along the acromion where, at its midpoint, it curves inferiorly along the midlateral aspect of the shaft of the humerus (see posterior exposure, Chap. 3). The use of self-retaining retractors immediately after the skin incision will control bleeding. Thereafter, dissection is carried with the cutting cautery down to the spine of the scapula. The deltoid muscle is retracted inferiorly, with the line of incision continuing into the substance of the muscle, but stopping short of the axillary nerve and circumflex humeral vessels, unless greater exposure is necessary along the shaft of the humerus. The tendons of the supra- and infraspinatus are divided transversely and tagged for later reapproximation in a manner that allows visualization of the posterior capsule and the glenohumeral joint. Larger self-retaining retractors hold the muscles out of the way and effect hemostasis. The posterior capsule is incised using cutting cautery or sharp dissection. A portion of the posterior capsule, along with as much of the glenoidal labrum as can be visualized posteriorly, is excised. With adequate muscular relaxation provided by the anesthesiologist, it is now possible to distract the articular surfaces and inspect them. Since the patient is in the lateral decubitus position, the humeral head will be superior. Accordingly, it is prudent to remove the glenoidal articular surface first, so that the field is not obscured by bleeding from the raw surface of the humeral head. The osteotomy should include the subchondral bone and the articular surface perpendicular to the axis of the neck of the scapula, and is best accomplished by the use of a very sharp 3 cm osteotome. The glenoid can easily be removed in one piece. The operator should then verify the desired position of the humerus prior to making the cut on the humeral head. If the position is anatomically appropriate, provisions can be made for translocating the humerus cephalad so that an addition site for arthrodesis can be gained by denuding and decorticating the undersurface of the acromion. In many cases, this will be possible as long as there is sufficient contact between the glenoid and the humeral head when the position is finalized. In some patients with small glenoidal surfaces, it is inadvisable.

When the proposed final position has been judged to be adequate, the plane of the glenoidal resection may be verified and duplicated on the humeral head by parallel placement of a second 3 cm osteotome. Usually less than 1.5 cm of head need be resected to achieve a tight fit of the articular surfaces that will permit compression. Obviously, if the articular surfaces have been distorted by trauma or arthritis, some modification of this procedure will be necessary, and occasionally it is desirable to produce a ball-in-socket configuration. In these cases, removal of the articular cartilage and subchondral bone can be done with a pneumatic drill and appropriate cutting burrs. However, the bony surfaces should be congruous and well-aligned prior to the insertion of the fixation devices, and the ultimate position of the fusion must be checked repeatedly.

Fixation

We use two methods of fixation, and the choice between them depends on the circumstances and the patient. The simpler of the two involves 6.5 mm cancellous screws inserted across the fusion site from the lateral aspect of the humeral head into the neck of the glenoid (Fig. 16-6). The 16 mm threads are preferable, since a lag effect and compression are desired. A 3.2 mm drill bit is used through the humeral head and into the neck of the glenoid. Inserting the fingers of both hands on either side of the humeral head and along the neck of the glenoid posteriorly allows the surgeon to direct an assistant in the placement of the screws and avoid either posterior or anterior protrusion. Particularly in a paralytic patient, the bone of the humeral head will be quite soft and that of the glenoid harder, but since it is cancellous bone a tap will not be required. If desired, the first drill bit introduced can be left in situ temporarily and will maintain the position while a second hole is drilled by the assistant. For most adults, a 70 to 80 mm long 6.5 mm cancellous screw with 16 mm thread will provide adequate compression if a washer is used to prevent the screw head from sinking into the bone. All of the threads should be beyond the surface of the glenoid, otherwise compression will not occur. The screw lengths can be predetermined by simple external measurement; it is important to direct them in different quadrants of the head and glenoid. Usually four or five screws are sufficient to achieve adequate fixation and compression. However, if external fixation such as a shoulder spica is not to be employed, this fixation, particularly if the bone is osteoporotic, will be insufficient and should not be trusted. The reliability and general condition of the patient will determine whether or not a spica will be required.

Because of the morbidity and inconvenience associated with having to wear a shoulder spica for 12 weeks, we tend to use this method less and less, although patients who might well not cooperate should not be offered the opportunity to dispense with the spica postoperatively. If one is to be used, the fixation portion of the operative procedure will have been completed. Operative radiographs can confirm the position of the screws, although it is difficult to be absolutely certain of the position of the fusion on a radiograph. Assuming the fixation is judged to be adequate and the fusion site is compressed tightly, the wound is irrigated copiously with antibiotic solution and simply closed in layers with a suction drain.

Because it is difficult or impossible to apply a comfortable plaster spica on an anesthetized patient, the arm is supported by either a commercially available adjustable splint or a sling and pillows with a Velpeau bandage. When the patient is sufficiently comfortable and able to stand (2 or 3 days after surgery) a full spica may be applied. It is vital that the cast rest on the padded iliac crests, lest an excessively long and heavy lever-arm be applied to the limb and jeopardize the integrity of the fusion.

Compression Plates

For those patients in whom sufficient trust exists to dispense with spica immobilization, it will be necessary to reinforce the fixation by means of compression plates (Fig. 16-7). If this method is chosen, the operator will have planned ahead to avoid placing the screws in positions that will interfere with either the location of the plates or the screws used to attach them. For most patients, a 10-hole narrow dynamic compression plate (DCP) can be applied to the spine of the scapula and across the acromion to the level of the surgical neck of the humerus. The use of a malleable template will facilitate the contouring of the plate, but in all cases it is a tedious job that must be done very carefully to avoid a major bend within a screw hole that would compromise its strength. Sometimes the plate must be twisted axially in addition to being bent. Where the plate overlies a cancellous bony area, cancellous screws can be used for fixation, although cortical screws are preferred and present less problems in insertion. The last few holes on the shaft of the humerus can usually accommodate cortical screws but those overlying the head, particularly when they pass through the arthrodesis site into the glenoid, will invariably be cancellous. A screw directed through the acromion into the humeral head can be cancellous with a 32 mm thread. As many cortical screws as can be used in the scapular fixation are inserted. In some places the spine of the scapula will provide insufficient bone for fixation of a cortical screw. Here a lock nut may be used with the cortex screw.

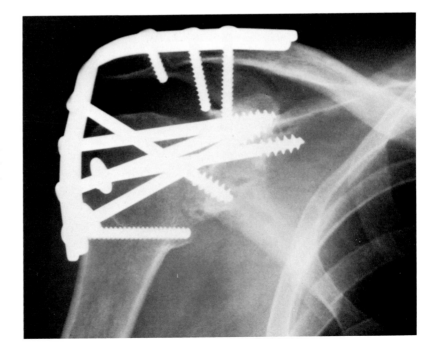

Fig. 16-7. Compression plate shoulder fusion for a brachial plexus injury with a flail shoulder. It was not necessary to use a plaster spica in this case.

Placement of the cancellous screws through the DCP can be a problem. Therefore, they should be placed in the head before the fixation to the scapula is done. If possible, the plate should be attached in such a way that it and the screw heads will not compromise the soft tissues that will need to be closed over them. In fact, patients who are extremely thin and have poor subcutaneous tissues are not good candidates for this method of fixation because of the possibility of erosion of the metal through the thin tissues.

A second plate may be applied along the posterior aspect of the scapula and humerus, and we have used either a second DCP or a buttress plate, depending on the local anatomy. The problem with this plate is the thickness of the bone of the scapula, which makes fixation difficult. In addition, there is danger from overly long screws that could conceivably penetrate the thorax.

Ordinarily, a bone graft is not necessary unless there has been loss of bone stock. However, the resected humeral head may be used to reinforce the area of fusion between the acromion and the subjacent humeral head. Rarely is additional bone graft from the iliac crest needed.

Closure is in layers with the use of a suction drain. Although only a sling is used in some patients, in others a premade orthoplast gunslinger splint is applied in the operating room or can be made in the immediate postoperative period.

Radiographic assessment of the fusion site in the operating room is confined to judging the position of the fixation and the gross opposition of the bony surfaces, since with compression technique, they should appear tightly opposed. Any appearance of lucency between the bones indicates significant malposition.

If a spica is used, a radiograph is taken after it has been applied to ensure that no change in the position has occurred. At 6 weeks, the midpoint for spica immobilization, an additional radiograph is taken. The cast is windowed at 2 weeks for removal of the sutures.

Postoperative Care

For patients in whom the orthoplast splint and compression plate technique is used, immobilization may be discontinued at 6 weeks in most cases, but no heavy use of the arm is permitted for at least 12 weeks. The spica cast is removed at 12 weeks and plain films as well as tomograms are obtained. However, the amount of metal in the area makes interpretation of the tomograms difficult. Most patients' shoulders are clinically fused by 12 weeks, as demonstrated by lack of motion at the fusion site. Even if radiographic consolidation is not complete, they are generally begun on gentle mobilization exercises without stress. For some patients, particularly those who have had significant loss of bone stock because of a prosthesis, or who have had special situations such as a fusion done for a neuropathic joint, the plaster immobilization may be required for as long as 5 months. This has only occurred very rarely.

In some patients, as described by Milgram, the range of motion of the fused shoulder complex may be increased by resection of the lateral clavicle distal to the coracoclavicular ligaments as a secondary procedure if deemed necessary.

COMPLICATIONS AND THEIR MANAGEMENT

The biomechanics of an arthrodesed shoulder in an active patient will, of necessity, may predispose to fracture of the humerus if forces of great magnitude are applied, such as in a heavy fall or severe twisting injury. The arthrodesis site usually does not disrupt, although it may, particularly if the bony remodeling has not been completed. When they do occur, the fractures are usually not difficult to treat, although one should be alerted to the possibility of rotational or angular deformity that would alter the initial position of the shoulder fusion. Ordinarily, the use of a shoulder spica for 6 to 8 weeks provides sufficient healing to allow remobilization. Dr. Leffert has noted three humeral fractures in 20 years of doing shoulder fusions.

As previously stated, skin complications due to the presence of hardware may occur. These are likely in very thin patients, in whom it is hard to achieve sufficient soft tissue coverage for plates and the screws used to fix them to bone. Should erosion of a single screw head occur, the screw can be removed with little difficulty. The emergence of a portion of the plate through a skin ulceration is distressing, but ordinarily not disastrous if infection does not supervene. On the two occasions when this has occurred, the complication has been handled by daily sterile dressings and no antibiotics unless there is evidence of cellulitis. If the problem arises shortly after surgery, it is mandatory to maintain the plate until significant healing has occurred. If it then becomes necessary to remove the plate, this can be done and fixation supplemented with a spica. Usually 8 weeks will allow sufficient healing to permit plate removal if it becomes necessary. Fortunately, this has not been a common problem.

Some patients will be distressed by the cosmetic appearance of the shoulder due to continued atrophy of the soft tissues about the arthrodesis site. Although it is possible to fill the contour by the subcutaneous placement of Silastic implants, we have not recommended that approach to our patients.

In summary, the orthopaedic surgeon should be knowledgeable about several approaches to and techniques for arthrodesis of the shoulder. Except in instances of a weak elbow, and specific position of the arm for muscle transplants, we strongly recommend the functional and comfortable position of the arm recommended here which avoids excess abduction.

When needed and when properly performed, an arthrodesed shoulder may prove far more satisfactory to the patient than it has been given credit for in the past.

REFERENCES

1. Bateman JE: The Shoulder and Neck, 2nd ed. WB Saunders, Philadelphia, 1978
2. Carroll RE: Wire loop arthrodesis of the shoulder. Clin Orthop 9:185, 1957
3. Cofield RH, Briggs BT: Glenohumeral arthrodesis, operative and long term functional results. J Bone Joint Surg 61A:668, 1979
4. Davis JB, Cottrell GW: A technique for shoulder arthrodesis. J Bone Joint Surg 44A:657, 1962
5. DePalma AF: Surgery of the Shoulder, 3rd ed. JB Lippincott, Philadelphia, 1983
6. Research Committee of the American Orthopaedic Association: The survey of end results on stabilization of the paralytic shoulder. J Bone Joint Surg 24:699, 1942
7. Rowe CR: Re-evaluation of the position of the arm in arthrodesis of the shoulder in the adult. J Bone Joint Surg 56A:913, 1974

The Role of Physical Therapy in Rehabilitation of the Shoulder

17

Bette Ann Harris
Robert D. Leffert

Rehabilitation of the patient with shoulder dysfunction is a challenging task for the physical therapist because of the complex biomechanics of this joint. Pathologic conditions of the shoulder often result in pain, stiffness, and muscle weakness causing functional limitation. The role of physical therapy is to facilitate restoration of functional use of the involved extremity.

To achieve this goal, the physical therapist should begin with a thorough evaluation that will serve as the basis for an appropriate rehabilitation program. This process enables one to identify the major problems and to decide in what order they should be managed. Throughout the rehabilitation course, soft tissue healing and postoperative precautions need to be considered and may alter the ideal treatment program.

Although the wide range of shoulder dysfunctions will require different specific exercise programs, several guidelines apply to all rehabilitation programs:

1. The exercise program should not cause pain. There is never an indication for forced passive motion.
2. The scapular musculature should be included in an exercise program for the treatment of any shoulder disability.
3. Restoration of normal functional movement patterns should be the ultimate aim of treatment.
4. Realistic goals should be based on the diagnosis and restrictions that may result from the disability or surgery (treatment).
5. The quantity and quality of the exercises should be selected carefully. Exercising three times a week with the physical therapist or performing exercises at home two times a day may not be the most effective methods. The patient needs to be actively involved in his or her rehabilitation, including a diligent home program. The idea that physical therapy is something done *to* the patient should be discouraged. It is important that the patient accept the responsibility for his or her own care in order to make progress.

Physical therapy is based on each patient's physical findings and takes into consideration past treatments and interventions. All patients begin their visit to a physical therapist with an initial evaluation. The problems are then identified, realistic short- and long-term rehabilitation goals are set, and an exercise program is developed. Responses to the program are constantly evaluated and modifications are made as necessary.

521

At our clinic, the problem-oriented approach to management is used. The next section briefly outlines the key areas to concentrate on when evaluating a patient with shoulder dysfunction. The first step is to perform an evaluation to gather the necessary information (Fig. 17-1).

EVALUATION

History

The interview should consist of a review of the medical record, physical therapy referral, the history of the present complaint, pertinent other medical history, current diagnosis, hand dominance, and other treatment (past and current) including surgical procedures for the present shoulder problem. The patient's social and work environment and description of his or her functional limitations should be assessed as well as goals and expectations from treatment. If surgery has been done, the physical therapist should communicate with the surgeon and obtain a copy of the operative note if possible. There should be a clear understanding as to the ultimate objective of the surgery (for example, realizing that a patient with severe rheumatoid arthritis and a disrupted rotator cuff, who has a total shoulder replacement, is not going to regain normal strength), as well as contraindications and precautions, including length of immobilization. For patients who are not treated surgically, there should be clear treatment objectives and a defined time frame in which these objectives are to be achieved.

General Inspection

An evaluation of the patient with shoulder dysfunction should begin as soon as the patient enters the examining room. Important information about function and level of discomfort can be gained by observing the patient's posture and movement. Specific activities to observe include the following.

GAIT

Does the arm swing normally or does the patient hold the arm stiffly at the side? If so, this could be indicative of pain with motion.

DRESSING

When the patient removes his shirt does he move cautiously? Does he "undress" the affected arm last, or when he puts on his shirt does he have to "dress" the affected arm first? If so, this could indicate limited range of motion, pain, weakness, or a combination of symptoms.

CHANGING POSITIONS

Can the patient move from standing to sitting to lying down easily or does changing positions appear labored? Can the patient use her affected arm for support when sitting up or coming to standing? If not, this could be an indication of joint pain.

For the general inspection of the shoulder girdle including the neck and upper back, the patient should be adequately disrobed so these areas can be easily observed. Figure 17-2 illustrates the evaluation of scapular symmetry and shoulder girdle weakness.

Specific Objective Tests

These include an evaluation of pain, soft tissue integrity, specific range of motion, strength, endurance, posture (including palpation of bony landmarks), and function.[3,9,10,13,14,17-19,28,29] Assessment should include screening of the cervical spine and distal joints of the involved extremity. From these findings, the therapist then establishes the problem list. All the factors contributing to the patient's decreased shoulder function are listed in order of primary importance. In assessing or identifying the problems to be managed by physical therapy, the critical questions to consider are the following:

1. What is the most important problem to manage immediately? For example, is muscle tightness limiting range of motion, or is it acute pain?
2. Do the factors interrelate? Is the pain inhibiting muscle function?

DATA BASE

1.00 PATIENT PROFILE

FOR POSITION ONLY

MASSACHUSETTS GENERAL HOSPITAL
DEPARTMENT OF REHABILITATION MEDICINE

PHYSICAL THERAPY

Date: _____

PRIMARY DIAGNOSIS: (for which Physical Therapy Requested)
(Include date of onset, date(s) of surgery)

PRECAUTIONS: yes ☐   no ☐

REFERRAL: _____

Requested by: _____ M.D.
            (Signature)
                              _____ M.D.
            Print name below signature

DO NOT WRITE BELOW THIS LINE

DATE ONSET NOTED	PHYSICAL THERAPY PROBLEM LIST	DATE RESOLVED

DATE: _____ THERAPIST: _____ EXT: _____

TREATMENT RECORD

Month	1	2	3	4	5	6	7	8	9	10	11	12	13	14	15	16	17	18	19	20	21	22	23	24	25	26	27	28	29	30	31
1																															
2																															
3																															
4																															
5																															
6																															

	NORMAL LIMITS	ABNORMAL	NOT EVALUATED
GENERAL STATUS			
2.00 COMMUNICATION			
2.10 CARDIOVASCULAR			
2.20 PULMONARY			
2.30 METABOLIC			
2.40 GI/GU			
2.50 VISION			
2.60 BEHAVIOR			
2.70 APPLIANCES			
3.00 PAIN AND TENDERNESS			
PHYSIOLOGICAL/ANATOMICAL SYSTEMS			
4.00 SKIN AND SOFT TISSUE			
4.10 SKELETAL AND JOINT CONDITION			
4.20 RANGE OF MOTION AND MUSCLE LENGTH			
4.30 NEUROMUSCULAR			
FUNCTIONAL MOTOR PERFORMANCE			
5.00 BALANCE AND EQUILIBRIUM			
5.10 POSTURE			
5.20 FUNCTIONAL MOBILITY			
5.30 ENDURANCE			
5.40 GAIT PATTERN			
THERAPIST			

Fig. 17-1. Form used to gather and record baseline information.

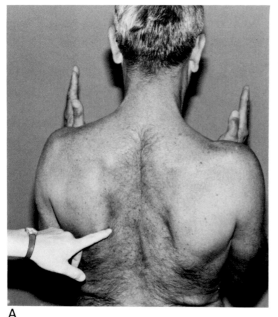

A

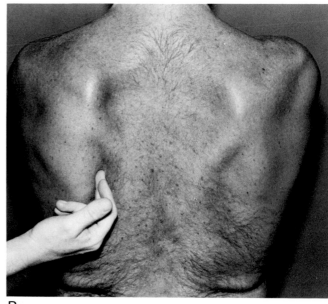

B

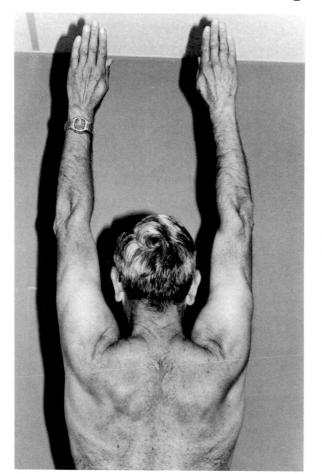

C

Fig. 17-2. (A–C) When checking the shoulder girdle, asymmetry of the scapula should be noted.

3. What problems can be managed later? For example, in a patient with a diagnosis of adhesive capsulitis, decreasing pain and gaining range of motion are immediate goals. Increasing strength and endurance would become part of the exercise program as pain decreases and range of motion improves.
4. What is the patient's lifestyle? To establish a realistic practical exercise program (i.e., one that the patient will follow), the patient's resources, work routine, and motivation must be considered.

TREATMENT

Once the priorities and the problem list have been established, an individualized treatment plan can be designed. Many exercise techniques and modalities have been described in the literature, but solid evidence as to which treatment is most effective is still lacking.[1,2,5,6,12,15,20–28] We believe that the most logical progression in treating a patient with shoulder dysfunction is as follows.

The overall goal is to establish normal scapulohumeral rhythm and normal biomechanics when the arm is elevated. All our exercises are geared to restoring a normal movement pattern through the available range of motion.

We do not believe in treating pain as a separate entity from a pathologic process. In our experience, pain is usually caused by a specific problem. Usually correcting the problem, such as relieving the inflammation or stretching out the tight muscle, will relieve the symptoms rather than mask them.

Our basic progression focuses on gaining mobility (range of motion) then stability. Unless contraindicated, we prefer to work on gaining active and passive range of motion concurrently. We also integrate the exercises into the patient's daily activities and encourage good posture habits. All patients are given a home program as well. The building up of strength and endurance are end goals, with attention on skill.

Table 17-1 is a flow chart that may be used as a guide for developing a physical therapy program for patients with shoulder dysfunction. This decision process is based on defining the patient's level of reactivity when performing specific motions, according to a classification system developed by Paris.[26] There are five levels of reactivity:

Acute Stages
Level I Pain at rest
Level II Pain with motion before soft tissue and/or joint resistance is felt

Subacute Stages
Level III Pain simultaneously as soft tissue/or joint resistance is felt

Level IV Pain as movement is attempted beyond soft tissue and/or joint resistance

Rehabilitation or Chronic Stage
Level V Pain-free

Criteria for advancing the exercise program are listed in Table 17-2.

Some modifications may be necessary depending on the patient's specific diagnosis and treatment. Obviously, if a specific motion is contraindicated, this motion is deferred until it is safe to begin it. For example, following a Bankart procedure for recurrent anterior shoulder dislocation, the patient's range of motion should be restricted in combined external rotation, abduction, and flexion as well as combined internal rotation and extension during the initial healing phase. Patients with recurrent shoulder instability should avoid unstable positions. By adding the specific contraindications to the diagnosis and evaluating where each patient belongs within this flow chart, an intelligent exercise program can be developed according to the patient's needs. The physical therapy program should also consider each patient's functional requirements.

Physical therapy treatment needs a specificity of training component tailored for the individual patient. An elderly patient will require exercises that are much less strenuous for strengthening than a young, healthy athlete who wishes to throw with his injured arm. Therefore, the rehabilitation goal for the athlete will have a higher level function and skill component. For the elderly patient, the specificity of training component may include functional retraining in dressing and kitchen activities. For the young baseball pitcher, component drills in throwing might be included.

Table 17-1. Physical Therapy Flow Chart[a]

Component Motions	Acute Stages		Subacute Stages		Chronic/ Rehabilitation Stage
	I	II	III	IV	V
	Too Painful for Exercise	Pain Felt Before Soft Tissue/Joint Resistance	Pain Felt Simultaneously with Soft Tissue/Joint Resistance	Soft Tissue/Joint Resistance Felt	Pain-free
Flexion/extension		Mobilizations: grade 1–2	Mobilizations: grade 2–3	Mobilizations: grade 3–4	
Abduction/adduction		PNF techniques	*1	*1	*1
External/internal rotation		Active assisted range of motion	Active exercise		
Horizontal abduction/adduction			Upper extremity weight-bearing: modified prone on elbows or modified plantigrade activities	Strength and endurance exercise	Progressive resistance exercise
Scapular motions			Stall bar activities		Functional training
	Breathing exercises for relaxation				
	Soft tissue massage	*2	*2	*2	*2
		Oscillations	*3	*3	*3
		Modalities such as ice, ultrasound, tens[b]		Heat	

See Table 7-2 for meaning of numbers and asterisks.

[a] Specific exercises are based on where the specific motions are restricted and which muscles are weak. Precautions and contraindications are based on the patient's diagnosis and, if applicable, any surgical intervention.

[b] Tens, transcutaneous electrical nerve stimulation.

In developing a successful rehabilitation program, choosing the correct exercise for the patient is only part of the treatment. The correct execution of the exercise by the patient along with postural education must be part of the total rehabilitation process. Table 17-3 is an example of the guidelines we use to instruct patients who have adhesive capsulitis, or frozen shoulder.

Table 17-2. Criteria for Advancing Exercise Program

1. Ability to perform exercise without pain
2. Ability to perform exercise in a normal movement pattern
*1. Exercises would be performed through increased pain-free range of motion, with greater amount of resistance at progressive levels
*2. Massage intensity increased as patient's pain level decreases
*3. Oscillations performed at increased range of motion at progressive levels

As stated previously, we believe that successful rehabilitation requires that the patient perform the exercises using normal body mechanics, avoiding substitution patterns. The following section will briefly outline physical therapy techniques for gaining range of motion, increasing strength, and improving function.

Range of Motion

One of the most widely used low-level exercises for gaining glenohumeral motion is the pendulum exercise. This passive exercise, as originally described by Codman,[4] utilizes the momentum gained by moving the trunk. Figure 17-3 illustrates the correct method of performing pendulums. The shoulder musculature is in a gravity-minimized position and the weight of the arm exerts gentle traction on the gleno-

Table 17-3. Guidelines for Exercise in Patients with Shoulder Dysfunction

Dos	Don'ts
Do the exercises given to you by your therapist! It's good to feel your muscles stretching	Don't push yourself beyond your pain limit!
	Don't just exercise once a day
Move your shoulder hourly	Don't overwork and overtire your shoulder
Listen to what your shoulder is trying to say to you	Don't life objects that are too heavy for you
Use good body mechanics	Don't work overhead for extended periods of time: Use a step ladder if reaching overhead brings on pain!
Use good posture! Straight and relaxed standing	
Take part in natural rhythmic activities such as rowing, swimming, bowling, golf	Avoid abnormal exercises such as push-ups and lifting weights at 90° abduction

humeral joint. When done properly, this exercise should be relatively pain-free and can be used successfully in postsurgical patients to gain flexion, extension, abduction, and adduction. This exercise will gently mobilize the glenohumeral joint.

Gaining range of motion in the early stages of shoulder rehabilitation depends on how the patient is positioned during exercise. Active assisted range of motion using the therapist or the uninvolved arm to support the affected extremity is most comfortably performed with the patient supine. This position requires the least effort because the scapula is adequately stabilized. Because a patient often has accompanying scapular weakness during the acute rehabilitation phase, the affected arm often has greater active and/or active assisted range of motion supine than in sitting or standing. As the patient's level of reactivity decreases and the shoulder becomes less acute, the exercise can become more active. When the patient regains adequate scapular muscle stability, the positions to exercise can then progress to gravity-eliminated positions. Wall climbing is often used as a home exercise in an effort to gain glenohumeral range of motion in patients with adhesive capsulitis, tendonitis, bursitis, or who have had shoulder surgery. However, if this exercise is given before the patient has adequate scapulohumeral muscle control, the patient will perform wall climbing using substitute motions such as elevating the scapula. This will not achieve glenohumeral motion and may cause further impingement at the glenohumeral joint. The ability to hyperextend the lumbar spine and give a false appearance of shoulder motions makes wall climbing a poor choice of exercise.

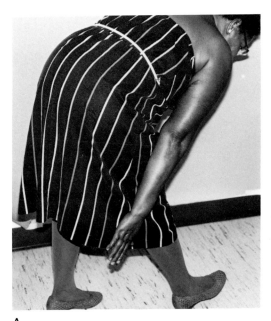 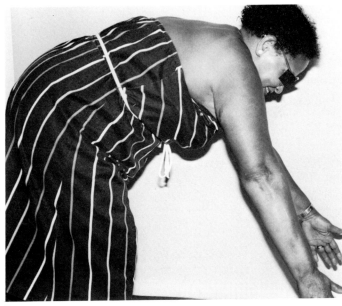

A   B

Fig. 17-3. (A,B) Pendulum exercises used in a patient with total shoulder replacement.

An alternative early home exercise for gaining glenohumeral range of motion is to teach the patient to roll a large beach ball on a waist-high table while standing. The patient can roll the ball forward and backward (to gain flexion and extension), side to side (to gain adduction and abduction) and in circles (for combined motions including rotations). The patient should be instructed to move the glenohumeral joint and to avoid substitute motions (Fig. 17-4).

A variety of facilitation techniques to increase range of motion may be helpful. If the limitation is primarily caused by muscle and other soft tissue tightness, massage techniques, proprioceptive neuromuscular facilitation (PNF) and modalities may be of use. Superimposing the PNF techniques of rhythmic stabilization, hold relax, or contract relax on active assisted range of motion in diagonal planes has been demonstrated to be helpful.[28,31] The use of modalities such as ultrasound, heat, and cold have also been shown to be effective as adjuncts to exercise.[21]

When restriction is primarily due to joint tightness, mobilization techniques have been recommended by Paris, Maitland, Karltenborn, and others.[6,16,20,26] These techniques include traction and glides in varying intensity (Fig. 17-5). The theory of mobilization is to restore normal physiological motion to the specific joints affected. For example, if the glenohumeral joint capsule is tight, the head of the humerus is unable to glide caudally (downward) when the patient elevates the arm. Performance of this motion passively by the therapist is intended to help restore the normal biomechanical movement to this joint. Although these techniques are widely used in physical therapy clinics today with apparently good results, little documentation in the literature confirms their effectiveness over the more traditional methods.[22,24]

Recently, continuous passive motion (CPM) machines to gain early range of motion, promote joint nutrition, and aid in joint healing have been used as part of the early rehabilitation process in the immediate postoperative period following joint replacement and reconstructive surgery. To date, CPM has been used successfully as part of the rehabilitation process in patients who have had total knee replacements[7] and those who have had reconstructive surgery of the shoulder.[8] In a preliminary report by Craig,[8] 48 patients who had undergone various shoulder procedures, such as rotator cuff repair, anterior acromioplasty, coracoacromial ligament excision with bursec-

tomy, or total shoulder replacement, used CPM to provide forward flexion and external rotation immediately postoperatively in addition to the routine rehabilitation protocol. This group was compared with 28 similar patients who did not use CPM. The CPM group achieved target range of motion significantly earlier, experienced less pain, and had, on the average, a shortened length of hospital stay. No adverse effects from use of the CPM were noted. It appears from these early reports that use of continuous passive motion may play an important role in the early postoperative management of appropriate shoulder patients. We have not yet incorporated it into our regular therapeutic management.

Muscle Performance

To increase upper extremity function following a shoulder injury, exercise to restore muscular strength and endurance should be part of the rehabilitation process. As shoulder mobility increases, active muscle control needs to be obtained in the newly gained range of motion for stability. A variety of techniques and modalities are available for increasing both strength and endurance of the shoulder girdle musculature.[11,12,15,17,28,31] Correct execution of the exercises utilizing normal rhythmic motion is important to avoid further damage to the injured shoulder.

In the early stages of increasing strength, active exercises and isometrics within the available range of motion are employed. As the muscles are ready to take resistance, surgical tubing or Theraband for graded resistance can be used by the patient at home (Fig. 17-6). We gauge the correct amount of resistance to be the force one's muscles can take when performing the desired motion with a normal movement pattern. If the patient uses a substitute motion to complete the desired task, too much demand is being placed on the muscle (Figs. 17-7, 17-8).

Another valuable technique in the early stages of gaining stability is the use of isometric contractions at different points in the range of motion. Rhythmic stabilization, which is controlled isometric contractions of both the agonist and antagonist, is a useful technique for gaining stability.

Positioning the patient's upper extremity in weight-bearing positions of the development sequence is also helpful in facilitating activity in the shoulder muscula-

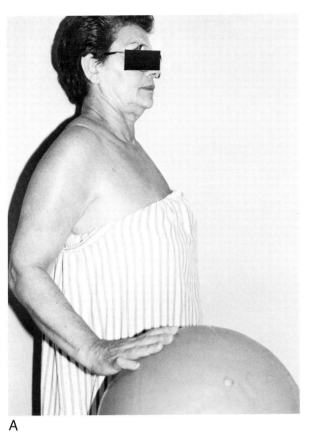

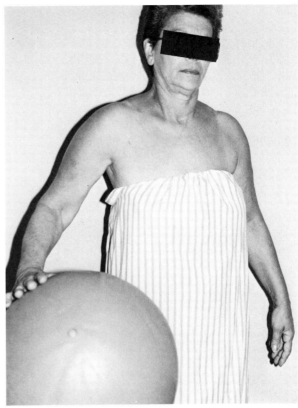

Fig. 17-4. (A–C) A patient with limited shoulder motion using a beach ball to gain glenohumeral flexion, extension, rotation, and abduction.

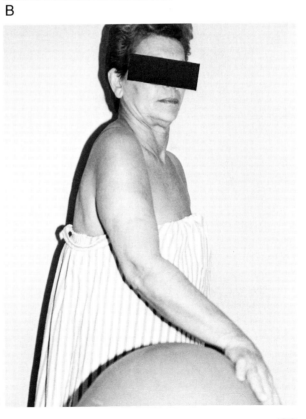

C

529

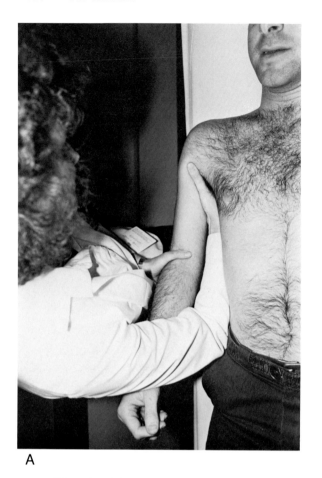
A

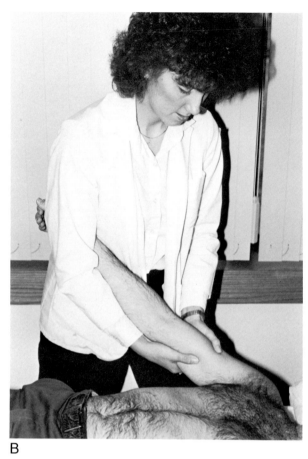
B

Fig. 17-5. (A) A physical therapist applying gentle traction to the glenohumeral joint. **(B)** The mobilization technique of distraction is used to facilitate forward flexion.

ture. The quadruped position—on hands and knees—requires muscle activity of the entire shoulder girdle complex.

In the end stages of rehabilitation of the active individual, formal weight training programs may be of use. However, using the proper amount of resistance and using the arm in a normal movement pattern to avoid impingement is of utmost importance. For example, lateral raises on the exercise machine, which is an exercise designed to increase deltoid strength, has the patient positioned with the arms abducted to 90° and internally rotated. This exercise can cause impingement of the supraspinatus or the long head of biceps or even bony impingement of the greater tuberosity against the acromion. If a patient is to undergo weight training on machines, care

must be taken to modify the exercises to avoid further injury.[11] Use of isokinetics can be helpful in building strength and endurance. Isokinetic exercise is different from exercising with free weights because dynamic muscle activity is performed at a constant angular velocity (Fig. 17-9). This allows a muscle or muscle group to work maximally throughout the full arc of motion.[30] However, the same caution in avoiding poor biomechanics must be observed when using isokinetic machines. The most important disadvantage of all these instruments is that the exercising levers of these devices are uniaxial, permitting movement only in a single cardinal plane, whereas normal shoulder function combines glenohumeral and scapular movement and the resultant movement is multiplanar.

The PNF techniques may also be used for pro-

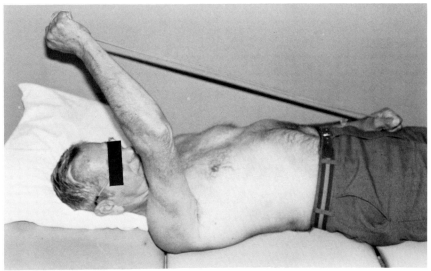

A

Fig. 17-6. (A,B) A patient after rotator cuff repair using Thera-band for early muscle strengthening during the rehabilitation phase.

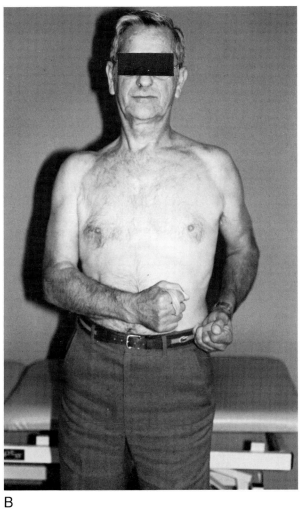

B

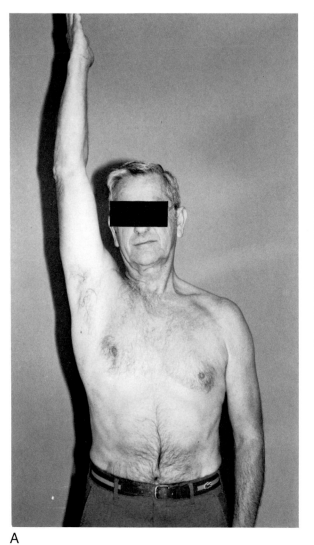
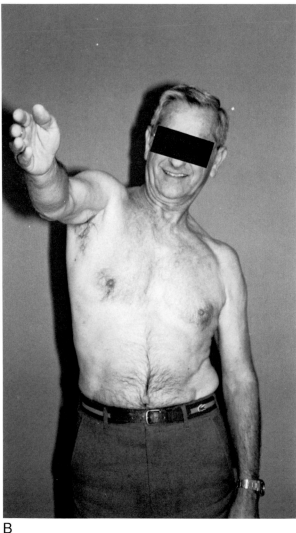

A   B

Fig. 17-7. (**A**) The same patient performing shoulder flexion with a normal movement pattern. (**B**) Substitute scapular motion and lateral trunk flexion to elevate the arm, to compensate for true glenohumeral motion.

gressive resistance exercise. Their patterns are diagonal: spiral combinations of movements similar to normal movement patterns.[31] Maximal resistance training can be carried out by the therapist applying the resistance manually (Fig. 17-10), by the patient using elastic strapping such as Theraband or having the patient exercise on a triplicate pulley system (Fig. 17-11A,B). An incorrect position for resistive exercising is shown in Figure 17-11C: as this is the position of impingement.

In a recent study designed to examine the effects of proprioceptive neuromuscular facilitation techniques versus conventional weight training programs (bench press and leg press) on muscular strength and athletic performance, Nelson and his colleagues found both techniques successful in increasing strength. However, PNF was demonstrated to be significantly more effective in improving the functional activities of distance throwing and vertical jumping.[23] Therefore, PNF patterns might be more advantageous to use in rehabilitation programs for two important reasons: first, because of the functional carry over; and

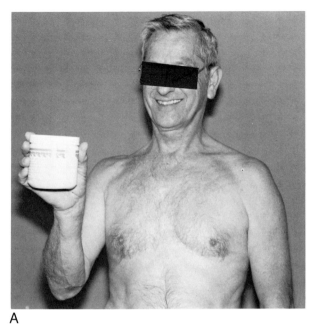
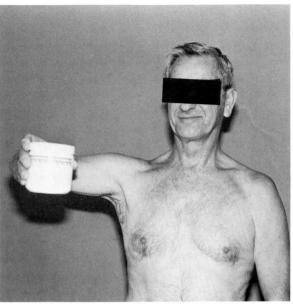

A B

Fig. 17-8. Proper body mechanics should be utilized during functional activities. (**A**) Correctly lifting an object. (**B**) Incorrectly lifting the same object. Positioning the arm out in 90° of abduction can cause impingement. Do not let the elbow "fly" when reaching upward.

Fig. 17-9. A patient performing isokinetic shoulder flexion and extension exercise during the chronic/rehabilitation phase.

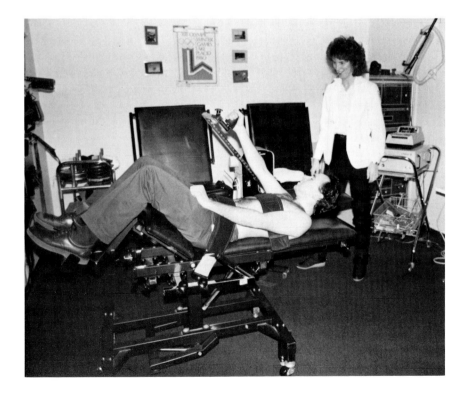

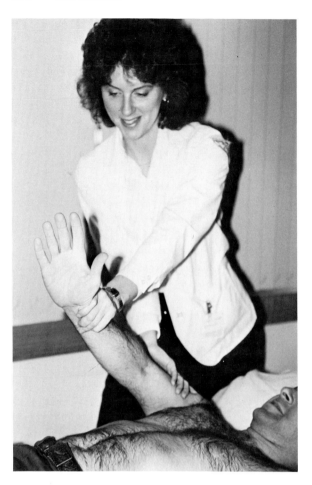

Fig. 17-10. A physical therapist applying manual resistance in the PNF diagonal motion of flexion, abduction, and external rotation.

second, because of safety The PNF patterns are more easily adapted to normal scapulohumeral motion because simultaneous combinations of rotation and elevation are permitted.

Gaining strength is only one aspect of restoring muscle performance. Increasing muscle endurance must also be considered. Exercises utilizing low resistance with a high number of repetitions are used to achieve this goal. Endurance exercises can be done using isokinetic machines or through repetitive exercises in functional positions.

Functional Training

An important component of any rehabilitation program is functional exercise based on the patient's spe-cific needs. In the early stages of physical therapy, exercises should be integrated into the patient's daily routine for carry over from the formal exercise periods. Activities to promote normal rhythmic arm swing when walking can provide gentle range-of-motion exercise to the injured shoulder. As the patient progresses to a strengthening program, incorporating exercises into a functional activity is beneficial. In athletes, component drills of a sport can be chosen to help build strength and endurance. In designing the specific activity, the therapist needs to consider the patient's strength, endurance, range of motion, and any contraindications, in order to obtain the desired effect.

SUMMARY

Although this chapter is an overview of the rehabilitation of the shoulder girdle, the information presented here provides a framework applicable to all patients. The specific choice of how and when to progress individual patients will be dependent on the diagnosis, intervention, evaluation findings, and the desired outcome. The general progression should be consistent.

Acute Phase

The treatment goals are to teach joint protection, maintain joint kinematics, and decrease pain and inflammation. Specific techniques to use at this stage include active and passive range-of-motion exercises, gentle mobilization, joint protection and pacing activities, and the use of physical agents such as ice and transcutaneous electrical nerve stimulation.

Subacute Phase

During the subacute phase, the treatment goals shift more to restoration of range of motion, increasing soft tissue flexibility, and increasing muscle strength. Added exercise techniques at this stage include stretching and gentle strengthening.

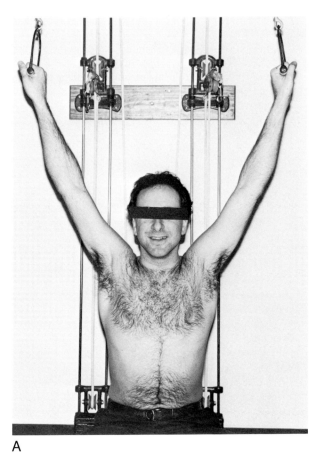

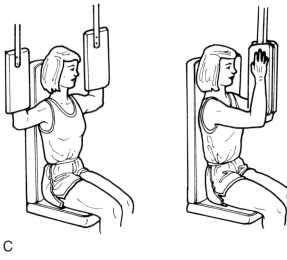

Fig. 17-11. (**A,B**) A patient performing progressive resistance exercises in PNF patterns using a triplicate pulley system. (**C**) An example of *how not* to perform progressive resistance exercise. The patient's poor body mechanics and the arms' abducted at 90° may cause impingement.

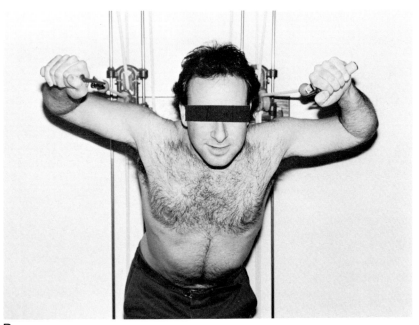

Rehabilitation or Chronic Phase (Pain-free)

At this stage, increasing strength, power, and endurance become the priorities. Restoration of normal functional activity is part of the therapy program.

The timing of these phases is dependent on the reason for the shoulder dysfunction. The specific exercise progression and the frequency, intensity, and duration of therapy will be dependent on the patient's age, diagnosis, associated medical problems, and functional goals. These are discussed in connection with the various pathologic conditions of the shoulder.

REFERENCES

1. Aronen JG, Regan K: Decreasing the incidence of recurrence of first time anterior shoulder dislocations with rehabilitation. Am J Sports Med 12:283, 1984

2. Bulger DY, Binder AI, Hazelman BL et al: Frozen shoulder: prospective clinical study with an evaluation of three treatment regimens. Ann Rheum Dis 43:353, 1984

3. Calliet R: Shoulder Pain, 2nd ed. FA Davis, Philadelphia, 1981

4. Codman EA: The Shoulder: Rupture of the Supraspinatus Tendon and Other Lesions in or about the Subacromial Bursa. G. Miller & Co., Brooklyn, New York, 1934

5. Connolly, J, Regen R, Evans AB: The management of the painful stiff shoulder. Clin Orthop 84:97, 1972

6. Cookson JC, Kent BE: Orthopaedic manual therapy—an overview. Part I: The extremities. Phys Ther 59:136, 1979

7. Couts RD, Toth C, Karta J: The role of CPM in the rehabilitation of the total knee patient. In Total Knee Arthroplasty—A Comprehensive Approach. Hungerford D, Krakow K, Kenna R (eds): Williams & Wilkins, Baltimore, 1984

8. Craig EV: Continuous passive motion in the rehabilitation of the surgically reconstructed shoulder. A preliminary report. Second Open Meeting of the American Shoulder and Elbow Surgeons, New Orleans, Louisiana, February 1986

9. Cyriax JH, Cyriax PJ: Illustrated Manual of Orthopaedic Medicine. Butterworth, London, 1983

10. Davis GJ, Goves JA, Larson RL: Functional examination of the shoulder girdle. Phys Sports Med 4:82, 1981

11. Einhorn AR: Shoulder rehabilitation: equipment modifications. J Sports Phys Ther 6:247, 1985

12. Elsmer RC et al: Protocol for strength testing and rehabilitation of the upper extremity. J Orthop Sports Phys Ther 4:229, 1983

13. Hoppenfeld S: Physical Examination of the Spine and Extremities. Appleton-Century-Crofts, Norwalk, Ct, 1976

14. Inman VT, Saunders JB, Abbot LC: Observations of the function of the shoulder joint. J Bone Joint Surg 26:1, 1946

15. Jobe FW, Moynes DR: Delineation of diagnostic criteria and a rehabilitation program for rotator cuff injuries. Am J Sports Med 10:336, 1982

16. Kaltenborn FM: Mobilization of the Extremity Joints: Examination and Basic Treatment Techniques. Olaf Norlis, Bokhandel, Oslo, 1980

17. Kegerreis ST: The construction and implementation of functional progressions as a component of athletic rehabilitation. J Orthop Sports Phys Ther 4:14, 1983

18. Kendall FP, McCreary EK: Muscles Testing and Function, 3rd ed. Williams & Wilkins, Baltimore, 1983

19. Luttgens K, Wells K: Kinesiology: Scientific Basis of Human Motion, 7th ed. WB Saunders, Philadelphia, 1982

20. Maitland GD: Treatment of the glenohumeral joint by passive movement. Physiotherapy 69:3, 1983

21. Michlovitz S: Thermal Agents. FA Davis, Philadelphia, 1986

22. Moutz V: Evaluation of manipulation and other manual therapy. Sc and J Rehab Med 11:173, 1979

23. Nelson AG, Chambers RS, McGown, CM, Penrose KW: Proprioceptive neuromuscular facilitation versus weight training for enhancement of muscular strength and athletic performance. J Orthop Sports Phys Ther 7:250, 1986

24. Nicholson GG: The effects of passive joint mobilization on pain and hypomobility associated with adhesive capsulitis of the shoulder. J Sports Phys Ther 6:238, 1985

25. O'Donoghue DH: Treatment of Injuries to Athletes. WB Saunders, Philadelphia, 1984

26. Paris SV: Extremity Dysfunction and Mobilization. Institute Press, Atlanta, GA, 1980

27. Radin E: Relevant biomechanics in the treatment of musculoskeletal injuries and disorders. Clin Orthop 146:2, 1980

28. Sullivan PE, Markos PD, Minor MA: An Integrated Approach to Therapeutic Exercise—Theory and Clinical Application. Reston Publishing, Reston, VA, 1982

29. Tank R, Halbach J: Physical therapy evaluation of the

shoulder complex in athletes. J Orthop Sports Phys Ther 3:108–119, 1982

30. Thistle HG, Hislop HG, Moffroid M et al: Isokinetic contraction: A new concept of resistive exercise. Arch Phys Med Rehab 48:279, 1967

31. Voss DE, Ionta MK, Meyers BJ: Proprioceptive Neuromuscular Facilitation: Patterns and Techniques, 3rd ed. Harper & Row, Philadelphia, 1985

18

SHOULDER INFECTIONS

Principles of Antibiotic Therapy

Newton E. Hyslop, Jr.

Optimal treatment of bacterial infection of the structures making up the shoulder requires consideration of the anatomy; analysis of the organism(s) isolated from clinical specimens; selection of antibiotics based on comparison of the actions, pharmacologic properties, and adverse effects of antibiotics active against the organism; and determination of the merits and risks of operative procedures (e.g., aspiration, irrigation, debridement) in achieving treatment goals.

While complete descriptions of available antibiotics are presented elsewhere and are subject to change, the general principles of treatment remain constant.[8,18,20,23,24]

IDENTIFICATION OF THE PATHOGEN(S)

It is a truism that making the appropriate choice of antimicrobial therapy first requires isolation of the pathogen(s). Unfortunately, it is also true that cultures of *sterile* fluids and tissues collected under clinical conditions will yield a bacterial isolate sufficiently frequently that cautious interpretation of the significance of certain bacterial isolates is always required, even when the specimen was obtained from what is believed to be an infected site.

The first and foremost safeguard against misinterpretation of culture results, whether positive or negative, is comprehensive microbiological evaluation of clinical specimens. The slight additional cost is minute compared to the consequences of failure to identify and isolate the pathogen(s). Anaerobes and other fastidious bacteria, fungi, and mycobacteria will be overlooked unless specimens are specifically examined for them. Failure to do so may lead to erroneous treatment based on "negative" cultures, or on recovery of only one agent from a polymicrobial infection.

Therefore, *routine evaluation* should always include blood cultures and evaluation of clinical specimens for a range of organisms. Any tissues submitted for histologic study should also be cultured. Fluids and pus should be examined microscopically with Gram and acid-fast bacilli (AFB) stains and potassium hydroxide (KOH). Unless specimen material is scant, normally all specimens should also be cultured for bacteria, fungi, and mycobacteria. Specimens for bacterial isolation should be plated for incubation under routine and anaerobic conditions, and special media

541

should be used where appropriate (e.g., chocolate agar plates or slants) in addition to the usual broth inoculation.

Comprehensive microbiological evaluation requires a generous sample: the equivalent of 2 to 3 ml when possible. When pus is not present, tissue specimens are preferred to intraoperative swabs alone. Ideally, pus and fluids should be transferred to a prereduced carrier vial to maintain anaerobic conditions, but submission in a syringe is acceptable. Since irrigation fluids dilute the concentration of organisms, they are generally less satisfactory culture specimens than a smaller undiluted specimen, although they are still useful.

Normal skin flora (e.g., coagulase-negative staphylococci, "diphtheroids," *Proprionobacter* species) and respiratory flora (e.g., viridans streptococci) are often isolated from difficult-to-obtain low-volume aspiration specimens and from tissue specimens that require grinding (e.g., bone) before inoculation. Microbiology laboratories normally inoculate specimens onto culture plates and into liquid media. Since survival and replication of even one organism is possible in liquid media, a discrepancy between finding normal flora organisms growing only in liquid culture and not on plates is usually explained as minute contamination of specimen at the time of collection, or during handling in the laboratory.

Consequently, *normal flora isolates* are usually dismissed even when obtained from a presumably infected site. However, when the site contains a foreign body, such as a prosthesis, the true pathogen may be a member of the normal flora (e.g., coagulase-negative staphylococci), especially in subacute infections. If so, it is usually present on the primary plates, and may also be seen in Gram stains.[2]

Misinterpretation of recovery of a common contaminant only from liquid media may be avoided by including *colony counts* as part of the routine bacteriologic evaluation of tissue aspirates and of specimens requiring grinding, especially when patients have special risk factors for infection with a member of the normal flora. Since colony counts use larger inocula than routine plates, growth of an organism in liquid media together with multiple colonies in colony counts lends credence to its pathogenic significance when a "common contaminant" is recovered from a properly collected and handled specimen.

FACTORS IN CHOOSING ANTIBACTERIAL AGENTS

Effective treatment of bone and joint infections caused by the most common bacterial pathogens as a rule requires that *bactericidal* (cidal) antibiotic concentrations reach the organism. Although *bacteriostatic* (static) antibiotics may cure skin and soft tissue infections caused by the same organisms, treatment of bone and joint infections with static agents frequently results in relapse, and occasionally even fails to suppress an active infection.

Cidal Versus Static Antibiotics

Cidal antibiotics as a general rule are antibiotics capable of binding covalently to cell wall or cell membrane targets (e.g., β-lactams, vancomycin) at concentrations which are achievable in vivo. With the exception of the aminoglycosides, which are also cidal, intracellular-targeted agents (e.g., chloramphenicol, lincomycins, macrolides, sulfonamides, tetracyclines) are static: the growth of the organism is only inhibited in the presence of antibiotic and resumes on transfer to antibiotic-free medium.

Division of antibiotics into static and cidal categories is not quite so simple, however. While chemical class is a clue, at lower concentrations even cidal agents have static effects (e.g., β-lactams). Conversely, antibiotics that are static when acting alone can be cidal in combination (e.g., trimethoprim–sulfamethoxazole). Finally, a particular agent may be static for most classes of organisms but still be bactericidal with a few: for example, chloramphenicol is cidal against *Hemophilus influenzae* and *Streptococcus pneumoniae* in vitro and in vivo, whereas it is static against most other gram-negative and gram-positive bacteria.

Thus the conventional division of antibiotics into cidal and static categories has certain important exceptions and qualifications. In particular, members of the β-lactam class differ in antibacterial effect as a result of minor chemical differences. Both penicillins and cephalosporins exert their antibacterial effect by chemically reacting through the β-lactam function with specific cell wall proteins, many of which are enzymes involved in synthesis of bacterial cell walls and whose function is subsequently modified. Because of chemical differences among the β-lactams, not all of the enzymes are equal targets for each β-lactam.

Not all the enzymes are necessary for the organism's survival. To have a lethal effect, an antibiotic must either have a high affinity for a key enzyme (*lethal hit*), or it must inactivate several nonlethal enzymes whose collective inactivation is lethal. Partial inactivation of a key enzyme or inactivation of too few nonlethal enzymes produces only growth inhibition and generates aberrant bacterial forms. Since such partially and fully inhibited organisms are able to recover on removal to antibiotic-free media, the result is a static effect paradoxically produced by a cidal class of antibiotics.

Tolerance to Cidal Antibiotics

A static effect on interaction between β-lactam and susceptible organism can occur by any one of three mechanisms: (1) too low a concentration to achieve sufficient chemical alteration of the target protein(s) to affect function; (2) an intrinsic resistance to a cidal effect, termed tolerance, usually limited to particular strains belonging to a species otherwise normally susceptible to cidal action when exposed to a clinically attainable concentration of antibiotic; (3) altered binding affinity for target proteins or reduced access, as a result of differences in sidechain bulk or lipophilicity.

The concentration-dependence of β-lactams' effects on bacteria is highly relevant to choosing dosing regimens for specific disease states, in which cure is related to constant exposure of organisms to cidal concentrations of antibiotics (e.g., endocarditis). It is not surprising that a cidal action requires exposure to a higher concentration than those that partially inhibit (*subinhibitory*) or completely inhibit (*inhibitory*) growth. The minimal concentrations required for bactericidal (MBC) and inhibitory (MIC) effects on a clinical isolate are determined by inoculating fixed numbers of bacteria into broths containing serial concentrations of antibiotic, incubating for a constant interval, and then reading turbidity to assess growth inhibition. Cidal action is checked by subculturing aliquots of inhibited broths onto plates that are then incubated and observed for growth.

The *MBC/MIC ratio* for β-lactams is generally 5 to 10. When it is 20 or greater, an isolate is considered to be tolerant to the cidal action at clinically attainable concentrations, even if a cidal effect can be demonstrated at higher, nonphysiological concentrations.[19] While the full clinical relevance of tolerant strains in clinical infections remains to be determined, with more laboratories determining MICs and MBCs of clinical isolates in recent years, a number of such strains have been recovered from serious *Staphylococcus aureus* infections. In several instances of endocarditis, strains deemed tolerant by in vitro assay seemed clinically resistant to treatment with the corresponding β-lactam and did not improve until therapy was shifted to vancomycin.

The "generations" of cephalosporins illustrate the alterations in binding affinity and access among chemical congeners that in turn affect their cidal activity against a diverse range of bacteria. While reactivity of β-lactam function remains virtually identical, sidechain and nuclear structural alterations that broaden antibacterial spectrum by promoting binding to cell wall proteins from a greater variety of species often are bought at the expense of changed affinity for old targets. For example, the efficacy of cephalosporins against *Staphylococcus aureus* diminishes progressively on passing from first- to third-generation cephalosporins, while the efficacy against gram-negative rods markedly improves. Consequently, third-generation cephalosporins, as a rule, are ineffective in staphylococcal infections but very effective against susceptible gram-negative organisms.

Synergy Between Static Antibiotics and Phagocytes in Disposal of Organisms

A static action of β-lactams does appear to increase susceptibility of organisms to complement activation and to phagocytosis and intracellular killing by neutrophils and macrophages. This enhanced disposal of antibiotic-treated bacteria by phagocytes is, in fact, probably the dominant mechanism of successful treatment of common less serious infections, such as cellulitis, pneumonia, and certain soft tissue infections, with static-class antibiotics or low doses of cidal-class antibiotics.

The concept of the synergistic role of phagocytes in the efficacy of static antibiotics is reinforced by their complete failure in treating bacterial infections that complicate granulocyte disorders (e.g., leukemia, agranulocytosis). These patients require cidal-class antibiotics maintained at cidal concentrations in vivo to control invasive infection.

If the successful use of static antibiotics and static concentrations of cidal antibiotics in treating common pathogens in skin and soft tissue infections depends on enhanced susceptibility of antibiotic-inhibited bacteria to phagocytic disposal, the high failure rate when bone and joint infections are treated only with static agents, or with low concentrations of cidal antibiotics, points to an intrinsic failure of phagocyte synergy in these infections, as in endocarditis. Failure of phagocyte synergy probably reflects problems of access for antibiotics and for phagocytes to bacteria sequestered in the dead bone, necrotic tissue, and loculated pus characteristic of osteomyelitis. This hypothesis is also consistent with the proven need for debridement and for prolonged treatment with high doses of cidal antibiotics.[17,18]

COMBINATIONS OF ANTIBIOTICS

While simultaneous administration of two or more antibiotics is often essential in treating *polymicrobial* infection, *single-organism* infections have usually been treated with only one antibiotic. As described above, a cidal agent has been shown to be always required for particular infections, such as endocarditis.

Synergy Between Two or More Antibiotics

Studies on mechanisms by which antibiotics kill bacteria, such as in vitro analysis of *kill rates*, have demonstrated that certain combinations of antimicrobials acting together may be more potent than either acting alone, or else may kill faster (synergy). So far, these laboratory findings have received their greatest application in the treatment of bacterial endocarditis caused by single organisms, especially viridans streptococci, enterococci, coagulase-positive and coagulase-negative staphylococci, and gram-negative rods, where the role of combination therapy has been most clearly established.[10]

The most obvious role for synergistic therapy is exemplified by the *Enterococcus*, for which there is no single cidal antibiotic, but which is killed by the combination of gentamicin in low concentration with high concentrations of either penicillin G or ampicillin. A second indication is exemplified by the case of viridans streptococci, which are usually exquisitely sensitive to penicillin G. Combination therapy with gentamicin or streptomycin permits a shorter course of parenteral treatment of S. *viridans* endocarditis, since short-course dual therapy is as effective as prolonged treatment with penicillin alone.

Staphylococci represent another situation where synergistic therapy often is considered. First, strains tolerant to the cidal action of β-lactams may require combined treatment to obtain a cidal action at clinically attainable concentrations. Second, even organisms susceptible to the cidal action of β-lactams may not all be in the growth phase and will therefore be relatively resistant to a β-lactam alone. This differential susceptibility of log and plateau growth phases may explain the slow killing effect of penicillins and cephalosporins in clinical studies of endocarditis. Blood cultures treated with antibiotic removal devices show that bacteremia can continue for 2 to 3 days after treatment has started.

Finally, faster kill rates may be important in controlling infection because of the adverse clinical consequences of continued survival of bacteria, such as in the treatment of staphylococcal endocarditis. In treating *methicillin-sensitive* staphylococcal endocarditis with penicillinase-resistant penicillins, the combination of nafcillin with rifampin and/or gentamicin has been used. For *methicillin-resistant* staphylococci, a similar potentiation of vancomycin's cidal effect has been demonstrated with some stains of S. *aureus* and S. *epidermidis*, provided that the isolate is sensitive to each of the agents in the combination. However, since antagonism has also been observed with combined therapy of certain staphylococcal stains, *in vitro analysis of combinations is imperative*.

In the case of gram-negative rods, tolerance to β-lactams (a high MBC/MIC ratio) is probably more common than is generally recognized, but under most conditions it is not clinically important. However, where bactericidal activity is required, such as in gram-negative infection in agranulocytosis, endocarditis, or meningitis, a cidal action may be achieved with some of the newer β-lactams alone, by combination with a second β-lactam, or by adding an aminoglycoside.

Testing for Synergy, Indifference, and Antagonism: Serum Bactericidal Assay

Formal demonstration of antibiotic synergy is a research laboratory procedure. Since synergy cannot be predicted, with the exception of synergistic action of penicillins with gentamicin against enterococci, it is essential that some clinical approximation be made if treatment with antibiotic combinations seems indicated.

The serum bactericidal assay, given proper controls, methodology, and experienced personnel, is a reasonable means of clinically assessing the synergistic effect of combination therapy. It also allows detection of two other possible outcomes: *indifference*, in which there is no qualitative or quantitative improvement in antimicrobial activity beyond the sum of the effects of the agents individually; and *antagonism*, where the cidal action or the potency of the agents singly is reversed when they are combined.[10] Blood samples should be drawn at multiple times to reflect the various peak and trough combinations, and the several samples should be assayed simultaneously using the same suspension of the organism to ensure comparable data. Also, drug assays (e.g., gentamicin levels) should be performed on each of the serum samples to document the presence and concentration of those drugs that can be measured chemically. Finally, before beginning combination therapy the serum cidal and static concentrations for the principal antibiotic alone should be determined against the clinical isolate to interpret the effects of the in vivo combination.

Results of serum bactericidal activity are expressed as the highest serum dilution still capable of killing the organism. Thus, in a typical synergistic result for the combination of nafcillin (10 g/day) with rifampicin (600 mg/day), the peak serum cidal activity shifts from 1:16 on nafcillin alone (10 g/day) to 1:1024 with the combination.

Since there is considerable strain specificity among organisms in the responses to antibiotic combinations, it is absolutely essential that the *clinical isolate obtained at the beginning of treatment be saved* by the laboratory for later studies during the course of treatment. Alterations in treatment may be required by the development of hypersensitivity or by other adverse responses to single drug or combination drug therapy.

Other Reasons for Using Combinations of Antibiotics in Treatment of Single-Organism Infections

Other justifications for multiple drug therapy of single-organism infections, besides synergy, are: (1) better tissue distribution of antimicrobial activity through selection of cidal agents with different pharmacologic properties; and (2) prevention of emergence of resistant mutants as a result of selective pressure during prolonged drug treatment.

These two objectives underlie the multiple-drug treatment of tuberculosis. Prevention of emergence of resistance is also used to justify two-drug treatment of gram-negative rod bacteremia in the leukopenic patient. Selection of drug-resistant mutants as a result of treatment with single cidal antimicrobials fortunately is not a common problem in osteomyelitis and septic arthritis. However, when osteomyelitis is treated with static agents, such as erythromycin, chloramphenicol, and tetracycline, selection of resistant organisms is a very common outcome, and illustrates yet again the important role of cidal antibiotic regimens in the management of bacterial infections of bones and joints.

COMBINED THERAPY WITH ONE AGENT THAT IS NOT AN ANTIBIOTIC: AUGMENTATION

Potentiation of the effect of an antimicrobial by addition of a second nonantibiotic drug is limited principally to the β-lactam family, and involves two separate mechanisms of potentiation.

Probenecid: Modification of In Vivo Half-Lives

Probenecid enhancement of blood levels of penicillins and cephalosporins has been well studied and is used commonly in outpatient settings (e.g., treatment of sexually transmitted diseases). The role of probenecid-enhanced antibiotic blood levels in treatment of bone and joint infections is limited to special circumstances in which oral treatment is appropriate.[17]

A sulfonamide analogue, probenecid competes for tubular secretion of organic acids, including those β-lactams with significant renal excretion by this mechanism: penicillin, ampicillin, amoxacillin, other charged penicillins, and cephalexin. Note that highly protein-bound β-lactams have little tubular secretion and therefore their excretion patterns are unaffected by the administration of probenecid.

Simultaneous administration of probenecid and an appropriate β-lactam prolongs the half-life and raises the average blood levels of the antibiotic. With high doses of oral antibiotic plus probenecid, it is possible to reach blood levels comparable to those achieved with parenteral therapy. However, *patient compliance must be complete to ensure effective treatment*, and compliance and absorption should be monitored occasionally by measurement of serum cidal levels.

Probenecid promotes uric acid secretion, and therefore initiation of treatment requires stepwise increase to full dosage to avoid crystalluria and stone formation. Probenecid is also a potent immunogen. Consequently, long-term combination therapy is frequently complicated by hypersensitivity reactions, especially fever and rash, which confuses the issue of which drug is responsible. Short-course treatment is much less likely to result in allergic reaction.

Inhibitors of Microbial Beta-Lactamases: Augmentation of Antibiotic Potency

Enzymatic hydrolysis of the β-lactam rings of penicillins and cephalosporins is the most common mechanism of antibiotic resistance to β-lactams. Although the responsible enzymes (β-lactamases) vary somewhat in structure and specificity from species to species, they can be grouped into approximately six categories based on the types of β-lactam structures that are susceptible and resistant, and on whether the enzyme is a product of plasmid or chromosomal DNA.

Recently, chemical analogues of β-lactams have been synthesized that have no antimicrobial activity but bind tightly to the enzyme-combining site of one or more β-lactamases. When present in excess, analogues such as clavulenic acid and sulbactam bind up all β-lactamase produced and protect β-lactam antibiotics that are otherwise susceptible to enzymatic hydrolysis. Inactivation of β-lactamases permits intact antibiotic to reach and bind to the cell wall target proteins. Thus, a β-lactamase-susceptible penicillin, such as ampicillin, becomes bactericidal for penicillinase-producing *Staphylococcus aureus*, which otherwise would have destroyed the drug and been totally resistant.

The in vivo efficacy of combinations of β-lactam antibiotics with an augmenting drug that itself is without antimicrobial activity requires two conditions: (1) nearly identical pharmacologic properties with regard to distribution, half-life, etc., and (2) accumulation of the augmenting agent at the infecting site in high enough concentrations to parallel in vitro competition for microbial β-lactamase.

Augmentation therapy is not equivalent to a synergistic action of two antimicrobials acting in concert. Combinations of clavulinic acid with ampicillin and with ticarcillin have only recently been introduced into general use. Until their reliability in the treatment of penicillinase-positive, methicillin-sensitive Staphylococcus aureus infections of bones and joints is established, this type of combined treatment should be considered experimental. Finally, it remains to be seen what incidence of hypersensitivity reactions and other adverse effects will complicate the use of β-lactamase inhibitors in clinical practice.

PHARMACOLOGIC CONSIDERATIONS UNIQUE TO BONE AND JOINT INFECTIONS

The structures most commonly involved in shoulder infections, whether by direct inoculation or hematogenous spread, are the synovium, cartilage, periosteum, bone, lymphatics, and occasionally fat.[3,12,14,15]

Fibrous capsular material, tendons, and muscle are normally highly resistant to infection, even operative infections. However, postoperative hematomas represent important nonanatomical compartments for bacterial replication. The role of *prophylactic antibiotics* in preventing operative wound infections results largely from adequate blood levels of antibiotics during the period of hematoma formation, intraoperatively and postoperatively.

Choice of Antibiotic

As a general rule, if a drug or drug combination has been shown to be effective in the treatment of bacterial endocarditis, it is a potential candidate for use in treating osteomyelitis and septic arthritis.

However, the pharmacologic characteristics that make an antibiotic or combination of antibiotics so effective in endovascular infection do not always parallel the special requirements of bone and joint infections. Not only do tissue congestion and necrosis impede diffusion of antibiotic to the site, but also low pH of pus may inhibit the drug's effect on the organism, and antibiotic uptake by surrounding normal bone may be important in controlling the spread of infection. Based on animal studies, highly protein-bound antibiotics demonstrate the highest uptake in bone, but no clinical data yet establish the relevance of drug hydrophobicity to outcome.

Furthermore, unlike endocarditis, in which clinical outcome is clear and easily measured (cure, relapse, or failure to respond), treatment regimens for bone and joint infections are not easily compared, because they have gradations of severity and involvement, are multifactorial in pathogenesis, multifocal in location, and generally incorporate a broader range of causative organisms.[1,2,4,5,7–9,11,16,20–22,25] Moreover, relapse after a delay of months or even years is a feature unique to osteomyelitis.

As a result of this clinical heterogeneity and the long follow-up required to assess treatment outcome, definition of appropriate therapy of acute and chronic osteomyelitis still remains controversial, because therapeutic trials are so difficult.[8,17,18,19,23,24]

The objectives of the antimicrobial component of treatment of bone and joint infections described here are based on analysis of reasons for failure with older regimens and of the many successes obtained with

newer drugs and current management programs. It is also likely that as new classes of antimicrobials are introduced, even better results will be obtained, as has already occurred in the management of tuberculous bone and joint disease.

Route of Delivery

Optimal antibiotic therapy of established infections ideally should deliver, at a minimum, an inhibitory concentration of cidal antibiotics to each of the structures affected. Since repeated surgical access to irrigate, debride, and reduce bacterial load is neither feasible nor desirable because of the associated risks, methods of antibiotic delivery are limited to two: direct instillation and passive diffusion from circulating blood.

DIRECT INSTILLATION

Direct instillation of antibiotics is really only applicable to the joint space, since any other form of local irrigation does not reach the other structures. Attempts to irrigate deep tissue spaces by placing catheters intraoperatively is unsuccessful because channels are formed after only a few days of irrigation through closed catheter systems. Moreover, the presence of a foreign body that exits to the skin is a well-described risk factor for superinfection and therefore should be avoided.[13]

Antibiotics normally enter joint fluid reasonably well, even from infected synovium, although they only reach values ranging from one-third to one-half peak blood levels. However, there is a role for direct instillation of antibiotics in conjunction with use of the arthroscope in the management of septic arthritis.[6]

Arthroscopy combined with irrigation is an effective way of gently debriding joint spaces and particularly in removing fibrin and purulent barriers to diffusion. Irrigation also washes out enzymes and other products of inflammation and bacteria that are destructive to cartilage. Repeated arthroscopy, as often as daily in the first 3 to 4 days of a particularly aggressive suppurative arthritis, may be most advantageous in preserving joint function due to its cleansing effect. Failure to include antibiotic in the irrigation solution, however, will dilute out existing antibiotic in the joint space, which will only reaccumulate to therapeutic levels after the next parenteral dose.

Therefore, once samples have been obtained for culture, the irrigant should be changed to one containing the therapeutic antibiotic in concentrations approximately twice the peak blood level (e.g., 100 μg/ml of a β-lactam), which are nonirritating to the joint and establish a higher concentration in the joint than is otherwise possible. Direct instillation in this manner is especially applicable when the organism has a relatively high MBC requirement (e.g., *Enterococcus*, which requires high penicillin or ampicillin concentrations even for synergy with gentamicin).

The use of *chemically stable antibiotics* in irrigants, such as vancomycin, aminoglycosides, or bacitracin, has been advocated for irrigating infected sites intraoperatively and does have some merit. However, back diffusion out of the joint space will occur if the same antibiotic is not part of the parenteral program, and concentrations will fall below therapeutic levels.

DIFFUSION FROM BLOOD

Diffusion of antibiotic from blood into infected tissues is a basic requirement for effective treatment. Antibiotics do not reach avascular areas, and hypovascular tissues often present insurmountable barriers to the accumulation of effective concentrations.

In situations in which avascularity or hypovascularity is reversible by ingrowth of vessels during healing, antibiotic treatment must be continued until revascularization occurs. In the meantime, continued treatment acts to promote healing by killing and inhibiting organisms at the boundary of the watershed and by preventing extension of active infection into vascularized areas.

When major vessel occlusion is present or when the infectious process propagates itself by small vessel thrombosis, antibiotic therapy alone will fail. Consequently *a cardinal rule in managing deep tissue infections is early assessment of its vascular status* and the likelihood of spontaneous reversal of any abnormal perfusion. Finally, both physician and patient should be aware that *prolonged antibiotic therapy has a significant risk for causing one or more adverse effects,* and therefore revascularization procedures, debridement, or amputation should be done in the beginning of the course of antibiotic therapy.

Joint space infections are generally free of major vascular complications, except in the hip. Also, because the synovium responds to infection with hypervascularity and hyperpermeability, antibiotic concentrations in effusions and exudates compare favorably with blood levels. However, as described previously, antibiotic concentrations may not be uniform throughout the joint because of fibrin clot and purulent barriers to diffusion.

Also, the normal avascularity of cartilage and of cemented protheses[26] and other foreign bodies can be important factors in outcome. When cartilage is devitalized by virulent infection, or organisms successfully invade the avascular cement–bone interface of protheses, these sites accumulate, at best, only inhibitory concentrations of antibiotic and are sources of posttreatment relapse.

Osteomyelitis is normally complicated by reduced perfusion of subperiosteal bone, whereas surrounding tissues are hyperemic and highly permeable, allowing rapid accumulation of antibiotic by diffusion. The hypovascular bone itself accumulates little or no antibiotic, but the subsequent process of revascularization–resorption eventually delivers effective concentrations, provided the involved bone has not been devitalized by fragmentation nor progressed to sequestrum formation. The empirically observed difference in optimal duration of treatment between infections of bone (4 to 6 weeks) and joints (2 to 3 weeks) is presumably due to this need to revascularize and remodel infected bone to eradicate organisms.

REFERENCES

1. Anderson RB, Dorwart BB: Pneumoarthrosis in a shoulder infected with *Serratia liquefasciens:* case report and literature review. Arthritis Rheum 26:1166, 1983

2. Archer G: *Staphylococcus epidermidis:* the organism, its diseases and treatment. P. 25. In Remington JS, Swartz MN (eds): Current Clinical Topics in Infectious Diseases. McGraw-Hill, New York, 1984

3. Armbuster TG, Slivka J, Resnick D et al: Extraarticular manifestations of septic arthritis of the glenohumeral joint. Am J Roentgenol 129:667, 1977

4. Berges O, Gibod-Boccon L, Berger JP, Faure C: Case report: BCG–osteomyelitis of the proximal end of the

humerus with an abscess dissecting into the deltoid muscle. Skel Radiol 7:75, 1981

5. Burdge DR, Scheifele D, Speert DP: Serious *Pasturella multocida* infections from lion and tiger bites. JAMA 253:3296, 1985

6. Cofield RH: Arthroscopy of the shoulder. Mayo Clin Proc. 58:501, 1983

7. Dawes DT, Hothersall TE: Septic polyarthritis due to *Bacteroides fragilis* in a patient with rheumatoid arthritis. Clin Rheumatol 3:381, 1984

8. Gelberman RH, Menon J, Austerlitz MS, Weisman MH: Pyogenic arthritis of the shoulder in adults. J Bone Joint Surg 62A:550, 1980

9. Hikes DC, Manolil A II: Wound botulism. J Trauma 21:68, 1981

10. Jawetz E: The doctor's dilemma. Have I chosen the right drug? An adequate dose regimen? Can laboratory tests help in my decision? P. 109. In Remington JS, Swartz MN (eds): Current Clinical Topics in Infectious Diseases. McGraw-Hill, New York, 1981

11. Kraft SM, Pamish RS, Longley S: Unrecognized staphylococcal pyoarthrosis with rheumatoid arthritis. Semin Arthritis Rheum 14:196, 1985

12. Lawson JP, Steere AC: Lyme arthritis: radiologic findings. Radiology 154:37, 1985

13. Maki DG: Infections associated with intravascular lines. P. 309. In Remington JS, Swartz MN (eds): Current Clinical Topics in Infectious Diseases. McGraw-Hill, New York, 1982

14. Master R, Weisman MH, Armbuster TG et al: Septic arthritis of the glenohumeral joint. Unique clinical and radiographic features and a favorable outcome. Arthritis Rheum 20:1500, 1977

15. McKusick KA: Radionucleide imaging in the management of skeletal infections. P. 316. In Remington JS, Schwartz MN (eds): Current Clinical Topics in Infec-

tious Diseases. McGraw-Hill, New York, 1983

16. Miller KD, Moore ME: Tuberculous arthritis of the shoulder: delayed diagnosis aided by arthrography. Clin Rheum 2:61, 1983

17. Nelson JD: A critical review of the role of oral antibiotics in the management of hematogenous osteomyelitis. P. 64. In Remington JS, Schwartz MN (eds): Current Clinical Topics in Infectious Diseases. McGraw-Hill, New York, 1983

18. Norden CW: Osteomyelitis. P. 697. In Mandell GL, Douglas RG, Bennett JE (eds): Principles and Practice of Infectious Diseases, 2nd ed. Wiley, NY, 1985

19. Sabath LD, Mokhbat JE: What is the clinical significance of tolerance to β-lactam antibiotics. P. 358. In Remington JS, Swartz MN (eds): Current Clinical Topics in Infectious Diseases. McGraw-Hill, New York, 1983

20. Schmidt D, Mubarack S, Gelberman R: Septic shoulders in children. J Pediatr Orthop 1:67, 1981

21. Seradge J, Anderson MG: Clostridial myonecrosis following intra-articular steroid injections. Clin Orthop 147:207, 1980

22. Small CB, Slater LN, Lowry FD et al: Group B streptococcal arthritis in adults. Am J Med 76:367, 1984

23. Smith JW: Infectious arthritis. P. 697. In Mandell GL, Douglas RG, Bennett JE (eds): Principles and Practice of Infectious Diseases, 2nd ed., Wiley, NY, 1985

24. Steigbigel NH: Diagnosis and management of septic arthritis. P. 1. In Remington JS, Swartz MN (eds): Current Clinical Topics in Infectious Diseases. McGraw-Hill, New York, 1983

25. Tang SC, Chow SP: Tuberculosis of the shoulder. Report of five cases treated conservatively. J R Coll Surg Edinb 28:188, 1983

26. Weissman BN: The radiology of total joint replacement. Orthop Clin North Am 14:171, 1983

The Management of Common Shoulder Infections

Richard A. Marder
Thomas Bilko

With the exception of malignant tumors, no disease or disorder of the shoulder is capable of inflicting as serious morbidity as infection. Although the advent of antibiotic therapy has had significant impact, immunosuppressed patients, in particular, continue to be at risk. Sepsis of the glenohumeral joint can precipitate irreversible degeneration of the articular surfaces and compromise the intricate bursal gliding mechanisms responsible for motion, leading to residual restriction of movement and chronic pain.

A significant advance in the diagnosis and treatment of acute as well as chronic sepsis has been the use of arthroscopy. Assessment of articular damage, selective synovial biopsy, vigorous joint lavage, and debridement of necrotic and inflammatory tissues can be performed without the potential scarring associated with arthrotomy.

While prompt identification and institution of treatment are essential to the successful resolution of sepsis, prevention must be foremost in the planning of invasive diagnostic and therapeutic procedures about the shoulder. An understanding of the microbiology and antibiotic treatment of common shoulder infections is instrumental in achieving both objectives.

PROPHYLAXIS

Prevention of postoperative infection requires an understanding of the causative factors. Sepsis results when host defenses are unable to eradicate the unavoidable local bacterial contamination that occurs during surgery. Bacteria can gain access to a surgical wound by airborne spread, direct implantation from a break in sterile technique, or endogenous seeding from a focus of distant host infection.[8,61] As few as 1,000 staphylococcal organisms can be expected to produce infection in 50 percent of joints experimentally inoculated.[66] Despite contamination, postoperative infection in the normal host is not common. The incidence is generally less than 5 percent in elective orthopaedic cases without prophylactic antibiotics.[33,56]

Impairment of host defenses by local or systemic factors may promote the unchecked proliferation of inoculated bacteria. Important local factors that are potentially avoidable include hematoma formation and devascularization of tissues by prolonged traction, crushing, or extensive dissection at surgery. The use of methyl methacrylate has been associated with reduction in leukocyte functions of phagocytosis and killing of bacteria.[57] Recently, Petty has experimentally demonstrated an increased incidence of infection associated with common orthopaedic implant materials.[58] Chronic debilitating illnesses, malnutrition, malignancy, primary immune deficiency, and administration of steroids and other drugs are systemic causes of immunosuppression associated with higher risks of postoperative infection.[1,9,16,23,29]

Countermeasures against infection include strict attention to sterile draping and surgical technique; atraumatic surgery, emphasizing hemostasis and reduction in operating time; double gloving when using implants; prophylactic antibiotics; ultraviolet light; and laminar flow.[5,14,38,39,64,71] For purposes of discussion and use, these prophylactic measures can be classified into three levels (Table 18-1).

Level 1 measures are inexpensive, easily incorporated into the surgeon's routine, and applicable to all types of shoulder surgery. Careful and thorough preparation of the skin before admission and prior to surgery is essential. The patient is forewarned to avoid excessive sun exposure and is instructed to gently wash the shoulder with soap during the 2 to 3 days before surgery. Patients with active or recent upper respiratory or genitourinary infection are not operated on electively. Although hexachlorophene and providone–iodine soaps are widely employed with success for skin preparation, the use of 1 percent iodine and 70 percent alcohol has proved efficacious at the Massachusetts General Hospital. Attention to sterile techniques during draping should include sealing the operative site with adhesive transparent drape to reduce bacterial contamination of the wound from exposed skin. There is no substitute for limiting dissection when possible, handling tissues with gentleness, avoiding prolonged traction, irrigating the wound frequently to prevent desiccation, and obtaining meticulous hemostasis. During the operation, the surgeon should frequently wash his or her hands with sterile water, which is kept covered and changed by the scrub nurse every hour to avoid contamination. Closed suction drainage is helpful in large wounds, and its use for no more than 24 to 48 hours is not associated with possible retrograde infection.[52]

Roles and Indications

The efficacy of prophylactic antibiotics in orthopaedic surgery is well established; their role and indications continue to evolve. Antibiotic use in prosthetic joint and fracture implant surgery is well accepted, largely because of the significant sequelae of postoperative sepsis and the accumulating data showing a marked reduction in occurrence of postoperative infection following antibiotic prophylaxis.[5,7,33] Controversy exists, however, regarding the role of antibiotics in clean, elective soft tissue surgery. Because infection rates in this type of surgery are traditionally very low, and no well-designed studies exist to date documenting significant reduction in infection in such cases, many surgeons oppose the use of prophylactic antibiotics in these instances.[40,75] Our rationale for advocating prophylactic antibiotics in shoulder surgery, except arthroscopy, is based on several observations. First, administration of an antibiotic medication prior to the procedure and discontinuation after 24 to 36 hours is effective and has not been associated with the emergence of drug-resistant superinfection.[7,53] Second, the risk of drug-related side effects from cephalosporin agents is minimal, and short-term use may lower the occurrence of toxicity. Finally, first-generation cephalosporins are effective against staphylococcal organisms and, when used for a short duration, are relatively inexpensive compared to the cost of postoperative infection. Cefazolin is currently our drug of choice for prophylaxis because of its greater activity against staphylococcal organisms. Cefazolin has the longest half-life of the first-generation cephalosporins as well as the highest bone and synovial levels following intravenous administration.[14,65] The first dose is administered in

Table 18-1. Prophylactic Measures against Operative Infection

Level 1
  Careful preoperative skin preparation
  Strict attention to draping
  Sterile, atraumatic techniques
  Double gloving
  Reduction in operating room traffic and conversation
  Closed suction drainage
Level 2
  Prophylactic antibiotics
Level 3
  Laminar flow
  Ultraviolet light

the induction room 30 minutes prior to incision, and subsequent doses are given postoperatively every 8 hours for 24 to 36 hours.

Open fractures and joint injuries constitute a different problem because bacterial organisms have been implanted prior to beginning antibiotic therapy. This has been likened to treatment of an incipient infection. Use of a cephalosporin agent alone can result in an increase in gram-negative infections.[31,55] Pending initial culture results, treatment of open injuries should begin with both a cephalosporin and an aminoglycoside, with the realization that antibiotics are not a substitute for thorough debridement and copious irrigation.

Laminar Flow and Ultraviolet Light

Laminar flow and ultraviolet light have generally been reserved for use in prosthetic joint surgery. Although no studies exist to date, unidirectional horizontal flow in shoulder surgery could be associated with a paradoxical increase in postoperative infection related to operating team position similar to what Salvati noted in knee replacement surgery.[63] Some authors have failed to observe a reduction in infection using laminar flow compared with prophylactic antibiotics alone.[22] Ultraviolet light systems require careful protection of the eyes and exposed skin of the operating team. We do not advocate ultraviolet systems or laminar flow in routine shoulder surgery. Because of the grave consequences of postoperative infection in allograft and prosthetic joint reconstruction, however, such measures are probably worthwhile in these cases.

ACUTE HEMATOGENOUS OSTEOMYELITIS

Acute hematogenous osteomyelitis represents a bacteremic-induced pyogenic infection of bone marrow. With infrequent exception, this is a disorder of childhood. The proximal humeral metaphysis is one of the most commonly involved sites. Predeliction for the metaphyseal region of long bones has been attributed to trauma, growth rate, and local vascular anatomy.[11,36,54] An experimental model has related metaphyseal localization to sluggish blood flow at the capillary venous junction.[18] In infants under the age of 1 year, infection may traverse patent transepiphyseal vessels to involve the epiphysis.[73] Spontaneous decompression into the glenohumeral joint is a possibility. With involution of the physeal vessels, the physis functions as a barrier to the spread of infection.

Staphylococcus aureus is the most common pathogen irrespective of patient age.[74] Streptococcal infection is frequent in neonates and young infants, while infection with gram-negative organisms has a higher incidence in older patients.[17,43] *Pseudomonas* infection should be suspected in intravenous drug users.[62]

Pathogenesis

The pathogenesis of acute hematogenous osteomyelitis has been well described by Trueta.[73] Local proliferation of bacteria results in a metaphyseal focus of acute inflammatory exudate. Cytotoxic material combined with increasing pressure within the closed compartment lead to cellular death and occlusion of nutrient arterial branches supplying the cortex. Driven by pressure, pus extends through the cortex, forming a subperiosteal abscess. Therapeutic intervention at this point can resolve the infection without sequela. If the infection continues unchecked, further compromise of cortical blood supply occurs, leading to formation of sequestra. Involucrum results from periosteal reaction and may spread the entire length of bone. Irreversible damage to the physis and joint is a possible complication.

Manifestations

The clinical manifestations of acute hematogenous osteomyelitis typically involve general and local host responses. Fever, chills, malaise, and nausea together with shoulder pain, swelling, and tenderness to palpation and movement should alert the surgeon to the likelihood of either osteomyelitis or septic arthritis. Erythema may be present, but a diagnosis of cellulitis should not be made in any case if pain with movement of the upper extremity exists. A recent history of trauma and upper respiratory or other infection may be obtained.

Evaluation

Laboratory evaluation begins with a complete blood count and differential, sedimentation rate, and blood cultures. Although leukocytosis is unreliably present, most cases will demonstrate a left shift, and the sedimentation rate is consistently elevated.[49] Blood cultures are positive in approximately one-half of cases.[3,48]

It is well recognized that plain radiographs will require more than 1 week or more to demonstrate any bony changes.[10,28] Nonetheless, initial films may show soft tissue swelling.

Radionuclide scans can be helpful in the work-up of a patient with suspected acute hematogenous osteomyelitis. Initial reports of technetium scans noted nearly 100 percent sensitivity rates, but within the past 5 years several studies have revealed cases with normal scans despite culture-proven infection.[32,69] The accuracy of technetium scans is approximately 90 percent.[37] The advantage of technetium is that a delayed scan for bony uptake requires only 4 hours, while gallium scanning requires 24 to 48 hours. Because of this we do not employ radionuclide scanning when infection is strongly suspected. Instead, we proceed directly to biopsy to establish the diagnosis and initiate appropriate antibiotic therapy.

Biopsy should be performed in the operating room with the patient under general anesthesia. After sterile preparation of the extremity, an 18-gauge needle is introduced into the subperiosteal abscess under fluroscopic control and aspiration is performed. If no material is obtained, lavage with nonbacteriostatic saline is done. If this fails, intracortical biopsy is undertaken with a Craig biopsy needle or an 18-gauge spinal needle with obturator. If septic arthritis is suspected, joint aspiration is performed first to avoid cross-contamination. Sufficient fluid (1 ml) is sent for culture and sensitivity first. If additional fluid is available, a Gram stain and cell count are performed.

Treatment

Treatment with an antistaphylococcal agent, usually nafcillin or oxacillin, is begun pending culture results. Additional supportive measures are instituted and include intravenous hydration and immobilization of the shoulder in a sling until the signs of infection have resolved. Gentle use of the shoulder and pendulum exercises are encouraged thereafter.

If infection has been diagnosed early, antibiotic therapy alone can be curative.[11,25] If the process is undetected for more than 5 days, open drainage is indicated, and in older children and adults drilling of the cortex and sequestrectomy may be advisable.

Recent reports have shown successful treatment in children using short-term parenteral antibiotics followed by oral therapy.[11,50] Intravenous antibiotics are administered until clinical infection has resolved and then oral therapy is used for a total of 6 weeks. We prefer a 6-week course of intravenous antibiotic in older children and adults. Efficacy of treatment can be determined by performing frequent serum assays to maintain a 1:8 serum dilution bactericidal titer.[60]

Prognosis is related to any physeal injury, concurrent septic arthritis, or residual sequestra. The latter may require additional surgery and antibiotic therapy to effect cure.

SEPTIC ARTHRITIS

Pyogenic infection of the synovium can result in rapid joint destruction by chemical and mechanical means. Articular cartilage can be irreparably damaged either by the action of proteolytic enzymes released from leukocytes and synovial cells during the inflammatory response or by the rise in intraarticular pressure from accumulation of purulent material within the joint.[15,59] Expansion of the intraarticular volume can stretch the capsule and ligaments, leading to subluxation or dislocation. Infection may activate an autoimmune response that results in continued articular destruction despite eradication of the invading organism.[4] These potential sequelae underscore the importance of immediate attention to the patient with suspected joint infection.

Pathogenesis

Sepsis of the glenohumeral joint other than from trauma or surgery is most frequently the result of hematogenous spread of extraarticular infection. Important primary sites include skin, respiratory, and genitourinary infections as well as bacteremia from intravenous drug use.[47] In children, direct spread of an adjacent focus of metaphyseal osteomyelitis may be responsible. Factors that predispose to infection include impaired host immunity and underlying degenerative or inflammatory diseases of the shoulder.

Although *Staphylococcus aureus* is the most frequent cause of suppurative arthritis, age-related differences in causative organisms have been noted.[35,70] *Hemophilus influenzae* is the most common organism causing septic arthritis in children under the age of 2 years, while the incidence of gram-negative infection is increased in older patients. The clinical manifestations may include fever and chills, pain and limited shoulder motion, local warmth, erythema, and swelling. Especially in patients with impaired immunity, the systemic response to infection may be absent. This may lead to a delay in diagnosis unless the examiner's suspicion is aroused by the finding of a painful shoulder with limited motion. Osteomyelitis, acute calcific tendinitis, gout, pseudogout, and rheumatoid flare may be confused with septic arthritis. Differentiation may require joint aspiration.

Evaluation

Routine laboratory studies and radiographs are performed in every case, but diagnosis requires synovial fluid aspiration for Gram stain and culture. The blood leukocyte count with differential and sedimentation rate is helpful in monitoring the response to treatment. Blood cultures are positive in approximately 50 percent of cases. Other studies, including chest radiographs, urinalysis and culture, and cerebrospinal fluid analysis, may be indicated by history and examination. The earliest radiographic changes in septic arthritis are limited to the soft tissues. Capsular distention and loss of muscle planes may be noted with swelling. The initial bony change is subchondral resorption, which is not usually evident before 1 week. This is followed by periarticular subchondral erosions and eventually joint space narrowing. While radionuclide scans may demonstrate periarticular uptake, this is not helpful in establishing the diagnosis and may only contribute to a delay in the institution of appropriate diagnostic and therapeutic measures.

If the diagnosis of septic arthritis is considered,

we perform arthrocentesis. Strict sterile conditions are mandatory for joint aspiration. Any overlying area of cellulitis should be avoided. Generally, an anterior approach to the glenohumeral joint is used. A wide area is prepared with 70 percent alcohol and allowed to dry. Sterile disposable drapes are used to avoid contamination, and a mask and gloves are worn by the surgeon. After minimal subcutaneous infiltration with 1 percent lidocaine, an 18-gauge spinal needle with obturator is inserted through the capsule. If difficulty is encountered in aspiration, lavage with non-bacteriostatic saline is employed. Immediate examination of the aspirate is undertaken, and if no pathologic material is identified on Gram stain, either arthroscopy or formal arthrotomy is carried out in the operating room. If clinical evidence of infection exists, a negative aspiration in the office must be aggressively managed by either method without undue delay because failure to obtain aspirate may be due to thickened purulent material. Young children and infants usually require aspiration under general anesthesia. If aspiration is negative, consideration should be given to the possibility of acute hematogenous osteomyelitis of the proximal humerus.

Treatment

Treatment of pyogenic arthritis of the shoulder involves the application of well-established principles of adequate drainage, antibiotic administration, immobilization, and rehabilitation of the joint following resolution of the infectious process.

Surgical drainage was the mainstay of treatment prior to antibiotics, but recent studies have demonstrated the efficacy of frequent needle aspiration and arthroscopy.[24,26] This has proven satisfactory in our experience except in cases when infection has been present more than 3 to 5 days, allowing formation of adhesive loculi that prevent thorough evacuation of the joint by needle aspiration; or when a rapid clinical response to treatment is not apparent or serial analysis of joint fluid reveals continuing infection by cell count and culture. In such cases, arthroscopy can be used to evacuate purulent material from the joint. This allows direct evaluation of any articular damage, debridement of adhesions and fibrinous accumulations, synovial biopsy when needed, placement of suction irrigation and drainage systems when desired, and elimination of purulent material from joint recesses by thorough lavage. Any fluid reaccumulation thereafter can generally be managed by needle aspiration. With the exception of traumatic and surgical infections, whereby multiple tissue planes are involved simultaneously and open debridement is generally necessary, arthroscopic lavage is a safe, reliable means of achieving joint decompression while avoiding the scarring and adhesions that may complicate arthrotomy.

Following aspiration, we begin treatment based on the result of Gram stain; we make certain that an antistaphylococcal agent is employed in every case. Once culture reports are returned, definitive antibiotic therapy is selected.

Until pain and swelling have subsided the shoulder should be immobilized in a sling to facilitate healing. Once the infection is under control, gentle active assisted and active range-of-motion exercises are initiated without overstressing the joint. Well-motivated patients usually require no formal assistance. Pendulum-type exercises are particularly helpful in reestablishing glenohumeral motion. Isometric exercises may be added to regain muscle tone once the full range of motion is achieved.

Antibiotic therapy of septic arthritis remains nonuniform, due in large part to the lack of well-designed prospective studies to evaluate the duration of treatment. While successful treatment of joint infections with oral antibiotics in children has been reported, no such studies exist for adults.[72] Treatment of nongonococcal infection for 2 to 4 weeks is recommended in the literature.[13,27] Our concern about the refractory nature and virulence of *Staphylococcus aureus* or gram-negative bacterial infection has led us to employ 6-week or longer courses of parenteral antibiotics to eradicate infection as determined by clinical response, synovial fluid analysis, and sedimentation rate. For sepsis due to *Streptococcus* and *Hemophilus*, 4 weeks of parenteral treatment is usually sufficient if infection is recognized and treated early. We have no experience with oral antibiotics in the treatment of serious bone and joint infections; we are concerned primarily with unreliable serum levels that may result from noncompliance or poor absorption.

Prognosis following septic arthritis is related to a number of key factors: virulence of the infecting organism, preexisting joint disease, host immunosuppression, and, most importantly, a significant delay in the eradication of infection.[26,35,41] Some have reported adverse results if more than 1 week has elapsed before treatment is instituted, while Gelberman noted that a satisfactory outcome was obtained in cases treated within 4 weeks.[24,34] The following case illustrates the result when infection is not recognized and treatment is delayed. A 72-year-old man developed right shoulder pain after sustaining closed soft tissue trauma in an automobile accident. Three weeks after injury, the patient's arthrogram demonstrated a rotator cuff tear. Conservative treatment was elected. The patient developed increasing pain in the shoulder especially with movement and was referred to our office 3 months after the date of injury. No systemic or local signs of infection were present. Radiographs and tomograms (Fig. 18-1A,B) revealed articular destruction of both the glenoid and humeral head with moderate osteopenia. An arthroscopy was performed with the findings of synovitis and articular erosion (Fig. 18-1C,D) and a Gram stain revealed gram-positive cocci. All cultures were positive for *Staphylococcus aureus*. The patient was treated for 6 weeks with parenteral vancomycin because of a penicillin allergy. Cultures of joint fluid at the end of treatment were negative. At 6 months follow-up, the patient still had significant pain and marked restriction of motion despite vigorous physical therapy (Fig. 18-1E). This case underscores the importance of suspecting infection because of worsening symptoms after an invasive procedure as well as the poor outcome when treatment is delayed for a significant period of time.

POSTOPERATIVE INFECTION

Incidence

Sepsis complicating shoulder surgery is, fortunately, rare. In more than 300 shoulder arthroscopies performed at the Massachusetts General Hospital, no infections have occurred. The editor has personally performed and supervised 700 Bankart repairs and has had only 1 postoperative infection. The largest experience with total shoulder replacement is reported by Neer, who noted only 1 infection after 276

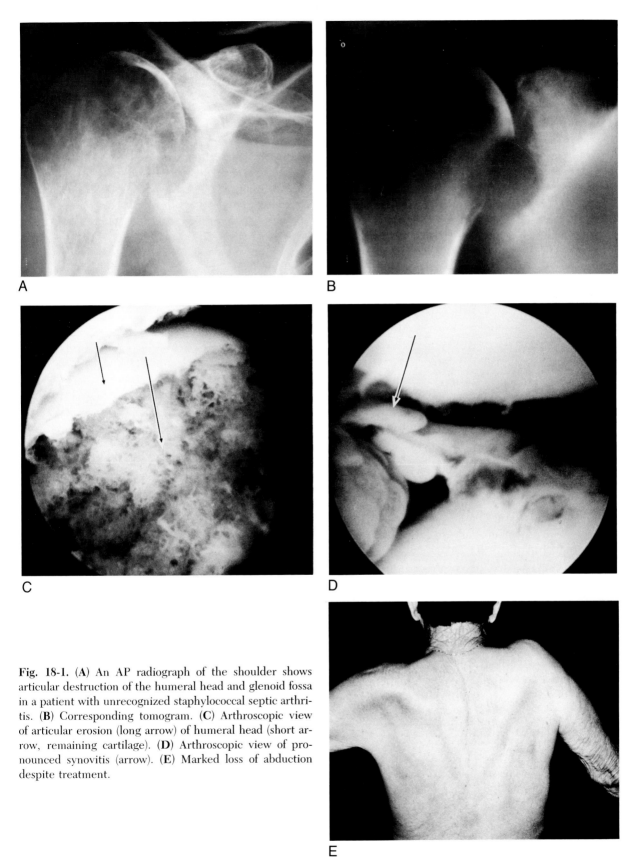

Fig. 18-1. (A) An AP radiograph of the shoulder shows articular destruction of the humeral head and glenoid fossa in a patient with unrecognized staphylococcal septic arthritis. (B) Corresponding tomogram. (C) Arthroscopic view of articular erosion (long arrow) of humeral head (short arrow, remaining cartilage). (D) Arthroscopic view of pronounced synovitis (arrow). (E) Marked loss of abduction despite treatment.

557

procedures.[5] The abundant vascular supply to the shoulder area may be partly responsible, but other factors are important as well. The shoulder is unlike the hip, which lies in close proximity to the contaminated perineal region, or the knee, which occupies a very superficial position with little protection.

Traditionally, infection has been classified as superficial or deep relative to the fascial layer. While the septic process may be confined to a localized area, involvement of the entire extent of the surgical wound is a serious possibility. The possibility of concurrent deep infection requires careful evaluation of any postoperative cellulitis or serous wound drainage, especially after any type of implant surgery.

Superficial Infection

Cellulitis is manifest within the first week of surgery as erythema, warmth, and induration around the incision. Direct tenderness is a prominent feature, but shoulder motion is not painful. Mild fever, lymphangitis, and regional lymphadenopathy may be present. If painful motion or incisional drainage develops, deep infection should be suspected.

Laboratory evaluation is of little help in diagnosing cellulitis because the leukocyte count and sedimentation rate are often elevated after major surgical procedures. Radiographs and radionuclide scanning reflect operative changes only in the immediate postoperative period, although the early blood pool scan may be positive because of soft tissue uptake.

Treatment includes immobilization of the shoulder, antibiotics, and application of moist heat. The most common pathogens are *Staphylococcus* and *Streptococcus*. Either a first-generation cephalosporin or penicillinase-resistant penicillin can be utilized. Oral therapy is usually adequate but if marked improvement is not forthcoming within 24 to 36 hours, a parenteral antibiotic is implemented. With resolution of clinical signs, gradual shoulder motion is begun.

Deep Infection

The majority of deep infections complicating soft tissue reconstructive surgery occur within the first few weeks of operation. Delayed infection after internal fixation and prosthetic replacement may develop from several months to 2 years following surgery. Hematogenous infection may occur as late as 9 years after surgery.[68] Staphylococci continue to account for the majority of infections but anaerobic, gram-negative, and mixed infections are being reported with increasing frequency.[21,67] Regardless of the time of presentation, infection may become chronic.

The clinical expression of deep infection can be variable depending upon the host resistance, virulence of infecting organism, and type of surgery. Following soft tissue reconstruction such as Bankart and rotator cuff repairs, the manifestations of postoperative infection are usually apparent within the first 2 weeks after surgery. Spiking fevers and chills, increasing shoulder pain, swelling, warmth, erythema, and drainage from the incision form a striking constellation of findings.

An unusual form of postoperative infection, toxic shock syndrome, has recently been described as a complication of elective musculoskeletal surgery.[2] Patients exhibit a generalized toxic reaction with multiple organ involvement as a result of infection with a toxin-producing strain of *Staphylococcus aureus*. The following case illustrates this peculiar form of postoperative sepsis. A 21-year-old man underwent a right shoulder Bankart repair for recurrent anterior dislocation. Within 24 hours of surgery, he developed a temperature of 105°F. No localizing signs of infection were noted, and blood, urine, and sputum cultures were negative. Total white cell count was 9,000 mm^3. The patient developed acute progressive azotemia and was transferred to the Massachusetts General Hospital 3 days postoperatively. At that time no overt evidence of wound infection was present. Repeat cultures were negative and supportive therapy with peritoneal dialysis was instituted. At 7 days postoperatively, the patient continued febrile with spiking temperatures to 101°F and polyarthralgias were noted, but the operated shoulder continued to appear benign. By 2 weeks, renal function had improved, and fluctuance in the operated shoulder developed. Radiographs demonstrated generalized periarticular osteopenia (Fig. 18-2A). Aspiration revealed infection with *Staphylococcus aureus*. Surgical exploration revealed an extraarticular abscess, which was debrided and irrigated. The Bankart repair was found to be intact, and no intraarticular extension of infection was noted. The wound was packed open and frequent dressing changes performed until secondary healing

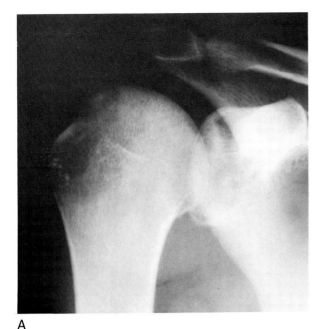

A

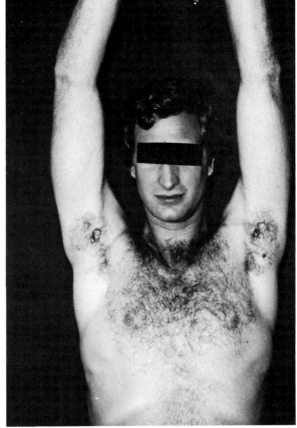

B

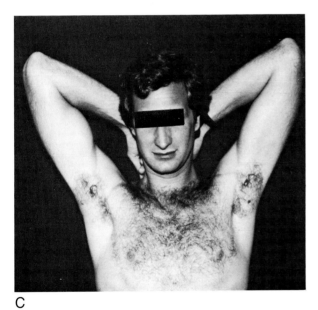

C

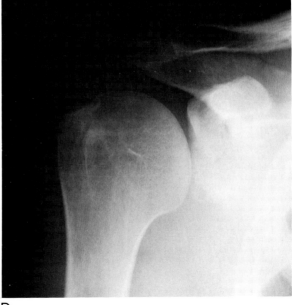

Fig. 18-2. (A) An AP radiograph of the right shoulder shows diffuse periarticular subchondral resorption in response to acute infection after a Bankart repair. (B) Elevation of the right shoulder at follow-up. (C) Full external rotation at follow-up. (D) Normal-appearing glenohumeral joint at 10-year follow-up.

D

occurred. Ten-year follow-up revealed full range of motion, no shoulder laxity, and normal glenohumeral articulation (Fig. 18-2B).

Depending on the virulence of the infecting organism, sepsis following fracture fixation or joint replacement may present as an acute, fulminant process or a subtle, chronic finding. Normally, following cemented joint replacement or stable fixation of a fracture, the shoulder is relatively painless after 48 hours. Persistence of extremity pain after this time may be a harbinger of developing infection. Absence of swelling, redness, and warmth does not eliminate the possibility of infection; low-grade sepsis may be manifested as persistent pain and a shoulder that is somewhat tender to palpation and passive movement but otherwise benign in appearance. Failure to recognize this presentation of infection may lead to a chronic condition with draining sinuses, infected nonunion, or prosthetic loosening with severe bone stock destruction.

Diagnostic Tests

A compendium of ancillary tests and studies including blood leukocyte count and differential, erythrocyte sedimentation rate, roentgenograms, tomograms, sinograms, arthrograms, and radionuclide scans is available to establish the probability of infection. Definitive diagnosis relies on recovering culture-positive tissue or fluid. Recognition of certain limitations of the aforementioned studies is important to the orthopaedic surgeon who is evaluating postsurgical infection. Surgery itself frequently elevates the sedimentation rate and leukocyte count for several weeks. It has been observed that the sedimentation rate may remain elevated for several months following arthroplasty. Conversely, sedimentation rate has been noted to be normal in as many as one-quarter of infected arthroplasties.[19] Roentgenograms may reflect only swelling in the immediate period following surgery. A period of 1 to 2 weeks is required before nonspecific subchondral rarefaction may be seen, and erosions, joint narrowing, sequestra formation and sclerosis, fixation failure, and implant loosening take much longer to become visible. Technetium and gallium bone scans are nonspecific for infection and uptake can be demonstrated in normal arthroplasties for periods up to 6 months after surgery. According

to early reports, indium 111 white cell scanning does appear more sensitive in detecting infection.[44]

Diagnosis of infection may prove difficult even by standard culture techniques. Gristina has noted a unique adaptation of bacteria affixing themselves to biomaterials by means of a polysaccharide membrane, which reduces their elution into periprosthetic tissues and fluid, resulting in failure of detection in standard culture media.[12] In these cases, diagnosis must be inferred from the histologic examination of infected tissues and enriched media used to attempt laboratory isolation of the pathogenic organism.[46]

Treatment

Acute infection after Bankart repair or other soft tissue reconstructive surgery may prove difficult to differentiate from sterile hematoma. Moreover, a deep infection need not communicate with the joint. If blind aspiration of a suspected infection or hematoma is carried out, purulence may be introduced intraarticularly. If the patient's condition permits an anesthetic, we proceed directly to surgical debridement.

The layers of the wound are carefully and atraumatically reopened until purulent material is encountered. Cultures are taken before irrigating the wound to avoid diluting the concentration of organisms. Some material is transferred to a prereduced carrier vial to maintain anaerobic conditions. Additional material is obtained for Gram stain. All visible necrotic tissue is debrided and the wound is irrigated copiously. This allows inspection of the capsule, which has not been disturbed to this point. To avoid disrupting the repair, needle aspiration is performed. If infection is encountered within the joint, a 2 cm vertical incision lateral to the repair can be made for irrigation and drainage without jeopardizing the repair. The wound is then packed open utilizing daily or more frequent dressing changes as needed until secondary healing occurs. Initial antibiotic therapy is based on the Gram stain and an antistaphylococcal agent is used until the final culture result is available. Parenteral antibiotics are administered for 6 weeks or longer until tenderness is absent and the sedimentation rate has returned towards normal. When clinical signs of infection have subsided, rehabilitation of the shoulder is initiated as outlined previously.

Initial treatment of postoperative infection should be thorough to avoid development of chronic sepsis. The following case illustrates how failure of initial therapy required multiple efforts to eradicate infection. A 21-year-old man developed an infected hematoma afer a Bankart repair of his right shoulder. The hematoma was aspirated, and oral Keflex was used for 2 months to treat a *Staphylococcus aureus* infection. The patient presented to this office 10 months later, with pain, fever, and chills. The wound appeared benign but motion was painful at the extremes. Leukocyte count was normal but the sedimentation rate was 52. Radiographs revealed osteopenia with subchondral erosion of the humeral head and periosteal reaction about the scapular neck (Fig. 18-3A). A gallium scan revealed periglenoid uptake. An arthroscopy was performed. Seropurulent material was recovered and marked synovitis noted. *Staphylococcus aureus* was cultured and the patient treated with vancomycin for a total of 6 weeks. Repeat

cultures from arthroscopy 1 week later were negative and the joint appeared benign. The patient did well for 7 months, when swelling, erythema, and spontaneous drainage of the old incision occurred. Surgical debridement revealed a sinus tract originating at the neck of the scapula where a large Tevdek suture was found. The wound was irrigated and closed over suction drainage. *Staphylococcus aureus* was again cultured. The patient was treated with 6 weeks of vancomycin. Follow-up at 5 years showed a painless shoulder with full range of motion and a normal joint radiographically (Fig. 18-3B).

Surgical Methods

Early deep infection following internal fixation of fractures requires immediate surgical attention. After the usual sterile preparation, the incision is reopened. A Gram stain is performed and cultures are obtained.

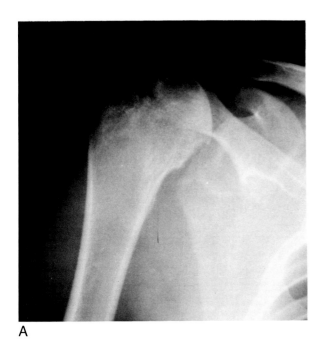

A

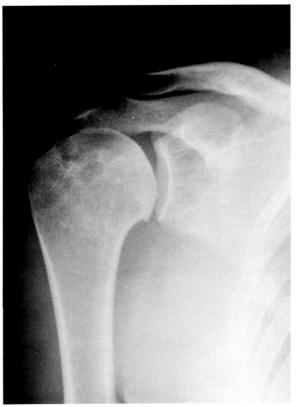

B

Fig. 18-3. (A) An AP radiograph shows articular erosion of the humeral head and periosteal reaction of the scapular neck in a patient with recurrent infection after a Putti-Platt repair. **(B)** Good preservation of glenohumeral joint at 5-year follow-up after eradication of infection.

Any necrotic tissue or devascularized bone is excised. Copious irrigation with 10 L of sterile saline followed by 2 L of a saline solution with bacitracin (50,000 units/L) is performed. Fracture reduction and stability are checked and, if found secure, the implant is recovered with a deep layer but the skin and subcutaneous tissue are packed open. The patient is returned to the operating room in 24 to 36 hours for reinspection and further debridement if required. Thereafter, frequent dressing changes are performed on the wound using sterile technique. Secondary healing of the wound is allowed to occur. We do not employ suction–irrigation systems because, in our experience, the affluent quickly exceeds the effluent. If fixation is insecure at the initial debridement, the fragments are repositioned and either external fixation or a larger implant is used to achieve stability. Intramedullary nailing should be avoided because of the risk of refractory intramedullary osteomyelitis.[45] We utilize antibiotics as recommended by Gustilo.[30] If infection is discovered within 3 weeks after surgery, 3 weeks of intravenous antibiotic followed by 3 weeks of oral therapy are usually sufficient. At 3 weeks following surgery, the fracture must be assumed to be infected. Hence, parenteral treatment is used for pain to 6 weeks and an additional 3 to 6 months of oral antibiotics are indicated.

The traditional treatment of sepsis complicating hemiarthroplasty and total replacement of the glenohumeral joint is debridement of all infected tissues, removal of the prosthesis and methylmethacrylate, and a 6-week course of intravenous antibiotic. While good success in eradicating infection can be expected, the functional result of excisional arthroplasty is often poor, with patients continuing to experience pain and having limited motion. Arthrodesis may be successful but is technically difficult because of the absence of the humeral head. Other methods of treatment may yield improved function, such as the Lawrence Jones procedure (see Chap. 6), which, in our hands, has proven reliable when replacement arthroplasty has failed or sepsis has occurred.

Recent experiences with exchange arthroplasty in septic hip replacements offer the possibility of similar success in treating infected shoulder prostheses.[6,20] Both one- and two-stage procedures can be performed. We believe, based on the results of delayed reimplantation of hip arthroplasties following a therapeutic course of parenteral antibiotic administration, that two-stage exchange arthroplasty would be preferable. Success with either method is more likely when one is dealing with less virulent organisms.

If infection is acute, that is, within the first 12 weeks of surgery, the implant may remain well fixed. In these cases, arthroscopic synovial debridement followed by a 6-week course of parenteral antibiotic may have some chance of salvaging the implant. The patient must be forewarned that this method is unproven and that removal of the prosthesis may be eventually if it is unsuccessful. A potential disadvantage of this form of treatment is the development of chronic infection that results in severe bone stock destruction preventing future prosthetic reimplantation.

The treatment of infected prosthetic joints is continuing to evolve.

REFERENCES

1. Bagdade JD, Root RK, Bulger RJ: Impaired leukocyte function in patients with poorly controlled diabetes. Diabetes 23:9, 1974
2. Bartlett P, Reingold AL, Graham DR et al: Toxic shock syndrome associated with surgical wound infections. JAMA 247:1448, 1982
3. Blockey NJ, Watson JT: Acute osteomyelitis in children. J Bone Joint Surg 52B:77, 1970
4. Bobechko WP, Mandell L: Immunology of cartilage in septic arthritis. Clin Orthop 108:84, 1975
5. Boyd RJ, Burke JF, Colton T: A double blind clinical trial of prophylactic antibiotics in hip fractures. J Bone Joint Surg 55A:1251, 1973
6. Bucholz HW, Elson RA, Engelbrecht E et al: Management of deep infection of total hip replacement. J Bone Joint Surg 63B:342, 1981
7. Burnett JW, Gustilo RB, Williams DN, Kind AC: Prophylactic antibiotics in hip fractures. A double blind, prospective study. J Bone Joint Surg 62A:457, 1980
8. Charnley J: Postoperative infection after total hip replacement with special reference to contamination in the operating room. Clin Orthop 87:167, 1972
9. Cierny G, Mader JT: Management of adult osteomyelitis. P. 15. In Evarts CM (ed): Surgery of the Musculoskeletal Systems, vol. 4. Churchill Livingstone, New York, 1983
10. Clawson DK, Dunn AW: Management of common bac-

terial infections of bones and joints. J Bone Joint Surg 49A:164, 1967

11. Cole WG, Dalziel RE, Leitl S: Treatment of acute osteomyelitis in childhood. J Bone Joint Surg 64B:218, 1982

12. Cristina AG, Costerton JW, Leake E, Kolkin J: Bacterial colonization of biomaterials. Clinical and Laboratory studies. Orthop Trans 4:355, 1980

13. Cunha BA: The use of penicillins in orthopaedic surgery. Clin Orthop 190:36, 1984

14. Cunha BA, Gosling HR, Pasternak HS: The penetration characteristics of cefazolin, cephalothin, and cephradine into bone in patients undergoing total hip replacement. J Bone Joint Surg 59A:856–9, 1977

15. Curtiss PH, Jr., Klein L: Destruction of articular cartilage in septic arthritis. I. In vivo studies. J Bone Joint Surg 47A:1595, 1965

16. Dale DL, Petersdorf RG: Corticosteroids and infectious diseases. Med Clin North Am 57:1277, 1973

17. Edwards MS, Baker CJ, Wagner ML et al: An etiologic shift in infantile osteomyelitis: the emergence of the Group B streptococcus. J Pediatr 93:578, 1978

18. Emslie KR, Nade SML: Acute haematogenous staphylococcal osteomyelitis: a description of the natural history in an avian model. Am J Pathol 110:333, 1983

19. Fitzgerald RH: The infected hip arthroplasty: current concepts in treatment. Hip 347, 1984

20. Fitzgerald RH, Jones DR: The infected hip transplant. Treatment with resection arthroplasty and late total hip arthroplasty. Am J Med 78:225, 1985

21. Fitzgerald RH, Rosenblatt JE, Tenney JH, Bourgault AM: Anaerobic septic arthritis. Clin Orthop 164:141, 1982

22. Freeman MAR, Challis JH, Zelezonski J, Jarvis ID: Sepsis rates in hip replacement surgery with special reference to the use of ultra clean air. Arch Orthop Unfall Chir 90:1, 1977

23. Gardner ID: The effect of aging on susceptibility to infection. Rev Infect Dis 2:801, 1980

24. Gelberman RH, Menon J, Austerlitz MS, Weisman MH: Pyogenic arthritis of the shoulder in adults. J Bone Joint Surg 62A:550, 1980

25. Gillespie WJ, Mayo KM: The management of acute haematogenous osteomyelitis in the antibiotic era: a study of the outcome. J Bone Joint Surg 63B:126, 1981

26. Goldenberg DL, Brandt KD, Cohen AS, Cathcart ES: Treatment of septic arthritis: comparison of needle aspiration and surgery as initial modes of joint drainage. Arthritis Rheum 18:83, 1975

27. Goldenberg DL, Cohen AS: Acute infectious arthritis: A review of patients with nongonococcal joint infections. Am J Med 60:369, 1976

28. Griffin PP: Bone and joint infections in children. Pediatr Clin North Am 14:533, 1967

29. Gristina AG, Rovere GD, Shoji H: Spontaneous septic arthritis complicating rheumatoid arthritis. J Bone Joint Surg 56A:1180, 1974

30. Gustilo RB: Management of infected fractures. P. 117. In Evarts CM (ed): Surgery of the Musculoskeletal System, vol. 4. Churchill Livingstone, New York, 1983

31. Gustilo RB, Mendoza RM, Williams DN: Problems in the management of type III (severe) open fractures. J Trauma 24:8, 1984

32. Hamilton S, Hurley GD: Radio-isotope bone scanning in suspected osteomyelitis in children. Eur J Nucl Med 4:325, 1976

33. Hill C, Flamant R, Mazas F, Evrad J: Prophylactic cefazolin versus placebo in total hip replacement. Report of a multicenter double-blind randomized trial. Lancet 1:795, 1981

34. Ho G, Su EY: Therapy for septic arthritis. JAMA 247:797, 1982

35. Ho G, Toder JS, Zimmermann B: An overview of septic arthritis and septic bursitis. Orthopaedics 7:1571, 1984

36. Hobo T: Zur Pathogenese der akuten hametogenen osteomyelitis, mit Berucksichfigung der Vitaltar-bungslehre. Acta Schol Med Kioto 4:1, 1921

37. Howe DW, Savage JP, Wilson TG, Paterson D: The technetium phosphate bone scan in the diagnosis of osteomyelitis in childhood. J Bone Joint Surg 65A:431, 1983

38. Letts RM, Doermer E: Conversation in the operating theater as a cause of airborne bacterial contamination. J Bone Joint Surg 65A:357, 1983

39. Lowell JD: The ultraviolet environment. Orthop Rev 8:111, 1979

40. Mader JT, Cierny G: The principles and the use of preventive antibiotics. Clin Orthop 190:75, 1984

41. Master R, Weisman MU, Armbuster TG et al: Septic arthritis of the glenohumeral joint: Unique clinical and radiographic features and a favorable outcome. Arthritis Rheum 20:1500, 1977

42. McCue SF, Berg EW, Saunders EA: Efficacy of double-gloving as a barrier to microbial contamination during total joint arthroplasty. J Bone Joint Surg 63A:811, 1981

43. McHenry MC, Alfidi RJ, Wilde AH, Hawk WA: Haematogenous osteomyelitis: a changing disease. Cleve Clin Q 42:125, 1975

44. Merkel K, Brown ML, Dewainjee MK: Comparison of indium-labeled-leucocyte imaging with sequential technetium-gallium scanning in the diagnosis of low grade musculo-skeletal sepsis. J Bone Joint Surg 67A:465, 1985

45. Meyer S, Weiland AJ, Willenegger H: The treatment of infected non-union of fractures of long bones. J Bone Joint Surg 57A:836, 1975

46. Mina JM, Marder RA, Amstutz HC: The pathology of failed total joint arthroplasty. Clin Orthop 170:175, 1982

47. Miskew DBW, Lorenz MA, Pearson RL, Pankovich AM: *Pseudomonas aeroginosa* bone and joint infection in drug abusers. J Bone Joint Surg 65A:829, 1983

48. Mollan RAB, Piggot J: Acute osteomyelitis in children. J Bone Joint Surg 59B:2, 1977

49. Morrey BF, Peterson HA: Hematogenous pyogenic osteomyelitis in children. Orthop Clin North Am 6:935, 1975

50. Nade S: Acute haematogenous osteomyelitis in infancy and childhood. J Bone Joint Surg 65B:109, 1983

51. Neer CS, Watson KC, Stanton FJ: Recent experience in total shoulder replacement. J Bone Joint Surg 64A:319, 1982

52. Nelson CL, Evarts CM, Andrish J, Marks KE: Infected total hip replacement—results and complications. J Bone Joint Surg 57A:1025, 1975

53. Nelson CL, Green TG, Porter RA, Warren RD: One day versus seven days of preventive antibiotic therapy in orthopaedic surgery. Clin Orthop 176:258, 1983

54. Ogden JA: Pediatric osteomyelitis and septic arthritis: The pathology of neonatal disease. Yale J Biol Med 52:423, 1979

55. Patzakis MJ: Antibiotic and bacterial considerations in open fractures. Surg Gynecol Obstet 70:46, 1977

56. Pavel A, Smith RL, Ballard A, Larsen IJ: Prophylactic antibiotics in clean orthopaedic surgery. J Bone Joint Surg 56A:777, 1974

57. Petty W: The effect of methyl methacrylate on bacterial phagocytosis and killing by human polymorphonuclear leukocytes. J Bone Joint Surg 60A:752, 1978

58. Petty W, Spanier S, Shuster JJ, Silverthorne C: The influence of skeletal implants on incidence of infection. J Bone Joint Surg 67A:1236, 1985

59. Phemister DB: The effect of pressure on articular surfaces in pyogenic and tuberculous arthritides and its bearing upon treatment. Ann Surg 80:481, 1924

60. Prober CG, Yeager AS: Use of the serum bactericidal titer to assess the adequacy of oral antibiotic therapy in the treatment of acute hematogenous osteomyelitis. J Pediatr 95:131, 1979

61. Ritter MA: Surgical wound environment. Clin Orthop 190:11, 1984

62. Roca RP, Yoshikawa TT: Primary skeletal infections in heroin users: a clinical characterization, diagnosis and therapy. Clin Orthop 144:238, 1977

63. Salvati EA, Robinson RP, Zeno SM et al: Infection rates after 3175 total hip and total knee replacements performed with and without a horizontal unidirectional filtered inflow system. J Bone Joint Surg 64A:525, 1982

64. Sanderson MC, Bentley G: Assessment of wound contamination during surgery: a preliminary report comparing vertical laminar flow and conventional theatre systems. Br J Surg 63:431, 1976

65. Schurman DJ, Hirschman HP, Kajiyama G et al: Cefazolin concentrations in bone and synovial fluid. J Bone Joint Surg 60A:359–362, 1978

66. Schurman DJ, Johnson BL, Amstutz HC: Knee joint infections with *Staphylococcus aureus* and *Micrococcus* species. J Bone Joint Surg 57A:40, 1975

67. Speller DCE: Microbiology of infected joint prosthesis. Semin Orthop 1:1, 1986

68. Stinchfield FE, Bigliani LU, Neu HC et al: Late hematogenous infection of total joint replacement. J Bone Joint Surg 62A:1345, 1980

69. Sullivan DC, Rosenfield NS, Ogden J, Gottschalk A: Problems in the scintigraphic detection of osteomyelitis in children. Radiology 135:731, 1980

70. Swensen H: Septic arthritis and osteomyelitis. Orthop Surv 4:125, 1980

71. Tengue B, Kjellander J: Antibiotic prophylaxis in operations on trochanteric femoral fractures. J Bone Joint Surg 60A:97, 1978

72. Tetzloff TR, McCracken GH, Nelson JD: Oral antibiotic therapy for skeletal infections of children. II. Therapy of osteomyelitis and suppurative arthritis. J Pediatr 92:485, 1978

73. Trueta J: The three types of acute haematogenous osteomyelitis. A clinical and vascular study. J Bone Joint Surg 41B:671, 1959

74. Waldvogel FA, Vasey H: Osteomyelitis: the past decade. N Engl J Med 303:360, 1980

75. Williams DN, Gustilo RB: The use of preventive antibiotics in orthopaedic surgery. Clin Orthop 190:83, 1984

The Diagnosis and Management of Tumors About the Shoulder

19

Mark C. Gebhardt
Henry J. Mankin
Alan L. Schiller
Daniel I. Rosenthal

It is appropriate to point out at the outset that in terms of the various tumor diagnoses, staging studies, the extent of the patient's disease, and principles of management, the lesions that affect the bones and soft tissues around the shoulder joint do not differ materially from those encountered in other sites in the body. Hence the general discussions of the subject contained within the various older and many recent texts[36,52,62,86,98,105,128,196,219,225] devoted to these subjects are generally applicable. The interested reader may find the detail in these various texts and articles more valuable than the necessarily compacted review required for a book chapter such as this. Nevertheless, primary and metastatic tumors about the shoulder are an important component of the practice of the orthopaedist interested in shoulder problems, and a review of these principles and practices with special emphasis on the scapula, clavicle, and humerus is important and necessary for the sake of competency, as well as serving as a convenient guide to proper management of the benign and malignant neoplasms encountered.

Certain tumors, although not unique to the shoulder, have a higher frequency of presentation at that site than at many other sites and will probably account for the major component of the lesions reported in any series. Although metastatic carcinoma is by far the most frequent tumor seen in the bones of the shoulder region and thus does not differ from other sites, certain of the primary tumors, both benign and malignant, appear to prefer this region. Among the benign lesions are chondroblastoma, unicameral bone cysts, enchondroma, and osteocartilaginous exostoses; and for malignant or aggressive tumors, high on the list for the shoulder region are Ewing's sarcoma, chondrosarcoma, osteosarcoma (Tables 19-1, 19-2). Among the soft tissue tumors, the lipoma is clearly the most frequent lesion encountered of the benign group and among the malignant tumors, epitheloid sarcoma and malignant fibrous histiocytoma, liposarcoma, and synovioma may occur, although the latter two occur more often in the lower extremity.

In this discussion we attempt to describe the techniques of staging for benign and malignant tumors

Table 19-1. Primary Bone Lesions of which a High Percentage Occur in the Shoulder

	Percentage of Lesions Occurring in the Shoulder
Extremely likely (>25%)	
Simple cyst	35–50
Likely (15–25%)	
Osteochondroma	21–27
Chondroblastoma	16–26
Desmoplastic fibroma	21–24
Not rarely (5–25%)	
Enchondroma	5–16
Primary lymphoma of bone	5–19
Chondrosarcoma	13–19
Osteosarcoma	10–16
Parosteal osteogenic sarcoma	5–20
Ewing's sarcoma	2–15

(Data compiled from references 36, 98, 157, 196.)

Table 19-2. Primary Bone Lesions Likely to be Seen in Shoulder

	Percentage of Shoulder Lesions Represented by Diagnosis
Osteochondroma	23
Osteosarcoma	17
Chondroblastoma	13
Chondrosarcoma	10
Simple cyst	9
Ewing's sarcoma	5
Total	77

(Data compiled from four refs. 36, 98, 157, 196.)

of bone and soft parts; the clinical characteristics of the various lesions; their appearance on imaging studies; some features of the pathology; and finally the principles of treatment, not only as generally applied but specifically for tumors of the shoulder.

STAGING STUDIES FOR BENIGN AND MALIGNANT TUMORS OF BONE AND SOFT TISSUES

Staging Schema

Although staging methods and schema were proposed for various solid and lymphogenous tumors a number of years ago, tumors of connective tissue were not fully included in the original discussions, and have only recently been the subject of extensive discussion in the literature. Most tumor surgeons now utilize the staging systems described by Enneking et al.,[53,57] working with the Musculoskeletal Tumor Society for malignant neoplasms of bone. For primary soft tissue tumors, two systems are valuable: the Enneking system (which some find does not really take proper cognizance of the size of the lesion) and that advocated by the American Joint Commission[191,227] (Table 19-3). Comparison of the systems for malignant tumors

of the soft tissue readily disclose the deficiencies, but to date there has been no firm evidence to suggest that one system is better than the other. In view of this fact and since this volume is intended for the orthopaedist, for convenience of presentation we will utilize the same staging system (Enneking et al.[53,57]) (Table 19-3) for both bone and soft tissue tumors.

The staging systems for both bone and soft tissue tumors depend on the definition of three crucial components: the grade of the tumor (G), the anatomical location of the lesion (T), and the presence or absence of distant metastases.[53,57,191] The G is best defined according to malignancy, and generally lesions that are benign are either designated as G0 or excluded from the staging system. Low-grade lesions, regardless of tissue type, are classified as G1, and high-grade tumors as G2. A partial listing of the primary tumors and soft tissue tumors, most of which are encountered around the shoulder, are shown in Tables 19-4 and 19-5. Metastatic tumors are, of course, not staged by this method, nor are disseminated lymphomas, leukemias, or Ewing's sarcoma, but may still require assessment by the techniques described below.

The anatomical location (T) is assessed by imaging studies and is defined according to the preservation or violation of a well-defined anatomical compartment (Table 19-6). Thus, a lesion contained completely within an anatomical compartment is designated as T1; one that has broken out and extended beyond the confines of the compartment of origin to involve a second adjacent site is considered to be T2. In consideration of the anatomy of the shoulder, a lesion

Table 19-3. Staging Protocols

MSTS[a]		AJC[b]	
Stage IA	(G1, T1, M0)	Stage IA	(G1, T1, N0, M0)
IB	(G1, T2, M0)	IB	(G1, T2, N0, M0)
Stage IIA	(G2, T1, M0)	Stage IIA	(G2, T1, N0, M0)
IIB	(G2, T2, M0)	IIB	(G2, T2, N0, M0)
Stage III	(Any G, T, M1)	Stage IIIA	(G3, T1, N0, M0)
		IIIB	(G3, T3, N0, M0)
		IIIC	(G1–3, T1–2, N1, M0)
		Stage IVA	(G1–3, T3, N0–1, M0)
		IVB	(G1–3, T1–3, N0–1, M1)

[a] G1, low grade; G2, high-grade sarcoma; T1, intracompartmental; T2, extracompartmental; M, distant or nodal metastases.

[b] G1, well differentiated; G2, moderately well differentiated; G3, poorly differentiated sarcoma; T1, tumor < 5 cm; T2, tumor > 5 cm; T3, destruction of cortical bone, invasion of major artery or nerve; N1, histologically verified metastasis to lymph node; M1, distant metastases.

(Adapted from Enneking WF, Spanier SS, Goodman MA: A system for the surgical staging of musculoskeletal sarcoma. Clin Orthop 153: 106, 1980; and Suit HD, Mankin HJ, Schiller AL: Staging systems for sarcoma of soft tissue and sarcoma of bone. Cancer Treat Symposia 3: 29, 1985.)

Table 19-4. Classification of Bone Tumors Commonly Seen about the Shoulder

Tissue of Origin	Benign	Malignant
Bone	Osteoid osteoma Osteoblastoma	Juxtacortical osteosarcoma Central osteosarcoma Telangiectatic osteosarcoma Paget's sarcoma Radiation-induced sarcoma
Cartilage	Osteocartilaginous exostosis Enchondroma Juxtacortical chondroma Chondroblastoma Chondromyxoid fibroma	Exostotic chondrosarcoma Enostotic chondrosarcoma Juxtacort. chondrosarcoma Clear cell chondrosarcoma Dedifferentiated chondrosarcoma
Fibrous	Fibrous dysplasia Unicameral bone cyst Aneurysmal bone cyst Desmoplastic fibroma	Fibrosarcoma Malignant fibrous histiocytoma
Blood vessels	Hemangioma	Hemangiosarcoma Hemangiopericytoma Gorham's disease
Marrow elements	Histiocytosis	Hodgkin's lymphoma Non-Hodgkin's lymphoma Ewing's sarcoma Myeloma
Unknown		Giant cell tumor

(Adapted from Dahlin DC: Bone Tumors: General Aspects and Data on 6,221 Cases. Charles C Thomas, Springfield, Illinois, 1978; and Spjut HT, Dorfman HD, Fechner RE et al: Atlas of Tumor Pathology, Fascicle 5: Tumor of Bone and Cartilage. Armed Forces Institute of Pathology, 1971.)

Table 19-5. Classification of Soft Tissue Tumors Commonly Seen about the Shoulder

Tissue of Origin	Benign	Malignant
Fibrous	Fibroma Benign FH[a] Elastofibroma Dorsi Fibromatosis	Fibrosarcoma MFH[b]
Adipose	Lipoma Neurolipoma Angiolipoma Hibernoma	"Atypical" lipoma Liposarcoma Fibroblastic Liposarcoma Pleomorphic Liposarcoma
Muscle	Leiomyoma Rhabdomyoma	Leiomyosarcoma Embryonal Rhabdomyosarcoma Pleomorphic Rhabdomyosarcoma
Blood vessels	Hemangioma Angiomatosis Lymphangioma	Hemangiosarcoma Hemangiopericytoma Lymphangiosarcoma
Peripheral nerve	Neurofibroma Neurolemmoma	Neurofibrosarcoma Malignant schwannoma
Tendosynovium	Fibroma PVNS	Synovioma Epithelioid sarcoma Clear Cell sarcoma
Miscellaneous	Benign Granular Cell Tumor Myxoma	Malignant granular cell tumor Malignant mesenchymoma Undifferentiated sarcoma Alveolar soft parts sarcoma

[a] FH, Fibrous histiocytoma.
[b] MFH, Malignant fibrous histiocytoma.

that is totally confined to any of the component bones is considered to be T1, while one that has broken out to extend into the adjacent soft tissues or joints is T2. Tumors of the soft tissues that are entirely confined to a single muscle or muscle within a myofas-

Table 19-6. Surgical Sites (T)

Intracompartmental (T1)	Extracompartmental (T2)
Intraosseous	Soft tissue extension
Intraarticular	Soft tissue extension
Superficial to deep fascial	Deep fascial extension
Paraosseous	Intraosseous or extrafascial
Intrafascial compartments	Extrafascial planes or spaces

Anterior or posterior arm
  periscapular
	Axilla
	  Periclavicular
	  Paraspinal
	  Head and neck

(Adapted from Enneking WF, Spanier SS, Goodman MA: A system for the surgical staging of musculoskeletal sarcoma. Clin Orthop 153:106, 1980.)

cial space are designated as T1, while those that extend beyond fascial planes to involve either the adjacent compartment, the bone, or the neuromuscular bundle are considered to be T2. An example of a T1 lesion is a malignant tumor of the soft tissue confined within the posterior compartment of the arm. If the lesion dissects through the intramuscular system to involve either the anterior compartment or the medial space containing the vessels and nerves, the lesion is designated as T2. A tumor arising in the subscapularis that invades the body of scapula is a T2, while another of the same type totally contained within its fibrous envelope of the subscapularis is T1. There are some cloudy issues in the definition, particularly surrounding the deltoid muscle, which is separated from the humerus and rotator cuff by the subdeltoid bursa. A tumor of the humerus that breaks out into the subdeltoid bursa is considered to be T2, although the deltoid is not invaded; while a soft tissue sarcoma of the deltoid that breaks into the bursa is probably also T2, but this definition is perhaps a little less clear. Similarly, since the radial nerve traverses the posterior compartment, a large neurofibrosarcoma arising from the nerve is probably T2 by definition despite being confined to the posterior compartment anatomically, since it can extend both into the brachial plexus proximally or into the anterior compartment distally by perineural tracking.

Under the Enneking staging system the presence or absence of metastases (M0 or M1, respectively) does not recognize a difference between extension to regional nodes (a rare event for most bone tumors and less rare, but still uncommon, for soft tissue tumors) and pulmonary metastases. Most often staging data for M can be readily assessed by physical examination for enlarged nodes (but occasionally lymphangiography, computed tomography (CT), or biopsy of suspicious nodes is indicated) and full lung tomography or CT of the chest (the former is less accurate for young people, while the latter, because of its higher resolution, offers a sizable number of false positives in individuals over the age of 50).

Staging Algorithms

Table 19-7 shows the staging algorithms for the study of patients who present with lesions of the bones or soft tissues about the shoulder. The work-up plan for each depends on assessing the grade (G) of the tumor, usually on the basis of histologic and special stain and electron microscopic study of the tumor tissue obtained at biopsy; the anatomical extent of the lesion (T), usually determined by physical examination and appropriate imaging studies; and the presence or absence of metastases (M), as determined by physical examination and imaging studies of the lymph nodes and lungs.

Each patient must first undergo the "first-order screen," virtually identical for bone and soft tissue tumors. A careful history and complete physical examination are essential and should include evaluation and examination of not only the shoulder region but the entire patient. The physical examination must include examination of the thyroid, abdomen, breasts, gonads, rectum, and prostate.

Initial staging studies should include radiographs of the shoulder and entire humerus, usually at least three views, and sometimes tomography, especially

Table 19-7. Protocol for Staging of Bone and Soft Tissue Tumors of the Shoulder

I First-order screen
  History
  Physical plane radiographs (? xeroradiogram, magnification views)
  Chest radiograph
  Laboratory tests: CBC, ESR, calcium, phosphate, alkaline phospatase assays, SIEP, SGOT, BUN, blood sugar

II Diagnostic decision	→	III Second-order studies
Benign		Biopsy (open incision)
Primary malignant		Lung tomograms or angiograms; CT scans of lesion; biopsy (culture EM)
Round cell		Lung tomograms or lymphangiograms; liver/spleen scan; gallium scan; biopsy (culture, EM, surface markers)
Metastatic carcinoma		Lung tomograms or mammogram; TVP; thyroid; bone marrow; biopsy (culture, EM, estrogen/progesterone receptors)

CBC, complete blood count; ESR, erythrocyte sedimentation rate; SGOT, serum glutemate oxaloacetate transaminase; BUN, blood urea nitrogen; EM, electron microscope.

for the scapula, and xeroradiography or CT if a soft tissue tumor is suspected. Chest radiography (PA and lateral), a bone scan, and the laboratory data cited (designed principally to screen for metabolic bone disease, leukemia, or myeloma) are necessary. On the basis of these preliminary data, the orthopaedist and radiologist should have sufficient material to make a diagnostic decision as to whether the lesion is benign, a primary tumor of bone or soft tissue, a lymphoma or round cell tumor, or a metastatic deposit from some other site.

If the lesion is thought to be benign, an incisional biopsy, frozen section, and then an excision without further work-up is appropriate. This should provide the diagnosis on the basis of histologic study. Occasionally for small tumors that have a diagnostic radiographic pattern (such as a lipoma, chondroblastoma, or osteocartilaginous exostosis), the lesion may be excised or curetted without resorting to a frozen section. This approach should be discouraged if the lesion is large or if there is doubt about the diagnosis (see section on techniques of biopsy, below). Also some lesions such as fibrous cortical defects and certain unicameral bone cysts may not require biopsy or treatment and may simply be observed.

If the lesion is thought to be a primary malignant tumor of bone or soft tissue, additional studies, prior to biopsy, should include CT of the lesion, angiography and/or magnetic resonance imaging (MRI), all of which help to define the anatomical extent of the lesion (T); and either full lung tomograms or a CT scan of the chest (usually dependent on the age of the patient). If the tumor is thought to be a primary (or secondary lymphoma or round cell tumor of bone), additional work-up should include lymphangiography, a liver-spleen scan, a staging abdominal CT, and a bone marrow examination.[231] If myeloma is suspected, the bone scan may be less helpful in determining the presence of additional lesions and a skeletal survey, including a skull series, may be helpful.

If the lesion is thought to be a metastatic tumor to one of the bones of the shoulder, additional studies including mammography, intravenous pyelography, thyroid scanning, and acid phosphatase determination should be performed prior to biopsy.[214]

It should be evident that many of these staging studies could be performed after the biopsy, and perhaps in these days of limitations of resources, this is a wiser course. It should be evident, however, that if the biopsy is performed prior to bone scan, CT, MRI, angiography, or lymphangiography, it may increase the difficulty in interpreting these studies. In addition, the completion of the work-up prior to the biopsy allows for a more intelligent placement of the biopsy incision based on the anatomical location of the tumor.

The Biopsy

In recent years the technique of biopsy of bone and soft tissue lesions has been the subject of several studies, to which the interested reader is referred.[34,65,136,139,159,164,197,211] The general principles of biopsy of lesions about the shoulder do not differ materially from those for other anatomical sites, although the complexity of the anatomy must be carefully considered prior to performing the procedure.

The following general principles are critical to performance of the biopsy of any lesion about the shoulder, regardless of its diagnosis, size or extent of the disease.

1. The biopsy is an essential part of the procedure and should only be performed after review of the staging data with the radiologist and pathologist.
2. The operative procedure should be performed as carefully as the definitive surgery and by as senior a person, and should be done by the individual or individuals responsible for the total management of the patient.
3. Prior to performing the biopsy, the possible alternative procedures (resective or ablative) necessary for subsequent management should be carefully measured, and the incision and soft tissue dissection performed to offer the least likelihood of compromise of any subsequent procedures.
4. The tissue obtained should be studied not only for tumor (all special tests such as estrogen receptors, electron microscopy, special stains, flow cytometry, or surface markers should be discussed with the pathologist and planned for in advance of the surgery) but also for other types of lesions, including especially infection. All tissue obtained at biopsy should be sent for culture. A frozen section is helpful principally in assuring the surgeon and pathologist that sufficient pathologic tissue has been obtained.

In terms of technique of the biopsy, the following rules should be followed.

1. The incision should be small and longitudinal in the extremity. Transverse incisions about the shoulder, except over the clavicle, should be avoided. The incision should be placed in such a manner that the entire track of the biopsy procedure can be excised with the specimen at the time of definitive treatment.
2. Meticulous hemostasis should be performed and soft tissue dissection limited to avoid extension of the tumor cell within muscle compartment or the loose alveolar tissues of the shoulder.
3. Muscle planes should not be violated, since this possibly extends an intracompartmental (T1) lesion to a T2. The exception to this rule is in relation to the anatomy of the deltoid, which more or less makes it mandatory that a biopsy of the upper end of the humerus be performed through the deltopectoral groove. If one performs the biopsy through the deltoid muscle, the subsequent sur-

gery will require sacrifice of that portion of the muscle violated by the surgery and hence all muscle anterior and medial to the laterally placed incision will be denervated.

4. On biopsy of a bone tumor that has a soft tissue mass extending from it, it is not necessary to enter the bone. If a pathologic fracture occurs through the biopsy defect site, the case becomes much more complicated. If it is necessary to enter the bone, a small plug of methyl methacrylate may be helpful in avoiding a spill and preventing pathologic fracture.

5. Closure of the biopsy site should be in multiple layers of continuous sutures, after careful hemostasis is obtained. A drain should not be used, since this contaminates all of the tissues between the wound and the exit site of the drain tubing.

6. Needle biopsies may be appropriate for bone and soft tissue lesions about the shoulder, especially if the lesion is likely to bleed excessively or is in an anatomical location where biopsy is likely to violate an anatomical plane. The pathologist should be consulted prior to the biopsy to be certain that he or she concurs with the approach.

PRINCIPLES OF MANAGEMENT

In general, the principles of management of the various bone and soft tissue tumors that occur about the shoulder do not materially differ from those in other parts, except perhaps in relation to the surgical problems associated with the rather complex anatomical structures, and especially the rotator cuff. The principles have been enunciated in prior publications,[2,45,52,57,69,123,136,139,145,214,247] but are deserving of at least partial reiteration since they are critical to sound judgement regarding selection of an operative procedure and its performance.

Safety

Perhaps the foremost issue is that of safety for the patient. As orthopaedists, we are conditioned from our earliest residency to the concept that relief of pain and restoration of form and function are our principal goals in the management of any musculoskeletal disorder. Because so few of the disorders we treat are truly life threatening, we sometimes lose sight of the fact that as physicians we must also assume the awesome responsibility for preservation of life. In the management of patients with aggressive or malignant tumors about the shoulder or any anatomical part, the first consideration must be the safety of the surgical or nonsurgical plan; only after that is considered optimal, can we consider the other issues. Expressed more directly, an amputation in a live patient is better than a functional restoration of the shoulder in a dead one.

Enneking and co-workers[53,57] have described four types of surgical procedures commonly employed in the management of patients with bone or soft tissue tumors, based not on anatomical or functional factors, but on the proximity of the surgical margin to the tumor and its extensions into the adjacent tissues. Several studies[51,55,57] have now clearly demonstrated that the recurrence, and indeed survival, rates are heavily dependent on this factor, which, depending on the nature of the lesion, may determine the success or failure of the procedure and the ultimate outcome.

To understand this classification system more fully, one must appreciate how tumors, especially malignant ones, grow and affect the adjacent tissues. Neoplasms of the connective tissues whether demonstrating "pushing" (such as the chondrosarcoma) or "invasive" (as seen in the osteosarcoma) borders, spread by extension into the adjacent normal tissues and by vascular invasion rather than by entry into the lymphatic system.[52,53,57] The normal tissues adjacent to the advancing border of the neoplasm become compressed and at times display a cellular response, presumably as an attempt to "wall off" the malignant tissue. This zone of compressed tissue spoken of as the "reactive zone" or "pseudocapsule" is a discrete anatomical layer, often relatively easily separated from the tumor by blunt dissection during a surgical procedure, a process known as "shelling out." Careful histologic study of the margin of the tumor, however, demonstrates that the reactive zone is usually not a tumor-free envelope but often contains discrete microscopic "daughter nodules" and even more frequently shows invasive tongues of tumor continuous with the major neoplastic mass. Another phenomenon that occurs with both malignant tumors of bone and soft tissues is the presence of discrete nodules of tumors in the same anatomical compartment, but often far removed from the primary site: so called "skip" lesions or metastases.[54] This is uncommon with such lesions as the chondrosarcoma or low-grade tumors of any tissue type, but relatively frequent with higher-grade lesions such as the osteosarcoma.

Procedures

If one then considers the possible types of resective or ablative surgical procedures that could be performed to achieve local control of the tumor, there are four. Each can be defined in terms of its proximity to and the likelihood that they will eliminate the major tumor mass, the daughter extensions, or the skip metastases[52,53] (Fig. 19-1). The procedures include the following.

INTRALESIONAL

This amputation or resection cuts across or exposes the primary lesion and thus leaves macroscopic disease behind. All piecemeal, debulking, or curettage procedures are included in this category.

MARGINAL

These are operative procedures (either local resection or amputation) in which the plane of separation of the normal tissue from the tumor mass is in the reactive zone. Procedures such as the "shelling out" of soft tissue or bone tumors are in this category and, as discussed above, are likely to leave microscopic tumor or daughter nodules behind.

WIDE

In these operations the plane of resection includes a significant cuff of normal tissue (be it bone, soft tissue, or both) but does not include the entire anatomical compartment in which the tumor is located. Cross bone resections or amputations for bone tumors and treatment of soft tissue or bone tumors by local resection of the affected structures with a wide cuff of normal tissue are included in this type of procedure. In theory, at least, the threat of local recurrence from daughter lesions or local tongues of invasion of

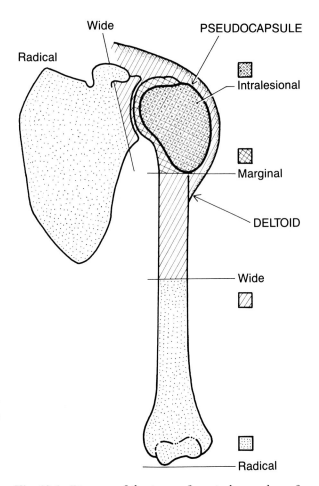

Fig. 19-1. Diagram of the types of surgical procedures for a stage IIB lesion of the proximal humerus (with presumed joint involvement). In this example a stage IIB bone tumor is diagrammed. Note that the definitions of radical, wide, marginal, and intralesional procedures can be applied to amputations as well as resections.

the reactive zone is eliminated by this type of surgery, but the problem of "skip" lesions remains.

RADICAL

These are amputations or resections in which the entire compartment(s) containing the tumor is (are) surgically excised en bloc. Theoretically, this type of procedure eliminates all possible forms of local recurrence of the lesion and, although the safest for the patient, is obviously the most costly in terms of restoration of normal form and function.

There are no set guidelines for deciding which of these four procedures should be applied to any lesion of bone or soft tissue about the shoulder or any other anatomical site. In terms of the staging system, many tumor surgeons believe that the protocols shown in Figure 19-2 are logical. However, as can be seen, there is considerable variation within the management of any particular lesion, dictated in part by the nature and grade of the tumor, the anatomical site, the possible roles of adjunctive chemotherapy or radiation, the age and condition of the patient, and, in no small measure, the wishes of the patient and his or her family. Ideally, however, benign lesions should be treated by intralesional or marginal surgery; stage IA lesions by marginal or wide procedures; stage IB by wide or sometimes marginal or radical procedures; and stages IIA or IIB tumors by wide or radical surgical procedures as circumstances dictate. In selected stage IIB tumors, in order to preserve limb function, it may be possible to peform a wide resection combined with adjunctive therapy such as radiation or chemotherapy in an attempt to prevent local recurrence.

Thus a unicameral bone cyst, chondroblastoma, or lipoma of the shoulder area is best treated by curettage or marginal resection; a giant cell tumor or low-grade chondrosarcoma of the upper end of the humerus by marginal or wide resection; and a high-grade malignant fibrous histiocytoma or osteosarcoma of the shoulder region by wide or radical resection or ablation including much or all of the compartment containing the tumor.

The actual performance of the surgery is also somewhat different from that utilized for the management of traumatic or degenerative lesions of the bones or soft tissues about the shoulder. The scars and soft tissue tracks of prior biopsies or surgical procedures must be included in the resection margin and should remain with the specimen.[139,211,221] *Gentle handling of tissues, meticulous hemostasis and avoidance of excessive soft tissue or skin devitalization are necessary to avoid wound complications such as skin slough, hematoma, and infection.* Rigid fixation of bone graft and protection of the part in the postsurgical period should be used to avoid pathologic fracture through bone weakened by the osseous part of the resection. Although preservation of function is important, the tumor surgeon must be prepared to sacrifice nerves or vascular structures close to the tumor margin and, if necessary, perform reconstructions for the vascular system at the time and for nerves at a second procedure. If bone autograft is to be used in the man-

Fig. 19-2. This chart outlines the ideal choice of surgical procedure for the various stages of disease.

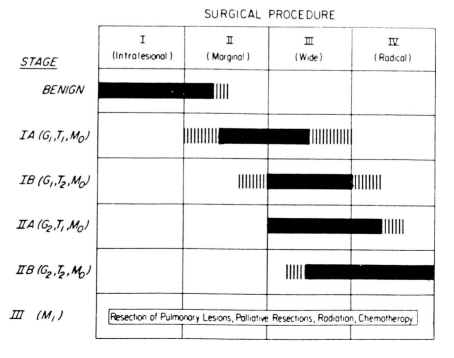

agement of the osseous reconstruction following resection of a malignant tumor, it should either be obtained first or as a separate procedure using fresh instruments, gloves, gowns, and drapes. Finally, and in reiteration, the entire procedure should be reviewed prior to the surgery and carefully planned out to be certain that the optimal margin is achieved; then, and only then, should the surgeon consider the restoration of the normal (or as near to normal as possible) form and function.

DIAGNOSIS AND MANAGEMENT OF TUMORS ABOUT THE SHOULDER

An inclusive and exhaustive description of the clinical, radiographic, and histologic characteristics and the various treatment strategies for all of the tumors that may occur around the shoulder is beyond the scope of this volume. Instead, we shall define some of the more common entities, describe some of the currently accepted methods of treatment, and append appropriate literature citations for the interested reader. This section of the chapter is divided into parts. Benign bone and soft tissue tumors is considered first; malignant primary lesions, second; and metastatic deposits included as a final portion. For each of the entities discussed, we provide a brief discussion of clinical description, imaging characteristics, pathologic features, and suggested protocols for management. A classification system for these lesions is shown in Tables 19-4 and 19-5.

Benign Tumors

TUMORS OF BONE

Osteoid Osteoma

Description. The lesion described by Jaffe and coworkers[107] over 50 years ago remains as enigmatic in cause now as then, but most pathologists agree that it is probably a benign neoplasm of bone, in which the vascular and nervous elements appear to share in the low-grade proliferative ac-

tivity.[36,52,93,98,105,196,202,219] Its characteristic location in the cortex of the bone, its capacity to evoke a sclerotic response in the surrounding osseous tissues, and the highly stereotypic pain pattern make this lesion relatively simple to diagnose. More frequent in male patients in the first four decades of life, the lesion has a highly characteristic clinical presentation dominated by complaints of dull aching pain that is worse at night and completely relieved by aspirin.[36,52,98,136,202]

Imaging Studies. The radiographic features of osteoid osteoma depend upon location. The typical intracortical osteoid osteoma is a round or oval lucent "nidus" measuring less than 1.0 cm in greatest dimension, surrounded by a markedly sclerotic periosteal and endosteal response. The nidus frequently contains calcification. Intramedullary osteoid osteoma is usually surrounded by a much smaller degree of ill-defined "cloud-like" medullary sclerosis and is, therefore, harder to identify on radiographs. Intraarticular or periosteal osteoid osteoma may provoke essentially no sclerotic response and can be very difficult to identify radiologically. Fortunately, radionuclide bone scans detect this lesion reliably. If more precise localization is needed, tomography or CT can be helpful. The lesions are markedly hypervascular, and in rare instances angiography will be useful.

Pathology. Microscopically the nidus is composed of a haphazard arrangement of woven bone spicules embedded in a prominent fibrovascular stroma (Fig. 19-3). Osteoblasts and osteoclasts are prominent along the surface of these spicules. Often the woven bone is heavily mineralized, which accounts for the radiographic image of the nidus. However, the nidus may be "lucent" on radiographs if these trabeculae are not well mineralized. The reactive bony shell that surrounds the nidus is often a mixture of lamellar and woven bone. Histologically, it is almost impossible to distinguish between the nidus of osteoid–osteoma and an osteoblastoma. The diagnostic features, therefore, include the histology coupled with the radiographic studies.

Treatment. Although one occasionally hears anecdotal accounts of the spontaneous disappearance of an osteoid osteoma,[52,76,98] the lesion usually persists and is relatively unresponsive to medications other than aspirin. Persistent discomfort, continued need

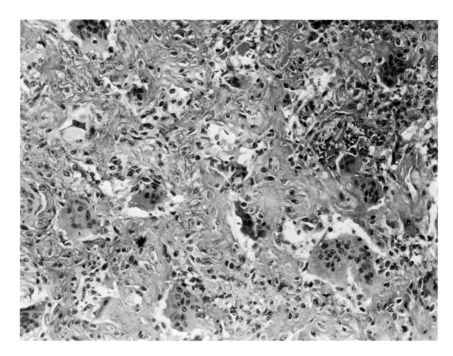

Fig. 19-3. The nidus of an osteoid–osteoma with an irregular arrangement of woven bone spicules surrounded by osteoblasts and osteoclasts. There is a rich vascular supply embedded in the fibrous stroma. This microscopic field is indistinguishable from an osteoblastoma. (Hemotoxylin and Eosin, H & E, × 200.)

for salicylates, limitation of the adjacent joint, and overgrowth of the bone all constitute an indication for surgical excision of the lesion and at least a shell of the surrounding dense bone. Incomplete removal or intralesional curetting of the nidus is often associated with a recurrence and thus en bloc marginal resection is recommended,[52,76,136,210] if this can be performed without sacrificing function of the part.

Osteoblastoma

Osteoblastoma is a rare "benign" tumor of bone that histologically resembles the osteoid osteoma, but presents in a different manner[130,142,148,154,238] and may, on occasion, behave in an aggressive or even malignant fashion.[93,148,200,238] The tumor also occurs most often in male patients, is most frequent in the posterior elements of the spine but may affect the long bones, and is most common in young adults.[43,200] The lesion is usually considerably larger than the osteoid osteoma, and the patients rarely present with the classic aspirin dependence. The tumor is sometimes "aggressive," in that it promptly recurs with simple curettage and can be quite destructive in radiographic appearance.

Imaging Studies. The radiologic appearance of osteoblastoma is extremely variable. In the extremities,

these lesions are frequently lytic and sometimes surrounded by an expanded shell of periosteal bone. They are typically demarcated by a well-defined boundary and contain variable amounts of internal calcification. When they occur in the axial skeleton, the lesions are often radiologically dense and frequently accompanied by massive sclerotic response from the adjacent bone.

Pathology. The histologic features of osteoblastoma are identical to the nidus of an osteoid–osteoma. The so-called "aggressive" osteoblastoma has plump atypical osteoblasts that are not morphologically different from the fibrovascular "stroma." Since such lesions often recur and may even metastasize, we believe that this entity should be classified as a low-grade osteosarcoma.

Management. As indicated above, the osteoblastoma may on occasion behave in an aggressive or even malignant manner so that, if possible, it would seem appropriate to excise the lesion completely. Of the lesions located around the shoulder in our series, this was possible in two: one in the glenoid and the other in the anatomical neck of the humerus.[238] In two others it was possible to curette the lesion thoroughly, burr the wall with a power drill, wash the cavity with 50 percent phenol in normal saline (no alcohol wash to follow), and then pack the cavity with allograft or autograft. None of the four lesions so treated in our series recurred, but our patients with lesions at other sites (especially the pelvis) have not been quite this fortunate.[43,238]

Fibrous Dysplasia

Fibrous dysplasia of bone is a disorder in which regions of the medullary cavity of the bones are replaced by a peculiar fibroosseous tissue.[84,105,223] The disease may be limited to one bone (monostotic)[96] or in many parts of the skeleton (polyostotic); a small number of the latter cases may be associated with a bizarre polyendocrinopathy and peculiar, flat, irregularly shaped, lightly pigmented skin lesions (cafe au-lait spots). The process more likely represents a developmental abnormality than a true neoplasm, but no consistent familial or genetic factors have been identified in the pathogenesis.[84,105] The diagnosis of florid polyostotic disease can often be made early in childhood, but recognition of less severe syndromes and especially the monostotic form may not occur until adult life.[84] Children with the florid polyostotic form of the disease may be dwarfed and show grotesque skeletal deformities affecting the skull, facial bones, and extremities, especially the hips and occasionally shoulder girdles.[84,92] The most prevalent endocrine disturbance is precocious puberty (Albright's syndrome), but hyperthyroidism, sever vitamin D-resistant rickets, and Cushing's disease have been described.[1,41,84]

Imaging Studies. The radiologic appearance of fibrous dysplasia depends on the histologic maturity of the lesion. "Young" lesions contain little bone and appear radiologically lucent. There may be an expanded appearance due to endosteal resorption and periosteal new bone formation. A thickly sclerotic "rind" often surrounds lesions in the extremities. Severe deformity is typical of the polyostotic form of the disease, but is less frequent in monostotic fibrous dysplasia.

Maturation of the lesions results in the formation of myriad microscopically visible "chinese characters" of bone. The "ground glass" appearance characteristic of fibrous dysplasia results from the summation of these structures. Particularly dense and prominent ground glass appearance is characteristic of lesions involving the facial bones. Fibrous dysplasia may also include cystic components, and other cell types, especially cartilage, which are recognizable on radiographs.

Pathology. Microscopically the diagnostic feature of fibrous dysplasia is the purposeless, haphazard mixture of woven bone spicules enmeshed in a benign collagenous spindle cell background. Furthermore, the bone spicules are not surrounded by prominent osteoblasts but, in fact, have their collagenous fibers contiguous with that of the adjacent stroma. The bone spicules have peculiar "C" and "U" shapes as they grow adjacent to nearby vessels (Fig. 19-4). Often osteoblasts are prominent and occasionally masses of hyaline cartilage may be embedded in the fibrous matrix. If the cartilage is abundant, it may be confused with a primary cartilage tumor. In large lesions, hemorrhagic foci occur that account for the radiographic "cyst" and may be confused histologically with an aneurysmal bone cyst. However, if such lesions are adequately sampled, diagnostic histologic features of fibrous dysplasia are seen.

Management. Treatment of the bony lesions of fibrous dysplasia are principally directed at prevention or correction of bony deformities, and sometimes represents a major challenge. Curettage of the lesional area is usually associated with a recurrence of the pathologic tissue and eventual erosion and destruction of implanted autograft.[92] Since allograft is replaced at a much slower rate, when the integrity of the bone is threatened or when a deformity is to be corrected, our current policy is to use cadaveric alloimplants as internal struts and supplement them as necessary with appropriate internal fixation devices. Malignant degeneration is fortunately rare and, for practical purposes, is not a consideration in these patients.[102]

Unicameral Bone Cyst

The unicameral or simple bone cyst is one of the most frequently encountered lesions of the humerus. It is most common in the first two decades of life and occurs equally in boys and girls.[19,36] The cause is unknown, but is presumed to be a disorder of the growth plate,[36] possibly a transient circulatory compromise resulting from a developmental anomaly of the veins of an affected bone,[17,28] or some alteration in the structure of the chondrocyte columns.[105] The

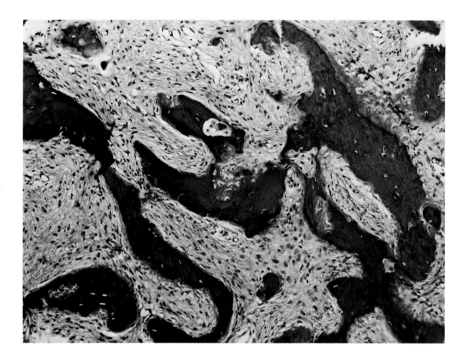

Fig. 19-4. Fibrous dysplasia with the characteristic woven bone spicules that lack osteoblasts enmeshed in benign fibrous tissue. Some osteoclasts are visible. The peculiar "c" shape of the bone is secondary to growth around vessels. (H & E, × 125.)

lesion consists of a symmetrically central thin-walled cystic cavity filled with a clear fluid (that is in communication with the serum), which initially abuts on the epiphyseal plate and, with advancing age, moves away.[28] The cysts are painless and are usually discovered incidentally on chest radiographs or when a pathologic fracture occurs through the weakened bone. Rarely a unicameral cyst penetrates the epiphyseal plate to enter the epiphysis and cause growth disturbance.[25]

Imaging Studies. A unicameral bone cyst is basically a fluid-filled sac. It has a simple geometric shape and contains no internal structure (Fig. 19-5). Occasionally, ridges on the surface of the cyst give the appearance of internal septations, which is a false impression readily disproven by tomography or CT. The cyst margins are well-defined. Periosteal reaction is not seen except in the event of pathologic fracture. The fluid-filled nature of the structure can occasionally be proven by demonstration of a "fallen fragment" of bone within the cyst. Computed tomography is often diagnostic in these lesions, because the uniform water density of the internal contents can be established. Occasionally, the fluid content of bone cysts will be partially or completely replaced by air.

Pathology. The histologic picture of a simple bone cyst consists of a benign fibrous wall that may have osteoclast-type giant cells, macrophages filled with hemosiderin, prominent vessels, and even bone spicules, often of the woven type. The internal surface does not have an endothelial lining. However, the lining is usuall extremely thin and wispy and may be obscured by the abundant hemorrhagic fluid evacuated by the surgeon (Figs. 19-6 and 19-7).

Management. Over the years a number of protocols have been advanced for the management of these lesions. If the cortical wall is thick enough to limit the likelihood of fracture, there is probably no reason to treat this lesion, since most will disappear by the time the child reaches maturity. A pathologic fracture through a unicameral cyst will heal, essentially at the same rate as a normal bone and on occasion appears to stimulate at least partial obliteration of the cyst. For those patients in whom the cyst continues to be a problem, the time-honored method of management is curettage and packing of the cavity with allograft or autograft[28,161] (we prefer the former), but care should be taken to avoid vigorous mechanical curettage of the region of the epiphyseal plate. The recurrence rate following such procedures has been esti-

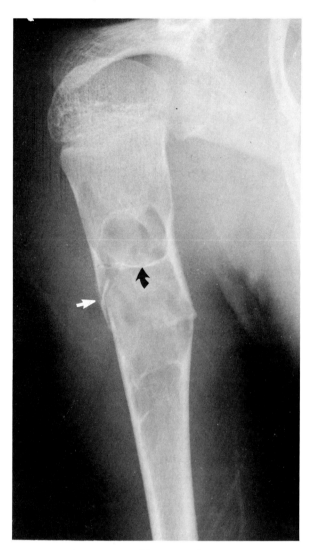

Fig. 19-5. This unicameral bone cyst first came to attention following a fracture (white arrow). The cyst margins are well defined by a thin sclerotic boundary. There is no evidence of active periosteal response. Transverse ridges arising from the endosteum on the surface of the cyst give the impression of internal septa (black arrow).

mated at 50 percent or more.[161] Subtotal resection of the cyst region has been advocated by Fahey and O'Brian and others with reported greater success rates.[67,153] In the past decade, the method proposed by Scaglietti of injecting the cyst with methylprednisolone has become the treatment of choice in many centers for uncomplicated cysts and seems to result

in a slow obliteration in up to 75 percent of the lesions so treated.[23,193,194]

Aneurysmal Bone Cyst

Aneurysmal bone cyst is a much less common lesion than its unicameral counterpart and is encountered even less commonly in the osseous structures around the shoulder.[36,98,157,196] Neither the cell of origin nor the intrinsic neoplastic nature of the process for this lesion is clearly defined, and there is some evidence to support the contention, now held by a number of pathologists, that the lesion is often a secondary one and in fact, represents an abnormal vascular response to an underlying process such as giant cell tumor, osteoblastoma, or chondroblastoma.[36,117,215] In support of that view is the occasional finding in one or another site within a lesion of a focus of tissue demonstrating some of the histologic characteristics of a more aggressive tumor such as the giant cell tumor or osteoblastoma. Nevertheless, the aneurysmal cyst appears to have a clinical pattern of presentation and natural history quite distinct from these other entities, which dictate that at least for purposes of classification it be treated as a discrete entity.

Most aneurysmal bone cysts present in individuals under the age of 25 and have a predilection for the shafts or metaphyses of the long bones or, less commonly, the vertebrae.[19,36,98,157,196,215] A traumatic episode is often associated with the onset of the lesion and the patient may note persistent pain at the site and a distinct swelling over the part. In relation to the shoulder, most of the aneurysmal cysts we have encountered have been in the upper end of the humerus, where they produce a circumferential, somewhat eccentric enlargement of that bone and may cause considerable pain, interference with normal function of the part, and serve as a site for pathologic fracture. Although the lesions may appear quite aggressive on radiographic imaging and sometimes resemble either an aggressive giant cell tumor or the highly malignant telangiectatic osteosarcoma (see below), they are benign in nature and should be treated relatively conservatively if possible.

Imaging Studies. As mentioned above, the radiographic appearance of aneurysmal cyst is similar to that of other lesions causing massive expansion of the bony profile (Fig 19-8). In the tubular bones the lesion tends to have an ovoid configuration and an expanded

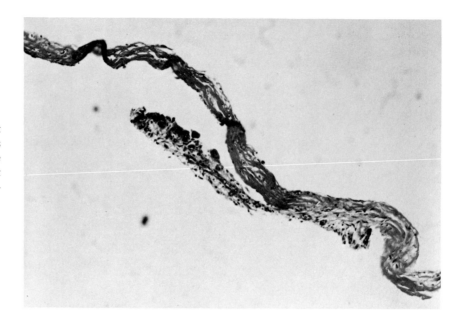

Fig. 19-6. A simple bone cyst with a wispy lining of fibrous tissue and some osteoclast-type giant cells. Such transparent tissue is often not seen at surgery. (H & E, × 125.)

or "blistered" appearance. The borders are well-demarcated and often sclerotic. Occasionally, the cyst walls will be unusually thick or dense, suggesting that expansion of the lesion has ceased.

Computed tomography of these lesions generally reveals the presence of a solid internal soft tissue component, a finding not present in a unicameral bone cyst. Occasionally, fluid–fluid levels may be demonstrated, particularly if the patient has had to lie on the CT couch for a prolonged period of time.

Despite the presence of numerous hemorrhagic spaces on pathologic examination, lesions appear hypovascular on angiography.

Pathology. Histologically, the diagnosis of an aneurysmal bone cyst is really made by excluding the following most common lesions that have cyst formation, listed in decreasing frequency: giant cell

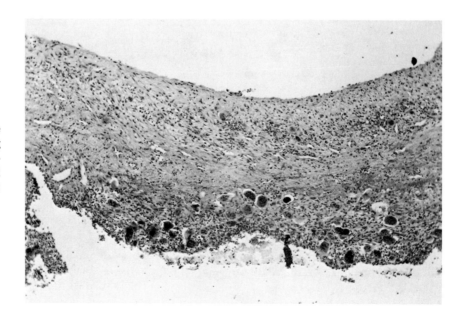

Fig. 19-7. Another simple bone cyst with a thicker lining of fibrous tissue, osteoclast-type giant cells, vessels, and macrophages. (H & E, × 79.)

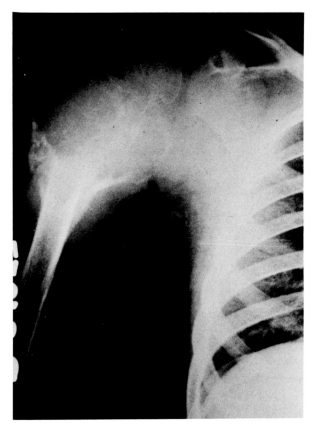

Fig. 19-8. A typical radiograph of an aneurysmal bone cyst of the proximal humerus in a 13-year-old girl; the cyst enlarged significantly following a steroid injection. The cortex has been destroyed but the lesion is surrounded by a shell of periosteal bone leading to an "aneurysmal" enlargement of the bone. The extent, although not well marginated, is well delineated but at times differentiation from a telangiectatic osteosarcoma can be difficult. The patient responded well to curettage and allograft bone packing.

tumor, osteoblastoma, chondroblastoma, osteosarcoma, and fibrous dysplasia, all of which may undergo hemorrhagic cyst formation. If all of the tissue is carefully examined, the majority of so-called aneurysmal bone cysts will fall into one of these categories. However, a small percentage of lesions will not have any diagnostic features of other entities and, therefore, may be called aneurysmal bone cysts. The histologic features are nonspecific but include a lining of benign fibrous tissue, often with spicules of woven of lamellar bone, scattered osteoclast-type giant cells, and hemosiderin-laden macrophages (Fig. 19-9). In essence,

the lining is similar to that of a unicameral bone cyst, except it is thicker and must "aneurysmally" balloon the bone on the radiograph.

Management. The principal problems in managing patients with aneurysmal bone cyst involve assessing the nature of the problem. As indicated above, these lesions are rare and although they do resemble to some extent more common unicameral cyst, they usually are more symptomatic, more eccentrically placed, and are much more aggressive and "blown-out" in appearance on radiographic studies. Differentiating the lesions from the giant cell tumor or telangiectatic osteosarcoma is more difficult on routine studies.[117] Both of the latter tumors may show extraosseous extension and are highly vascular on the angiogram, while the aneurysmal cyst is not. Of course the histologic studies, although occasionally confusing, are usually diagnostic for the two more aggressive neoplasms.

A second problem in relation to the diagnosis is the biopsy. Aneurysmal bone cysts can bleed with extraordinary briskness and sometimes can be quite frightening to the surgeon. Needle biopsies would ordinarily be more valuable as a diagnostic approach but are often unsatisfactory in obtaining sufficient tissue to assess the nature of the lesion. Despite the potential for excessive blood loss, the most appropriate course is an open biopsy, frozen section, and then definitive treatment if the tissue is diagnostic. If it is not, it is preferable to wait until the permanent sections are available before planning and performing the surgical management. This course, although more difficult for the patient, is safer in that the management of either the giant cell tumor or especially the telagiectatic osteosarcoma requires considerably greater attention to surgical margins than the more benign aneurysmal cyst.

The most appropriate course for the surgical management of aneurysmal cysts about the shoulder is thorough curettage and packing of the resultant cavity with either auto- or allograft bone.[27,117,215] This approach is most appropriate if no or only limited distortion of the joint surface is present. If the latter has occurred, some form of buttressing with allograft or autograft struts is probably a reasonable approach. Aneurysmal bone cysts may recur if all of the lesional tissue is not removed and, under these circumstances, may require a marginal resection and arthrodesis of

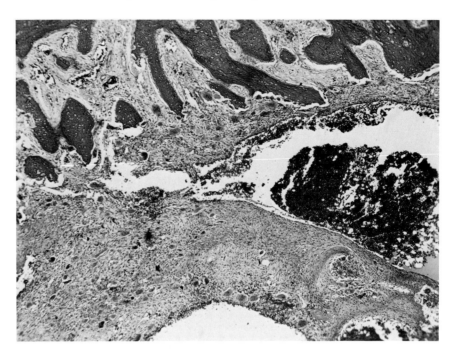

Fig. 19-9. The so-called aneurysmal bone cyst has a thick lining of benign fibrous tissue, spicules of woven bone, scattered osteoclast-type giant cells, and macrophages. The spaces filled with blood are *not* lined by endothelial cells. (H & E, × 50.)

the joint or replacement of the resected segment with graft, prosthesic implant, or both. If the lesion recurs, the patient should be subjected to restaging and a careful restudy of the tissue obtained at the time of primary resection to be certain that some more serious pathologic entity has not been overlooked. Radiation therapy, sometimes advocated for aneurysmal bone cysts of the spine, probably has no place in the management of lesions of the appendicular skeleton and especially the region around the shoulder.

Osteocartilaginous Exostosis

Solitary osteocartilaginous exostoses (called by some authors osteochondromas) are the most common tumors of the skeleton,[36] and probably of the bones of the shoulder girdle as well. The tumors are considered to result from a genetic defect in the embryonic cartilage anlage or the restraining periosteum surrounding the physis and ring of Ranvier.[105] They often present as sessile or (less commonly about the shoulder) pedunculated, cartilage-covered bony excrescences in the metaphyseal region of the humerus or the body of the scapula. The lesions grow by a disordered form of endochondral ossification and, just as for normal physes, cease to enlarge at the time of skeletal maturity.[114]

The tumors are probably present at birth, but do not usually become clinically manifest until the latter part of the first or early part of the second decade of life. The patient is usually noted to have a painless, nontender, eccentric enlargement of the metaphyseal region of the humerus often associated, if the lesion is large, with some shortening and/or bowing of that bone. If the exostosis presents in relation to the posterior aspect of the blade of the scapula, a prominent bony knob may be seen and felt; if it is on the vertebral face of the bone, winging of the scapula and crepitus with motion may be the principal findings. The tumors themselves usually cause no difficulty for the patient unless, as in the case of the scapular lesions, a bursa forms between the tumor and the subjacent ribs or, as in the case of the humerus, they press on adjacent neurovascular structures.[136] Rarely, particularly around the shoulder, a fracture of the stalk may cause significant acute symptoms.

The multiple hereditary form of osteocartilaginous exostosis is an autosomal dominant disturbance, slightly more common in male patients, characterized by often large numbers of cartilage-covered bony excrescences distributed throughout that portion of the skeleton that arises from cartilage by endochondral ossification.[105,106,136,201,216,217] The combination of the metaphyseal enlargement resulting from the presence of the lesions and the growth disturbances associated with their presence produce sometimes gross distortions in the skeleton. Shortening and bowing of the humerus, distortion of the normal shape of the scapula, narrowing of the thoracic outlet, and limitation of motion of the shoulder girdle are common findings in such patients. As in the solitary form of the disease, the lesions are in themselves asymptomatic, but may cause pain by development of bursal sacs or by pressure on adjacent neurovascular structures.

Of considerable importance is the much-debated incidence of "malignant degeneration" of the benign osteocartilaginous exostotic lesions, either solitary or in a patient with widespread disease.[98,105,136] The incidence of chondrosarcoma arising in solitary osteocartilaginous exostoses is probably far less than 0.1 percent and, for practical purposes, is not a significant threat.[136] The incidence according to some authors is considerably higher in the hereditary multiple form of the disorder, although we have observed it infrequently in our practice, and it is unlikely to occur more frequently than in 1 percent of patients so afflicted. More centrally placed large tumors that cause pain or are seen to enlarge after maturity is reached should be viewed with some suspicion. The bone scan is of some value in evaluating these patients in adulthood.[136]

Imaging Studies. Recognizing benign osteocartilaginous exostosis is generally not difficult. The lesions are exophytic. Since they arise by disordered growth of the growth plate, no cortex ever forms beneath an exostosis. Instead, there is smooth continuity of the adjacent normal cortex with the "stalk" of the exostosis (Fig. 19-10). Occasionally, the stalk may be very short and inapparent. When seen "en face," the cortical defect beneath the exostosis appears surrounded by the wall of the stalk, giving rise to the so called "chimney sign." Osteochondromas appear to be shaped and molded by the action of adjacent muscles, characteristically pointing away from the nearest joint.

The lesions may be topped by a cartilaginous cap of variable thickness. The cartilaginous component can be recognized by the typical radiographic appearance of scattered, dense, punctate, accurate, and circular calcifications and by the lobular contour suggesting a nodular growth pattern. Since the amount of cartilage covering an exostosis is thought to be rele-

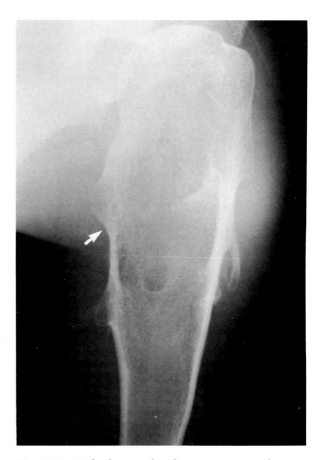

Fig. 19-10. Multiple osteochondromas are seen in the proximal humerus of a patient with familial osteochondromatosis. Notice that the stalk of the lesion shows a common medullary canal with the underlying bone and that there is continuity of the cortex of the bone with the cortex of the lesion (arrow).

vant to the diagnosis of malignancy, several efforts have been made to measure the thickness of cartilage, but success in predicting malignant transformation has been limited. Other features suggesting malignant transformation are large areas of nonmineralized cartilage (best seen with CT or MRI) and invasion of the stalk of the lesion.

Pathology. The osteochondroma has two diagnostic histologic features: a benign hyaline cartilage cap, usually undergoing endochondral ossification, which is covered on its external surface by a thin fibrous membrane, the residual perichondrium; and a direct communication with marrow cavity of the parent bone since no cortex ever formed embryologically. The cartilage cap is thicker and more cellular in children and teenagers and less so in adults (Fig. 19-11). However, even in the elderly the cartilage cap may still be active and should not be interpreted as a chondrosarcoma. The prominance of the endochondral ossification with formation of the primary trabeculae accounts for the dense mineralization on radiographs. If portions of the perichondrium remain in the patient, the lesion may recur and does not mean that a malignancy has occurred.

Management. For solitary osteocartilaginous exostoses, the lesion should be staged by appropriate studies to be certain that it does not represent a primary exostotic chondrosarcoma (see below). As indicated above, lesions that are small, painless, enlarging only slowly in children and not at all in adults, and show none of the characteristics of malignancy on imaging studies can be considered to be benign with very small likelihood of malignant degeneration.[136] The indications for resection are related to alterations in function or contour of the shoulder (deformity of the humerus or winging of the scapula, narrowing of the thoracic outlet) or pressure on adjacent structures (costal or neurovascular). Resection, particularly of large sessile lesions located on the medial or poste-

rior part of the proximal humerus, may be technically difficult. Wherever possible, the perichondrium covering the cartilage cap should be resected with the specimen and the tumor amputated through its base at the junction with the normal cortex.

The indications for surgery in patients with the multiple hereditary form of the disease are much less clear. In this circumstance, removing the lesion(s) does not "cure" the disease and the surgical procedures should be reserved for those patients who demonstrate sufficient evidence of interference with function or pressure on adjacent neurovascular structures.[201] In a rare patient with florid disease, a rapidly enlarging tumor, pain at the site, and increased activity on bone scan or imaging studies suggestive of malignant degeneration dictate that the patient should be staged for the possibility of chondrosarcoma and treated accordingly (see below).

Enchondroma

The solitary enchondroma is less common than its exostotic counterpart, but has an extraordinarily high incidence in the proximal humerus,[36,98,152,157,196] so that its frequency in patients who present with complaints about the shoulder may be quite high. As with the osteocartilaginous exostosis, the lesion possi-

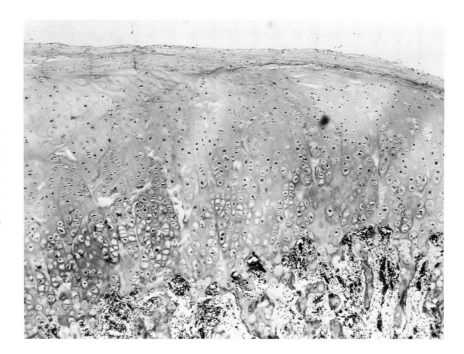

Fig. 19-11. The hyaline cartilage cap of an osteochondroma with the prominent surface layer of fibrous tissue representing the perichondrium. There is also active endochondral ossification. (H & E, × 50.)

bly represents persistence of a small remnant of the cartilage anlage of the embryonic skeleton, and hence may be present at birth and slowly enlarge during childhood.[105] The relationship of increase in lesional size to activity and cessation of physeal growth is far less clear however, since even proven benign enchondromas show histologic evidence of DNA synthesis and increased activity on bone scan even in individuals late in life.[136] The mean age of presentation in several series is in the third decade,[36,98,157,196] and in modest contrast to the exostotic tumor and to the lesions in other parts, enchondromas about the shoulder in our series were found to be more frequent in women. The tumor is almost always metaphyseal or metaphyseodiaphseal in location and centrally placed, causing in some cases some concentric enlargement of the bone. The tumors of the upper humerus, or more rarely of the scapula, are usually asymptomatic, being noted either on chest radiographs or on imaging studies performed for a painful or limited shoulder of other cause. Occasionally a patient is seen in whom the first finding is a pathologic fracture through an enchondroma of the upper end of the humerus.

The two syndromes that make up multiple enchondromatosis (Ollier's and Mafucci's syndromes) are much less frequent than the solitary form of the disease (particularly Mafucci's syndrome, in which the skeletal cartilage tumors are associated with venous malformations of the soft tissues) and far rarer than their exostotic counterpart, hereditary multiple osteocartilaginous exostosis.[127,133,147] The lesions usually affect many of the bones preformed in cartilage and, when widespread, cause severe deformities of the skeleton and considerable disability. Unlike the exostotic form of cartilage tumors, the evidence for genetic transmission is very limited and the disease appears to arise mostly as a spontaneous mutation.[147] Lesions are discovered at an early age and progress throughout the period of growth; in florid cases they may cause grotesque deformities of the limbs.

The major issue that must concern the orthopaedist caring for patients with solitary or multiple enchondromas is "malignant degeneration" or, as has been suggested by Unni et al.,[239] spontaneous onset of malignancy in patients with these tumors. Differentiation of a benign lesion from a low-grade malignancy is often difficult[72] on clinical, imaging, or even histologic grounds, and perhaps more than any other lesion, the enostotic cartilage tumors are either under- or

overtreated. General axioms we apply to these tumors are as follows:[136]

1. Chondrosarcomas are rare prior to the age of skeletal maturity.
2. Large tumors are malignant, small ones are benign.
3. The more proximally placed in the skeleton the lesion is the more likely it is to be malignant; the more distal and acral, the less likely.
4. Cortical erosion, lack of margination, and a soft tissue mass on imaging studies are findings consistent with malignancy.
5. Activity of the bone scan does not differentiate benign from malignant, but a lesion that shows no activity on bone scan is almost surely benign.
6. The more heavily calcified the lesion, the less likely it is to be malignant.
7. The incidence of malignancy in an central cartilage lesion is considerably greater in patients with Ollier's and especially Mafucci's syndromes.
8. Independent of all of the above, the patient who presents with persistent pain, and especially night pain, should be viewed with a strong suspicion that the lesion is malignant.

These axioms are obviously somewhat "soft" and require considerable experience to apply appropriately. Thus, a large painful tumor of the scapula in a middle-aged patient with Mafucci's syndrome that shows cortical erosion, lack of calcification, and is active on scan is obviously malignant; while a small, asymptomatic, solitary lesion in the distal parts of a teenager is almost surely benign. The difficulty lies in the middle ground, when considerable diagnostic acumen may be required to assess the grade of the lesion and determine the appropriate treatment.

Imaging Studies. The typical enchondroma is a centrally placed calcified lesion found within the metaphysis or diaphysis of a tubular bone (Fig. 19-12). If the tumor is well-demarcated by adjacent trabecular bone or if it erodes the endosteal margin of the cortex the boundaries will be sharply defined and lobular in configuration. Otherwise its margins may be difficult to discern. Mineral deposition occurs on the surface of individual cartilage lobules and between the lobules in a characteristic pattern that may be punctate or arranged in a series of tiny arcs and bro-

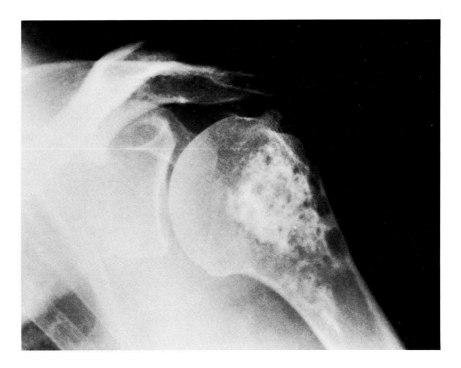

Fig. 19-12. A typical enchondroma of the proximal humerus showing ringlike areas and amorphous deposits of calcification centrally with a radiolucent halo peripherally. The cortex is thinned (scalloped) in areas but is intact. At times it is difficult to be sure that one is not dealing with a low-grade chondrosarcoma.

ken arcs. Since mineral deposition is a time-dependent process, the oldest portions of the lesion tend to calcify first and hence calcification begins centrally. The lesions are, therefore, often surrounded by a radiolucent halo when patients are seen as young adults. Progressive mineralization of the halo may give the incorrect impression that the lesion is enlarging. The distribution of mineral within a quiescent enchondroma tends to be relatively uniform and the lesion may be demarcated by an ossified wall. Noncalcified areas within a basically calcified lesion should suggest recent growth, and hence the possibility of malignant transformation. Enchondromas take the "path of least resistance" in their growth, enlarging along the shaft of the bone and hence resulting in a tumor longer than it is broad. Radiographically, they may be difficult to differentiate from medullary infarction of bone.

Pathology. Enchondromas are histologically composed of benign hyaline cartilage and resemble the cartilage anlage of the bone. Often the peripheral portion of the enchondroma is mineralized and may even undergo endochondral ossification. Therefore, the peripheral portions are rimmed by bone, either woven or lamellar (Figs. 19-13, 19-14). Enchondromas may be closely applied to the endosteal surface of the cortex but they never infiltrate between preexisting cancellous marrow bone. Although there may be binucleate chondrocytes, the nuclei are small black dots lacking pleomorphism and atypia (Fig. 19-15). In cases of Ollier's disease or Maffucci's syndrome the nuclei are plump but, more importantly, there may be foci of myxoid cartilage with stellate chondrocytes that have their cell processes touching one another (see Fig. 19-33). Therefore, if myxoid tissue is present in an otherwise typical enchondroma, these two diagnoses should be ruled out.

Management. As indicated above, the most important issue in relation to these lesions is careful and accurate staging studies to allow one to be certain of the diagnosis. If a lesion of the proximal humerus is asymptomatic, clearly benign, and is unlikely to result in pathologic fracture, there is little reason to perform a surgical procedure. The patient should be observed by serial radiographic studies, possibly at 6-month or yearly intervals until its lack of aggressive behavior is established. If the tumor is considered benign, but is of some concern to the physician and patient, the logical approach is an open biopsy, frozen section (to be certain that the lesion is benign), thorough curettage, burring of the cavity, instillation of

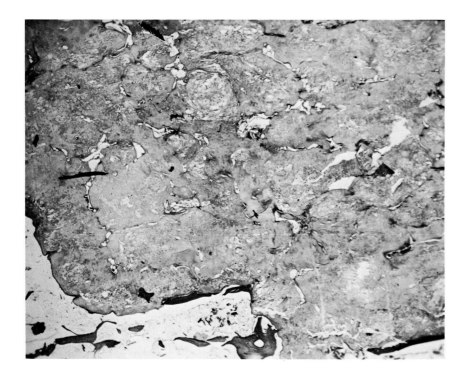

Fig. 19-13. A low-power view of an enchondroma illustrates the bony rim separating the lobular hyaline cartilage from the fatty marrow. Despite the relatively large size of the lesion, there is no intertrabecular invasion of the marrow. (H & E, × 12.)

50 percent phenol in saline, and packing of the cavity with auto- or allograft. If the pathologist is uncertain on the basis of the frozen section, it would be more logical to close the wound and wait for permanent sections before proceeding to the definitive surgical procedure.

In patients with Ollier's or Mafucci's syndromes, the physician should cultivate a high index of suspi-

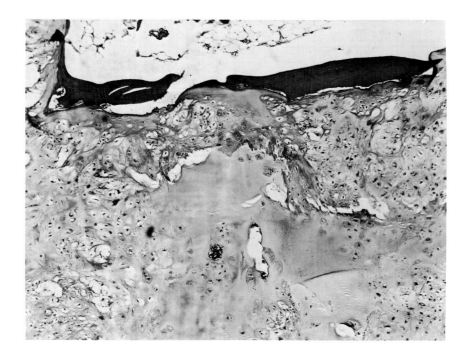

Fig. 19-14. An enchondroma with a prominent rim of lamellar bone. The relatively acellular focus in the center is that of calcified hyaline cartilage. These features of a bony periphery surrounding calcified hypocellular matrix are typical for a enchondroma. (H & E, × 50.)

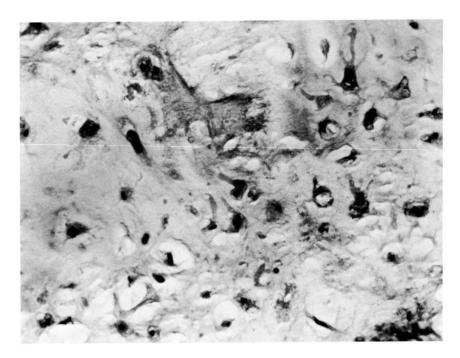

Fig. 19-15. The chondrocytes of an enchondroma have uniform dark nuclei surrounded by abundant hyaline matrix. The granulation in the matrix represents calcification. In this field, two binucleate cells are indicative of cartilage growth rather than malignancy. (H & E, × 313.)

cion for malignant change in the lesions,[22,33,72,127] and be concerned with the onset of pain or changes on bone scan. Occasionally in such patients operative procedures are necessary to correct alignment of the extremities or improve function of a part, but these are less common about the shoulder than in the lower extremity.[136]

Chondroblastoma

The chondroblastoma is a benign cartilage lesion, usually located in the epiphyseal or apophyseal center of the long bones (especially the proximal humerus), and considerably more prevalent in adolescent boys.[103,108,199] The lesion is often painful and tender and results in reduced function and atrophy of the musculature quite early in the course. Although benign, chondroblastomas may be quite destructive locally, sometimes penetrating the epiphyseal plate to enter the metaphysis and may recur after incomplete local treatment.[103,136]

Imaging Studies. Chondroblastoma can usually be readily recognized by its occurrence in secondary growth centers, a rare location for all other types of neoplasms. It is usually demarcated by a sclerotic boundary that may be quite thick (Fig. 19-16). Central

mineralization may be present, which may or may not be recognizably cartilaginous in nature. A curious feature of chondroblastoma is that the lesions sometimes provoke a response at a distance from the lesion, especially distally.

Pathology. Histologically the chondroblastoma is composed of sheets of polygonal cells (chondroblasts) with sharp cytoplasmic borders and a central nucleus. The diagnostic feature is the merging of these cells with islands of poorly formed hyaline cartilage, often bordered by osteoclasts. Furthermore, the chondroblasts are usually outlined by dense dark-staining granules representing the earliest pericellular matrix calcification. If calcification is abundant, the radiograph may have a stippled appearance (Figs. 19-17, 19-18). This tumor may undergo hemorrhagic cyst formation and mimic an aneurysmal bone cyst. Although osteoclasts may be prominent, the features that distinguish this tumor from a giant cell tumor are the presence of cartilage-like foci and the sharp cystoplasmic borders of the chondroblasts, which may be calcified.

Management. Patients with chondroblastoma are almost invariably symptomatic, and the tumor is sufficiently locally destructive to dictate surgery in almost

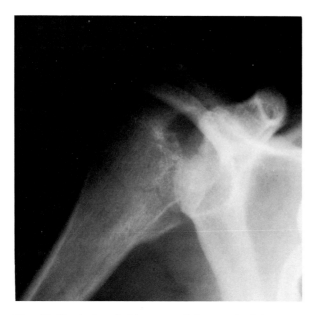

Fig. 19-16. A chondroblastoma of the proximal humerus is seen as a rounded lytic area arising in the head of the humerus, proximal to the closed growth plate. An ill-defined sclerotic boundary surrounds the lesion.

every case. Because most of the tumors are located in the epiphyseal center, and hence lie between the articular cartilage (proximally in the favorite site in the proximal humeral epiphysis) and the epiphyseal cartilage distally, curettage should be performed gently and carefully to avoid injuring either of these structures. For similar reasons, the use of adjuvant materials such as liquid nitrogen or phenol should be avoided.[136] The cavity should be packed with auto- or allograft bone, and the limb immobilized for a sufficiently long time to allow repair of the rotator cuff. The recurrence rate after such treatment approximates 25 percent,[103,136,220] but repeat curettage and packing is usually successful in eradicating the lesion.[220]

Less Common Benign Cartilage Lesions

Although the chondromyxoid fibroma may occur at any site, it is a rare tumor, most prevalent about the knee in individuals in the second and third decade.[71,177,198] The lesion is usually eccentric, well marginated, and shows an expanded portion of the bone with a thin cortical shell. The inner margin is usually scalloped and the lesion may show psuedo-

trabeculation.[136,198] The tumor, which consists of sheets of interspersed fibrous, myxoid, and cartilaginous elements, is clearly benign but has a high rate of recurrence after local curettage and packing with bone (up to 40 percent).[136,198]

Juxtacortical chondroma is a rare hyaline exostotic cartilage lesion that may affect the proximal humerus or scapula in teenagers and young adults. The tumor is often symptomatic and must be differentiated from a juxtacortical chondrosarcoma or osteosarcoma; usually biopsy (needle or open) is required. The lesion produces a scalloping from without and shows circumferential heaped-up periosteal reaction of the adjacent bone. Stippled calcification may be present in the substance of the lesion and helps to differentiate the tumor from other juxtacortical lesions.

TUMORS OF SOFT TISSUES

The listing of benign and malignant tumors of the soft tissues shown in Table 19-5 includes a number of lesions that are only occasionally or rarely encountered by even the orthopaedist interested in oncology. The likelihood of the average orthopaedist with a strong interest in neoplastic entities about the shoulder encountering some of these lesions is very small. As discussed in the introductory section, there is little reason to enlarge this chapter to include all of these various entities. The interested reader is referred to several recent texts that detail the clinical and histologic characteristics of these unusual tumors.[62,86,90,225] It nevertheless seems appropriate to select out a small number of the more frequently encountered tumors for brief description.

Of all the benign tumors that may affect the shoulder, most present with a painless mass, which in the case of the lipoma may have been present for many years or, for the hemangioma or lymphangioma, from birth. The ubiquitous (superficial, deep, or intramuscular) lipoma[42,60,64,112,124,245] usually feels soft and almost ballotable, suggesting that it is fatty in nature. The hemangioma[9] or lymphangioma[62,91,163,225,243] may feel soft and puffy, but is irregular in contour and structure and, if extensive, may produce edema of the extremity, discoloration, and clotting abnormalities. The tumors arising from nerve and fibrous tissue are usually quite firm to palpation. Neurilemomas or neurofibromas[156,176,244] are firm, discrete, and movable. If present in close juxtaposition to a major

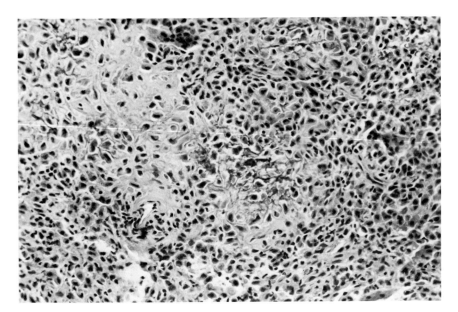

Fig. 19-17. A chondroblastoma with an island of cartilage-like matrix bordered by osteoclasts. The chondroblasts are polygonal with sharp will delineated cytoplasmic borders. (H & E, × 200.)

nerve trunk, they may give rise to pain when palpated or cause neurologic symptoms or signs. These neural tumors as well as the neurolipoma may arise as discrete solitary lesions, but also may occur in association with the syndrome of neurofibromatosis. In the latter case the patient may display all or some of the manifestations of that disease including the skin lesions (fibroma molluscum, axillary freckles, pachydermatocele, and café-au-lait spots), soft tissue tumors (plexi-

form neurofibromas and neurolipomas), and abnormalities of bone (scoliosis, psuedoarthrosis of the tibia, localized gigantism, and facial distortion) and viscera (dumbbell tumors, pheochromocytoma, mental retardation, and glioma).[179] Elastofibroma dorsi almost always presents as a firm mass in the deep soft tissues over the scapula or posterior chest wall of elderly individuals (more often women than men) and has a slow and indolent course of painless

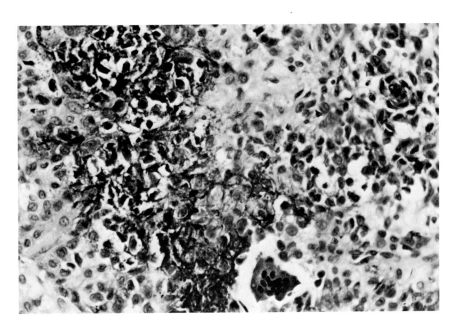

Fig. 19-18. A higher power view of the chondroblastoma with many cells outlined by a thin rim of mineralized matrix. An osteoclast is easily seen. (H & E, × 313.)

growth.[222,225] Fibromatosis (extraabdominal desmoid) is relatively uncommon in the upper extremity but is characterized by the presence of a firm painless mass without discrete borders, firmly fixed to the muscle or fascia and occasionally tightly adherent to the periosteum of the subjacent bone.[61,111,160,180]

As can be readily appreciated by this brief description of the clinical characteristics of some of the more common and especially the rarer lesions that usually present as a painless mass about the shoulder, there is little in the history or physical examination that can help in the differential diagnosis of these tumors. Perhaps the most readily distinguished are those in which an associated anomaly is present, such as multiple lipomas, neurofibromatosis, and hemangio- or lymphangiomatosis of a portion or all of the upper extremity.

Imaging Studies

Soft tissue tumors can be extremely difficult to identify based upon imaging studies. Fatty tumors are an exception to this rule. Lipomas are invariably lucent lesions with well-defined margins. On CT, the density of a lipoma will be approximately −50 Hounsfield units. The lesion may contain scattered strand-like opacities. Problems may arise in the variant forms of lipoma such as fibrolipoma, angiolipoma, and invasive lipoma. In such cases, tissue of higher density will be mixed with the lucent component, making it difficult to exclude the possibility of liposarcoma.

Benign tumors of neural origin are usually slightly less dense than muscle on CT scan and have oval or spherical contours. Fibromatosis presents as a nondescript soft tissue mass, sometimes with invasive margins. Differentiation from malignancy based on radiographic criteria is impossible.

Pathology (Lipoma, Hemangioma, Neurofibroma, Neurilemoma, and Desmoid)

The histologic examination of fibromatosis illustrates the invasive margins just mentioned. These tumors are composed of elongate spindle cells arranged in interdigitating fascicles, admixed with varying amounts of collagen fibers. Regardless of site, all the fibromatoses have the same histologic make up. The margins are often that of infiltrative lesions, namely tumor cells insinuating between preexisting structures such as skeletal muscle, fat, or tendon (Fig. 19-19). Although these tumors are cellular, they lack the mitotic activity, pleomorphism, and necrosis characteristic of fibrosarcoma or other malignancies (Figs. 19-20, 19-21).

Management

As indicated in the introductory sections of the chapter, the most important aspect of these lesions is to be certain that the tumor is, in fact, not a malignant tumor. With the exception of the desmoid the vast majority of these tumors, if their diagnosis could be determined by noninvasive means, would be best left untreated unless they cause cosmetic (as in the case of some large lipomas), functional (as occurs with some intramuscular hemangiomas), or neural complaints (neurilemoma or neurofibroma). Excising these benign lesions (excluding desmoids) surgically once the diagnosis is established is usually accomplished relatively easily by marginal surgery (shelling out), with special care taken for lesions that lie close to vital structures such as major nerve trunks or the brachial plexus.

As indicated in the section on imaging, the lipoma is, for practical purposes, the only one of these lesions that can be diagnosed easily by standard radiography, CT, and MRI. The radiographic findings of the remaining benign soft tissue lesions offer few clues to distinguish one of these lesions from the other or from a malignant tumor. Most often an open biopsy is required, but this should not be done until after the staging procedure has been completed. It is essential not to do an excisional biopsy on a lesion the nature of which is unknown, unless it is very small and located superficial to the deep fascia. The more prudent course is to perform an incisional biopsy through as small an incision as possible, or perhaps even a needle biopsy, and obtain a small segment of tissue for a frozen section. On the basis of the degree of assurance offered by the pathologist as to the nature and grade of the lesion, the surgeon should either perform a marginal excision if the lesion is clearly benign. If it is either malignant or indeterminate, close the wound and wait until the permanent sections are studied to define the grade of the lesion before planning and carrying out the definitive procedure.

The extraabdominal desmoid represents a special case. Although these lesions do not metastasize, the

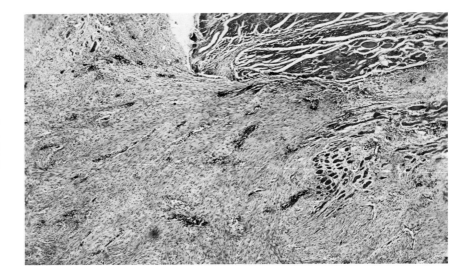

Fig. 19-19. fibromatosis with an infiltrative border since tumor dissects between skeletal muscle fibers. (H & E, × 31.)

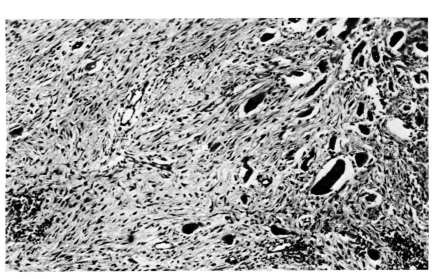

Fig. 19-20. The cells of the fibromatoses are elongate spindle cells enmeshed in collagen. Here isolated skeletal muscle fibers remain in various states of atrophy. (H & E, × 125.)

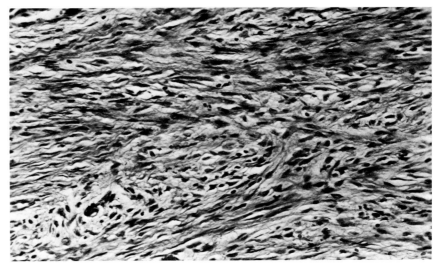

Fig. 19-21. In fibromatoses the spindle cells are arranged in interdigitating bundles. (H & E, × 200.)

591

tumors are locally aggressive: the recurrence rate is extraordinarily high with any but wide excision.[61,111,160,180] The lesions extend through the muscle bundles and it is very difficult to palpate the margin of the tumor during the resection. It is much safer to plan as wide an excision as is feasible[111] to avoid leaving tissue, which will ultimately recur as a secondary lesion, often more extensive and invasive than the primary mass. Such wide resections for "benign" processes pose some problems in terms of loss of function and, particularly for lesions involving the chest wall, the base of the neck, and brachial plexus, radiation therapy has sometimes been suggested as a reasonable approach.[111,124a] In general, such treatment should only be used when the surgical excision cannot be performed or if only an incomplete excision has been obtained. There is also a role for radiotherapy in recurrent lesions.

Malignant Tumors

TUMORS OF BONE

Osteosarcoma

Osteosarcoma is the most common primary malignant tumor of the bone, and the proximal humerus is the third most common site of occurrence.[36,135] Despite vast strides in the treatment of this group of entities over the past few decades, osteosarcoma remains the most malignant of the lesions with which the orthopaedist must deal. As can be noted by study of Table 19-4, a number of forms of osteosarcoma are now recognized as being distinct entities, each having somewhat different clinical presentations, imaging, and histologic characteristics. Differentiation among the various forms is more than academic, since the natural history and prognosis for some of these are quite different and, in some measure, dictate the method of treatment.

Juxtacortical osteosarcoma, a malignant tumor arising from the periosteal or external cortical surface of the bone, is classified as a low-grade (G1) lesion by most pathologists.[241] In the past several years, some pathologists have attempted to classify the lesions into periosteal and parosteal groups, based in part on the clinical characteristics and histologic appearance.[240,241] As far as the shoulder is concerned, the differentiation remains unclear and is probably of little

consequence since the presentation, prognosis, and treatment are essentially identical. The histologic grade of the lesion is much more important in determining prognosis than the name applied to the lesion; in fact, some juxtacortical osteosarcomas are high grade.[21] The lesion is considerably less common than the central form of osteosarcoma, and occurs in an older age cohort, with most of the patients in their third and fourth decades.[21,36] The lesions may be present for a considerable period of time, showing only slow progression and enlargement over months and years, and are slow to metastasize.

Parosteal osteosarcomas of the shoulder occasionally affect the humerus,[21,36] (the tumors rarely occur in flat bones such as the pelvis or scapula) and present as slowly enlarging, bony, hard, eccentrically placed, irregular excrescences on the metaphyseal and diaphyseal surfaces of the bone, extending out into the soft tissues and sometimes, late in the course, eroding the cortex to enter the medullary cavity.[21] The lesions are often painless at first, but later cause a dull aching pain and by their bulk or interference with the musculature cause a limitation of excursion of the adjacent joint. Although metastatic deposits in the lung are uncommon early in the course, they may occur and recur repeatedly after incomplete resections. When the lesion has violated the medullary cavity, the histologic appearance may take on a more malignant aura and show wide metastatic spread.[21]

Central osteosarcomas of the humerus, scapula, and clavicle are not uncommon (especially the first, which is the third most common site of occurrence of this lesion).[20,36,39,144,196] The tumors are more prevalent in male patients and principally affect individuals in their second and third decades,[126] but a second peak of incidence occurs in the elderly.[36,99] Osteosarcoma of the humerus has an intermediate prognosis (slightly better than lesions arising in the distal femur or proximal tibia but not as good as parosteal osteosarcoma or osteosarcoma of the jaw bones) and pulmonary metastases eventually occur in about 50 percent of the patients, even with appropriate surgical control of the primary tumor and adequate adjuvant chemotherapeutic treatment.[68,82,122]

Osteosarcoma of the humerus almost always arises from the proximal metaphysis and rapidly destroys the medullary cavity and cortex to break out of the bone. Because the subdeltoid bursa is less adjacent to the periosteal tissues at this site the tumor grows into this space rapidly, and at the time of presentation many of the patients have enormous soft tissue masses completely surrounding the bone and invading the musculature. The lesion will sometimes invade the epiphyseal center and break into the shoulder joint.[213] Pain with movement and later with rest, often worse at night, and limitation of motion and a noticeable enlargement of the shoulder are the usual presenting complaints. Occasionally the cortical destruction is so severe as to result in a pathologic fracture, a particularly ominous sign.[36,126] On physical examination, the bony, hard, somewhat tender enlargement of the shoulder region is sometimes associated with dilated veins over the site. Axillary adenopathy is rare. Because the neurovascular structures in the axillary sheath are separated from the primary tumor by a fibromuscular plane, neurologic complaints or findings (other than for the occasional involvement of the radial or axillary nerves) are uncommon. Laboratory evaluation may demonstrate an elevation of the serum alkaline phosphatase level[36,125,126,219,237] and, less commonly, a rapid erythrocyte sedimentation rate.

As noted above, the most common site of metastasis for osteosarcoma is to the lungs, but the lesions may also spread to distant bones and, less commonly, lymph nodes or brain. The natural history is such that the metastatic lesions in 80 percent of the patients who have distant spread are discovered in the first year or 2 following initial treatment.[80] This suggests that microfoci existed in the pulmonary or other osseous sites at the time of the presentation of the original tumor, but were either "suppressed" or so small that several months are required for the lesion to be noticeable on even the most sensitive imaging systems.

The other forms of osteosarcoma shown in Table 19-4 are far less common, but each has distinguishing characteristics that require some special consideration in their evaluation and management. Paget's sarcoma may arise in the proximal humerus of older individuals, usually with florid Paget's disease (the humerus is a less common site of origin than the femur, pelvis or, tibia), and histologically may show characteristics of high-grade fibrosarcoma, chondrosarcoma, or osteosarcoma (or often all three).[100] The lesion evolves rapidly, penetrating the cortex to cause a large soft tissue mass. The prognosis for this lesion is particularily baleful, with only a few survivors in all reported series.[100,246]

Telangiectatic osteosarcoma[104] is a particularly viru-lent form of central osteosarcoma, in which the lesion contains an enormous number of dilated vascular structures (as displayed on angiography or, to the great consternation of the surgeon, encountered at the time of biopsy). The prognosis for these lesions is said to be considerably worse than the standard central osteosarcoma, but several recent publications have raised some dispute regarding this contention.[104] Radiation-induced osteosarcoma may arise in bones that have received radiation in excess of 3000 cGy for another neoplastic process or because they lie within the field of radiation to the lymph nodes (such as the humerus in the treatment of breast carcinoma or Hodgkin's disease).[209] The latent period for radiation-induced sarcoma is usually greater than 4 years but may in some instances be as long as 30 years following the primary exposure to radiation. Radiation-induced sarcomas are considered to have a poor prognosis, with pulmonary metastases usually supervening within a few months.

Imaging Studies. The typical osteosarcoma is a large lesion with poorly defined margins. It characteristically destroys cortical bone and extends centrifugally from its point of origin, growing equally or almost equally in all directions (Fig 19-22). The lesion is frequently highly premeative in growth and extends through microscopic holes or preexisting vascular channels in bone. It can thus be seen in the soft tissues outside of a bony cortex that appears to be grossly intact. It often produces periosteal response, often with the typical "sun burst" appearance, but sometimes layered or interrupted. *"Codman's triangles"* are often seen at the junction between the cortex and periosteal elevation.

A variable amount of tumor new bone formation may be present. In some instances, the lesions are heavily mineralized, in others little or no tumor-bone is recognizable. In such instances, osteosarcoma may be difficult or impossible to differentiate from other malignant neoplasms based on imaging data. Parosteal osteosarcoma tends to be more heavily and uniformly mineralized. In some cases, it can simulate an exuberant periosteal response.

Angiographic studies done for surgical planning typically reveal a hypervascular mass. Computed tomography is important to define the extent of the soft tissue component and spread within the medullary canal of the bone. It is also the imaging modality

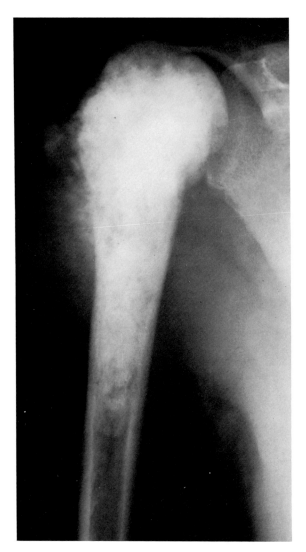

Fig. 19-22. An osteogenic sarcoma of the proximal humerus is seen as a large, densely bone-forming mass extending one-third of the way down the shaft of the humerus. The mineral pattern has an ill-defined "cloud-like" appearance. Mineralization in the soft tissue component of the tumor and an ill-defined "hair-on-end" appearance of the periosteal response are seen along the lateral surface of the metaphysis.

of choice for detection of pulmonary metastasis in young patients.

Pathology. Osteosarcoma is defined as a sarcoma that produces bone, invariably of woven type, as its cell product. It is not crucial what percent of tumor

is osseous; as long as bone is a product of the sarcoma cells, osteosarcoma is the correct diagnosis. Therefore, it is not surprising that osteosarcoma may have protean histologic patterns. The tumor may produce mixtures of cartilage, fibrous tissue, and bone in varying amounts with one tissue predominating almost to the exclusion of the others. *Any* high-grade sarcoma of bone should be carefully examined histologically to exclude a lurking focus of osteosarcoma. Various classifications based on the predominant tissue in osteosarcoma have been used by pathologists but the common denominator in all is the presence of bone tissue produced by the sarcoma. It is not surprising, therefore, that imaging studies can be so variable with respect to mineralization, cyst formation, and/or necrosis, with patterns suggestive of cartilage, soft tissue, and/or bone. The presence of necrosis and hemorrhagic cyst formation may also mimic an aneurysmal bone cyst, so great care must be taken to examine the wall of the cyst for malignant features (Figs. 19-23 to 19-25). Rarely, intramedullary osteosarcomas may have low-grade features with only a few mitoses, mild anaplastic, and little or no necrosis and must be distinguished from fibrous dysplasia. Juxtacortical osteosarcomas often have such features, which may account for their more favorable prognosis.

Management. As with any malignant primary tumor of bone or soft tissue, a critical feature of the management is a careful and accurate staging of the lesion.[53,57] The anatomical extent of the tumor (T) is best defined by the imaging studies (plain films, angiograms, CT, bone scan, and MRI); the presence or absence of distant metastases (M) by bone scan and full lung tomograms or CT of the chest; and the grade of the lesion (G) by study of the histologic data and, more recently, by the additional adjunct of flow cytometric analysis of DNA kinetics.[2,137] *Only after these procedures are performed can the orthopaedist and oncologist decide on the best approach to management.*

Two separate issues that must be addressed are local control and adjunctive chemotherapy for control of the distant micrometastases presumed to be present.[221] Local control is best achieved by either an amputation or excision that allows wide or radical margins. For lesions of the proximal humerus, radical margins dictate the necessity of an interscapulothoracic amputation, while wide margins would include

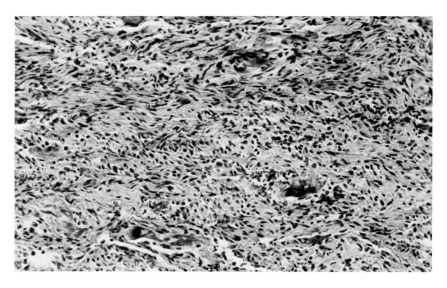

Fig. 19-23. An osteosarcoma with a predominating fibrosarcomatous pattern. However, admixed with the pleomorphic spindle cells are woven bone spicules, bordered focally by benign osteoclasts. (H & E, × 200.)

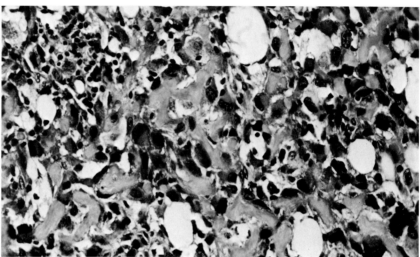

Fig. 19-24. A high-power view of an osteosarcoma with woven bone populated by large atypical osteocytes and surrounded by similar atypical osteoblasts with hyperchromatic nuclei and mononuclear bizarre giant cells (tumor giant cells). (H & E, × 313.)

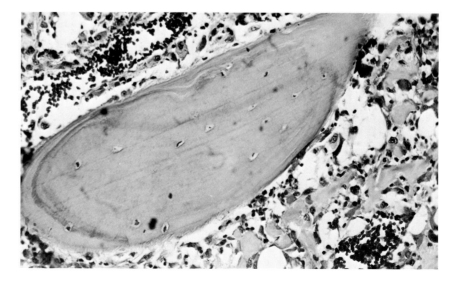

Fig. 19-25. The osteosarcoma invades between and surrounds a preexisting trabecula of lamellar bone. This feature is characteristic of any malignant tumor. (H & E, × 200.)

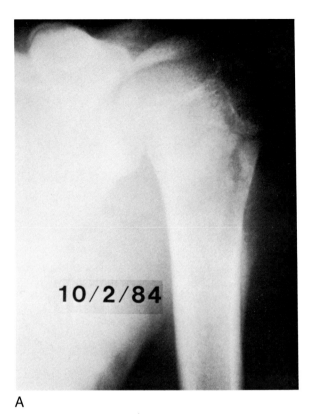

A

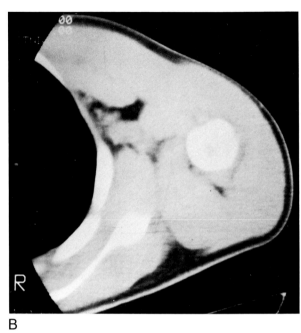

B

Fig. 19-26. (A) A 15-year-old boy with a high-grade osteosarcoma of the left proximal humerus. **(B)** The CT scan shows that there is a small soft tissue mass mostly confined by the deltoid muscle. (*Figure continues.*)

an excision of the upper end of the humerus, glenoid, deltoid, shoulder joint, and rotator cuff. If the neurovascular structures are sufficiently distant from the soft tissue extension, a wide resection can be achieved by a Tikhoff-Linberg conservative forequarter amputation, which leaves the patient with a flail shoulder but a functional elbow, forearm, and hand.[143] In recent years, we have substituted an allograft arthrodesis in which the stump of the humerus and the neck of the scapula are connected by an allograft segment and maintained in place by AO compression plates (Figs. 19-26 to 19-28).[69] This often offers a satisfactory shoulder joint (based on scapulothoracic motion) and, of course, retains the function of the elbow, forearm, and hand. The only two nerves that may be encountered during the resection are the axillary (which should be sacrificed anyway, if one takes the deltoid with the tumor) and the radial if the soft tissue extension lies posteriorly and distally. The local recurrence rates for either of these procedures are so low in the hands of most experienced surgical units as to

make it rarely necessary to perform the more disfiguring and disabling forequarter amputation, although an amputation may be necessary for very large lesions involving the brachial plexus and axillary artery[45,134,143] (Fig. 19-29). If the lesion affects the scapula, a total scapulectomy including a cloak of covering musculature is usually indicated (Fig. 19-30). Saving even a small portion of the glenoid and the neck of the scapula vastly improves the function of the shoulder joint, but this should not be done if it increases the risk of local recurrence.

For patients with a juxtacortical osteosarcoma, the type of resections for the more malignant tumors described above are rarely needed. Since many of these lesions are diaphyseal and often quite discrete, a wide resection of the shaft and the adjacent musculature and soft tissues is often adequate to achieve local control.[59] Under these circumstances, we have used allograft replacements of either a portion of the humerus (intercalary) or one in which the entire proximal humerus is replaced and function restored (at

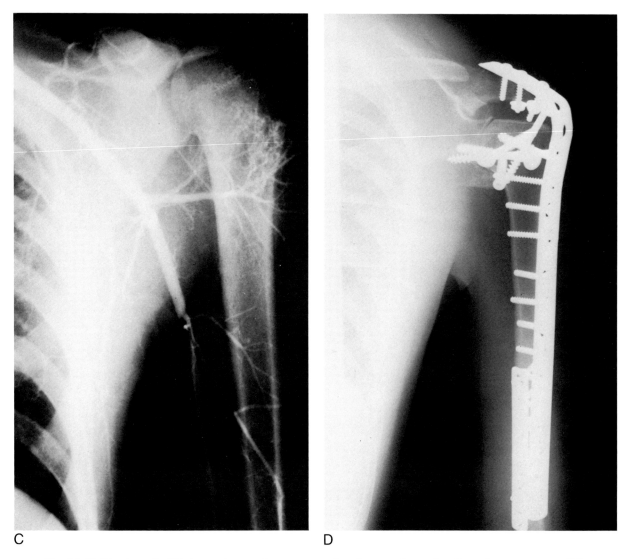

C   D

Fig. 19-26 (*Continued*). (**C**) An angiogram demonstrates that the vessels are free from the tumor mass. (**D**) Following resection, the patient's shoulder was reconstructed with an arthrodesis using an allograft bone (described in Fig. 19-27).

least in part) by reanastomosis of the deltoid, latissimus, pectoralis major, and rotator cuff to the insertions on the alloimplant.[138]

For some patients with telangietatic, radiation-induced, or especially Paget's sarcoma who present with pulmonary or bony metastases, it seems unreasonable to perform an extensive ablative surgical procedure. Under these rare circumstances where life expectancy is quite poor, radiation therapy may be used pallia-

tively to gain some control of the local lesion and decrease the patient's pain.

The second problem in relation to the management of osteosarcomas is to prevent the growth and, it is hoped, destroy the micrometastases presumed to be present in the lungs and possibly other sites. It is beyond the scope of this chapter to discuss the rationale for or variations between the various chemotherapeutic protocols advocated. There is little doubt that

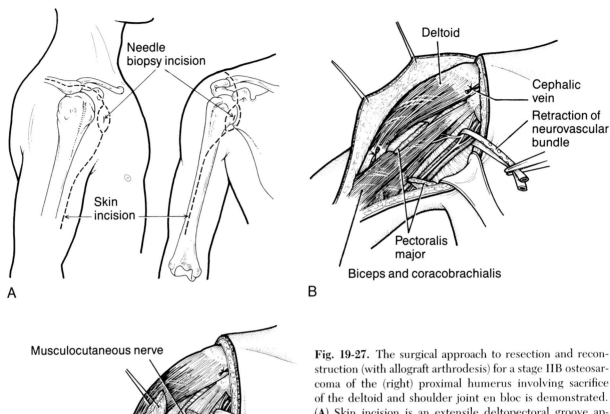

A

B

Deltoid

Cephalic vein

Retraction of neurovascular bundle

Pectoralis major

Biceps and coracobrachialis

Needle biopsy incision

Skin incision

Musculocutaneous nerve

Short head of biceps and coracobrachialis

C

Fig. 19-27. The surgical approach to resection and reconstruction (with allograft arthrodesis) for a stage IIB osteosarcoma of the (right) proximal humerus involving sacrifice of the deltoid and shoulder joint en bloc is demonstrated. **(A)** Skin incision is an extensile deltopectoral groove approach elipsing the biopsy tract. **(B)** A large posterior skin flap is raised, fascia and some fibers of the deltoid are saved (if possible) with the flap. The pectoralis major origin is divided away from the bone and the brachial artery, vein, and plexus are retracted medially. **(C)** The musculoskeletal nerve is identified and preserved if possible. The short head of the biceps and coracobrachialis muscle can usually be preserved, but the long head of biceps must be sacrificed. (*Figure continues.*)

such drugs are successful in increasing the continuous disease-free survival and, in combination with resection of nodules from the lungs, the total survival of patients with high-grade osteosarcomas.[13,24,30,31,47, 48,50,68,80,81,89,97,122,132,134,146,175,185,187,188,233,234] In recent years, the trend has been toward preoperative chemotherapy, followed by limb-sparing surgery and then postoperative drug administration for approximately 1 year following removal of the lesion.[45,121,183,184,248] The drugs found most useful to date include high-dose methotrexate with citrovorum rescue, Adriamycin, and cis-platinum, and all of the current protocols utilize one or several of these as the major agents.

Chondrosarcoma

The various forms of chondrosarcoma of bone, some of which are quite rare, as shown in Table 19-4, and all have been reported to occur in the shoulder. In

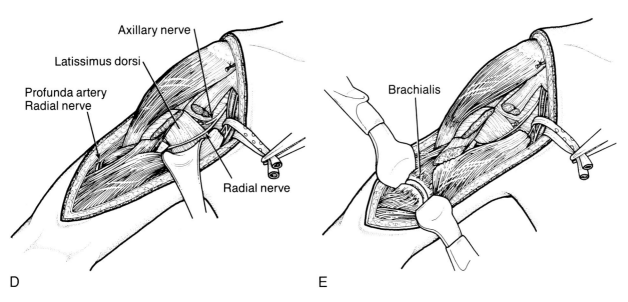

D

E

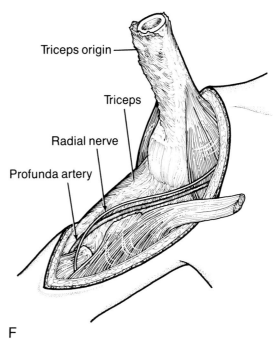

F

Fig. 19-27 (*Continued*). (**D**) The axillary nerve and circumflex vessels are exposed and divided. The radial nerve can often be preserved. The latter is also exposed distally prior to making the bone cut. (**E**) The level of the bone cut is determined by preoperative assessment of the bone scan, CT scan, and MRI. A marrow margin (7 to 10 cm) beyond the tumor is needed. The brachialis is kept with the specimen as a soft tissue cuff, whereas the biceps (short head) can often be preserved. (**F**) The arm is abducted and the triceps origin is divided with care to leave a cuff of muscle as a posterior tumor margin. The radial nerve and profunda artery are preserved if possible. (*Figure continues.*)

fact the bones that comprise the shoulder, along with the pelvis and proximal femur, appear to be favorite sites for cartilage tumors. As indicated in the discussion of benign cartilage tumors, differentiation of benign cartilage tumors from low-grade chondrosarcomas and low-grade from high-grade sarcomas is difficult and requires considerable care in evaluating the patient, a thorough and carefully performed series

of imaging studies, and an experienced and competent pathologist. The seven axioms provided in that section are helpful but, as indicated, cartilage tumors are more frequently under- or overtreated than any other lesions of bone. Since cartilage tumors are relatively uncommon (as compared with the osteosarcoma) unless the staging is performed in a center with considerable experience with these difficult le-

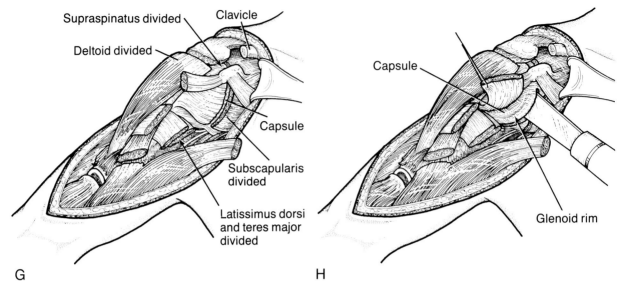

G

H

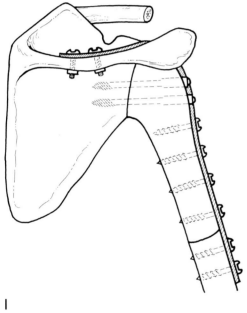

I

Fig. 19-27 *(Continued).* **(G)** Next the deltoid origin is divided and the distal 1 cm of clavicle is resected to gain exposure of the rotator cuff. The cult muscles are divided proximal to the glenoid and the latissimus dorsi and teres major insertions are also cut. **(H)** the glenoid osteotomy is made proximal to the shoulder capsule under direct vision anteriorly and posteriorly to ensure that the joint is removed en bloc. **(I)** A fresh frozen allograft bone segment is cut to fit the defect and fixed to the glenoid with compression screws in 60° abduction (relative to the axillary border of the scapula), 35° of forward flexion, and 25° of medial rotation. A long DC plate is used as a tension band for the proximal osteosynthesis and to achieve osteosynthesis distally.

sions, mistakes are common and unfortunately often serious.

The most common form of malignant cartilage tumor around the shoulder is the hyaline central chondrosarcoma, a lesion that occurs slightly more frequently in the humerus than the scapula and much less commonly in the clavicle or upper ribs.[7,36,73,94,95,136,173,196] The tumors arise most

frequently in individuals in the fourth decade or beyond and both sexes are affected equally. Chondrosarcoma is rare prior to the age of 25. In similar presentation to its benign counterpart, the enchondroma (pages above), the lesions of the humerus are usually metaphyseodiaphyseal and centrally placed within the bone. Depending in large measure on the grade of the tumor (G1 or G2), the tumors may be small and,

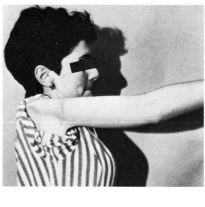
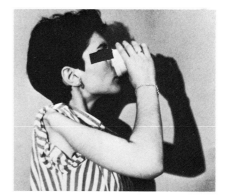
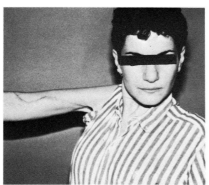
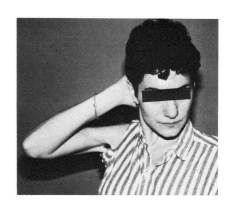

Fig. 19-28. This patient demonstrates the functional results of resection and arthrodesis. She is able to position her hand to her mouth and behind her head. Abduction and forward flexion approach the horizontal. She is able to get her hand into a front pocket.

although expansile, entirely confined to the bone or very large, destructive, and extending far beyond the cortical confines to invade the soft tissues and neurovascular structures. Since chondrosarcomas usually grow less rapidly and are less prone to early metastasis than the osteosarcoma or Ewing's tumor, the primary lesion (particularly if low grade) may reach enormous size with only modest pain and without serious impairment for the patient.

The most common presenting complaints for a patient with a chondrosarcoma about the shoulder are pain, often dull and nagging, present at rest and sometimes interfering with sleep, a slowly enlarging mass, and reduced function of the shoulder. Physical examination usually discloses a firm, often only slightly tender mass fixed to the underlying bone. Depending on the site, the lesion may cause some limitation of motion or altered neurologic function in the extremity.

Exostotic chondrosarcomas are in general, low grade (in contrast with the enostotic lesions, which may be either high or low grade) and grow only slowly

to assume sometimes enormous size prior to discovery. As a rule the lesions do not invade the medullary cavity, but may produce erosive lesions and sometimes an extensive response in the adjacent cortex (particularly for the juxtacortical chondrosarcoma). The complaints and findings, although often milder, are similar to those for the enostotic lesions but, because the lesion is usually eccentrically placed, may produce a greater distortion of the normal anatomy.[136]

Although there remains some dispute about the fact of and frequency with which "malignant degeneration" occurs in benign cartilage lesions in patients with hereditary multiple osteocartilaginous exostoses and the two forms of enchondromatosis (Ollier's and Mafucci's syndromes), there is little doubt that such patients are at greater risk for the development of a chondrosarcoma (exostotic for the former and enostotic for the latter) and that the grade of these lesions if often higher than those tumors arising as solitary lesions.[36,127,136,219,239]

Two variants of the hyaline chondrosarcoma are worthy of mention. The clear cell chondrosarcoma[242]

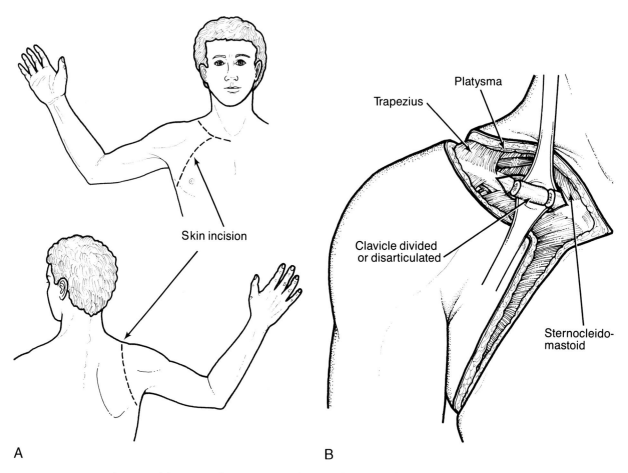

A   B

Fig. 19-29. This set of figures outline an approach to performing a forequarter amputation. (**A**) The skin incision is as marked in this diagram, but frequently must be modified according to the location of the tumor. At times, complex skin flaps or skin grafts may be needed. (**B**) The skin incisions are carried through the deep fascia to expose the clavicle. We prefer to expose the vessels first from an anterior approach, although other surgeons prefer a posterior approach. By resecting a small segment of the clavicle, or disarticulating the sternoclavicular joint, the vessels are easily visualized. (*Figure continues.*)

is a rare lesion that usually arises in the epiphyseal region of the bone in young adults, is low-grade in its behavior, and has a distinctive histologic appearance. Dedifferentiated chondrosarcoma[31,151,158] is rarely a primary event but usually occurs as a late sequel or recurrence of an inadequately surgically excised tumor. With rather extraordinary frequency (estimated as high as 20 percent), chondrosarcomas that recur even years after surgery may assume a highly malignant pattern much more closely resembling a high-grade fibrosarcoma or malignant fibrous histiocytoma than the primary hyaline lesion. The prognosis for patients with such lesions is poor; the

course is usually swift, unretarded by ablative surgery, radiation, or chemotherapy.

Imaging Studies. The features that declare the cartilaginous nature of a chondrosarcoma are the same as those seen in enchondroma and osteochondroma: growth in the form of nodules, calcification in arcs and broken arcs. The malignant nature of the lesion can be identified by large areas of noncalcified tumor, the less well-formed osseous margins, and penetration of the cortex (Fig. 19-31). The typical chondrosarcoma is less invasive than osteogenic sarcoma and results in a macroscopic area of cortical penetration rather

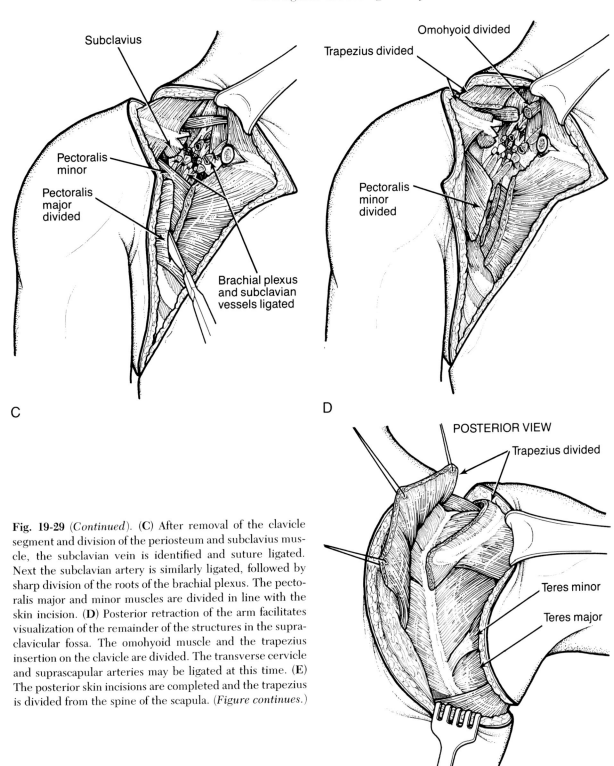

Subclavius

Pectoralis minor

Pectoralis major divided

Brachial plexus and subclavian vessels ligated

C

Omohyoid divided

Trapezius divided

Pectoralis minor divided

D

POSTERIOR VIEW

Trapezius divided

Teres minor

Teres major

E

Fig. 19-29 (*Continued*). (**C**) After removal of the clavicle segment and division of the periosteum and subclavius muscle, the subclavian vein is identified and suture ligated. Next the subclavian artery is similarly ligated, followed by sharp division of the roots of the brachial plexus. The pectoralis major and minor muscles are divided in line with the skin incision. (**D**) Posterior retraction of the arm facilitates visualization of the remainder of the structures in the supraclavicular fossa. The omohyoid muscle and the trapezius insertion on the clavicle are divided. The transverse cervicle and suprascapular arteries may be ligated at this time. (**E**) The posterior skin incisions are completed and the trapezius is divided from the spine of the scapula. (*Figure continues.*)

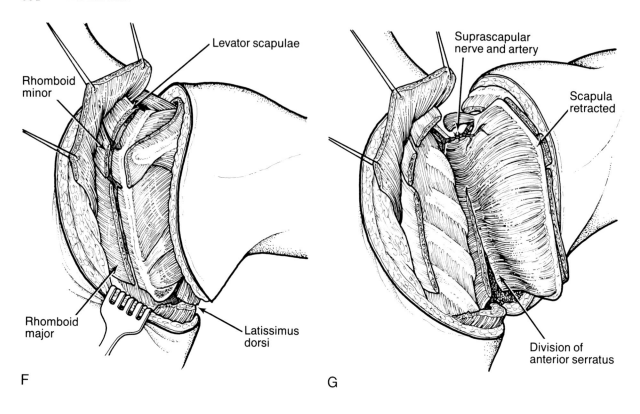

F

G

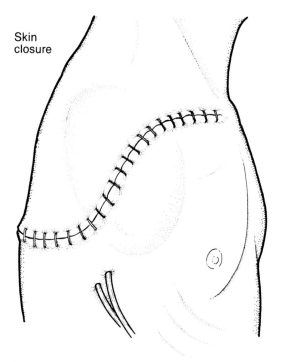

Skin
closure

H

Fig. 19-29 (*Continued*). (**F**) The muscles inserting on the vertebral border of the scapula (levator scapulae, rhomboideus major and minor) are divided, as is the latissimus dorsi near the inferior angle of the scapula. (**G**) The scapula can now be retracted anteriorly to expose the undersurface, which is covered by the subscapularis and serratus anterior. The latter is divided near its origin on the chest wall. The specimen can now be removed and the wound irrigated and checked for hemostasis. (**H**) Depending on the extent of the necessary resection of the chest wall muscles (pectoralis, latissimus dorsi, serratus anterior), it may be possible to close a deep layer of muscle. Otherwise, the skin edges are closed with adequate suction drainage of the flaps. A compression dressing is applied.

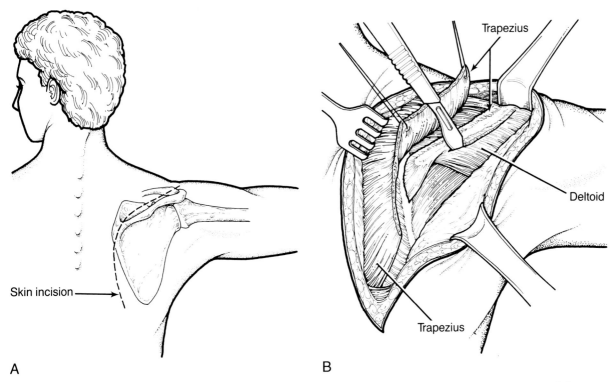

A   B

Fig. 19-30. (A) Lesions localized to the body of the scapula may be amenable to a wide resection of the scapula (scapulectomy). This is particularly beneficial if the glenoid can be spared. The skin incision parallels the spine of the scapula and continues along the vertebral border. **(B)** The trapezius and deltoid insertion are removed from the scapular spine. (*Figure continues.*)

than diffuse permeation. The soft tissue component mushrooms through the periosteum to produce a markedly eccentric soft tissue mass. The typical chondrosarcoma of low to moderate histologic grade is angiographically hypovascular. In lesions of the highest grade, the neoplasm bears less resemblance to its cell of origin, and all of these principles may be violated. In such instances the tumor resembles other high-grade malignancies of bone, such as osteosarcoma.

Pathology. Chondrosarcoma is a sarcoma that produces cartilage as its cell product. The cartilage is usually of hyaline type but often these tumors have mixtures of both hyaline and myxoid cartilage. The low-grade tumors are usually hyaline and, therefore, have extensive mineralization of the matrix indicative of slow growth. High-grade tumors may be of the myxoid variety and have minimal or no mineraliza-

tion. Therefore, the type of cartilage tissue correlates with grade and radiographic appearance. Malignant cartilage lesions invade between normal structures such as cancellous bone, cortical vascular channels, or into soft tissues, whereas benign lesions do not. If a chondrosarcoma is carefully sectioned and studied, a preexisting enchondroma may be found as the precursor lesion. Rarely, and particularly in the elderly, a high-grade chondrosarcoma, osteosarcoma, or fibrosarcoma arises in association with an enchondroma. Such tumors have also been termed "dedifferentiated chondrosarcoma."[37,151,158] Therefore, the biopsy site should be chosen carefully, and the most lytic, nonmineralized focus should be sampled since this area would most likely represent high-grade tumor.

Malignant cartilage is hypercellular with many binucleate cells. There is nuclear pleomorphism and atypia, focal chondrocyte necrosis, in the absence of

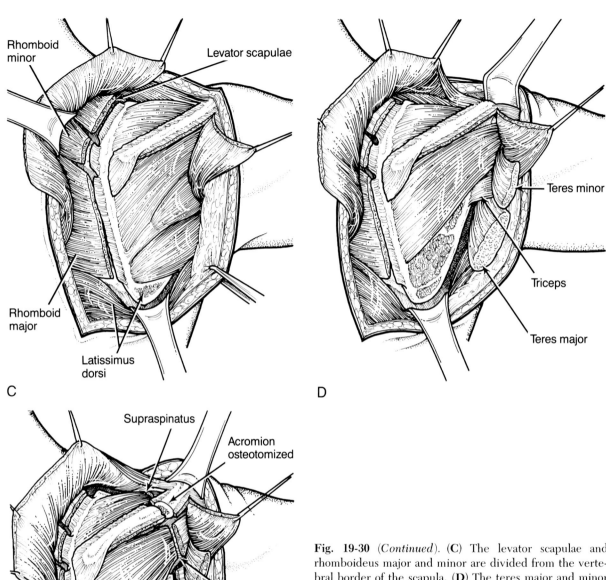

C

Rhomboid minor

Levator scapulae

Rhomboid major

Latissimus dorsi

D

Teres minor

Triceps

Teres major

E

Supraspinatus

Acromion osteotomized

Capsule

Triceps divided

Infraspinatus

Fig. 19-30 (*Continued*). (**C**) The levator scapulae and rhomboideus major and minor are divided from the vertebral border of the scapula. (**D**) The teres major and minor and triceps origins are divided. (**E**) The supraspinatus and infraspinatus are sectioned near the glenoid, and the lateral scapular spine is divided to expose the base of the glenoid and capsule of the shoulder. (*Figure continues.*)

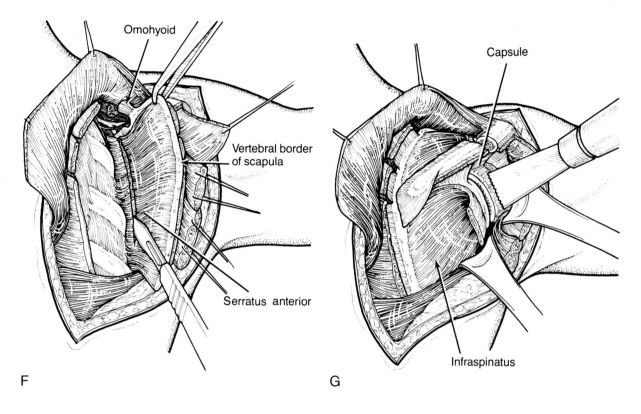

F

G

Fig. 19-30 (*Continued*). (F) The scapula is next retracted anteriorly to expose the underlying subscapularis and serratus anterior, which are divided near the base of the glenoid. (G) The lateral scapula is divided with an oscillating saw at the neck; the glenoid and acromion process are preserved. (H) After removal of the specimen, the remaining muscle groups are reapproximated to obtain a deep repair and the wound is closed over suction drains.

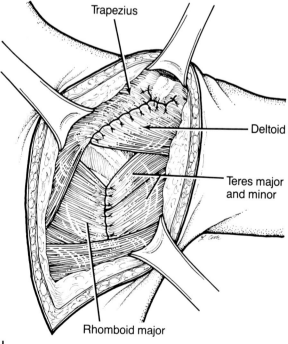

H

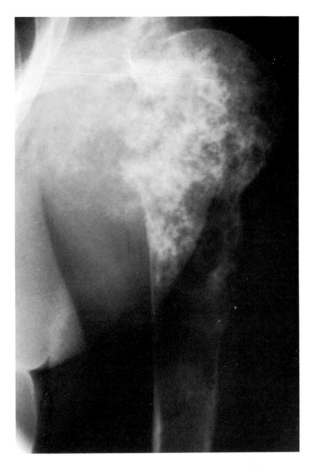

Fig. 19-31. A chondrosarcoma of the proximal humerus showing punctate and ringlike pattern of mineralization of the cartilage nodules. Focal penetration of the medial aspect of the humerus, results in an eccentrically placed, lobular soft tissue mass.

matrix mineralization, and infiltrative extension of the matrix into preexisting tissue. Cartilage lesions, therefore, possess a spectrum of changes and are the most difficult tumors to evaluate (Figs. 19-32 to 19-34).

Management. The principles of management for patients with chondrosarcomas of the shoulder do not materially differ from those with other low- or high-grade sarcomatous lesions about the shoulder.[63] The patient must be accurately staged to assess the extent of the lesion, the presence or absence of pulmonary metastases (lymph node metastases or spread to other bones or viscera is extremely uncommon except for the dedifferentiated chondrosarcoma), and the grade

of the tumor. The choice of the site to biopsy in patients with chondrosarcoma is particularly important, since considerable intratumor variation in pattern may be present; usually an open biopsy is required. Flow cytometric analysis of DNA kinetics has been found to be helpful in grading these lesions.[2,35]

The treatment of most forms of chondrosarcoma is almost entirely surgical; radiation and chemotherapy have been found to be of only limited value for the low-grade hyaline lesions but may be helpful for high-grade tumors or in palliation of the dedifferentiated chondrosarcoma. The first surgical procedure is the best opportunity to achieve a cure; subsequent efforts to eradicate recurrences are much more difficult and the threat of dedifferentiation looms higher with each such attempt. The surgical excision should include wide margins (marginal surgery is perhaps acceptable for very low grade lesions), except perhaps for the dedifferentiated lesion, which should be treated either by radical surgery if metastases have not occurred or palliative procedures if they have. In general, for low-grade and some high-grade tumors of the upper end of the humerus, we have performed resection and allograft replacement and, for tumors of the scapula, subtotal or complete scapulectomy with satisfactory results. The function of the shoulder is impaired, but most patients achieve a good restoration of movement in the lower ranges and avoid the problems of a flail shoulder associated with the Tikhoff-Linberg operation.

Giant Cell Tumor

The causes of the giant cell tumor of bone are poorly understood, but most pathologists and orthopaedic oncologists believe that the tumor arises from bone cells, either the osteoclast or osteoblast.[77,78,195] Evidence exists that the stromal cells of the tumor, at least in culture, show receptor sites for parathyroid hormone and calcitonin, confirming the osseous nature of the low-grade lesion.[77] Although receptors for estrogen and progesterone have not been found in several cases we studied, the tumors have been noted to evolve rapidly during pregnancy.[110] Giant cell tumors are on the "borderline" between benign and malignant tumors and have been classified as either by various authors. There is, however, little doubt that most are locally aggressive and that a small number (estimated to be less than 5 percent) will

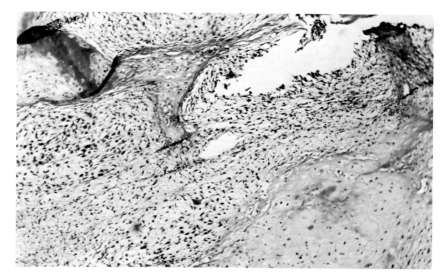

Fig. 19-32. A low-power view of a chondrosarcoma with myxoid and hyaline cartilage. This relatively high grade lesion (grade II/III) has pleomorphic cells. The radiograph would indicate that the myxoid area is radiolucent, whereas the hyaline focus is partially mineralized. (H & E, × 79.)

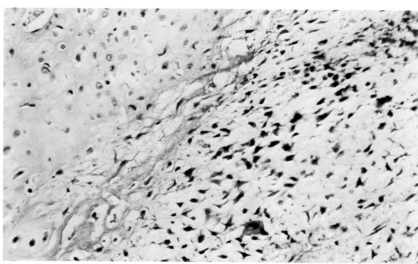

Fig. 19-33. The junction of myxoid and hyaline tissues in a grade II/III chondrosarcoma. The myxoid tissue (right) has stellate cells with pleomorphic nuclei. The cells processes touch those of other cells, whereas the hyaline cartilage (left) has chondrocytes isolated in lacunae without cell-to-cell contact. (H & E, × 200.)

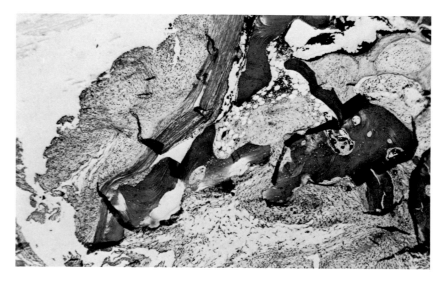

Fig. 19-34. A characteristic finding of chondrosarcoma is the infiltrative growth through cortex into soft tissue. This myxoid chondrosarcoma also permeates the marrow space. (H & E, × 31.)

609

eventually metastasize[11,75,181,201] if inadequately treated. Although rare, metachronous multicentric giant cell tumors may occur, and one of the more common sites for such lesions is the upper end of the humerus.[166] The existence of a primary "malignant giant cell tumor" with a distinctive sarcomatous histologic pattern is reported by some authorities, but is apparently very rare.[190,192]

Giant cell tumors of the upper end of the humerus are not rare lesions (the site is the fourth most common, preceded in frequency by the distal femur, proximal tibia, and distal radius) and occur in young adults (18 to 40 years of age), more often in women than men.[46,75,196] The lesions are almost always epiphysiometaphyseal in location and, when small, are located eccentrically.[38,105] Because of the location in juxtaposition to the subchondral cortex of the proximal humerus, distortion and sometimes fracture of the cartilaginous surface occurs. Because the bone is markedly thinned by the often aggressive lesion, pathologic fracture[77] is common and may result in a soft tissue extension into the joint or subperiosteal space subjacent to the subdeltoid bursa.

Patients with giant cell tumor of the proximal humerus usually complain of aching pain in the shoulder, often exacerbated following minor trauma, which presumably has caused a pathologic fracture in the markedly thinned cortex. Function of the shoulder may be impaired and examination often shows deltoid atrophy and a symmetrical enlargement of the upper end of the humerus.[38,77,105]

Imaging Studies. Giant cell tumor has a characteristic radiographic appearance that allows the diagnosis to be suggested in the majority of cases. The lesion is purely lytic, occupying both the epiphyseal (or apophyseal) and metaphyseal parts of the bone, in most instances coming within several millimeters of articular cortex (Fig. 19-35). No central mineralization is seen and the lesion is generally not surrounded by a sclerotic wall, although its boundaries with adjacent cortical and trabecular bone are moderately well defined. In the upper end of the humerus, the distal margin often appears indistinct and irregular, perhaps reflecting the relative absence of trabecular bone to demarcate the edge of the lesion. The bone often has an expanded or aneurysmal appearance due to periosteal bone formation around the periphery of the expanding lesion. Gaps in the mineralized periosteal shell may occur without necessarily indicating that the lesion is extraosseous. Computed tomography, sometimes with intraarticular contrast, is the best radiographic means of demonstrating intraarticular spread of the lesion. A radionuclide bone scan invariably shows increased uptake in the lesion, and angiography reveals a markedly hyperemic appearance similar to what is seen in renal cell carcinoma.

Pathology. The diagnostic histologic appearance of giant cell tumor has three main features: "stromal" cell, which is round or oval with poorly defined cytoplasmic borders; a central vesicular nucleus and a few mitoses (usually less than 5/10 hpf); a random distribution of osteoclast-type giant cells; and nuclei of the giant cells and stromal cells are identical. Other features include reactive fibrosis and/or bone formation, hemosiderin- and lipid-laden macrophages, and hypereosinophilic giant cells with dark pyknotic nuclei that are presumably dying cells. Characteristic of these tumors, they invade into the subarticular cartilage bone plate and into periosteal vessels. These tumors commonly undergo hemorrhage with necrosis and cyst formation (Fig. 19-36).

Management. Following careful staging studies (which must include CT of the chest, a bone scan, and biochemical studies to rule out the easily confused brown tumor of hyperparathyroidism), a biopsy (either by needle, if a marginal or wide resection is contemplated, or open, if an intralesional procedure is to be performed) surgical eradication of the tumor should be performed.[136] Although of some value for giant cell tumors of the spine, radiation has no place in the management of patients with lesions of the humerus and the recently advocated use of transarteriographic embolization is probably excessively dangerous in the upper extremity. If the lesion is small and has not greatly eroded the subchondral cortex, curettage, burring, and phenolization of the cavity and packing with auto- or allograft bone form the standard and accepted method of therapy.[150] Substitution of liquid nitrogen for the phenol cautery has been advocated, but is likely to result in osteonecrosis, pathologic fracture, and collapse of the joint.[140] Substitution of polymethyl methacrylate for the bone appears to be associated with a decreased rate of local recurrence of the lesion in patients with giant cell tumors about the knee, but experience with this procedure for the upper end of the humerus is limited.[169,170] Using the standard intralesional approach described above, the recurrence rate particularly for proximal humerus lesions is high, approaching 60 percent in some series.[77] If the patient presents with a recurrence; a very thin, perforated, or distorted subchondral cortex; a pathologic fracture; or an extensive soft tissue mass, the advisable course is of marginal or wide resection (Fig. 19-37). The defect so created may be treated by arthrodesis using autogenous fibular grafts as proposed by Enneking,[52,56] allograft implantation[138] (Figs. 19-35E, 19-37F–H) or insertion of metallic devices.[18,247] None of these techniques is likely to result in a normal shoulder, but the primary goals of eradicating the tumor and restoring stability and partial function can usually be achieved.

Round Cell Tumors

The generic term "round cell tumors" is used to describe several lesions which for the most part arise from the marrow elements (Table 19-4). Included in this group are the Ewing's sarcoma, various types of Hodgkin's lymphomas, and myeloma. Although there are significant differences in clinical presentation, imaging characteristics, and prognosis among these lesions, all are characterized histologically by the presence of a pattern of small, uniformly sized round cells with prominent nuclei and scant cytoplasm.[171]

Ewing's sarcoma is a highly malignant lesion principally affecting white patients (the disease is rare in blacks) in their teens or early 20.[36,115,172,194] Male patients are more frequently affected than female pa-

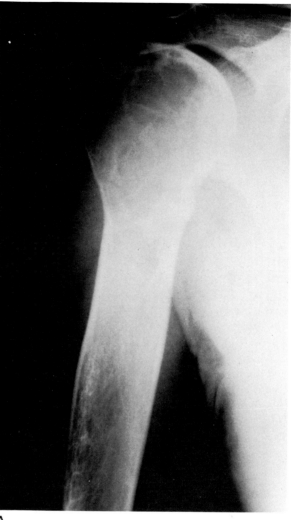

A

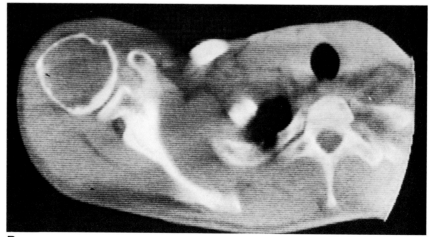

B

Fig. 19-35. (A) The AP radiograph of a giant cell tumor of the proximal humerus in a 34-year-old classical guitar player, which recurred following curettage and "cryosurgery" with liquid nitrogen. **(B)** The CT scan shows that the humeral cortex is markedly thinned but there is no soft tissue mass. (*Figure continues.*)

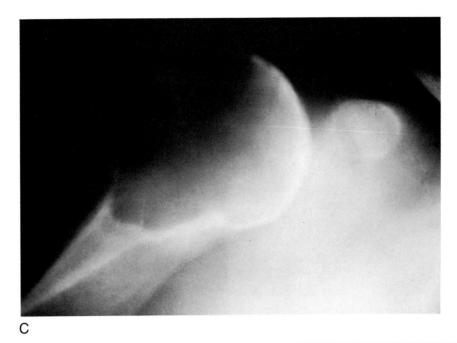

C

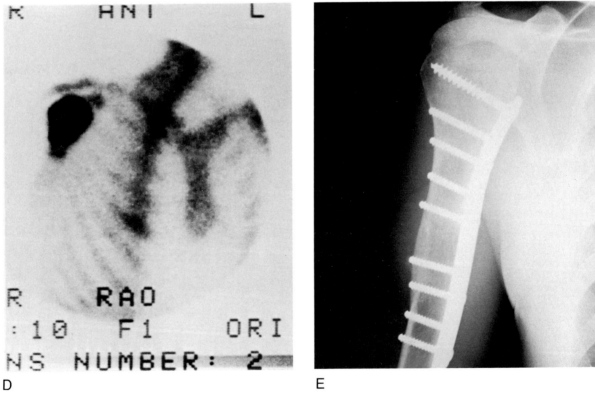

D

E

Fig. 19-35 (*Continued*). (**C**) A plane tomogram shows the extremely thin subchondral bone plate. (**D**) A radionuclide bone scan demonstrates the characteristic increased uptake. (**E**) This patient underwent a wide resection and reconstruction with an osteoarticular allograft bone. The deltoid muscle was spared. The articular cartilage was preserved in DMSO and the host rotator cuff muscles were sutured to the allograft tendons. This radiograph was obtained 2 years postoperatively. He had good motion (90° abduction, 90° forward flexion) and has resumed his guitar playing as well as his employment as an executive.

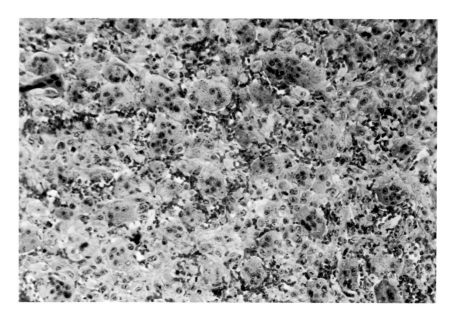

Fig. 19-36. A giant cell tumor with abundant randomly scattered osteoclast-type giant cells and round to oval "stromal" cells. The nuclei of both cell types are identical. Some giant cell nuclei are dark, squeezed, and distorted representing the dying giant cell. (H & E, × 125.)

tients. Involvement of the axial skeleton (especially the pelvis and scapula) is frequent and the humerus is also a common site. The tumors most frequently occur in the metaphysis or diaphysis of a long or flat bone. Although they arise centrally from the medullary cavity, the tumor tissue rapidly breaks out in concentric fashion to produce an often sizable soft tissue mass at the time of presentation.[98,219] Metastases to the lungs (and occasionally other bones—a particularly ominous prognostic sign) occur early in the course and are present in as many as 30 percent of patients at the time of initial discovery.[74] Patients with Ewing's sarcoma of the bones of the shoulder usually present with pain and a tender, diffuse, poorly localized swelling of the affected part. They may appear chronically ill and show signs suggestive of hematogenous osteomyelitis. Fever, an elevated leukocyte count, and rapid sedimentation rate are commonly seen in patients with Ewing's sarcoma and may indicate a poorer prognosis.[70,171,172]

Primary lymphoma of bone is most often classified as non-Hodgkin's lymphoma (primary Hodgkin's disease of bone is exceedingly rare) and histologically resembles the more common and familiar diffuse disease (affecting the lymph nodes, liver, spleen, and other viscera as well as the bones).[14,88,171,184,206] The disease occurs in a somewhat older age group than the Ewing's sarcoma, with the peak incidence in young adults. The tumor is rare in teenagers (in contrast with Ewing's sarcoma) and is somewhat more frequent in male patients. The peculiar immunity to Ewing's sarcoma observed in blacks is not as evident for primary lymphoma of bone.

The clinical complaints and findings in the patient with primary lymphoma of bones about the shoulder are considerably less dramatic than for Ewing's sarcoma and are usually more indolent in evolution. The pain is relatively mild, the swelling and tenderness less noticeable, and the patient is usually afebrile and has no systemic signs of diffuse disease (with the exception of an occasional moderate rise in the erythrocyte sedimentation rate). The incidence of dissemination of primary non-Hodgkin's lymphoma of bone at the time of discovery of the primary lesion is so low as to suggest that if tumor is discovered in other sites (such as lymph nodes, lungs, viscera, or other bones) the patient has stage 4 diffuse lymphoma, rather than a primary disorder localized to one bone. Since the diffuse process is more common than the primary osseous disease, the orthopaedist treating such patients must be constantly concerned with the issue of whether the bony tumor represents primary or secondary disease, at least for the first several years after completion of treatment.[231]

Myeloma of a single bone such as the humerus or scapula is almost without exception a manifestation of multiple myeloma, which is a malignant member of a group of disorders known as monoclonal

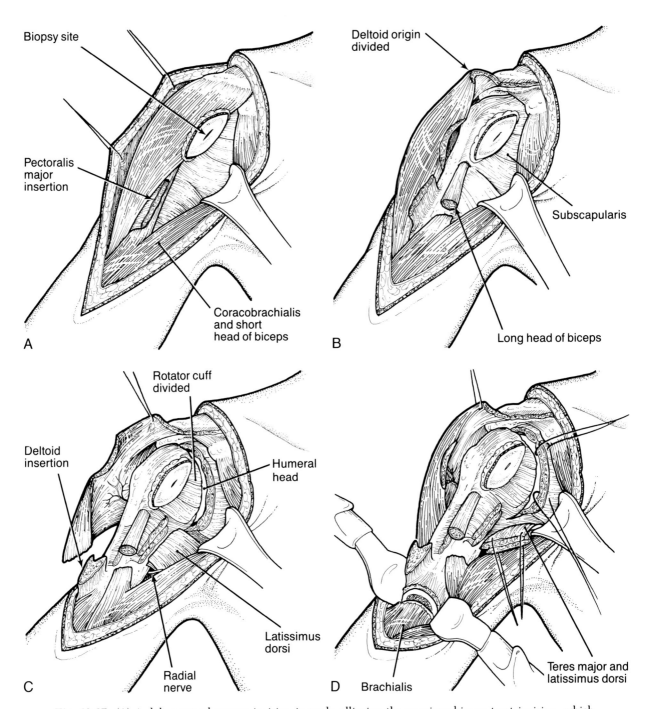

Fig. 19-37. (**A**) A deltopectoral groove incision is made ellipsing the previous biopsy tract incision, which is excised en bloc with the specimen. The importance of placing the biopsy incision in the deltopectoral groove is apparent because any deltoid muscle anterior to this will either be removed or denervated. The coracobrachialis and short head of biceps are retracted medially after the insertion of pectoralis major is divided. (**B**) The deltoid is elevated extraperiosteally to expose the proximal humerus; a portion of the origin is retained if necessary. The long head of the biceps is divided. (**C**) The staging studies are used to determine the bone cut, which is usually made 3 to 5 cm beyond the radiographic extent of the lesion. The insertion of the deltoid may need to be divided. The latissimus dorsi and teres major insertion are divided and the radial nerve is protected. The rotator cuff and capsule are marked with tagging sutures prior to division. (**D**) The brachialis is split after the biceps are retracted and the bone is divided at the appropriate level. (*Figure continues.*)

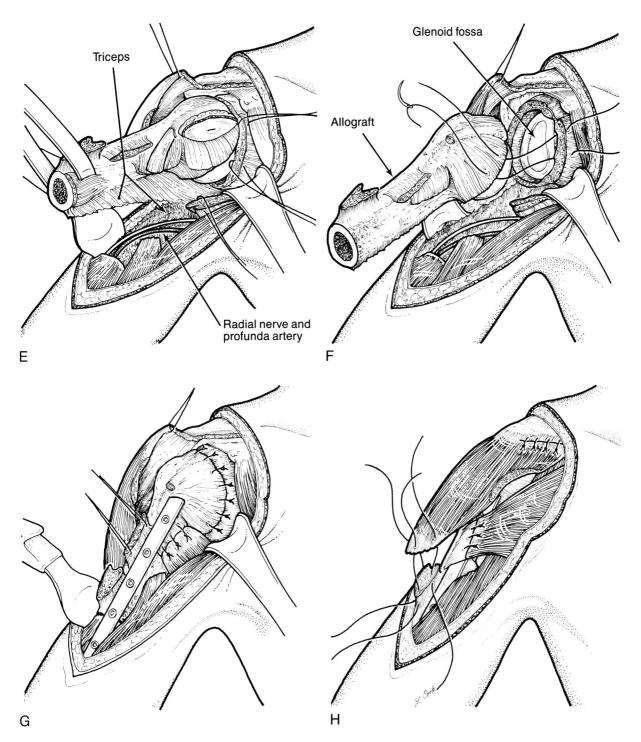

Fig. 19-37 (*Continued*). (**E**) If one abducts the proximal fragment, the triceps origin can be divided and the specimen is removed and checked by a pathologist for margins. (**F**) An osteoarticular allograft is thawed and cut to fit the measured defect. Careful attention is directed toward achieving a tight repair of the rotator cuff and capsule, holding the allograft in 46° to 60° of abduction. (**G**) The osteosynthesis is achieved with a DC plate and the teres major, latissimus dorsi, and pectoralis major insertions are sewn to the corresponding areas on the allograft. (**H**) The deltoid insertion and origin are repaired and the wound closed with attention toward providing good soft tissue coverage of the allograft. The patient is immobilized in Velpeau splint that holds the arm in abduction.

gammopathies.[79,120] The syndrome is a diffuse neoplasm of plasma cells, presumed to arise from a single clone of malignant cells that proliferate in the marrow over time to involve eventually many of the skeletal parts, as well as the viscera. Very rarely one encounters a patient with a lesion in one bone (plasmacytoma) in whom no signs of disseminated disease are found (see below) and in whom effective treatment of the primary site results in a prolonged remission.[85] Patients with myeloma are usually over 50 years of age and the disease occurs equally in men and women. Any bone may be affected, but the presenting site is most often in the axial skeleton (including the scapula), ribs, or proximal appendicular parts.

Myelomatous infiltrates in the skeleton arise from the marrow and produce at first multiple small destructive areas in the medullary bone (giving rise to the permeative pattern seen on radiograph), but soon become confluent to produce a large often rounded defect in skeleton. This thins the cortex and renders the bone very susceptible to pathologic fracture. The lesions are often painless until fracture supervenes, which is the way most cases are discovered.[171]

Patients with plasma cell myeloma may display some significant abnormalities in the blood, urine, and bone marrow that make the diagnosis relatively simple and often eliminate the need for a biopsy.[98,120] The neoplastic plasma cells usually produce an abnormal globulin, readily detected and identified by plasma or urine immunoelectrophoresis (positive and virtually diagnostic in over 90 percent of the patients and far more specific than the standard protein electrophoresis) and analysis of the urine for Bence Jones protein by electrophoretic technique (likely to be positive in about 45 percent of the patients). Bone marrow aspiration in patients with diffuse myeloma will frequently show over 20 percent plasma cells (up to about 8 percent is normal) and this test is diagnostic. Over 90 percent of the patients with multiple myeloma will have a normocytic normochromic anemia and a marked elevation of the erythrocyte sedimentation rate (ESR). A complete blood count, ESR, and plasma immunoelectrophoresis are useful as screening studies to rule out multiple myeloma (with about 90+ percent certainty) and, as discussed above, should be performed as part of the staging process for all adults with bone tumors.

The natural history for inadequately treated Ewing's sarcoma is one of a rapid and relentless downhill course, with the patient dying of the disease in a relatively short period of time.[171,172] For primary lymphoma, the course is slower, but most untreated patients develop the disseminated variety of the process within a few years.[171] Fortunately, as will be discussed below, the appropriate use of radiation and chemotherapy has been successful in achieving a high salvage rate for patients with these malignant neoplasms.[14,151] As indicated above, almost all patients with a plasmacytoma of the region of the shoulder have multiple myeloma, for which remission can often be achieved by the appropriate use of chemotherapy and radiation. However, the patients almost always relapse and the disease is generally considered universally fatal.[119,120]

Imaging Studies. Ewing's tumor and lymphoma have similar radiographic manifestations and are often indistinguishable on imaging studies. Solitary plasmacytoma and multiple myeloma have radiographic appearances that may differ both from each other and from the previously mentioned round cell neoplasms.

The typical lesion of Ewing's sarcoma/lymphoma is highly permeative on imaging studies (Fig. 19-38). Growth of the lesion occurs through preexisting vascular channels and Haversian systems such that large quantities of bone are left behind the advancing edge of the tumor. As a result, the margins between involved and uninvolved bone may be difficult or impossible to discern on radiographs. A large soft tissue mass is frequently present, extending circumferentially around the bone of origin, and often appearing to be outside of a grossly intact cortex due to spread of the neoplasm through microscopic pathways. The lesions have an approximately equal predilection for the metaphysis and diaphysis of tubular bones. Since other neoplasms are uncommon in the diaphysis, demonstration of a diaphyseal lesion should suggest the diagnosis of a round cell tumor. A periosteal response is frequent, often having a layered or lamellar appearance. When seen in flat bones, recognizable periosteal response is less frequent and the lesions tend to be accompanied by a diffuse sclerotic response.

Solitary plasmacytoma produces a radiographic appearance that may closely resemble giant cell tumor, although not sharing the propensity for subarticular location seen in that lesion. The lesions are well defined and frequently expand the contour of the af-

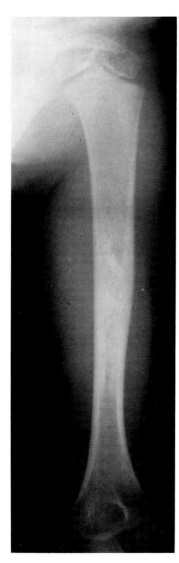

Fig. 19-38. Ewing's sarcoma of the humerus is seen as an ill-defined region of permeative bone destruction extending over the middle one-third of the humeral shaft. There is reactive sclerosis in the medullary cavity. An ellipsoidal soft tissue mass surrounds the arc of abnormal bone.

panied by periosteal response and do not distort or expand the contour of the involved bone. These features result in the "punched out" appearance of the myelomatous lesion. A profound systemic osteopenia frequently accompanies myeloma, perhaps resulting from osteoclastic activating factor secreted by the tumor cells. Blastic lesions due to myeloma may be seen, but are exceedingly rare. The lesions of multiple myeloma are often not detectable on radionuclide scan, making this condition one of the few diseases for which radiographic skeletal survey is still indicated.

Pathology. The histologic appearance of round cell tumors of bone is often subtle, distorted, and difficult to diagnose. Myeloma is a tumor of plasma cells. Lymphoma, whether Hodgkin's or non-Hodgkin's type, may be identified by a number of parameters including cell surface markers and electron microscopy. Ewing's sarcoma is described as a tumor of unknown origin, having abundant cytoplasmic glycogen and producing little or no collagen (Fig. 19-39). Unfortunately, all these tumors may undergo severe cellular distortion and squeeze artifact, which preclude a definitive diagnosis. Therefore, when a suspected round cell tumor is to be biopsied, great care should be taken to handle the tissue gently, obtain samples for electron microscopy, immunoperoxidase, and cell surface markers. Furthermore, some tissues should be fixed in alcohol for later staining for glycogen. Bacterial cultures should also be done.

Histologically, these tumors are composed of sheets of small round cells with little or no cytoplasm and oval nuclei. In myelomas, plasma cells should be easily recognizable. Squeeze artifact may so distort cells that even osteomyelitis may not be able to be diagnosed with light microscopy. As of now there is no specific immunoperoxidase test for Ewing's sarcoma and the definitive test is therefore still electron microscopy.

Management. The round cell tumors, perhaps more than any other group of tumors discussed in this chapter, demand careful staging studies not only to define the extent of the local lesion but also more importantly to determine the presence of widespread systemic disease. In addition to the standard imaging studies (including a skeletal survey if one suspects a myeloma) a patient thought to have a round cell lesion should have staging chemical studies (as defined

fected bone. Multiple myeloma has a more aggressive appearance. Multiple small areas of bone destruction, partly coalescent in areas, may be seen in many bones. In general, the distribution of lesions follows the distribution of bone marrow in the adult. Thus, peripheral bones are generally spared until the marrow of the central skeleton has been largely replaced. Individual lesions are purely lytic, usually not accom-

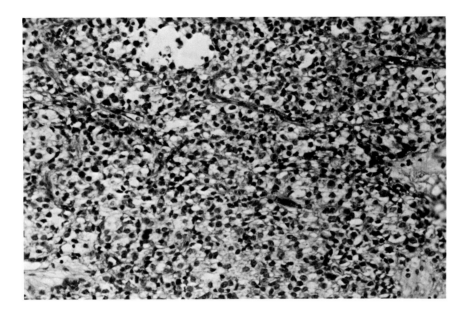

Fig. 19-39. An example of Ewing's sarcoma with sheets of small round cells containing clear cytoplasm (glycogen) and round or oval nuclei. The monotonous uniform appearance of the cells is more characteristic of Ewing's sarcoma than lymphoma or infection. (H & E, × 200.)

above), a bone marrow aspiration, CT of the lungs, and, if lymphoma is suspected, a liver–spleen scan, a lymphangiogram (if lymph nodes are palpable), and a staging CT scan of the abdomen. At the time of biopsy, tissue should be obtained for electron microscopy, special stains (especially for glycogen and reticulin), and surface markers to attempt to identify the type of lymphoma.[171] An oncologist and pathologist with experience in dealing with these unusual entities should be consulted early in the course to help with interpretation of the data.

The round cell lesions of bone are generally sensitive to radiation therapy and many chemotherapeutic agents; hence, the treatment of all of these lesions is primarily nonsurgical. Most patients with Ewing's sarcoma can be effectively treated and essentially "cured" in over 60 percent of cases by radiation to the local site in combination with chemotherapy, principally Adriamycin and actinomycin D.[4,114,168,186,235] The treatment of primary lymphoma of bone is similar in its dependence on radiation as the primary tumoricidal agent with adjunctive drugs of major value in preventing development of disseminated disease. Depending on the type of cell involved, the long remission rate varies from 50 to over 80 percent.[14,98,136,178,206] Myeloma is also radiosensitive but the chemotherapeutic agents such as Alkeran (melphalan) and cyclophosphamide appear to be less effective in reducing the body's burden of abnormal

plasma cells and all but a very few of the patients die of the disease in a few years.[29,119,120]

It should be noted, however, that there is considerable weight of evidence to suggest that a secondary surgical resection of the site of Ewing's sarcoma or primary lymphoma after completion of the treatment is appropriate if it can be done with little risk or disability (such procedures include acromionectomy or subtotal scapulectomy).[141,162,171,172] Such a procedure reduces the rate of local relapse and eliminates, for practical purposes, a late developing radiation-induced sarcoma at the site.[224] If this is to be done, it should be planned in advance and discussed with the radiation therapist and oncologist so that the skin over the local site will be treated to reduce the likelihood of complications of wound healing.[109]

Other Malignant Lesions of Bone

As noted in Table 19-4, a variety of very rare primary lesions of bone are included, mainly for the sake of completeness. The interested reader can review the characteristics of these unusual tumors in texts and articles as cited. It should be noted that both the fibrosarcoma of bone[66,174] (which may be high- or low-grade) and the malignant fibrous histiocytoma[5,40,218,232,249] (almost always high-grade) appear to arise from fibroblastic elements and most often occur in middle-aged or elderly individuals. Recent reports have suggested that the malignant fibrous histiocytoma of bone may arise at the site of a prior bone infarct or focus of old osteomyelitis, while the fibrosarcoma may rarely be associated with an underlying fibrous dysplasia.[44,66,196] Both are primarily diaphyseal or metaphyseal in location and are extraordinarily destructive on the radiograph, with a large soft tissue mass often present at the time of discovery. The fibrosarcoma has a better prognosis than the malignant fibrous histiocytoma and both are best treated by wide or radical resection unless the lesion is determined to be low-grade at the time of biopsy.[101,136,232,249]

Malignant vascular tumors are rare entities that may occur as solitary tumors or in multiple sites in one or several bones.[36] The lesions are lytic and destructive, with only a small extraosseous component noted on imaging studies. The prognosis varies with the grade and the extent of the disease. Hemangiopericytoma of bone is exceedingly rare but usually solitary and highly malignant. All of these tumors are best treated by wide or radical procedures, and chemotherapy should be instituted for the high-grade lesions.

Gorham's disease, otherwise known as "disappearing bone disease," falls into a special category in that the angiomatous process that ultimately causes the destruction of the entire bone and sometimes extends to adjacent skeletal parts may not be truly neoplastic, never metastasizes, and is histologically benign. There is no effective treatment for this disorder.[49,83]

MALIGNANT SOFT TISSUE TUMORS

As indicated in the introductory statement, and as shown in Table 19-5, the range of malignant tumors of the somatic soft tissues that affect the shoulder are not significantly different from those seen in other body parts; nor are the clinical characteristics, imaging studies, or histologic appearance sufficiently distinct to warrant special mention. Since orthopaedists are in general less involved in the management of patients with soft tissue tumors than of bone, this section will be considerably abbreviated. The reader interested in expanding his or her knowledge regarding these lesions is referred to some recent texts and review articles that detail the presentations, histologic characteristics, and methods of treatment for the various entities.[3,15,26,58,62,86,90,113,131,165,189,204,212]

The malignant lesions of the soft tissues that may present around the shoulder can arise from any of the elements present in the musculotendinous, supporting connective tissues, or neural and vascular elements at the site.[62,86,90,225] Fibrosarcomas and malignant fibrous histiocytomas (now the most popular diagnosis) appear to arise from fibroblastic tissues; low-grade liposarcomas (including the locally invasive but nonmetastasizing invasive lipoma) and the higher-grade fibroblastic and pleomorphic liposarcomas arise from lipoid elements; the various rhabdomyosarcomas (usually highly malignant) and leiomyosarcoma (all grades) arise from a muscular primordium; the neurofibrosarcoma and malignant schwannoma arise from the nerve sheaths, the hemangiosarcoma, lymphangiosarcoma, and hemangiopericytoma from the vascular elements; and the synovioma, clear cell sarcoma, and epithelioid sarcoma arise, at least putatively, from tendosynovial elements. Although there are clear histologic differences among these lesions, as far as the biological behavior, presentation, appearance on imaging studies, and approaches to management are concerned, with only rare exception, the major prognostic factors are the size and site of the tumor and the histologic grade.[53,57,227] There is little evidence to suggest that a high-grade liposarcoma will present or behave differently than a similarly graded malignant fibrous histiocytoma, neurofibrosarcoma, angiosarcoma, synovioma, or undifferentiated sarcoma. All are deeply placed, grow rapidly, invade adjacent structures, and metastasize primarily to lungs and occasionally to lymph nodes (with the exception of the synovioma and epithelioid sarcoma, in which lymph node metastases occur in about 15 and 25 percent, respectively).[25,87] Similarly, the low-grade lesions such as the low-grade fibrosarcoma, liposarcoma, and leiomyosarcoma tend to be smaller, more slowly growing, less invasive, and much less prone to metastasize. A major exception is the rhabdomyosarcoma, which tends to resemble the Ewing's sarcoma in its behavior both locally and in its pattern of early metastasis.[6,23] Another exception is represented by the epithelioid sarcoma, which, on the basis of its often superficial location and bland histologic appearance, appears to be low-grade but, in fact, is highly malignant in biological behavior.[25,87]

Malignant soft tissue tumors may occur in all age ranges and occur equally in both sexes.[116,165] Sarcomas may be present at birth but, with the exception of the rhabdomyosarcoma, are generally rare in the first and second decades of life. The incidence increases in the middle years and with advancing age. As indicated in the section above on benign soft tissue tumors, the clinical differentiation between benign and malignant tumors of the soft tissues about the shoulder may be difficult. In general, malignant tumors are large, lie deep to the deep fascia, are less than discrete in outline, and tend to be firm, slightly, or nontender and fixed to adjacent structures. The patient's principal complaint is of a mass, usually painless and often only slowly enlarging. In the case of the synovioma, the history may be misleading since the lesion may have been present for some years prior to a sudden increase in size. If the lesion is of neural origin and involves a major nerve trunk, sensory or motor deficits may be present.

The natural history and prognosis for the various lesions are also more or less directly related to size of the tumor at the time of discovery and the grade.[227] Small tumors of low grade are likely to do well with only marginal or wide excision, while large high-grade tumors generally have a poor prognosis for both avoidance of local recurrence after marginal and sometimes even wide surgery and distant metastases. As noted above, the exceptions to these rules are the epithelioid sarcoma,[25,87] which, despite its bland appearance, is always a "bad actor," and all forms of rhabdomyosarcoma, regardless of how small, can be expected to metastasize rapidly if untreated.[6,230]

Imaging Studies

Most soft tissue sarcomas cannot be differentiated from one another by imaging studies. Liposarcomas can sometimes be recognized by the characteristic lucency of their fat component. However, high-grade liposarcomas may contain little or no recognizable fat. Calcifications are relatively more frequent in liposarcoma and in synovioma than in other lesions. Areas of macroscopic cystic necrosis are more frequent in high-grade lesions than in low-grade lesions.

These general principles notwithstanding, the major purpose of imaging studies in soft tissue sarcomas is to define the extent and anatomical relationships of the lesion rather than to diagnose the lesion. Computed tomography is probably the single most useful tool for this purpose, although recent experience with MRI suggests that it will shortly surpass CT for this purpose.

Pathology

Soft tissue sarcomas are not always identifiable on histologic grounds. Most pathologists use a system based on histogenesis; lipoblasts giving rise to liposarcoma, fibroblasts, fibrosarcoma and so on. However, a number of tumors are pleomorphic and unclassified other than being defined as high-grade malignancies. Therefore, light microscopy, electron microscopy, and immunoperoxidase stains are powerful adjuncts for soft tissue tumor classification, and care must be taken to prepare all biopsy samples appropriately for these tests. The common denominator for all these tumors seems to be the size of the tumor and histologic grade. The larger the tumor and the higher the grade, the worse the prognosis (Fig. 19-40).

Management

The key to any decision regarding appropriate management of patients with soft tissue sarcoma of the region of the shoulder is obtaining accurate staging data.[53,57,212] Regardless of which system one uses (Table 19-3), it is essential to define the grade of the lesion (G), the size and extent of the tumor (T), and the presence and absence of distant metastases (M, N). As indicated above, grading of some tumors is difficult and some pathologists prefer a three- or four-part scoring system for the soft tissue lesions.[32] If the Enneking system is to be used, 1/3 or 1–2/4 is considered low-grade and 2–3/3 or 3–4/4, high-grade.[53,137] For most biopsies of soft tissue tumors it is usually appropriate to obtain specimens for electron microscopy and special stains.[211] Determination of intra- and extracompartmental location of the tumor is best done by CT or MRI and the same technique can be used to estimate the size and proximity to adjacent structures, if the American Joint Commission staging system is to be used.[191,227] Information on the presence or absence of metastases can best be obtained by CT of the chest and, in some circumstances, lymphangiogram. For synovioma and epithelioid sarcoma, we have usually sampled the axillary lymph nodes at the time of biopsy (performed as a preliminary procedure prior to contamination of the field with the tumor.[167]

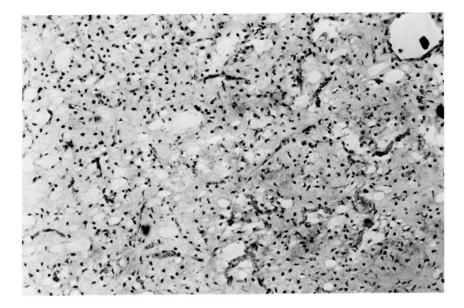

Fig. 19-40. A low-grade myxoid liposarcoma (grade I/III) with scattered fat-laden lipoblasts admixed with small myxoid cells and abundant matrix production. The presence of lipoblasts helps classify this tumor as a myxoid variant of liposarcoma. (H & E, × 125.)

Because most soft tissue sarcomas grow by invasion of the compressed reactive zone surrounding it or by the development of daughter nodules in close proximity but not necessarily in continuity with the main tumor mass, surgical treatment requires at least wide margins to achieve local control.[212] If this cannot be done safely, it would seem wisest to amputate the limb, although for most tumors about the shoulder it should be possible to perform limb-sparing surgery. Even low-grade lesions should never be "shelled out," particularly as an excisional biopsy, if one does not know the nature of the lesion. For high-grade lesions (IIA or IIB using the Enneking staging system), we generally advocate preliminary radiation therapy followed by wide resection. The preoperative radiation must be carefully planned to use diminishing fields and, if possible, to spare the site of the subsequent surgery. Depending on the site and the extent of the lesion, 4800 to 5400 cGy are administered over 5 to 6 weeks followed in 2 weeks by a wide local resection.[226,228,236] Two weeks later, after preliminary healing of the wound has been achieved, the radiation dosage is "boosted" to 6000 to 6600 cGy. Although there have been some problems with wound healing using this technique, they usually yield to appropriate local care or, in special cases, plastic surgical procedures. The local recurrence rate has been low, however, and study of the tissues after the radiation has shown a high percentage of tumor "kill," particularly for synovioma, liposarcoma, and malignant fibrous histiocytoma. For lower-grade tumors (IA and IB) if the lesion is small, surgery alone may suffice. When in doubt, we tend to suggest preliminary radiation rather than risk a local recurrence.

If the patient is referred to us following an excisional biopsy in which the lesion has been inappropriately shelled out, we proceed with the staging and treat the local site with the radiation according to the technique described above. Following completion of the first preliminary period of radiation treatment, the patient is restaged and a decision made as to whether the bed of the prior resection should be excised or the radiation boost administered without surgery. This second protocol has been less satisfactory in achieving local control in our hands, and we much prefer to deal with the lesion primarily rather than after an incomplete local excision.[229]

Some investigators have indicated improved survival data for patients with high-grade soft tissue sarcomas treated postoperatively with adjuvant Adriamycin.[189] This issue remains in contention at the present time.[3] If metastases occur (as they do in approximately 30 percent of the patients with high-grade tumors in which local control is achieved), thoracotomy and resection of the metastases and treatment with Adriamycin and/or cis-platinum is advised.[97]

Two special cases should be mentioned. For non-metastatic childhood rhabdomyosarcoma, multidrug chemotherapy has been proven to be of value in conjunction with surgical eradiation of the primary tumor or primary irradiation in unresectable cases.[6,230] Epithelioid sarcoma, despite its bland appearance, has a very high local recurrence and metastatic rate, and the tumors are relatively unaffected by either adjuvant radiation or chemotherapy. Radical surgery with lymph node dissection is usually advocated, although there may be a role for adjunctive radiation therapy in selected cases.[25,87,229]

Metastatic Carcinoma

Metastatic carcinoma to the bones of the shoulder girdle in middle-aged adults is far more prevalent than primary malignant tumors of bone if one excludes myeloma. Thus the orthopaedist in general adult practice is likely to see as many as 100 cases of metastatic disease for every primary malignant tumor. The primary sites from which the metastatic deposit to the shoulder girdle is likely to have originated in female patients include breast, lung, gastrointestinal tract, kidney, and thyroid (in approximately that order); in male patients it will be from the lung, prostate, gastrointestinal tract, kidney, and thyroid (note that carcinoma of the prostate is normally highest on this list for the pelvis, lower extremities, and spine but is somewhat less likely to present as a metastatic lesion to the shoulder than carcinoma of the lung).[10,118,155,182,207] The majority of these tumors present as destructive lesions, usually in the scapula, clavicle, or head and shaft of the humerus. About 90 percent of metastases from the prostate, 50 percent of carcinomas from the breast, and 20 percent of tumors from the lung or gastrointestinal tract seem to evoke a sclerotic response on the part of the host bone and may appear as an area of increased density on imaging studies. All of these lesions will be active on bone scan. Renal cell carcinoma and carcinoma of the thyroid are usually purely lytic and the latter may not show activity on bone scan (but, depending on the type of primary, may be very active on radioiodine scanning).[16,149,208]

Patients with metastatic carcinoma to the bones of the shoulder usually complain of pain at the site, made more severe by activity, but not usually relieved by rest. At times the initial onset of symptoms is sudden after minor trauma, usually indicating the occurrence of a pathologic fracture. Local tenderness is often present. A careful history and physical examination are likely to uncover evidence for the presence of either an occult primary tumor or other sites of metastatic spread. All patients in whom a malignant process of a bony site is suspected should have a careful examination of the breasts, rectum, pelvic organs, prostate, abdomen, lymph nodes, and thyroid.

SCREENING

Following the finding of a lesion on routine radiographic examination of the shoulder, the patient should be screened for the presence of malignant disease prior to biopsy (Fig. 19-1). In addition to the routine laboratory studies an acid phosphatase level should be obtained for male patients and mammogram for female patients. Both should have bone scans, CT scans of the chest, intravenous pyelography or ultrasound of the kidneys, and thyroid scans (this should be done prior to pyelography, since the contrast used for the latter study contains iodine and will necessitate a 2-week delay). If thyroid carcinoma is suspected, a skeletal survey and radioiodine scan may be valuable. As a general rule, we do not do bowel studies prior to biopsy but may, if suspicion of such a lesion exists, perform a liver spleen scan and CT examination of the abdomen.

The biopsy should be performed as atraumatically as possible. If the bone appears so weakened on radiographs as to be likely to fracture or if a pathologic fracture has already occurred, it is appropriate to perform some form of internal fixation of the site or implant polymethyl methacrylate if the frozen section shows the nature of the lesion to be metastatic carcinoma. For lesions of the humerus, simple rodding is often the treatment of choice. It is essential to obtain sufficient tissue at the time of biopsy for study of estrogen and progesterone receptors, particularly if breast or prostatic carcinoma is suspected. Special stains may be very helpful in differentiating thyroid, renal cell, and bowel carcinoma, and the pathologist should be consulted in advance of the biopsy procedure.

If renal cell carcinoma is suspected, it is sometimes best to use a needle biopsy technique, since these lesions can be extremely vascular (they may be found to be pulsatile on physical examination.)

MANAGEMENT

After the diagnosis has been made, the problem of management is usually the responsibility of the oncologist.[12] Decisions as to the necessity of treating the primary site, the use of hormones, chemotherapy, and radiation therapy are often beyond the purview and experience of the orthopaedist. Appropriate management of the local lesion is certainly the responsibility of the orthopaedist, however, and he or she should work closely with the radiation therapist and oncologist to obtain the best possible palliation. When pathologic fracture of a metastatic site seems imminent, prophylactic internal fixation with or without polymethyl methacrylate is an appropriate operative procedure and may significantly reduce pain and limitation of function.[203,205] Contrary to some suggestions by radiation therapists, the use of internal fixation does not materially interfere with the use of radiation therapy and may, in fact, make the treatment protocol less painful and difficult for the patient.

Two special cases exist in the management of patients with metastatic carcinoma. Occasionally one encounters a patient with either thyroid or renal cell carcinoma who appears to have a solitary metastasis. If the secondary deposit remains as the solitary focus of disease after adequate treatment of the primary lesion, it may be appropriate to plan a wide or marginal resection to eliminate the disease completely and, in a small percentage of the cases, induce a lasting remission. Although this circumstance is rare, it occurs sufficiently often to warrant serious consideration and discussion with the oncologist caring for the patient.

REFERENCES

1. Albright F, Butler AM, Hampton AO, Smith P: Syndrome characterized by osteitis fibrosa disseminata, areas of pigmentation and endocrine dysfunction, with precocious puberty in females. Report of five cases. N Eng J Med 216:727, 1937

2. Alho A, Connor JF, Mankin HJ et al: Assessment of malignancy of cartilage tumors using flow cytometry. J Bone Joint Surg 65A:779, 1983

3. Antman K, Amato D, Lerner H et al: Adjuvant doxorubicin for sarcoma: data from the Eastern Cooperative Group and the Dana-Farber/Massachusetts General Hospital studies. Cancer Treat Symposia 3:109, 1985

4. Bacci G, Picci P, Gitelis S et al: The treatment of localized Ewing's sarcoma: the experience of the Instituto Ortopedico Rizzoli in 163 cases treated with and without chemotherapy. Cancer 49:1561, 1982

5. Bacci G, Springfield DS, Campana R et al: Adjuvant chemotherapy for malignant fibrous histiocytoma in the femur and tibia. J Bone Joint Surg 67A:620, 1985

6. Bale PM, Parsons RE, Stevens MM: Diagnosis and behavior of juvenile rhabdomyosarcoma. Hum Pathol 14:596, 1983

7. Barnes R, Catto M: Chondrosarcoma of bone. J Bone Joint Surg 48B:729, 1969

8. Bauer TW, Dorfman HD, Latham JT Jr: Periosteal chondroma: a study of 23 cases. Am J Surg Pathol 6:631, 1982

9. Bendeck TE, Lichtenberg F: Cavernous hemangioma of striated muscle: review of the literature and report of two cases. Ann Surg 146:1011, 1957

10. Berrettoni BA, Carter JR: Current concepts review. Mechanisms of cancer metastasis to bone. J Bone Joint Surg 68A:308, 1986

11. Bertoni F, Present D, Enneking WF: Giant-cell tumor of bone with pulmonary metastases. J Bone Joint Surg 67A:890, 1985

12. Bhardwaj S, Halland JF: Chemotherapy of metastatic cancer in bone. CORR 169:28–37, 1982

13. Bleyer WA, Haas JE, Feigl P et al: Improved three-year disease-free survival in osteogenic sarcoma: efficacy of adjunctive chemotherapy. J Bone Joint Surg 64B:233, 1982

14. Boston HC, Dahlin DC, Ivins JC, Cupps, RE: Malignant lymphoma (so-called reticulum cell sarcoma) of bone. Cancer 34:1131, 1974

15. Bowden L, Booher RJ: The principles and technique of resection of soft parts for sarcoma. Surgery 44:963, 1958

16. Bowers TA, Murray JA, Charnsangare JC et al: Bone metastases from renal carcinoma. J Bone Joint Surg 64A:749, 1982

17. Broder HM: Possible precursor of unicameral bone cyst. J Bone Joint Surg 50A:549, 1982

18. Burrows HJ, Wilson JN, Scales JT: Excision of tumors of humerus and femur, with restoration by internal prosthesis. J Bone Joint Surg 57B:148, 1975

19. Campanacci M, Campanna R, Picci P: Unicameral

and aneurysmal bone cysts. Clin Orthop 204:25, 1986

20. Campanacci M, Cervellati G: Osteosarcoma: a review of 345 cases. Ital J Orthop, 1:5, 1975

21. Campanacci M, Picci P, Gherlinzoni F et al: Parosteal osteosarcoma. J Bone Joint Surg 66B:313–321, 1984

22. Cannon SR, Sweetnam R: Multiple chondrosarcomas in dyschondroplasia (Ollier's disease). Cancer 55:836, 1985

23. Capanna R, Dal Monte A, Gitelis S, Campanacci M: The natural history of unicameral bone cyst after steroid injection. CORR 166:204, 1982

24. Carter SK: Adjuvant chemotherapy in osteogenic sarcoma: the triumph that isn't? J Clin Oncol 2:147, 1984

25. Chase DR, Enzinger FM: Epithelioid sarcoma. Diagnosis, prognostic indicators, and treatment. Am J Surg Pathol 9:241, 1985

26. Clark RE, Jr., Martin RG, White EC, Old JW: Clinical aspects of soft-tissue tumors. Arch Surg 74:859, 1957

27. Clough JR, Price CHG: Aneurysmal bone cyst: pathogenesis and long term results of treatment. CORR 97:52, 1973

28. Cohen J: Unicameral bone cysts. A current synthesis of reported cases. Orthop Clin North Am 8:715, 1972

29. Cornwell GG, III, Pajak TF, Kochwa S et al: Comparison of oral melphalan, CCNU and BCNU with and without vincristine and prednisone in the treatment of multiple myeloma. Cancer 50:1669, 1982

30. Cortes EP, Holland JF, Glidewell O: Adjuvant therapy of operable primary osteosarcoma—cancer and leukemia group B experience. Rec Results Cancer Res 68:16, 1979

31. Cortes EP, Holland JF, Wang JJ et al: Amputation and adriamycin in primary osteosarcoma. N Eng J Med 291:998, 1974

32. Costa J: Histologic classification and grading of sarcomas. Cancer Treat Symposia 3:27, 1985

33. Cowan WK: Malignant change and multiple metastases in Ollier's disease. J Clin Pathol 18:650, 1965

34. Craig FS: Metastatic and primary lesions of bone. Clin Orthop 73:33, 1970

35. Cuvelier CA, Roels HJ: Cytometric studies of the nuclear content in cartilaginous tumors. Cancer 44:1463, 1979

36. Dahlin DC: Bone Tumors: General Aspects and Data on 6,221 Cases. Charles C Thomas, Springfield, Illinois, 1978

37. Dahlin DC, Beabout JW: Dedifferentiation of low grade chondrosarcoma. Cancer 28:461, 1971

38. Dahlin DC, Capps, RE, Johnson EWJ: Giant cell tumor: a study of 195 cases. Cancer 25:1061, 1970

39. Dahlin DC, Coventry MB: Osteogenic sarcoma. A study of six hundred cases. J Bone Joint Surg 49A:101, 1967

40. Dahlin DC, Unni KK, Matsuno T: Malignant (fibrous) histiocytoma of bone—fact or fancy. Cancer 39:1508, 1977

41. Danon M, Robboy MO, Kim S et al: Cushings' syndrome, sexual precocity and polyostotic fibrous dysplasia (Albright's syndrome) in infancy. J Pediatr 87:917, 1975

42. Dionne GP, Seemayer TA: Infiltrating lipomas and angiolipomas revisited. Cancer 33:732, 1974

43. Dorfman HD: Case records of the Massachusetts General Hospital. N Eng J Med 303:866, 1980

44. Dorfman HD, Norman A, Wolft H: Fibrosarcoma complicating bone infarction in a Caisson worker. J Bone Joint Surg 48B:528, 1966

45. Eckardt JJ, Eilber FR, Dorey FJ, Mirra JM: The UCLA experience in limb salvage for malignant tumors. Orthopaedics 8:612, 1985

46. Eckardt JJ, Grogan TJ: Giant cell tumor of bone. Clin Orthop 204:45, 1986

47. Edmonson JH, Green SJ, Ivins ET et al: Methotrexate as adjuvant treatment for primary osteosarcoma. N Engl J Med 303:642, 1980

48. Edmonson JH, Green SJ, Ivins JC et al: A controlled pilot study of high-dose methotrexate as post-surgical adjuvant treatment of primary osteosarcoma. J Clin Oncol 2:152, 1984

49. Edwards WH, Thompson RC, Varsa EW: Lymphangiomatosis and massive osteolysis of the cervical spine. A case report and review of the literature. Clin Orthop 177:222, 1983

50. Eilber FR, Eckhardt J, Morton DL: Advances in the treatment of sarcomas of the extremity. Cancer 54:2695, 1984

51. Eilber FR, Guiliano AE, Huth J et al: Limb salvage for highgrade soft tissue sarcomas of the extremities: experience at the University of California, Los Angeles. Cancer Treat Symposia 3:49, 1985

52. Enneking WF: Musculoskeletal Tumor Surgery. Churchill Livingstone, New York, 1983

53. Enneking WF: Staging of Musculoskeletal Neoplasms. Current Concepts of Diagnosis and Treatment of Bone and Soft Tissue Tumors. Springer-Verlag, Berlin-Heidelberg, 1984, pp 1–21

54. Enneking WF, Kogan A: The implications of "skip" metastases in osteosarcoma. Clin Orthop 11:33, 1975

55. Enneking WF, McAuliffe: Adjuctive preoperative radiation therapy in treatment of soft tissue sarcomas: a preliminary report. Cancer Treat Symposia 3:37, 1985

56. Enneking WF, Shirley PD: Resection-arthrodesis for malignant and potentially malignant lesions about the knee using an intramedullary rod and local bone grafts. J Bone Joint Surg 59A:223, 1977

57. Enneking WF, Spanier SS, Goodman MA: A system

for the surgical staging of musculoskeletal sarcoma. Clin Orthop 153:106, 1980

58. Enneking WF, Spanier SS, Malawer MM: The effect of anatomic setting on the results of surgical procedures for soft parts sarcoma of the thigh. Cancer 47:1005, 1981

59. Enneking WF, Springfield DS, Gross M: The surgical treatment of parosteal osteosarcoma in long bones. J Bone Joint Surg 67A:125, 1985

60. Enzinger FM: Benign lipomatous tumors simulating a sarcoma. In Dybala LW, Freitag SB, Culhane DC (eds): Managment of Primary Bone and Soft Tissue Tumors. Year Book Medical Publishers, Chicago, 1977, pp. 11–24

61. Enzinger FM, Shiraki M: Musculo-aponeurotic fibromatosis of the shoulder girdle (extra-abdominal desmoid). Analysis of thirty cases followed up for ten or more years. Cancer 20:1131, 1967

62. Enzinger FM, Weiss SW: Soft Tissue Tumors. C.V. Mosby, St. Louis, 1983

63. Eriksson AI, Schiller A, Mankin HJ: The management of chondrosarcoma of bone. CORR 153:44, 1980

64. Evans HL, Soule EH, Winkelmann RK: Atypical lipoma, atypical intramuscular lipoma, and well differentiated retroperitoneal liposarcoma: a reappraisal of 30 cases formerly classified as well defferentiated liposarcoma. Cancer 43:574, 1979

65. Evarts CM: Diagnostic techniques: closed biopsy of bone. Clin Orthop 107:100, 1975

66. Eyer-Brook AL, Price CHG: Fibrosarcoma of bone. Review of fifty consecutive cases from the Bristol Bone Tumour Registry. J Bone Joint Surg 51B:20, 1969

67. Fahey J, O'Brien E: Subtotal resection and grafting in selected cases of solitary unicameral bone cyst. J Bone Joint Surg 55A:59, 1973

68. Friedman MA, Carter SK: The therapy of osteogenic sarcoma: current status and thoughts for the future. J Surg Oncol 4:482, 1972

69. Gebhardt MC, McGuire MH, Mankin HJ: Resection and allograft arthrodesis for malignant bone tumors of the extremity. In Enneking WF (ed): Limb Salvage in Musculoskeletal Oncology. Churchill Livingstone, New York, 1987

70. Gehan EA, Nesbit MEJ, Vietti TJ et al: Prognostic factors in children with Ewing's sarcoma. Natl Cancer Inst Monogr 56:273, 1981

71. Gherlinzoni F, Rock M, Picci P: Chondromyxoid fibroma. The experience at the Instituto Ortopedico Rizzoli. J Bone Joint Surg 65A:198, 1983

72. Gilmer WS, Jr., Kilgore W, Smith H: Central cartilage tumors of bone. Clin Orthop 23:81, 1963

73. Gitelis S, Gertoni F, Chieti PP, Campanacci M: Chondrosarcoma of bone. The experience at the Instituto Ortopedico Rizzoli. J Bone Joint Surg 63A:1248, 1983

74. Glaubiger DL, Makuch R, Schwarz J et al: Determination of prognostic factors and their influence on therapeutic results in patients with Ewing's sarcoma. Cancer 45:2213, 1980

75. Goldenberg RR, Campbell CJ, Bonfiglio M: Giant cell tumor of bone. An analysis of two hundred and eighteen cases. J Bone Joint Surg 52A:669, 1970

76. Golding JST: The natural history of osteoid osteoma with a report of 20 cases. J Bone Joint Surg 36B:218, 1954

77. Goldring SR, Dayer J-M, Russell RGG et al: Cells cultured from human giant cell tumor of bone respond to parathyroid hormone. Calcif Tissue Res (Suppl) 22:269, 1977

78. Goldring SR, Schiller AL, Mankin HJ et al: Characterization of cells from human giant cell tumors of bone. Clin Orthop 204:59, 1986

79. Goodman MA: Plasma cell tumors. Clin Orthop 204:86, 1986

80. Goorin AM, Abelson HT, Frei E III: Osteosarcoma: fifteen years later. N Eng J Med 313:1637, 1985

81. Goorin AM, Delorey MJ, Lack EE et al: Prognostic significance of complete surgical resection of pulmonary metastases in patients with osteogenic sarcoma. J Clin Oncol 2:425, 1984

82. Goorin AM, Frei E III, Abelson AT: Adjuvant chemotherapy for osteosarcoma. A decade of experience. Surg Clin North Am 61:1379, 1981

83. Gorham LW, Stout AP: Massive osteolysis (acute spontaneous absorption of bone, phantom bone, disappearing bone). Its relation to hemangiomatosis. J Bone Joint Surg 37A:985, 1955

84. Grabias SL, Campbell CJ: Fibrous dysplasia. Ortho Clin North, 8:771, 1977

85. Griffiths DL: Orthopaedic aspects of myelomatosis. J Bone Joint Surg 48B:703, 1966

86. Hadju SI: Pathology of Soft Tissue Tumors. Lea and Febiger, Philadelphia, 1979

87. Hadju SI, Shiu MH, Forter JG: Tendosynovial sarcoma. A clinicopathologic study of 136 cases. Cancer 39:1201, 1977

88. Hait WN, Farber L, Cadman E: Non-Hodgkin's lymphoma for the nononcologist. JAMA, 253:1431, 1985

89. Han MT, Telander RL, Pairolero PC et al: Aggressive thoracotomy for pulmonary metastatic osteogenic sarcoma in children and young adolescents. J Pediatr Surg 16:928, 1982

90. Harkin JC, Reed RJ: Atlas of Tumor Pathology, Fascicle 3: Tumors of the Peripheral Nervous System. Armed Forced Institute of Pathology, Washington, D.C., 1969

91. Harkins GA, Sabiston DC: Lymphangioma in infancy and childhood. Pediatr Surg 47:811, 1960

92. Harris WH, Dudley R, Barry RJ: The natural history

of fibrous dysplasia. J Bone Joint Surg 44A:207, 1962

93. Healey JH, Ghelman B: Osteoid osteoma and osteoblastoma: current concepts and recent advances. Clin Orthop 204:76, 1986

94. Healey JH, Lane JM: Chondrosarcoma. Clin Orthop 204:119, 1986

95. Henderson ED, Dahlin DC: Chondrosarcoma of bone—a study of two hundred and eighty-eight cases. J Bone Joint Surg 45A:1450, 1963

96. Henry A: Monostotic fibrous dysplasia. J Bone Joint Surg 51B:300, 1969

97. Huth JF, Holmes EC, Vernon SE et al: Pulmonary resection for metastatic sarcoma. Am J Surg 140:9, 1980

98. Huvos AG: Bone Tumors. Diagnosis, Treatment and Prognosis. W.B. Saunders, Philadelphia, 1979

99. Huvos AG: Osteogenic sarcoma of bones and soft tissues in older persons. A clinicopathologic analysis of 117 patients older than 60 years. Cancer 57:1442, 1986

100. Huvos AG, Butler A, Bretsky SS: Osteogenic sarcoma associated with Paget's disease of bone: a clinicopathological study of 65 patients. Cancer 52:1489, 1983

101. Huvos AG, Higginbotham NL: Primary fibrosarcoma of bone. A clinicopathologic study of 133 cases. Cancer 35:837, 1975

102. Huvos AG, Higginbotham NL, Miller TR: Bone sarcomas arising in fibrous dysplasia. J Bone Joint Surg 54A:1047, 1972

103. Huvos AG, Marcove RC: Chondroblastoma of bone. A critical review. Clin Orthop 95:300, 1973

104. Huvos AG, Rosen G, Bretsky SS et al: Telangiectatic osteogenic sarcoma: a clinicopathologic study of 124 patients. Cancer 49:1679, 1982

105. Jaffe H: Tumors and Tumorous Conditions of the Bones and Joints. Lea & Febiger, Philadelphia, 1958

106. Jaffe HL: Hereditary multiple exostosis. Arch Pathol 36:398, 1973

107. Jaffe HL: "Osteoid osteoma." A benign osteoblastic tumor composed of osteoid and atypical bone. Arch Surg 31:709, 1935

108. Jaffe HL, Lichtenstein L: Benign chondroblastoma of bone. A reiteration of the so called calcifying or chondromatous giant cell tumor. Am J Pathol 18:909, 1942

109. Jentzsch K: Leg function after radiation therapy for Ewing's sarcoma. Cancer 47:1267, 1981

110. Johnston GA, Simon MA, Azizi F: Giant cell tumors of bone in pregnancy. J Reprod Med 24:43, 1980

111. Khorsand J, Karakousis CP: Desmoid tumors and their management. Am J Surg 149:215, 1985

112. Kindblom LG, Angervall L, Stener B et al: Intermuscular and intramuscular lipomas and hibernomas. A clinical, roentgenologic, histologic and prognostic study of 46 cases. Cancer 33:754, 1974

113. King DR, Clatworthy HW Jr.: The pediatric patient with sarcoma. Semin Oncol 8:215, 1981

114. Kinsella TJ, Lichter AS, Miser J et al: Local treatment of Ewing's sarcoma: radiation therapy versus surgery. Cancer Treat Rep 68:695, 1984

115. Kissane JM, Askin FB, Foulkes M et al: Ewing's sarcoma of bone: clinicopathologic aspects of 303 cases from the Intergroup Ewing's Sarcoma Study. Human Pathol 14:773, 1983

116. Kissane JM, Askin FB, Nesbit ME et al: Sarcomas of bone in childhood: pathologic aspects. NCI Monogr 56:29, 1981

117. Koskinen VS, Visuri TI, Holstrom T, Roukkula MA: Aneurysmal bone cyst. Evaluation of resection and curettage in twenty cases. Clin Orthop 118:136, 1976

118. Krishnamurthy GT, Tubis M, Hiss J Blahd WH: Distribution pattern of metastatic bone disease. A need for total body skeletal image. JAMA 237:2504, 1977

119. Kyle RA: Long-term survival in multiple myeloma. N Eng J Med 30B:314, 1983

120. Kyle RA: Multiple myeloma. Review of 869 cases. Mayo Clin Proc 50:29, 1975

121. Lane JM, Hurson B, Boland PJ, Glasser DB: Osteogenic sarcoma. Clin Orthop 204:93, 1986

122. Lange B, Levine AS: Is it ethical not to conduct a prospectively controlled trial of adjuvant chemotherapy in osteosarcoma? Cancer Treat Rep 66:1699, 1982

123. Lawrence WC: Limb-sparing treatment of adult soft-tissue sarcomas and osteosarcomas. Cancer Treatment Symposia, National Institutes of Health Consensus Development Conference Statement, Bethesda, MD, 3:1–161, 1984

124. Leffert RD: Lipomas of the upper extremity. J Bone Joint Surg 54A:1262, 1972

124a. Leibel SA, Wara WM, Hill DR et al: Desmoid tumors: local control and patterns of relapse following radiation therapy. Int J Radiation Oncol 9:1167, 1983

125. Levine AM, Rosenberg SA: Alkaline phosphatase levels in osteosarcoma tissue are related to prognosis. Cancer 44:2291, 1979

126. Levine AS: Cancer in the Young. Masson, New York, 1982

127. Lewis RJ, Ketcham AS: Maffucci's syndrome: functional and neoplastic significance. J Bone Joint Surg 55A:1465, 1973

128. Lichtenstein L: Bone Tumors. CV Mosby, St. Louis, 1977

129. Lichtenstein L, Hall JE: Periosteal chondroma: a distinctive benign cartilage tumor. J Bone Joint Surg 34A:691, 1952

130. Lichtenstein L, Sawyer WR: Benign osteoblastoma. Further observations and report of twenty additional cases. J Bone Joint Surg 46A:755, 1964

131. Lieberman Z, Ackerman LV: Principles in manage-

ment of soft tissue sarcomas. A clinical and pathological review of one hundred cases. Surgery 35:350, 1954

132. Link M, Goorin AM, Miser A et al: The role of adjuvant chemotherapy in the treatment of osteosarcoma (OS) of the extremity: preliminary results of the Multi-Institutional Osteosarcoma Study (MIOS). Proc Am Soc Clin Oncol 4:237, 1985

133. Mainzer F, Minagi H, Steinbach HL: The variable manifestations of multiple enchondromatosis. Radiology 99:377, 1971

134. Malawar M: Surgical technique and results of limb sparing surgery for high grade bone sarcomas of the knee and shoulder. Orthopaedics 8:597, 1985

135. Mankin HJ: Advances in the diagnosis and treatment of bone tumors. N Eng J Med 300:543, 1979

136. Mankin HJ: Bone and soft tissue tumors, p 11:3. In Evarts CM (ed): Surgery of the Musculoskeletal System, vol. 4. Churchill Livingstone, New York, 1983

137. Mankin HJ, Connor JF, Schiller AL et al: Grading of bone tumors by analysis of nuclear DNA content using flow cytometry. J Bone Joint Surg 67A:404, 1985

138. Mankin HJ, Doppelt SH, Tomford WW: Clinical experience with allograft implantation. The first ten years. Clin Orthop 174:69, 1983

139. Mankin HJ, Lange TA, Spanier SS: The hazards of biopsy in patients with primary bone tumors and soft tissue tumors. J Bone Joint Surg 64A:1121, 1982

140. Marcove R: a 17-year review of cryosurgery in the treatment of bone tumors. Clin Orthop 163:231, 1982

141. Marcove R, Rosen G: Radical en bloc excision of Ewing's sarcoma. Clin Orthop 153:86, 1980

142. Marcove RC, Alpert M: A pathologic study of benign osteoblastoma. Clin Orthop 30:175, 1963

143. Marcove RC, Lewis MM, Huvos AG: En bloc upper humeral interscapulo-thoracic resection. The Tikoff-Linberg procedure. Clin Orthop 124:219, 1977

144. Marcove RC, Mike V, Hajek JV et al: Osteogenic sarcoma under the age of twenty-one. A review of one hundred and forty five operative cases. J Bone Joint Surg 52A:411, 1970

145. Marcove RC, Rosen G: En bloc resections for osteogenic sarcoma. Cancer 45:3040, 1980

146. Marion J, Buyers V, Bruer K et al: Role of metastatectomy without chemotherapy in the management of osteosarcoma in children. Cancer 45:1664, 1980

147. Maroteaux P: Bone Diseases in Children. J.B. Lippincott, Philadelphia, 1979

148. Marsh BW, Bonfiglio M, Brady LP et al: Benign osteoblastoma. Range of manifestations. J Bone Joint Surg 37A:1, 1975

149. McCormack KR: Bone metastases from thyroid carcinoma. Cancer 19:181, 1966

150. McDonald DJ, Sim FH, McLeod RA et al: Giant cell tumor of bone. J Bone Joint Surg 68A:235, 1986

151. McFarland GBJ, McKinley LM, Reed RJ: Dedifferentiation of low-grade chondrosarcoma. Clin Orthop 112:157, 1977

152. McFarland GBJ, Morden ML: Benign cartilaginous lesions. Orthop Clin North Am 8:751, 1977

153. McKay D: Treatment of unicameral bone cysts by subtotal resection without grafts. J Bone Joint Surg 59A:515, 1978

154. McLeod R, Dahlin DC, Beabout JW: The spectrum of osteoblastoma. Am J Roentgenol 126:321, 1976

155. Meyor PC: A statistical and histological survey of metastatic carcinoma in the skeleton. Br J Cancer 11:509, 1957

156. Minor CL, Koop CE: Experience with the management of plexiform neurofibroma. Pediatrics 24:482, 1959

157. Mirra JM: Bone Tumors: Diagnosis and Treatment. J.B. Lippincott, Philadelphia, 1980

158. Mirra JM, Marcove RC: Fibrosarcomatous dedifferentiation of primary and secondary chondrosarcoma. J Bone Joint Surg 56A:285, 1974

159. Moore TM, Meyers MH, Patakis MJ, et al: Closed biopsy of musculoskeletal lesions. J Bone Joint Surg 61A:375, 1979

160. Musgrove JE, McDonald JR: Extra-abdominal desmoid tumors. Their differential diagnosis and treatment. Arch Pathol 45:513, 1948

161. Neer CS, Francis KC, Marcove RC et al: Treatment of unicameral bone cyst. A follow-up study of one hundred seventy-five cases. J Bone Joint Surg 48A:731, 1966

162. Neff JR: Nonmetastatic Ewing's sarcoma of bone: the role of surgical therapy. Clin Orthop 204:111, 1986

163. Nix JT: Lymphangioma. Am Surgeon 20:556, 1954

164. Ottolenghi CE: Aspiration biopsy of the spine. J Bone Joint Surg 51A:1531, 1969

165. Pack GT, Areil IM: Sarcomas of the soft somatic tissues in infants and children. Surg Gynecol Obstet 98:675, 1954

166. Peimer CA, Schiller AL, Mankin HJ et al: Multicentric giant cell tumor of bone. J Bone Joint Surg 62A:652, 1980

167. Peimer CA, Smith RJ, Sirota RL et al: Epithelioid sarcoma of the hand and wrist: patterns of extension. J Hand Surg 2:275, 1977

168. Perez CA, Tefft M, Nesbit ME et al: Radiation therapy in the multimodal management of Ewing's sarcoma of bone: report of the Intergroup Ewing's Sarcoma Study. Natl Cancer Inst Monogr 56:263, 1981

169. Persson BM, Ekelund L, Lovdahl R et al: Favourable results of acrylic cementation for giant cell tumors. Acta Orthop Scand 55:209, 1984

170. Persson BM, Wouters HW: Curettage and acrylic ce-

mentation in surgery of giant cell tumors of bone. C.O.R.R., 126:125, 1976

171. Pritchard DJ: Small Cell Tumors of Bone. p. 26. Instructional Course Lectures. CV Mosby, St. Louis, 1984

172. Pritchard DJ, Dahlin DC, Dauphine RT et al: Ewing's sarcoma. A clinico-pathological and statistical analysis of patients surviving five years or longer. J Bone Joint Surg 55A:10, 1975

173. Pritchard DJ, Lunke RJ, Taylor WF et al: Chondrosarcoma: a clinicopathologic and statistical analysis. Cancer 45:149, 1980

174. Pritchard DJ, Sim FH, Ivins JC et al: Fibrosarcoma of bone and soft tissues of the trunk and extremities. Orthop Clin North Am 8:869, 1977

175. Putnam JBJ, Roth JA, Wesley MN et al: Survival following aggressive resection of pulmonary metastases from osteogenic sarcoma: analysis of prognostic factors. Ann Thorac Surg 36:515, 1983

176. Raffensperger J, Cohen R: Plexiform neurofibromas in childhood J Pediatr Surg 7:144, 1972

177. Ralph LL: Chondromyxoid fibroma of bone. J Bone Joint Surg 44B:7, 1962

178. Reimer RR, Chabner BA, Young RC et al: Lymphoma presenting in bone. Results of histopathology, staging and therapy. Ann Intern Med 87:50, 1977

179. Riccardi VM: Von Recklinghausen neurofibromatosis. N Eng J Med 305:1617, 1981

180. Rock MG, Pritchard DJ, Reiman HM et al: Extra-abdominal desmoid tumors. J Bone Joint Surg 66A:1369, 1984

181. Rock MG, Pritchard DJ, Unni KK: Metastasis from histologically benign giant cell tumors of bone. J Bone Joint Surg 66A:269, 1984

182. Rosai J: Tumors and tumorlike conditions in bone. p. 2008. In Anderson WAD, Kissane JM (eds).: Pathology. CV Mosby, St. Louis, 1977

183. Rosen G: Preoperative (neoadjuvant) chemotherapy for osteogenic sarcoma: a ten year experience. Orthopaedics 8:659, 1985

184. Rosen G, Caparros B, Huvos AG et al: Preoperative chemotherapy for osteogenic sarcoma. Selection of postoperative adjuvant chemotherapy based on the response of the primary tumor to preoperative chemotherapy. Cancer 49:1221, 1982

185. Rosen G, Huvos AG, Mosende C et al: Chemotherapy and thoracotomy for metastatic osteogenic sarcoma. Cancer 4:841, 1978

186. Rosen G, Juergens H, Caparros B et al: Combination chemotherapy (T-6) in the multidisciplinary treatment of Ewing's sarcoma. Natl Cancer Inst Monogr 56:289, 1981

187. Rosen G, Marcove RC, Huvos AG et al: Primary osteogenic sarcoma: an investigative method, not a recipe. Cancer Treat Rep 66:1687, 1982

188. Rosen G, Nirenberg A: Chemotherapy for osteogenic sarcoma: an investigative method, not a recipe. Cancer Treat Rep 66:1687, 1982

189. Rosenberg SA, Chang AE, Glastein E: Adjuvant chemotherapy for treatment of extremity soft tissue sarcoma: review of National Cancer Institute experience. Cancer Treat Symposia 3:83, 1985

190. Russell DS: Malignant osteoclastoma and the association of malignant osteoclastoma with Paget's osteitis deformans. J Bone Joint Surg 31B:281, 1949

191. Russell WO, Cohen J, Enzinger F et al: The clinical and pathological staging system for soft tissue sarcomas. Cancer 40:1562, 1977

192. Sanerkin NG: Malignancy, aggressiveness and recurrence in giant cell tumors of bone. Cancer 46:1641, 1980

193. Scaglietti O, Marchetti PG, Bartolozzi P: Final results obtained in the treatment of bone cysts with methylprednisolone acetate (Depo-Medral) and a discussion of results achieved in other bone lesions. CORR 165:33, 1982

194. Scaglietti O, Marchetti PG, Bartolozzi P: The effects of methylprednisolene acetate in the treatment of bone cysts. Results of three years' followup. J Bone Joint Surg 61B:200, 1979

195. Schajowicz F: Giant-cell tumors of bone (osteoclastoma). A pathological and histochemical study. J Bone Joint Surg 43A:1, 1961

196. Schajowicz F: Tumors and Tumorlike Lesions of Bones and Joints. Springer-Verlag, New York, 1981

197. Schajowicz F, Derudi JC: Puncture biopsies in lesions of the locomotor system. Review of results in 4,050 cases including 941 vertebral lesions. Cancer 21:531, 1968

198. Schajowicz F, Gallardo H: Chondromyxoid fibroma (fibromycoid chondroma) of bone. A clinico-pathologic study of thirty-two cases. J Bone Joint Surg 53B:198, 1971

199. Schajowicz F, Gallardo H: Epiphyseal chondrosarcoma of bone. A clinico-pathological study of sixty-nine cases. J Bone Joint Surg 52B:205, 1970

200. Schajowicz F, Lemos C: Malignant osteoblastoma. J Bone Joint Surg 58B:202, 1976

201. Shapiro F, Simon S, Glimcher MJ: Hereditary multiple exostoses. J Bone Joint Surg 61A:815, 1979

202. Sherman MS: Osteoid osteoma. Review of the literature and report of thirty cases. J Bone Joint Surg 29A:918, 1947

203. Sherry HS, Levy RN, Siffert RS: Metastatic disease of bone in orthopaedic surgery. Clin Orthop 169:44, 1982

204. Shiu MH, Hadju SI: Management of soft tissue sarcoma of the extremity. Semin Oncol 8:172, 1981

205. Shocken JD, Luther WB: Radiation therapy for bone metastasis. Clin Orthop 169:38, 1982

206. Shoji H, Miller TR: Primary reticulum cell sarcoma of bone. Significance of clinical features upon the prognosis. Cancer 28:1234, 1971

207. Silverberg E: Cancer statistics. CA 34:7, 1984

208. Silverberg SG, Evans RH, Koehler AL: Clinical and pathological features of initial metastatic presentations of renal cell carcinoma. Cancer 21:1126, 1969

209. Sim FH, Cupps RE, Dahlin DC et al: Postradiation sarcoma of bone. J Bone Joint Surg 54A:1479, 1972

210. Sim FH, Dahlin DC, Beabout JW: Osteoid osteoma: diagnostic problems. J Bone Joint Surg 57A:154, 1975

211. Simon MA: Biopsy of musculoskeletal tumors. J Bone Joint Surg 64A:1253, 1982

212. Simon MA, Enneking WF: The management of soft-tissue sarcomas of the extremities. J Bone Joint Surg 58A:317, 1976

213. Simon MA, Hecht JD: Invasion of joints by primary bone sarcomas in adults. Cancer 50:1649, 1982

214. Simon MA, Karluk MB: Skeletal metastases of unknown origin. Diagnostic strategy for orthopaedic surgeons. Clin Orthop 166:96, 1982

215. Slowick FA, Campbell CJ, Kettelkamp DB: Aneurysmal bone cyst. An analysis of thirteen cases. J Bone Joint Surg 50A:1142, 1968

216. Solomon L: Bone growth in diaphyseal acalsis. J Bone Joint Surg 43B:700, 1961

217. Solomon L: Hereditary multiple exostosis. J Bone Joint Surg 45B:292, 1963

218. Spanier SS, Enneking WF, Enriquez P: Primary malignant fibrous histiocytoma of bone. Cancer 36:2084, 1975

219. Spjut HJ, Dorfman HD, Fechner RE et al: Atlas of Tumor Pathology, Fascicle 5: Tumors of Bone and Cartilage. Armed Forces Institute of Pathology, 1971

220. Springfield DS, Campana R, Gherlinzoni F et al: Chondroblastoma. A review of seventy cases. J Bone Joint Surg 67A:748, 1985

221. Springfield DS, Enneking WF, Neff JR, et al: Principles of tumor management. AAOS Instructional Course Lectures, 33:1–25, 1984

222. Stemmermann GN, Stout AP: Elastofibroma dorsi. Am J Clin Pathol 37:499, 1962

223. Stewart MJ, Gilmer WS, Edmonson AS: Fibrous dysplasia of bone. J Bone Joint Surg 44B:302, 1962

224. Strong LC, Herson J, Osborn BM et al: Risk of radiation-related subsequent malignant tumors in survivors of Ewing's sarcoma. J Natl Cancer Inst 62:1401, 1979

225. Stout AP, Lattes R: Atlas of Tumor Pathology, Fascicle I: Tumors of the Soft Tissues. Armed Forces Institute of Pathology, Washington, D.C., 1967

226. Suit HD, Mankin HJ Schiller AL et al: Results of treatment of sarcoma of soft tissue by radiation and surgery at Massachusetts General Hospital. Cancer Treat Symp 3:43, 1985

227. Suit HD, Mankin HJ, Schiller AL: Staging systems for sarcoma of soft tissue and sarcoma of bone. Cancer Treat Symposia 3:29, 1985

228. Suit HD, Mankin HJ, Wood KH et al: Preoperative, intraoperative and postoperative radiation in the treatment of primary soft tissue sarcoma. Cancer 55:2659, 1985

229. Suit HD, Russell WO, Martin RG: Sarcoma of soft tissue: clinical and histopathologic parameters and response to treatment. Cancer 35:1478, 1975

230. Sutow WW, Maurer HM: Chemotherapy of sarcomas—a perspective. Semin Oncol 8:207, 1981

231. Sweet DL, Mass DP, Simon MA et al: Histiocytic lymphoma (reticulum-cell sarcoma) of bone. J Bone Joint Surg 63A:79, 1981

232. Taconis WK, Van Rijssel TG: Fibrosarcoma of long bones. A study of the significance of areas of malignant fibrous histiocytoma. J Bone Joint Surg 67B:111, 1985

233. Taylor WF, Ivins JC, Dahlin DC et al: Trends and variability in survival from osteosarcomas. Mayo Clin Proc 53:695, 1978

234. Taylor WF, Ivins JC, Pritchard DJ et al: Trends and variability in survival among patients with osteosarcoma: a 7-year update. Mayo Clin Proc 60:91, 1985

235. Tepper J, Glaubiger D, Lichter A et al: Local control of Ewing's sarcoma of bone with radiotherapy and combination chemotherapy. Cancer 46:1969, 1980

236. Tepper JE, Suit HD: Radiation therapy of soft tissue sarcoma. Cancer 55:2273, 1985

237. Thorp WP, Reilly JJ, Rosenberg SA: Prognostic significance of alkaline phosphatase measurements in patients with osteogenic sarcoma receiving chemotherapy. Cancer 43:2178, 1979

238. Tonai M, Campbell CJ, Ahn GH et al: Osteoblastoma: classification and report of 16 patients. Clin Orthop 167:222, 1982

239. Unni KK, Dahlin DC: Premalignant tumors and conditions of bone. Am J Surg Pathol 3:47, 1977

240. Unni KK, Dahlin DC, Beabout JW: Periosteal osteogenic sarcoma. Cancer 37:2476, 1976

241. Unni KK, Dahlin DC, Beabout JW et al: Parosteal osteogenic sarcoma. Cancer 37:2466, 1976

242. Unni KK, Dahlin DC, Beabout JW et al: Chondrosarcoma: clear-cell variant. J Bone Joint Surg 58A:676, 1976

243. Watson WL, McCarthy WD: Blood and lymph vessel tumors. Surg Gynecol Obstet 71:569, 1940

244. White NB: Neurilemomas of the extremities. J Bone Joint Surg 49A:1605, 1967

245. White WL: Troublesome lipomata of the upper extremities. J Bone Joint Surg 44A:1363, 1962

246. Wick MR, Siegal GP, Unni KK et al: Sarcomas of bone complicating osteitis deformans (Paget's disease). Fifty years' experience. Am J Surg Pathol 5:47, 1981

247. Wilson PD, Lance EM: Surgical reconstruction of the skeleton following segmental resection for bone tumors. J Bone Joint Surg 47A:1629, 1965

248. Winkler K, Beron G, Kotz R et al: Neoadjuvant chemotherapy for osteogenic sarcoma: results of a cooperative German-Austrian study. J Clin Oncol 2:617, 1984

249. Yuen WWH, Saw D: Malignant fibrous histiocytoma of bone. J Bone Joint Surg 67A:482, 1985

Evaluation of the Shoulder 20

Carter R. Rowe

A standard, agreed upon method of assessing shoulder function, similar to that developed for the hip by Harris,[3] is needed. Efforts to develop a standard form are being made by the American Shoulder and Elbow Surgeons,[4] Constant and Murley in Cambridge, England, Welsh in Canada,[8] and the author.[6,7] An agreement has not, as yet, been reached. We hope that the final rating method will be clear, accurate, flexible, and not too complicated.

A summary of each method is given below.

THE AUTHOR'S METHOD

The method we have used is based on a total of 100 units. Five categories are evaluated: pain, stability, function, motion, and strength, depending on the aim of the surgical procedure.

Option I

In order to give flexibility to the rating method, the value of the rating units may be left open, so that the surgeon may adjust the rating criteria of shoulder function in relation to the aim of the surgical procedure. For instance, to evaluate the surgical pro-

cedures for recurrent dislocation of the shoulder, *pain* would be given 15 units, *stability* 25 units, *function* 25 units, *motion* 25 units and *strength* 10 units. Both pain and strength would be reflected in the other parameters. If the surgical procedure is performed primarily for pain (as for rheumatoid arthritis), then more rating units would be given for pain, than, for instance, for power or stability. If arthrodesis of the shoulder is being rated, then greater unit value is given for stability, strength, and pain, as these would be the aims of the surgical procedure.

Option II

If flexibility of the rating system is not preferred, and a standard rating for all conditions is recommended, we would elect the rating values shown in Figure 20-1.

THE AMERICAN SHOULDER AND ELBOW SURGEONS METHOD

The Society points out the inadequacies of a numeral rating system, and that it may, in fact, be misleading. This is true, as a painless shoulder, with no

631

Diagnosis:
Aim of Procedure:
Operation:
Shoulder: right: left:
Arm Dominance: right: left:

The rating in each category can be adjusted according to the AIM of the procedure.

Patient's Name:
Hospital Unit #:
Date of Operation:
Date of Followup:
Surgeon:
Preoperative rating:
Postoperative rating:
Patient's Evaluation (circle):
Exc.   Good   Fair   Poor

Unit Rating
(circle one in each category)

Unit Rating
(circle one in each category)

I. PAIN (15)
1. None   15
2. Slight during activity   12
3. Increased pain during activities   6
4. Moderate/severe pain in activity   3
5. Severe pain, dependent on medication   0

4. Severe limitations. Unable to perform usual work or lifting. No athletics. Sedentary occupation. Unable to perform body care without aid. Can feed self and comb hair.   5
5. Complete disability of extremity.   0

II. STABILITY (25)
1. Normal. Shoulder stable and strong in all positions.   25
2. Mild apprehension in normal use of arm. No subluxation or dislocation.   20
3. Avoids elevation and external rotation. Rare subluxation.   10
4. Recurrent subluxations. ("Dead arm syndrome.") Positive apprehension test or recurrent dislocation.   5
5. Recurrent dislocation.   0

IV. MOTION (25)
Abduction	151–170	15
& Forward	120–150	12
Flexion	91–119	10
	61-90	7
	31-61	5
	Less than 30	0

IR	Thumb to scapula	5
	Thumb to sacrum	3
	Thumb to trochanter	2
	Less than trochanter	0

ER	(with arm at side)	
	80°	5
	60°	3
	30°	2
	Less than 30°	0

III. FUNCTION (25)
1. Normal function. All activities of daily living. Performs all work, sports/recreation prior to injury. Lifting 30 + lb. Swimming, tennis, throwing. Combat.   25
2. Mild limitation in sports and work. Can throw, but limited in baseball. Strong in tennis, football, swimming, lifting (15–20 lb) and combat. Performs all personal care.   20
3. Moderate limitation in overhead work and lifting (10 lb) and athletics. Unable to throw or serve in tennis. Swims sidestroke. Difficulty with body care (perineal care, back pocket, combing hair, reaching back). Aid necessary at times.   10

V. STRENGTH (10) (compared to opposite shoulder) (specify method = manual, spring gauge, cybex)
Normal   10
Good   6
Fair   4
Poor   0

TOTAL UNITS   100

Excellent   (100–85 units)
Good   (84–70 units)
Fair   (69–50 units)
Poor   (49 units or less)

Fig. 20-1. The author's shoulder evaluation form. (*IR*, internal rotation; *ER*, external rotation.)

Name _____ Hosp. # _____ Date _____ Shoulder: R/L

I. PAIN: (5 = none, 4 = slight, 3 = after unusual activity, 2 = moderate, 1 = marked, 0 = complete disability, NA = not available) _____

II. MOTION:
  A. Patient Sitting
    1. Active total elevation of arm: _____ degrees*
    2. Passive internal rotation:
    (Circle segment of posterior anatomy reached by thumb)
    (Note if reach restricted by limited elbow flexion)

1 = less than trochanter	5 = L5	9 = L1	13 = T9	17 = T5
2 = Trochanter	6 = L4	10 = T12	14 = T8	18 = T4
3 = Gluteal	7 = L3	11 = T11	15 = T7	19 = T3
4 = Sacrum	8 = L2	12 = T10	16 = T6	20 = T2

    3. Active external rotation with arm at side: _____ degrees
    4. Active external rotation at 90° abduction: _____ degrees
    (Enter "NA" if cannot achieve 90° of abduction)

  B. Patient Supine:
    1. Passive total elevation of arm: _____ degrees*
    2. Passive external rotation with arm at side: _____ degrees

*Total elevation of arm measured by viewing patient from side and using goniometer to determine angle between <u>arm</u> and <u>thorax</u>.

III. STRENGTH: (5 = normal, 4 = good, 3 = fair, 2 = poor, 1 = trace, 0 = paralysis)

  A. Anterior deltoid _____   C. External rotation _____
  B. Middle deltoid _____   D. Internal rotation _____

IV. STABILITY: (5 = normal, 4 = apprehension, 3 = rare subluxation, 2 = recurrent subluxation, 1 = recurrent dislocation, 0 = fixed dislocation, NA = not available)

  A. Anterior _____   B. Posterior _____   C. Inferior _____

V. FUNCTION: (4 = normal, 3 = mild compromise, 2 = difficulty, 1 = with aid, 0 = unable, NA = not available)

  A. Use back pocket . . . . _____   I. Sleep on affected side . . . . _____
  B. Perineal care . . . . _____   J. Pulling . . . . _____
  C. Wash opposite axilla . . . . _____   K. Use hand overhead . . . . _____
  D. Eat with utensil . . . . _____   L. Throwing . . . . _____
  E. Comb hair . . . . _____   M. Lifting . . . . _____
  F. Use hand with arm at shoulder level . _____   N. Do usual work . . . . _____
  G. Carry 10–15 lb with arm at side . . . . _____   O. Do usual sport . . . . _____
  H. Dress . . . . _____

Fig. 20-2. American Shoulder and Elbow Surgeons shoulder evaluation form. (Courtesy of the American Shoulder and Elbow Surgeons.)

motion, could achieve a similar numerical score to a painful shoulder, with moderate motion. Rather than using unit numbers, the Committee elected to use five distinct sets of parameters (Fig. 20-2):

1. Pain
2. Motion
3. Strength
4. Stability
5. Function

Each is evaluated, but a total rating for the procedure is omitted. However, specific pre- and postoperative comparisons can be given for each of the above categories.

THE CONSTANT–MURLEY ASSESSMENT OF THE SHOULDER

The Constant–Murley rating system is offered with the option of using either a 100-point scoring method or assessing individual parameters on a descriptive basis (Fig. 20-3). The authors prefer the 100-point scoring system consisting of four categories: pain, activities of daily living, range of motion, power, total. They suggest that the functional assessment be independent of diagnoses and/or treatment and that the rating system be standard for all conditions and surgical procedures. They recommend the use of 35 subjective and 65 objective points to obtain the most reliable functional score. An outline of their proposed system is shown in Table 20-1 for a 60-year-old man with osteoarthritis of his right shoulder, as compared to his left shoulder.

	Points
INDIVIDUAL PARAMETERS (100):	
Pain	15
Activities of Daily Living	20
Range of Motion	40
Power	25
PAIN (15):	
None	15
Mild	10
Moderate	5
Severe	0
ACTIVITIES OF DAILY LIVING (20):	
A Activity Level: Full Work	4
Full Recreation/Sport	4
Unaffected Sleep	2
B Positioning: Up to Waist	2
Up to Xiphoid	4
Up to Neck	6
Up to Top of Head	8
Above Head	10
FORWARD AND LATERAL ELEVATION (EACH) (10):	
0°–30°	0
31°–60°	2
61°–90°	4
91°–120°	6
121°–150°	8
151°–180°	10
EXTERNAL ROTATION (10):	
Hand Behind Head—Elbow Forward	2
Hand Behind Head—Elbow Back	2
Hand on Top of Head—Elbow Forward	2
Hand on Top of Head—Elbow Back	2
Full Elevation from Top of Head	2
INTERNAL ROTATION (10):	
Dorsum of Hand to Lateral Thigh	0
Dorsum of Hand to Buttock	2
Dorsum of Hand to Lumbosacral Junction	4
Dorsum of Hand to Waist (3rd Lumbar Vertabra)	6
Dorsum of Hand to 12th Dorsal Vertabra	8
Dorsum of Hand to Intercapsular Region (7th Dorsal Vertabra)	10
POWER (25):	
(With a spring balance or a Cybex II)	

Fig. 20-3. The Constant–Murley Clinical Method of Functional Assessment of the Shoulder. (Courtesy of Dr. CR Constant and Dr. AHG Murley.)

SUMMARY

Thus, we have three methods of assessing shoulder function in use today. A single accepted standard method can be expected and hoped for in the future. For the present, the surgeon should identify his rating system, with its supporting criteria, which will help to make reasonable evaluations and comparisons available.

Table 20-1. Shoulder Function in a 60-Year-Old Man with Osteoarthritis of the Right Shoulder and a Normal Left Shoulder

		Right	Score	Left	Score
Pain		Moderate	(5)	None	(15)
ADL	Work:	Full	(4)	Full	(4)
	Recreation:	Nil	(−)	Full	(4)
	Sleep:	Poor	(1)	Unaffected	(2)
	Position:	Top of head	(8)	Above head	(10)
Range	Abduction:	90	(4)	180	(10)
	Flexion:	105	(6)	180	(10)
	Internal Rotation:	LV 5	(4)	DV 12	(8)
	External Rotation:	Limited	(4)	Full	(10)
Power		10 lb	(10)	20 lb	(20)
Total		Right:	46%	Left	93%

ADL, activities of daily living; LV, lumbar vertabra; DV, dorsal vertabra.

ESTIMATE OF (PERMANENT) PHYSICAL IMPAIRMENT

At the present time, there is need for an accurate and specific method of determining permanent physical impairment. The methods of rating impairment in the past have been based primarily on loss of motion. Other criteria, such as strength, stability, coordination, agility, and anatomical factors (e.g., deformity and sensation), are not rated.

The following is a review of evaluation methods used in the past:

1. In 1958, the American Medical Association published a *Guide to the Evaluation of Permanent Impairment of the Extremity.*[2] This was up-dated in 1984 and 1986.[1] However, the rating criteria are based only on *loss of motion.* An unstable, weak recurrent dislocation of the shoulder would get a normal rating, as it would have 100 percent motion, although the patient may have marked incapacity of his arm and shoulder due to weakness, instability and loss of coordination.

2. In 1960, the American Academy of Orthopaedic Surgeons appointed a committee to study impairment and issued a manual entitled *Manual for Orthopaedic Surgeons in Evaluating Permanent Physical Impairment.* Although the evaluating criteria are based chiefly on loss of motion, the committee went a step further and evaluated instability, length of the extremity, and a few postoperative conditions. Instability of the shoulder is evaluated only by "recurrent dislocation as frequently as every 4 to 6 months." Recurrent dislocation once a year is not included, nor are such categories as recurrent subluxation, function, strength, agility, coordination, and alignment, which are primary disabling criteria.

3. Finally, McBride's[5] rating system, although complete in many respects, is too detailed to be used by the average orthopaedic surgeon.

We recommend the form in Figure 20-4, as a complement to that of the American Medical Association, as we feel it is a more complete guide for determining physical impairment. The impairment may be noted as "permanent" or "temporary."

NAME _____ OCCUPATION _____ DATE _____

SHOULDER: RIGHT ☐   LEFT ☐   DOMINANCE: RIGHT ☐   LEFT ☐

HISTORY:

        DETAILS OF ONSET OR INJURY
        PATIENT'S COMPLAINTS
        PREVIOUS SURGICAL PROCEDURES, RESPONSE, COMPLICATIONS
        LIST OF DIAGNOSES
        PAIN (SUBJECTIVE AND NOT RATED), BUT SHOULD BE NOTED AND
           GRADED IN RELATION TO PATIENT'S PAIN THRESHOLD.

PHYSICAL EXAMINATION

MOTION
(According to AMA Guide to Physical Impairment)

	RIGHT	LEFT	PERCENTAGE OF IMPAIRMENT OF THE EXTREMITY
FORWARD FLEXION	_____	_____	_____
ABDUCTION	_____	_____	_____
BACKWARD EXTENSION	_____	_____	_____
ADDUCTION	_____	_____	_____
EXTERNAL ROTATION	_____	_____	_____
INTERNAL ROTATION	_____	_____	_____

FUNCTION
Rate 1 (poor) to 10 (normal)

STABILITY OF JOINT (Recurrent dislocation or subluxation)	_____	_____	_____
STRENGTH (manual)	_____	_____	_____
COORDINATION	_____	_____	_____
AGILITY, QUICKNESS	_____	_____	_____

ANATOMICAL (1 to 10)

DEFORMITY (Alignment, disfigurement)	_____	_____	_____
LOSS OF SENSATION	_____	_____	_____

        TOTAL PHYSICAL IMPAIRMENT _____

Fig. 20-4. The author's form for estimating physical impairment of the shoulder.

REFERENCES

1. American Academy of Orthopaedic Surgeons: Manual for Orthopaedic Surgeons in Evaluating Permanent Physical Impairment, Chicago, 1986
2. American Medical Association: A Guide to the Evaluation of Permanent Impairment of the Extremities and Back. Journal of the American Medical Association, 2nd Ed., 1958
3. Harris WH: Traumatic arthritis of the hip after dislocation and acetabular fractures. Treated by mold arthroplasties. J Bone Joint Surg 51A:737, 1969
4. Matsen FA: Chairman of Research Committee. American Shoulder and Elbow Surgeons, Park Ridge, IL, 1986
5. McBride ED: Disability evaluation. Journal of the International College of Surgeons, Vol. XXIV, No. 3, 1955, p. 341
6. Rowe CR, Patel D, Southmayd WW: The Bankart procedure. J Bone Joint Surg 60A:1, 1978
7. Rowe CR, Zarins B: Recurrent transient subluxation of the shoulder. J Bone Joint Surg 63A:863, 1981
8. Welsh P: Standardized assessment of shoulder function. Presented at the meeting of the American Shoulder and Elbow Surgeons, Los Angeles, Oct 24, 1985 (including the Constant–Murley assessment method)

Unusual Shoulder Conditions 21

Carter R. Rowe

As an epilogue, I have gathered together a number of unusual conditions of the shoulder, which have been observed by me, and my colleagues, and which may be of interest to the reader.

ABNORMAL INSERTION OF THE PECTORALIS MINOR MUSCLE

On two occasions, when exploring the shoulder, I noticed an abnormal insertion of the pectoralis minor muscle. The first shoulder was being explored for subacromial impingement (Fig. 21-1A). On the second occasion the shoulder was explored for recurrent dislocation (Fig. 21-1B). Instead of the pectoralis minor inserting on the medial aspect of the coracoid process, the entire tendon extended over the coracoid, passed through the two arms of the coracoacromial ligament, and inserted into the coracohumeral ligament and the greater tuberosity of the humerus. A bursa was present under the tendon in the patient shown in Figure 21-1A, who was completely relieved by reattachment of the tendon to its normal insertion. Seib[7] has studied the anatomical variations of the pec-

toralis minor in detail. His study covers 1,000 specimens. There was a 15 percent partial insertion of the pectoralis minor to the coracoid process and a 1 percent occurrence of the entire tendon crossed over the coracoid through the coracoacromial ligament, to attach 65.5 percent into the coracohumeral ligament, 25 percent into the joint capsule, and 12.5 percent into both the ligament and capsule. An interesting finding was a symptomatic bursa and a grooving of the coracoid process in those instances in which the entire tendon crossed the coracoid. This may account for an occasional patient with impingement syndromes that has not responded to surgery, because the tendon and secondary bursa were not recognized.

ABSENCE OF THE GLENOID FOSSAE

A colleague (Dr. Richard Freiberg, Cincinnati, Ohio) sent us the radiographs of a patient with absence of both glenoid fossae (Fig. 21-2). The patient had full range of motion and stable shoulders. Figure 21-2C, showing the arm in full elevation, is an excellent illustration of the supportive function of the joint

639

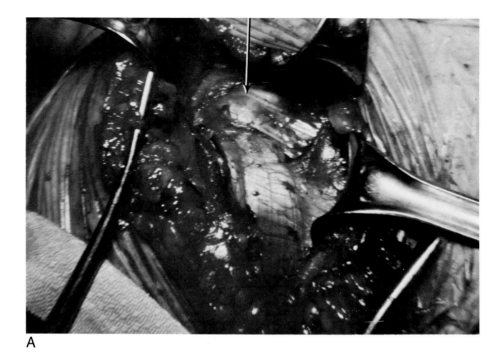

A

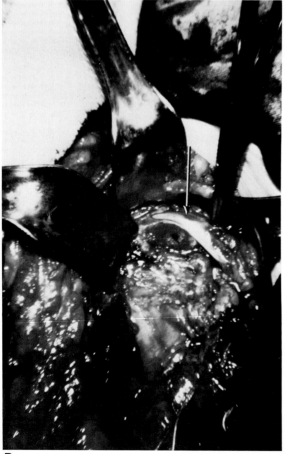

B

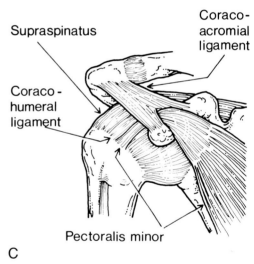

Supraspinatus

Coraco-
acromial
ligament

Coraco-
humeral
ligament

Pectoralis minor

C

Fig. 21-1. Abnormal insertion of the pectoralis minor muscle. (**A**) The arrow points to the entire tendon of the pectoralis minor passing over the coracoid process, through the coracoacromial ligament, to insert into the coracohumeral ligament and the lesser tuberosity. (**B**) The arrow points to the entire tendon of the pectoralis minor tendon passing over the osteotomized coracoid process. The exposure was for a Bankart procedure. (**C**) Artist's sketch of the course of the abnormal insertion of the pectoralis minor.

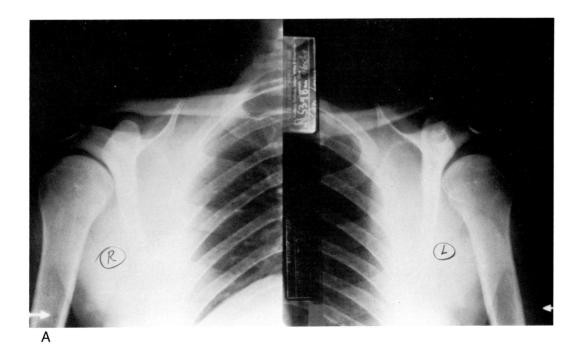

A

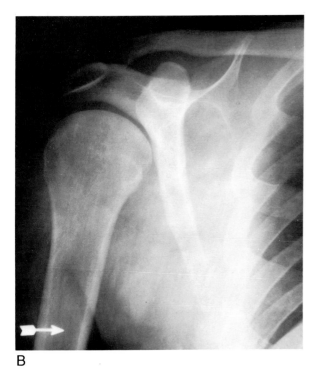

B

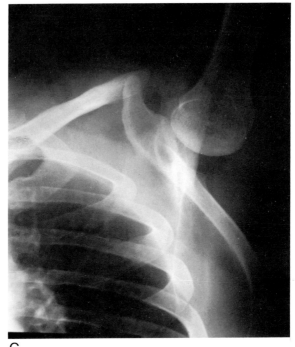

C

Fig. 21-2. Absence of the glenoid fossae. (**A**) Anteroposterior view of the shoulders, showing bilateral absence of the glenoid fossae. (**B**) Enlarged film of the right shoulder. Note the absence of inferior displacement of the humeral head. (**C**) Film of the left shoulder in full elevation. Again note the absence of inferior subluxation, which indicates the strength of the inferior capsule and capsular ligament. (Courtesy of Dr. Richard A. Freiberg.)

capsule, which prevents inferior subluxation of the humeral head.

ABSENCE OF THE CLAVICLES

Although not so rare as absence of the glenoid fossa, absence of the clavicles occurs frequently enough for one to be on the lookout for them (Fig. 21-3). They usually occur in patients with cleidocranial dysostasis. These patients do not complain of physical dysfunction due to absence of their clavicles, nor do the patients in whom I have performed a claviclectomy. In fact, they have a physical advantage in being able to move through narrower spaces than individuals with both clavicles.

VOLUNTARY WINGING OF THE SCAPULA

Voluntary dislocation of the glenohumeral joint is well established (Chap. 7). We have observed also several patients with voluntary superior dislocation

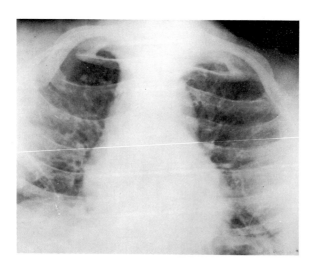

Fig. 21-3. Bilateral absence of the clavicles.

of the sternoclavicular joint (Chap. 7). These patients, as a rule, respond poorly to surgical correction. To complete the shoulder trio of voluntary dysfunctions, we have seen four patients with isolated voluntary winging of the scapula (Fig. 21-4), all of whom have responded conservatively to a careful explanation of their ability to wing their scapula, and instructions not to tighten or contract their shoulder muscles when elevating the arm. Other causes of winging of the scapula should be ruled out, such as involvement of the long nerve of Bell, subscapular osteochondroma, or contracture of the deltoid muscle.

ABSENCE OF THE PECTORALIS MAJOR MUSCLE

Absence of the sternocostal portion of the pectoralis major is seen occasionally by orthopaedists (Fig. 21-5). It is well to keep this in mind when a patient appears with a traumatic rupture of the pectoralis major. The traumatic rupture can be identified by a careful history and, if seen early, hematoma or ecchymosis of the insertion to the humerus. Also, the traumatic rupture does not produce as marked an anatomical defect, as seen with the congenital absence of the muscle. Another distinguishing point as demonstrated by Grant[4] is that with the congenital absence of the pectoralis major, the latissiumus dorsi will have hypertrophied. This would not be present with a traumatic rupture.

CONTRACTURE OF THE DELTOID MUSCLE

The majority of deltoid muscle contractures are due to intramuscular injections into the deltoid (Fig. 21-6). They may be misdiagnosed as paralysis of the deltoid or traumatic rupture. Characteristically, the patient is unable to bring the arm down to the side. Chronic discomfort is present, which is usually absent in traumatic conditions. Ogawa[6] and Kutsuma et al.[5]

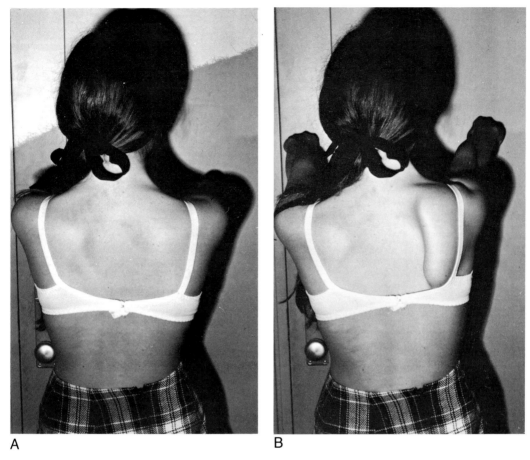

Fig. 21-4. Voluntary winging of the scapula. (**A**) Arms extended *without* winging of the scapula. (**B**) Arms extended *with* winging of the right scapula.

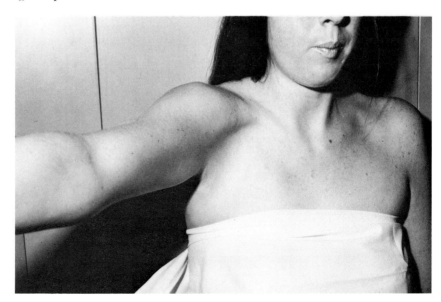

Fig. 21-5. Congenital absence of the right pectoralis major muscle.

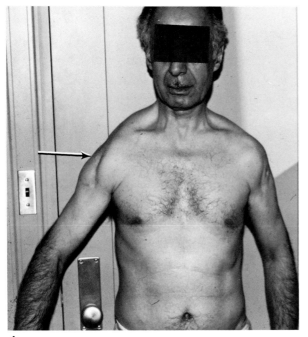

A

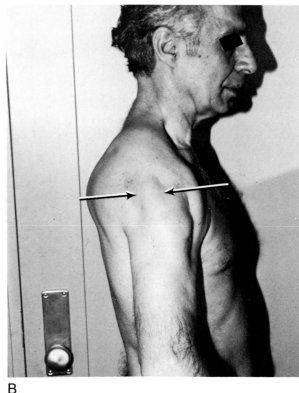

B

Fig. 21-6. Deltoid muscle contracture. (**A**) Anteroposterior view of right shoulder. (**B**) Lateral view of right shoulder.

summarize current investigations of this problem. Response to resection of the contracting band is usually good, but one should not expect 100 percent relief. Kutsuma recommends early surgical release, especially in those patients who have developed deformity of the humeral head.

SYMPTOMATIC CYSTS OF THE ACROMIOCLAVICULAR JOINT

The patient in Figure 21-7A was referred to us with the diagnosis of a possible fibrosarcoma. Exploration revealed a massive cyst of the acromioclavicular joint. This relieved the referring surgeon as well as the apprehensive patient (Fig. 22-7B). Pain is a differentiating factor. The pain of an acromioclavicular joint cyst is much more acute (Fig. 21-7C, D) than one would have from a soft tissue tumor. Both of our

patients were completely relieved with surgical resection of the cyst. Another unusual enlargement of the shoulder may be due to the massive chondromatosis of the subacromial bursa (Fig. 22-7E and F).

CORACOCLAVICULAR ARTICULATION

We are aware that the acromioclavicular articulation may vary from a well-developed joint with an articular disc to a poorly formed oblique unstable articulation. Occasionally the orthopaedic surgeon will see an articulation between the clavicle and the coracoid process (Fig. 21-8). This anatomical variant is usually asymptomatic. Other congenital anomalies may occasionally appear, such as a solid bony strut between the clavicle and coracoid process, or the bar may be incomplete.[3]

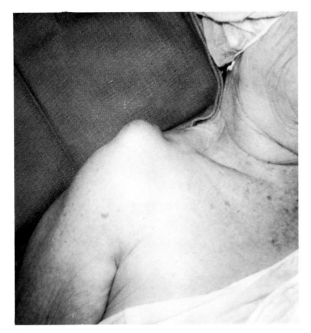

A

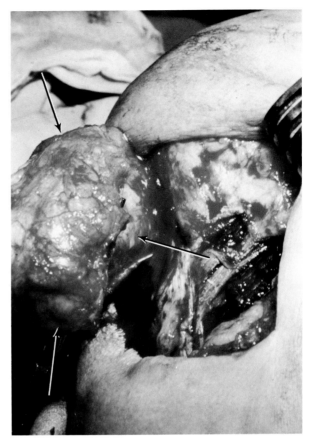

B

Fig. 21-7. **(A)** A large cyst of the right acromioclavicular joint, which was referred to us with the diagnosis of "fibrosacroma." **(B)** Resected specimen. **(C)** Cyst of the right acromioclavicular joint. **(D)** Pain on elevation of the arm. (*Figure continues.*)

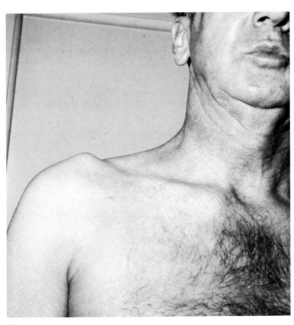

C

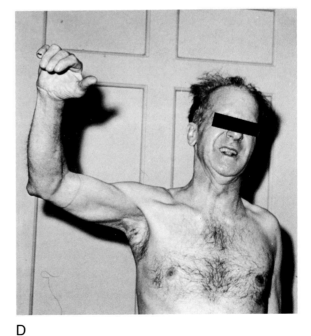

D

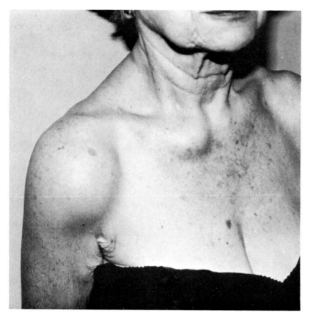

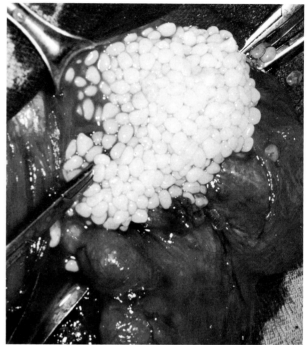

E

Fig. 21-7 (*Continued*). (**E**) Enlargement of right shoulder due to massive chondromatosis of right shoulder (**F**).

F

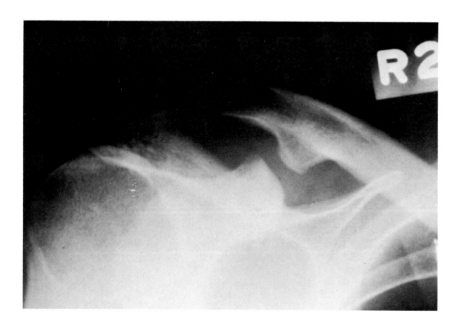

Fig. 21-8. Developmental articulation between the clavicle and coracoid process.

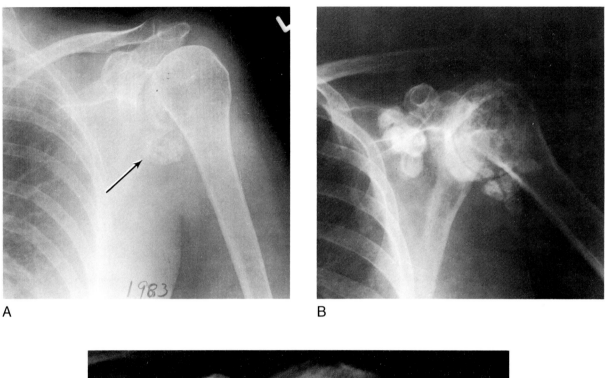

A

B

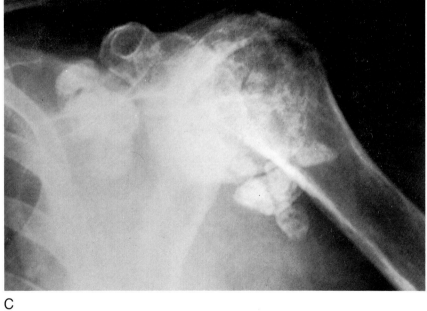

C

Fig. 21-9. (**A**) Solitary loose body in left shoulder. (**B**) Multiple loose bodies in left shoulder and severe subscapularis bursa. (**C**) Clinical appearance 2 years later.

EXCESSIVE LOOSE BODY FORMATION

Loose bodies in the glenohumeral joint may vary from an isolated body (Fig. 21-9A) to multiple disabling loose body formation (Fig. 21-9B and C).

AN UNUSUAL ASSIGNMENT

The following problem will be seen more frequently in the coming years; however, it was unusual for us. The young man shown in Figure 21-10, who had had successful cardiac surgery, was sent to us because of disabling recurrent anterior dislocations of his right shoulder. The complicating concern was that the line of his pacemaker was in his right cephalic vein (see arrow).

With the cooperation of our cardiac colleagues, a standby team was ready to put in a new line in case of injury to his present one during surgery. Needless to say, electrocautery was not used during surgery. Everything went well during surgery, without disturbance to his pacemaker or cardiac rhythm. For the past 10 years his Bankart procedure has been stable with an excellent range of motion.

BONE ABSORPTION AROUND THE SHOULDER

Perhaps the most common cause of bone absorption of the shoulder girdle is the distal clavicle in male weight-lifters (Fig. 21-11). Occasionally this may occur from direct trauma. This is a benign self-limiting condition. Figure 22-12B reveals reconstitution by eliminating weight lifting.

A much more serious condition is massive osteolysis ("disappearing" bone disease or "phantom bone"). A recent excellent review is given by Cannon,[1] in which he discusses seven cases seen at the Royal National Orthopaedic Hospital in London. Of the seven, three

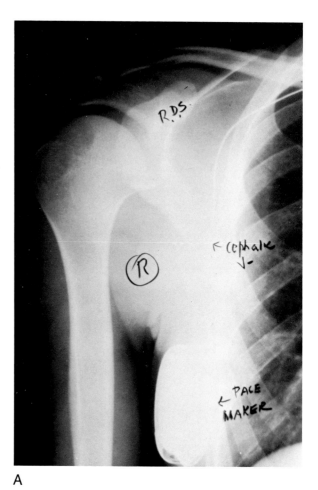

A

Fig. 21-10. **(A)** A patient with disabling recurrent anterior dislocation of the right shoulder, who had undergone major heart surgery. Note the pacemaker in the right cephalic vein. (*Figure continues.*)

involved the shoulder girdle (two of the humerus and one of the scapula) (Fig. 21-12).

CODMAN'S "PIVOTAL PARADOX" AND THE "ENVELOPE" OF MOTION OF THE GLENOHUMERAL JOINT

The coordinated rhythm and interplay of the four joints of the shoulder girdle have been carefully stud-

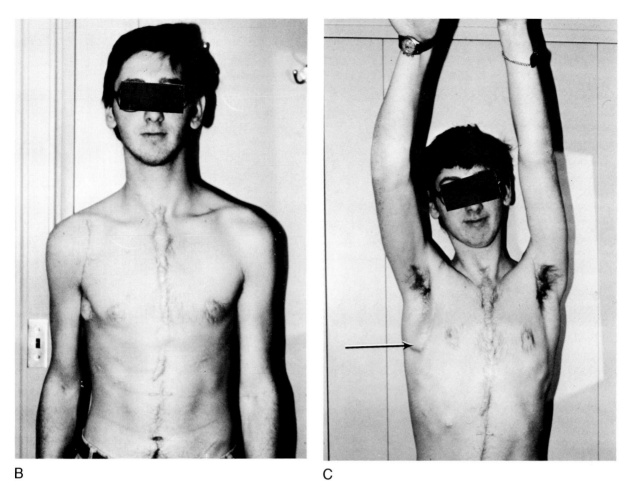

B   C

Fig. 21-10 (*Continued*). (**B, C**) Postoperative Bankart repair of the right shoulder with complete range of motion and a stable shoulder. Arrow points to pacemaker.

ied in all positions of the extremity. Little reference has been given in the past, however, to Codman's description of the "pivotal paradox" when the arm is raised to the overhead position[2] (Fig. 21-13). Codman points out that if the arm, with the elbow flexed 90° at the side of the body, is placed in 90° of external rotation (the solid line) and is raised in the coronal plane without rotation to 180°, the shoulder will be in 90° of internal rotation. If the arm is lowered to the side of the body in the coronal plane, again without rotation, it is in 90° of external rotation. He therefore contends that the arm in the overhead position must have been in 90° external rotation, as the arm was not rotated in moving into elevation. On the other hand, if the arm at the side of the body is placed in

90° of internal rotation (the dotted line) and elevated in the sagittal plane, without rotation to the overhead position, it will remain in 90° internal rotation. So Codman asks, was the arm in true internal or external rotation in the overhead position? However, in the last example, if the arm is lowered in the coronal plane to the side of the body it will be in 90° of external rotation, having rotated 180°.

A possible answer to Codman's "pivotal paradox" is the "envelope" of motion that occurs when the arm is elevated and is moved from one plane to another or from the sagittal to the coronal plane or vice versa. Rotation take place, even though the arm has not been actively rotated by the patient.

As shown in Figure 21-14 A–D, with the arm at

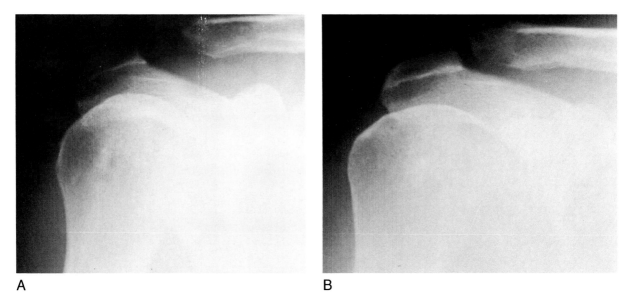

Fig. 21-11. (**A**) Osteolysis of distal of clavicle in a weight-lifter. (**B**) One year later, with reossification.

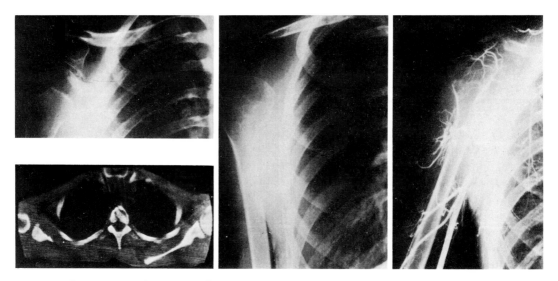

Fig. 21-12. "Disappearing bone disease" showing progressive osteolysis of the scapula and clavicle (Cannon SR: Massive osteolysis. J Bone Joint Surg 68B:24, 1986.)

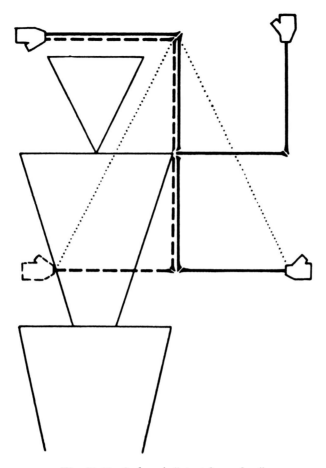

Fig. 21-13. Codman's "pivotal paradox."

the side of the body in 90° of internal rotation and elevated to 180° (the overhead position) in the saggital plane, it is still in 90° internal rotation. If it is lowered in the coronal plane to the side of the body, *without* rotating the arm, the shoulder will have rotated to 90° of external rotation, or 180° of rotation. The reverse is true (as pointed out by Codman) if the arm is placed in 90° of external rotation, elevated 180° to the overhead position, and lowered to the side of the body in the sagittal plane, it will be in 90° of internal rotation having rotated 180°.

As shown in Figure 21-14 E–H, if the arm at the side of the body in 90° of internal rotation is elevated only 90° in the sagittal plane and lowered to the side of the body in the coronal plane, it will have rotated only 90°, to the neutral position. This is an interesting phenomenon worthy of further study. Thus the degrees of rotation are equal to the degrees of elevation when the arm is moved or elevated from one plane to another. This is referred to as the envelope of motion. A beam of light attached to the humeral head will outline the degrees of rotation when moving from the sagittal to the coronal plane, or vice versa.

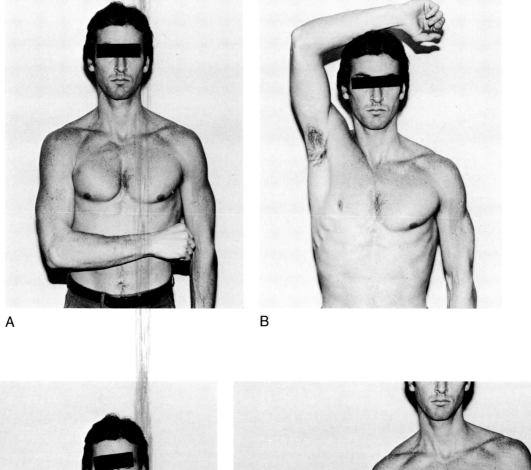

A   B

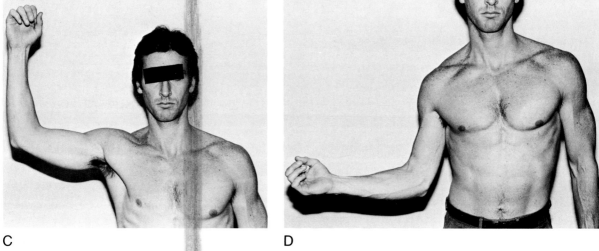

C   D

Fig. 21-14. (**A–D**) With the arm at the side of the body in 90° internal rotation, is elevated to 180° in the sagittal plane, and lowered to the side of the body in the coronal plane (without rotating the arm), the shoulder has rotated 180°, by passing from one plane to another (the sagittal to the coronal plane). The reverse is true. (*Figure continues.*)

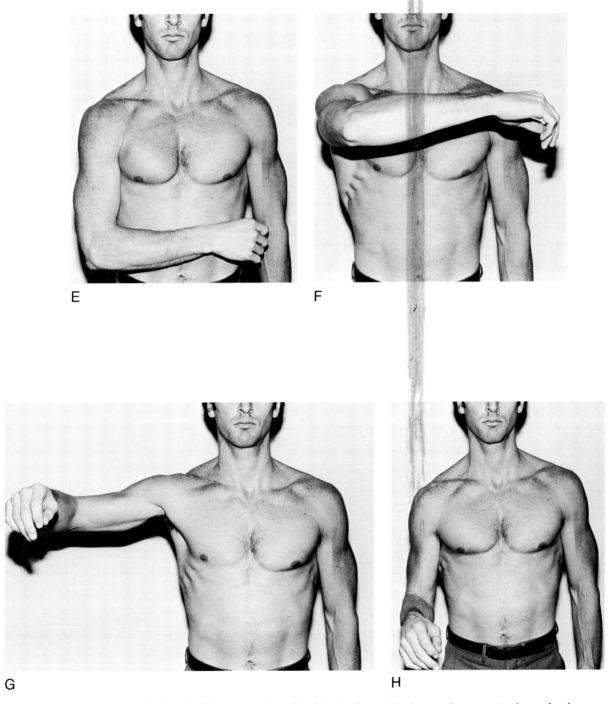

Fig. 21-14 *(Continued).* **(E–H)** If the arm at the side of the body in 90° of internal rotation is elevated only 90° in the sagittal plane, and lowered to the side of the body in the coronal plane (without rotating the shoulder), it will have rotated 90°. The degrees of rotation are equal to the degrees of elevation, when passed from one plane (sagittal) to another (coronal plane). This envelope of motion helps to explain Codman's pivotal paradox.

REFERENCES

1. Cannon SR: Massive osteolysis. J Bone Joint Surg 68B:24, 1986
2. Codman EA: The Shoulder. Reprinted by Robert E. Kreiger, Malabar, Florida, 1984
3. DePalma AF: Surgery of the Shoulder, 3rd ed. JB Lippincott, Philadelphia, 1983
4. Grant JCB: Grant's Anatomy (James E. Anderson, ed), 7th ed. Williams & Wilkins, Baltimore, 1978
5. Kutsuma T, Teroyama K: Results of surgical treatment for deltoid muscle contracture. p. 259. In Bateman and Walsh (eds): Surgery of the Shoulder. CV Mosby, Toronto, 1984
6. Ogawa K: Adult cases of deltoid contracture. Department of Orthopaedic Surgery, Saitama Medical School, Saitama, Japan (Received for publication June 16, 1982).
7. Seib GA: The musculus pectoralis minor in American whites and American negroes. Am J Phys Anthropol 4(23):389, 1938

Index

Page numbers followed by *f* represent figures; page numbers followed by *t* represent tables.